Highlights in Asthmology

Editors: Francois Bernard Michel, Jean Bousquet, Philippe Godard

With 102 Figures and 70 Tables

Springer-Verlag
Berlin Heidelberg New York
London Paris Tokyo

Professor François Bernard Michel, M.D.
Jean Bousquet, M.D., Ph.D.
Professor Philippe Godard, M.D.

Clinique des Maladies Respiratoires
Hôpital de l'Aiguelongue
Avenue du Major Flandre
F-34059 Montpellier Cédex

ISBN-13:978-3-642-70318-8 e-ISBN-13:978-3-642-70316-4
DOI: 10.1007/978-3-642-70316-4

Library of Congress Cataloging-in-Publication Data
Highlights in asthmology. Includes bibliographies. 1. Asthma. I. Michel, François-Bernard. II. Bousquet, Jean. III. Godard, Philippe. [DNLM: 1. Asthma. WF 553 H635] RC591.H53 1987 616.2'38
87-4604
ISBN-13:978-3-642-70318-8 (U.S.)

Softcover reprint of the hardcover 1st edition 1987

2329/543210

Table of Contents

Authors' addresses VII
Abbreviations XIII

A. Introduction 1
1. Preface (*F. B. Michel*) 3
2. Natural History of Asthma (*T. A. E. Platts-Mills, P. W. Heymann*) 7

B. Epidemiology 19
3. Epidemiology of Bronchial Asthma (*D. Charpin, J. Charpin*) . . 21
4. Genetic Factors of Allergy (*D. G. Marsh*) 31
5. Changing Prevalence of Asthma in Developing Countries (*K. J. Turner*) 37

C. Etiology 45
6. Viruses (*W. W. Busse*) 47
7. Allergic Bronchopulmonary Aspergillosis (*A. B. Tonnel, Ph. Gosset, B. Wallaert*) 58
8. Bacterial Asthma (*J. Pepys*) 66
9. Exercise-induced Asthma: Clinical Aspects (*S. D. Anderson*) 77
10. Asthma and Gastroesophageal Reflux (*M. Perrin-Fayolle*) 89

D. Immunology 97
11. The IgE Receptors (Introduction) . 99
11.1 IgE Receptors in Bronchial Asthma (*A. Kulczycki*) 100
11.2 IgE Receptors on Inflammatory Cells (*A. Capron, J.-P. Dessaint, A. B. Tonnel*) 107
12. Immunological Mechanisms (*C. W. Parker*) 117
13. Mechanisms of IgE-mediated Immediate Reactions (*A. L. de Weck*) 120
14. Properties of Short-term Sensitizing IgG Antibodies (IgG S-TS) in Asthma (*W. E. Parish*) 131
15. The Role of Lymphocytes and of their Abnormalities in Atopic Diseases (*M. Ricci, E. Maggi, G. F. del Prete, S. Romagnani*) 140
16. Delayed-type Hypersensitivity Responses to Inhalant Allergens: a Form of Cutaneous Basophil Hypersensitivity (CBH) (*E. B. Mitchell*) 147

E. Mediator Release and Bronchial Obstruction 153
17. Physiological and Pharmacological Control of Inflammatory Mediator Release in Bronchial Asthma (*S. T. Holgate*) 155
18. Mast Cells and Basophils (*S. P. Peters, J. A. Grant, A. M. Dvorak, L. M. Lichtenstein*) 167
19. Alveolar Macrophages (*Ph. Godard, M. Damon, Ph. Vago*) 186
20. Neutrophils and the Asthmatic Response (*A. B. Kay*) 195
21. Eosinophils in Bronchial Asthma (*E. Frigas, G. J. Gleich*) 201
22. Mediators of Asthma Derived from Arachidonic Acid (*R. A. Lewis, J.-L. Robin*) 212
23. PAF-acether (Platelet Activating Factor) (*B. Arnoux, C. Brink, J. Benveniste*) 221
24. Immediate-type Reactions (*B. Zweiman, P. C. Atkins*) 228
25. Late Phase Reactions (*W. Dorsch*) 237

F. Bronchial Pathophysiology 253
26. Bronchi of Asthmatic Patients (*Ph. Godard, Y. Maria, F. B. Michel*) 255
27. The Site of Bronchial Obstruction in Asthma (*Ch. Préfaut*) 260
28. Factors in Bronchial Hyperreactivity (*H. A. Boushey*) 265

29. Bronchial Hyperreactivity: Autonomic Nervous System Abnormalities (*M. A. Kaliner*) 276
30. Bronchial Hyperresponsiveness and Asthma: Unanswered Questions (*J. Orehek*) 285

G. Asthma due to Allergy Occupation, Food and Drugs 291
31. Preparation and Stability of Pollen Extracts (*H. Baer, M. C. Anderson*) 293
32. Allergen Standardization (*R. A. Goldstein*) 297
33. Allergen Avoidance (*D. Vervloet, A. Arnaud*) 301
34. Allergens Inducing Asthma (Introduction) 305
34.1 Pollen-induced Asthma (*J. Bousquet, P. Cour, F. B. Michel*) 306
34.2 Mite Allergens (*G. Pauli, J. C. Bessot*) 316
34.3 Molds (*M. Lopez, J. E. Salvaggio*) 322
34.4 Allergy to Domestic Animals (*B. Guérin, J. Bousquet*) 326
35. Agricultural Asthma (*J. Bousquet, A. Vergnenègre*) 331
36. Investigation of Occupational Asthma due to Low Molecular Weight Agents (*J.-L. Malo, A. Cartier*) 343
37. Occupational Asthma (*R. J. Davies, A. D. Blainey*) 351
38. Food-related Asthma (*D. A. Moneret-Vautrin*) 359
39. Drug-induced Asthma (*J. Bousquet, E. Fernandez, B. Guérin*) 364

H. Clinical Features and Diagnosis in Children and Adults 371
40. Clinical Aspects of Asthma (*P. S. Norman*) 373
41. Asthma in Childhood (*P. Scheinmann, J. Paupe*) 376
42. Diagnosis of Asthma in Childhood (*U. Wahn*) 380
43. Treatment of Childhood Asthma (*J. O. Warner*) 385
44. Asthma in Adults (*J. Bousquet, Ph. Godard, F. B. Michel*) 394
45. Skin Tests (*J. L. Ménardo, W. Skassa-Brociek, J. Bousquet*) .. 399
46. Diagnostic Value of IgE in Bronchial Asthma (*N. F. Adkinson Jr*) . 409
47. Pulmonary Function Tests in Asthma (*D. W. Cockcroft*) 412
48. Bronchial Provocation Tests (*S. L. Spector*) 421
49. Status Asthmaticus (*R. Pariente*) .. 431

I. Therapeutic Considerations 439
50. Physiopathological Data for the Treatment of Bronchial Asthma (*R. Pauwels*) 441
51. Possible Therapeutic Developments (*L. P. Craps*) 445

Index 449

Authors' addresses

N. F. Adkinson Jr., M.D.
The Johns Hopkins University
School of Medicine
The Good Samaritan Hospital
5601 Loch Raven Boulevard
Baltimore, Maryland 21239, USA

M. C. Anderson, M.S.
Immunopathology Branch
National Institute of Allergy
and Infectious Diseases (NIAID)
Westwood Building, Room 755
Bethesda, Maryland 20205, USA

S. D. Anderson, M.D.
Principal Scientific Officer
Department of Thoracic Medicine
Royal Prince Alfred Hospital
Missenden Road
Camperdown, NSW 2050, Australia

A. Arnaud, M.D.
Clinique de Pneumophtisiologie –
Prof. J. Charpin
Hôpital Sainte-Marguerite
Unité INSERM 174
B. P. 29
13277 Marseille Cédex 9, France

B. Arnoux, M.D.
INSERM U 200
Immunopharmacologie de l'Allergie
et de l'Inflammation
32 rue des Carnets
92140 Clamart, France

P. C. Atkins, M.D.
Associate Professor of Medicine
Allergy and Immunology Section
Department of Medicine
University of Pennsylvania
School of Medicine
Philadelphia, Pennsylvania 19104, USA

H. Baer, Ph.D.
Director, Allergenic Products Branch
Office of Biologics Research and Review
Center for Drugs and Biologics
Food and Drug Administration
Bethesda, Maryland 20205, USA

J. Benveniste, M.D., Ph.D.
Unité de Recherche
INSERM U 20
32 rue des Carnets
92140 Clamart, France

J. C. Bessot, M.D.
Service de Pneumologie – Pavillon Laënnec
Hospices Civils de Strasbourg
67091 Strasbourg, France

A. D. Blainey, M.B.
Academic Unit of Respiratory Medicine
St Bartholomew's Hospital
West Smithfield
London EC1A 7BE, United Kingdom

H. A. Boushey, M.D.
Associate Professor of Medicine
Cardiovascular Research Institute
University of California
School of Medicine
San Francisco, California 94143, USA

J. Bousquet, M.D., Ph.D.
Clinique des Maladies Respiratoires
Hôpital de l'Aiguelongue
Avenue du Major Flandre
34059 Montpellier Cédex, France

C. Brink, M.D.
Unité de Recherche
INSERM U 20
32 rue des Carnets
92140 Clamart, France

Professor W. W. Busse, M.D.
Head, Allergy and Clinical Immunology
University of Wisconsin
Department of Medicine
600 Highland Avenue
Madison, Wisconsin 53792, USA

Professor A. Capron, M.D.
Centre d'Immunologie
et de Biologie Parasitaire
Unité Mixte INSERM 167 – CNRS 624
Institut Pasteur
15 rue Camille Guérin
59019 Lille Cédex, France

A. Cartier, M.D.
Service de Pneumologie
Hôpital du Sacré-Coeur
5400 ouest, Boulevard Gouin
Montreal, Quebec, Canada H4J 1C5

D. Charpin, M.D.
Clinique de Pneumophtisiologie
Hôpital Sainte-Marguerite
B. P. 29
13277 Marseille Cédex 9, France

Professor J. Charpin, M.D.
Clinique de Pneumophtisiologie
Hôpital Sainte-Marguerite
B. P. 29
13277 Marseille Cédex 9, France

Professor D. W. Cockcroft, M.D.
Respiratory Clinic
Department of Medicine
University of Saskatchewan
Saskatoon, Canada S7N 0XO

P. Cour, Ph.D.
Laboratoire de Palynologie
Université des Sciences et Techniques
du Languedoc
34000 Montpellier, France

Professor L. P. Craps, M.D., Ph.D.
Sandoz Ltd
Pharmaceutical Division
4002 Basel, Switzerland

M. Damon, Ph.D.
INSERM U 58
Chemin de Navacelles
34000 Montpellier, France

R. J. Davies, M.D.
Academic Unit of Respiratory Medicine
St Bartholomew's Hospital
West Smithfield
London EC1A 7BE, United Kingdom

J.-P. Dessaint, M.D.
Centre d'Immunologie
et de Biologie Parasitaire
Unité Mixte INSERM 167 – CNRS 624
Institut Pasteur
15 rue Camille Guérin
59019 Lille Cédex, France

Priv.-Doz. W. Dorsch, M.D.
Kinderpoliklinik
Ludwig-Maximilians-Universität München
Pettenkoferstrasse 8 a
8000 München 2, GFR

A. M. Dvorak, M.D.
Divisions of Clinical Immunology
and Respiratory Medicine
The Johns Hopkins University
School of Medicine
The Good Samaritan Hospital
5601 Loch Raven Boulevard
Baltimore, Maryland 21239, USA

E. Fernandez, M.D.
Clinique des Maladies Respiratoires
Hôpital de l'Aiguelongue
Avenue du Major Flandre
34059 Montpellier Cédex, France

E. Frigas, M.D.
Department of Internal Medicine
Division of Allergy/Immunology
Mayo Clinic
Rochester, Minnesota 55905, USA

Professor G. J. Gleich, M.D.
Department of Internal Medicine
Division of Allergy/Immunology
Mayo Clinic
Rochester, Minnesota 55905, USA

Professor Ph. Godard, M.D.
Clinique des Maladies Respiratoires
Hôpital de l'Aiguelongue
Avenue du Major Flandre
34059 Montpellier Cédex, France

R. A. Goldstein, M.D., Ph.D.
Chief, Immunopathology Branch
National Institute of Allergy
and Infectious Diseases (NIAID)
National Institutes of Health
Westwood Building, Room 755
Bethesda, Maryland 20205, USA

Ph. Gosset, M.D.
Service de Pneumologie
et Immuno-Allergologie
Hôpital A. Calmette
59037 Lille, France

J. A. Grant, M.D.
Divisions of Clinical Immunology
and Respiratory Medicine
The Johns Hopkins University
School of Medicine
The Good Samaritan Hospital
5601 Loch Raven Boulevard
Baltimore, Maryland 21239, USA

B. Guérin, M.D.
Laboratoires des Stallergènes
160 quai de Polangis
94349 Joinville le Pont, France

P. W. Heymann, M.D.
Division of Allergy
and Clinical Immunology
University of Virginia
Department of Medicine
Charlottesville, Virginia 22908, USA

S. T. Holgate, M.D.
Senior Lecturer
and Honorary Consultant Physician
Southampton General Hospital, Medicine I
Level D, Centre Block
Tremona Road
Southampton SO9 4WY, United Kingdom

M.A. Kaliner, M.D.
Head, Allergic Diseases Section
National Institute of Allergy
and Infectious Diseases (NIAID)
National Institutes of Health
Building 10, Room 11C-205
Bethesda, Maryland 20205, USA

Professor A. B. Kay, M.D.
Director, Department of Allergy
and Clinical Immunology
Cardiothoracic Institute
Brompton Hospital
Fulham Road
London SW3 6HP, United Kingdom

A. Kulczycki Jr., M.D.
Howard Hughes
Medical Institute Laboratory
and Department of Internal Medicine
Division of Allergy and Immunology
Washington University School of Medicine
St. Louis, Missouri 63110, USA

R. A. Lewis, M.D.
Synthax Research
3401 Hill View Avenue
Palo Alto, California 94304, USA

Professor L. M. Lichtenstein, M.D., Ph.D.
Clinical Immunology Division
The Johns Hopkins University
School of Medicine
The Good Samaritan Hospital
5601 Loch Raven Boulevard
Baltimore, Maryland 21239, USA

M. Lopez, M.D.
Associate Professor of Medicine
Director
Clinical Immunology Laboratories
Tulane University
School of Medicine
1430 Tulane Avenue
New Orleans, Louisiana 70112, USA

E. Maggi, M.D.
Universita degli Studi di Firenze
Cattedra di Immunologia Clinica
Policlinico di Careggi
Viale Morgagni
50134 Firenze, Italy

J.-L. Malo, M.D.
Service de Pneumologie
Hôpital du Sacré-Coeur
5400 ouest, boulevard Gouin
Montreal, Quebec, Canada H4J 1C5

Y. Maria, M.D.
Clinique des Maladies Respiratoires
Hôpital de l'Aiguelongue
Avenue du Major Flandre
34059 Montpellier Cédex, France

D. G. Marsh, Ph.D.
The Johns Hopkins University
School of Medicine
The Good Samaritan Hospital
5601 Loch Raven Boulevard
Baltimore, Maryland 21239, USA

J.L. Ménardo, M.D.
Clinique des Maladies Respiratoires
Hôpital de l'Aiguelongue
Avenue du Major Flandre
34059 Montpellier Cédex, France

Professor F. B. Michel, M.D.
Clinique des Maladies Respiratoires
Hôpital de l'Aiguelongue
Avenue du Major Flandre
34059 Montpellier Cédex, France

E. B. Mitchell, M.D.
Clinical Research Centre
Division of Immunological Medicine
Northwick Park Hospital
Watford Road
Harrow, Middlesex HA1 3UJ,
United Kingdom

Professor D. A. Moneret-Vautrin, M.D.
Médecine "D" – Prof. J. P. Grilliat,
Prof. D. A. Moneret-Vautrin
Immuno-Allergologie
C. H. U. de Nancy-Brabois
Route de Neufchâteau
54511 Vandoeuvre les Nancy Cédex,
France

Professor P. S. Norman, M.D.
Clinical Immunology Division
The Johns Hopkins University
School of Medicine
The Good Samaritan Hospital
5601 Loch Raven Boulevard
Baltimore, Maryland 21239, USA

Professor J. Orehek, M.D.
Hôpital Salvator
Laboratoires d'Explorations Fonctionnelles
Respiratoires
13009 Marseille, France

Professor R. Pariente, M.D.
Service de Pneumologie et Reanimation
Hôpital Beaujon
100 boulevard du Général Leclerc
92110 Clichy, France

W. E. Parish, M.D.
Environmental Safety Laboratory
Unilever Research
Colworth House
Sharnbrook, Bedford MK44 1LQ,
United Kingdom

C. W. Parker, M.D.
Howard Hughes
Medical Institute Laboratory
and Department of Internal Medicine
Division of Allergy and Immunology
Washington University School of Medicine
St. Louis, Missouri 63110, USA

Professor G. Pauli, M.D.
Service de Pneumologie – Pavillon Laënnec
Hospices Civils de Strasbourg
67091 Strasbourg, France

J. Paupe, M.D.
Hôpital des Enfants Malades
Service d'Allergologie
149 rue de Sèvres
75730 Paris Cédex 15, France

Professor R. Pauwels, M.D.
Department of Respiratory Diseases
Academic Hospital
De Pintelaan 185
9000 Gent, Belgium

Professor J. Pepys, M.D.
34 Ferncroft Avenue
London NW3 7PE, United Kingdom

Professor M. Perrin-Fayolle, M.D.
Service de Pneumologie
C. H. U. Lyon Sud
69230 Saint Genis Laval, France

S. P. Peters, M.D., Ph.D.
Assistant Professor of Medicine
Divisions of Clinical Immunology
and Respiratory Medicine
The Johns Hopkins University
School of Medicine
The Good Samaritan Hospital
5601 Loch Raven Boulevard
Baltimore, Maryland 21239, USA

T. A. E. Platts-Mills, M.D.
Head, Division of Allergy
and Clinical Immunology
University of Virginia
Department of Medicine
Charlottesville, Virginia 22908, USA

Professor Ch. Préfaut, M.D.
Service d'Exploration Fonctionelle
Respiratoire
Hôpital de l'Aiguelongue
Avenue du Major Flandre
34059 Montpellier Cédex, France

G. F. del Prete, M.D.
Universita degli Studi di Firenze
Cattedra di Immunologia Clinica
Policlinico di Careggi
Viale Morgagni
50134 Firenze, Italy

Professor M. Ricci, M.D.
Universita degli Studi di Firenze
Cattedra di Immunologia Clinica
Policlinico di Careggi
Viale Morgagni
50134 Firenze, Italy

J.-L. Robin, Ph.D.
Rhône-Poulenc S.A.
Centre de Recherches de Vitry
13 quai Jules Guesde
94400 Vitry-Seine, France

S. Romagnani, M.D.
Universita degli Studi di Firenze
Cattedra di Immunologia Clinica
Policlinico di Careggi
Viale Morgagni
50134 Firenze, Italy

J. E. Salvaggio, M.D.
Department of Medicine
Tulane University
School of Medicine
1430 Tulane Avenue
New Orleans, Louisiana 70112, USA

Professor P. Scheinmann, M.D.
Hôpital des Enfants Malades
Service d'Allergologie
et de Pneumologie Infantiles
149 rue de Sèvres
75730 Paris Cédex 15, France

W. Skassa-Brociek, M.D.
Clinique des Maladies Respiratoires
Hôpital de l'Aiguelongue
Avenue du Major Flandre
34059 Montpellier Cédex, France

S. L. Spector, M.D.
Associate Clinical Professor of Medicine
Allergy Medical Clinic
11645 Wilshire Boulevard, Suite 600
Los Angeles, California 90025, USA

Professor A. B. Tonnel, M.D.
Service de Pneumologie
et Immuno-Allergologie
Hôpital A. Calmette
59037 Lille, France

K. J. Turner, Ph.D.
Associate Professor
Clinical Immunology Research Unit
Princess Margaret Children's
Medical Research Foundation
G. P. O. Box D 184
Perth, Western Australia 6001

Ph. Vago, M.D.
Clinique des Maladies Respiratoires
Hôpital de l'Aiguelongue
Avenue du Major Flandre
34059 Montpellier Cédex, France

A. Vergnenègre, M.D.
Service de Pathologie Respiratoire
Hôpital de Cluzeau
2 avenue Alexis Carrel
87042 Limoges Cédex, France

Professor D. Vervloet, M.D.
Clinique de Pneumophtisiologie –
Prof. J. Charpin
Hôpital Sainte-Marguerite
Unité INSERM 174
B. P. 29
13277 Marseille Cédex 9, France

Priv.-Doz. U. Wahn, M.D.
Krankenhaus Zehlendorf
Örtlicher Bereich Heckeshorn
Am Großen Wannsee 80
1000 Berlin 39, GFR

B. Wallaert, M.D.
Service de Pneumologie
et Immuno-Allergologie
Hôpital A. Calmette
59037 Lille, France

J.O. Warner, M.D.
Consultant Paediatrician
Brompton Hospital
Fulham Road
London SW3 6HP, United Kingdom

Professor A. L. de Weck, M.D.
Institute for Clinical Immunology
University of Bern
Inselspital
3010 Bern, Switzerland

Professor B. Zweiman, M.D.
Allergy and Immunology Section
Department of Medicine
University of Pennsylvania
School of Medicine
Philadelphia, Pennsylvania 90104, USA

Abbreviations

Ab	antibody
ABPA	allergic bronchopulmonary aspergillosis
ACTH	adrenocorticotrophic hormone
AD	adrenaline
ADCC	antibody-dependent cell-mediated cytotoxicity
AGEPC	acetyl-glyceryl-ether-phosphorylcholine
AM	alveolar macrophage
AMLR	autologous mixed lymphocyte reaction
AMP	adenosine monophosphate
APC	antigen presenting cell
ATCC	alloreactive T-cell clone
ATP	adenosine triphosphate
BAC	bronchoalveolar cell
BAL	bronchoalveolar lavage
BE	base excess
BH	bronchial hyperresponsiveness
BHR	bronchial hyperreactivity
BMRC	British Medical Research Council
CAMP	cyclic adenosine monophosphate
CBH	cutaneous basophil hypersensitivity
CDP	cytidine diphosphate
CF	cystic fibrosis
CIE	crossed immunoelectrophoresis
CLIE	cross-linear immunoelectrophoresis
COMT	catechol-O-methyltransferase
COPD	chronic obstructive lung disease
CRIE	crossed radioimmunoelectrophoresis
CV	closing volume
Df	dermatophagoides farinae
D_LCO	pulmonary diffusing capacity for carbon monoxide
Dpt	dermatophagoides pteronyssinus
DSCG	disodium cromoglycate
EAA	exogenous allergic alveolitis
ECF	eosinophil chemotactic factor
ECF-A	eosinophil chemotactic factor of anaphylaxis
ECP	eosinophil cationic protein
EIA	exercise-induced asthma
ELI	exercise lability index
ELISA	enzyme-linked immunosorbent assay
ENT	ear nose throat
EPO	eosinophil peroxidase

EPP	equal pressure point
ETYA	eicosatetraynoic acid
FA	food allergy
FACS	fluorescence-activated cell sorting
FDA	Food and Drug Administration
FEF	forced expiratory flow
$FEV_{(1)}$	forced expiratory volume (in one second)
FRC	functional residual capacity
FVC	forced vital capacity
Gaw	airway conductance
GC-MS	gas chromatography-mass spectrometry
GEFSA	Groupe d'Etudes Francais pour la Standardization des Allergenes
GER	gastroesophageal reflux
GMP	guanosine monophosphate
H & E	hematoxylin and eosin
HBDT	human basophil degranulation test
HD	Hodgkin's disease
HEPES	N_2-hydroxyethylpiperazine-N-prime-2-ethane sulfonic acid buffer
(5-)HETE	(5-)hydroxyeicosatetraenoic acid
HLA	human leukocyte antigen
HMW	high molecular weight
5-HPETE	5-hydroperoxyeicosatetraenoic acid
HPLC	high performance liquid chromatography
HR	heart rate
HRA	histamine releasing activity
HRP	horseradish peroxidase
HSA	human serum albumin
Id	idiotype
ID	intradermal
IDR	intradermal reaction
IEF	isoelectric focusing
IF-A	inflammatory factor of anaphylaxis
Ig	immunoglobulin
IL	interleukin
IPB	ipratropium bromide
Ir	immune response
Is	immune suppressor
ISH	isocapnic hyperventilation
IU	international unit
IUIS	International Union of Immunological Societies
LBO	late bronchial obstruction
LBR	late bronchial reaction
LCR	late cutaneous reaction
LDL	low density lipoprotein
LES	lower esophageal sphincter
LESP	lower esophageal sphincter pressure
LNR	late nasal reaction
LPR	late phase reaction; late phase skin response
LSP	low sphincter pressure
LT	leukotriene

MAO	monoamine oxidase
MBP	major basic protein
MHC	major histocompatibility complex
MIF	migration inhibiting factor
MLR	mixed leukocyte reaction
MMEFR, MMFR	maximum midexpiratory flow rate
MPE	monomethylphosphatidylethanolamine
NAD	noradrenaline
NCA	neutrophil chemotactic activity
NCF	neutrophil chemotactic factor
NCF-A	neutrophil chemotactic factor of anaphylaxis
NHLI	National Health and Lung Institute
NIAID	National Institute for Allergy and Infectious Diseases
NIBSC	National Institute for Biological Standards and Control
OA	occupational asthma
PAF	platelet activating factor
PB	peripheral blood
PBA	polyclonal B-cell activators
PC	phosphatidylcholine
PCA	passive cutaneous anaphylaxis
PE	phosphatidylethanolamine
PEFR	peak expiratory flow rate
PFR	peak flow rate
PG	prostaglandin
P.I.	inspiratory pressure
PIE	pulmonary infiltrations with eosinophilia
PLA_2	phospholipase A_2
PMN	polymorphonuclear
PRN	only if needed
PT	prick test
RAST	radioallergosorbent test
Raw	airway resistance
RBL	rat basophilic leukemia
RD	reflux disease
RIA	radioimmunoassay
RSV	respiratory syncytial virus
RV	residual volume
SA	status asthmaticus
SCG	sodium cromoglycate
SD	standard deviation
SDS	sodium dodecyl sulfate
SGaw	specific airway conductance
SRS	slow reacting substance
SRS-A	slow reacting substance of anaphylaxis
S-TS	short-term sensitizing
TAME	tosyl-L-arginine methylester
TCPA	tetrachlorophthalic anhydride

TCS	T-cell supernatants
TDI	toluene diisocyanate
THAM	tromethamine
TL	thermolabile
TLC	total lung capacity
TLV	threshold limit value
TS	thermostable
Tx	thromboxane
URI	upper respiratory infection
VC	vital capacity
VE L BTPS	expired ventilation
VIP	vasoactive intestinal peptide
V.T.	tidal volume
WFR	wheal and flare reaction
WHO	World Health Organization

A. Introduction

1. Preface

F. B. Michel

Asthmology is the neologism I suggested for the title of a book published in 1981 on bronchial asthma [4, 5].

Among a certain number of scientific publications on this subject, it is one of the few suggestions that I have the weakness to feel somewhat proud of. In fact, this word has had the career I hoped it would and, judging by the frequency with which it is used in both written and spoken language, it did answer a need. I had no intention of suggesting one more neologism but it seemed to me that the word *asthmology* had an element of novelty and, above all, produced the necessary awareness of the need to bring together, within a kind of subtopic in pulmonary disorders, many different researchers, such as specialists of molecular biochemistry and immunology, physiologists, pneumologists, allergists, pediatricians, specialists of internal or physical medicine and psychologists. This is our current practice within the framework of a multispeciality consultation in *asthmology*.

Thus, the person who is particularly interested in *bronchial asthma* cannot fail to be surprised by the extreme diversity in the points of view concerning this syndrome.

To take just one obvious example, lung specialists and allergists differ greatly in their approach of tackling the problem, each taking into account his own conception of the truth. That is to say, in the end, putting too much emphasis on his own point of view.

However, if there is one extremely multifactor syndrome in medicine, it is really bronchial asthma. Misunderstanding or minimizing one or several factors of asthma or, on the contrary, favoring one factor more than another immediately leads to possible mistakes. Besides, asthma is an excellent example of the overlapping of the *innate* with the *acquired*. In fact, contrary to ideas which were acceptable at the beginning of the 20th century, and in particular to Pasteur's concept of "one cause, one illness", many syndromes like high blood pressure or asthma are the result of the overlapping of hereditary factors and acquired factors. This is one reason why asthma is not really an illness in the real sense of the word but, a clinical and functional respiratory *syndrome* [1].

The **innate**, the "terrain", transmitted by heredity, can possibly concern two factors: The *bronchial hyperreactivity factor* (BHR), is often present in early childhood and its reality is a result of the studies of large groups of homo- and heterozygotic twins. What we know less about, is the way in which it is transmitted and the substratum of its transmission.

The *allergic factor* represents, in the case of allergic component asthma, another element of the "terrain". We know that it is transmitted by the major complex of histocompatibility, which is situated on the short arm of the 6th pair of chromosomes.

Whereas it retains all its value, supported by daily clinical practice, this notion of the *innate* must however be qualified by the possibility of an *acquired* BHR, of which professional and postviral asthma are precise examples. After having believed for a long time that a person could only become an asthmatic if he was congenitally endowed with BHR characteristics, we now know that, in certain circumstances, such as severe virosis of the respiratory airways or massive exposure to an inhaled industrial irritant, BHR may appear, as evidenced by asthma, without any allergic mechanism and it will disappear when exposure to the professional risk ceases.

The **acquired** is represented by all factors in the environment which may favor it. This rather imprecise word, in fact, groups together the personal environment whether it be familial, professional, material or psychological, climatic and atmospheric etc. It is possible to distinguish more precisely among the factors supporting asthma (Fig. 1.1).

The *allergic component* has its place and treatment as one of the decisive elements in the evolution of our conceptions of bronchial asthma.

Without questioning in any way the importance of this component it is quite certain that, at least in France, it has been and remains overestimated; or to put it in a caricatural way, it has become frequently customary to say *asthma = allergy*. The reality of the allergic component of asthma, as well as its "weight" of responsibility in the triggering of that type of asthma, must, therefore, always be examined.

Moreover, one tends to forget that, allergic or not, asthma is also, and more and more as it evolves, an inflammatory disease of the bronchi. The anatomical results of this inflammation have been known for a very long time, but we are now getting to know its mechanisms better and better. These come from the cellular secretion and release of inflammatory mediators; cells and mediators being linked together by numerous interactions. Arachidonic acid and PAF metabolites are now considered as responsible agents, just as histamine has been considered for a very long time.

Prostaglandins, thromboxanes, leukotrienes and platelet aggregating factor (see also Chapter 22) [2] are able to reproduce, either individually or together, all the pathological conditions which are characteristic of asthma. The effectiveness of the glucocorticoids, one of whose mechanisms is to inhibit phospholipase A_2, seems to underline the physiopathological importance of these arachidonic acid metabolites. However, seen from a clinical point of view, 90% of these patients were able to ingest aspirin (or any other nonsteroid anti-inflammatory drug) without feeling any side effect; this phenomenon and the physiopathological inferences it implies have yet to be explained. PAF, platelet activating factor, is also a derivative from the membrane phospholipids and has strong bronchomotor and pro-inflammatory effects both in animals and man.

This bronchial inflammation evolves with time, which explains the different kinds of asthma and, in particular, bronchial obstruction which, as time goes on, becomes less and less reversible as it is more and more connected with the anatomical lesions and no longer with the bronchospasm.

Finally, it must be pointed out that if many mechanisms are becoming explainable there is still a long way to go between clinical symptoms and the understanding of biological reality.

Thus, taking the example of aspirin-induced asthma, which is both a difficult clinical form and a fascinating physiopathological model, the responsibility of arachidonic acid metabolites, although strongly suspected, has still not been demonstrated in vivo (Fig. 1.1).

The *infectious component* does not really correspond to bacterial infection but mainly to viral infection, whose role in the triggering of childhood asthma has been shown in numerous studies.

The *interrelationship between upper airway diseases and asthma* is also a reality. Although we have long known that rhinitis and sinusitis can be associated with asthma and/or play a part in the responsibility of its genesis, the use of sinuscopy, making it possible to **see** the cavity of the maxillary sinuses, to effectively **treat** certain anomalies and to **drain** and **clear** it better, also contributes to the improvement of a good number of asthmatics.

The *digestive component:* Although the frequent association between asthma and gastroesophageal reflux does not allow us to establish a cause-and-effect relationship between the two ailments all the time, it is quite evident that starting antireflux treatment often influences favorably the evolution of asthma.

The *psychological component:* Asthma remains, at least in Europe, underdiagnosed and undertreated. There are many reasons for this; one of them concerns nosology. As it disturbs respiration, that is to say breathing, in other words life, asthma is frightening and the word asthma itself is taboo. Therefore one hesitates to use it, preferring to resort to more reassuring words such as *asthma-like bronchitis* or *asthmatic bron-*

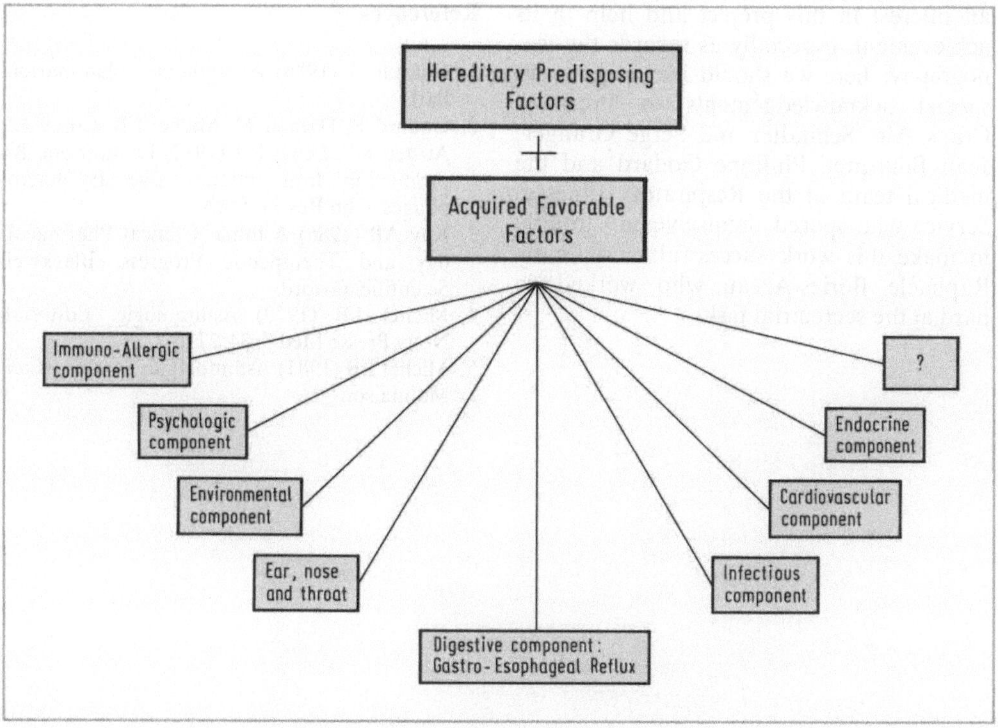

Fig. 1.1. Etiologic factors of bronchial asthma

chitis; it is also stated quite frequently, in order to reassure everybody but without any valid scientific argument, that "it will clear up on its own" at puberty.

Such an approach to asthma would not be serious, were it not detrimental to the asthmatic. On the contrary, it encourages people to leave things as they are whereas, in fact, it would be better to call a spade a spade, that is to say, give asthma its proper name, and to begin a complete assessment and a long-term therapeutic strategy. There are even some asthmatics who, after an evolution of between 3 and 5 years have not had their bronchial flow rate measured. All this in the hope, legitimate but unfounded, of distinguishing between asthmatic bronchitis, which is only temporary, and a so-called asthmatic illness which lasts a lifetime.

This is accompanied by a certain fatalistic, blasé pessimism which would have us believe that asthma is never cured. This is true if one speaks in terms of BHR, but incorrect if one speaks of asthmatic symptoms which are perfectly possible to control with adequate treatment.

Far from being a handicap, bronchial asthma treated, can be the beginning of a richer life, as certain Olympic athletes have shown it to be. Precisely because the respiratory functions and the person's development have been menaced by it.

Childhood asthma is no longer a permanent stigma but, on the contrary, with proper treatment, offers an opportunity to transform a handicap into a better life, just like those asthmatic children whose reeducation in the swimming pool took them to the Olympic stand.

This work would not have seen light of day without the active collaboration of many people whom we wish to thank: all the colleagues who accepted to write texts; the Publisher, represented in particular by Professor Clemens who coordinated the presentation of the work; the Sandoz-Laboratories who were so kind as to take an interest in this project and help in its achievement, especially as regards the iconography; here we should like to give our special acknowledgements to Professor Craps, Mrs Schindler and Serge Granger; Jean Bousquet, Philippe Godard and the medical team of the Respiratory Illnesses Service who spared themselves no trouble to make this work successful; and finally Raphaèle Bories-Azeau who worked so hard at the secretarial tasks.

References

1. Charpin J (1986) Allergologie. Flammarion, Paris
2. Godard P, Damon M, Michel FB, Corey EJ, Austen KF, Lewis RA (1983) Leukotriene B4 production from human alveolar macrophages. Clin Res 31:548A
3. Kay AB (1986) Asthma. Clinical Pharmacology and Therapeutic Progress. Blackwell Scientific, Oxford
4. Michel FB (1979) Asthmologie. Editorial. Nouv Presse Méd 8, 34:2725
5. Michel FB (1981) Asthmologie. Sandoz, Rueil Malmaison

2. Natural History of Asthma

T. A. E. Platts-Mills, P. W. Heymann

The characteristic symptoms of asthma are caused by reversible airway obstruction. This obstruction is largely due to smooth muscle spasm occurring in bronchi that are already hyperreactive. In addition to short-term episodes of wheezing, patients can often date the onset of their disease, i.e., the time when they started to have episodes of wheezing. Although very little prospective data is available, we assume that the onset of the disease coincides with the onset or increase in bronchial reactivity. Similarly, we assume that remissions (or cure) of asthma in most cases represent times at which there are falls in bronchial reactivity. When patients are asked about the causes of their asthma, they usually identify the *trigger factors* which cause their already hyperreactive airways to go into spasm. The underlying or *true* causes of the disease are the factors that lead to hyperreactivity, and most patients do not understand the causes of their bronchial reactivity. In trying to discuss the *natural history* of asthma, we will focus on what is known about the development and reversal of bronchial hyperreactivity rather than the short-term factors that influence episodes of bronchospasm.

There is good evidence that both experimental allergen exposure and seasonal natural exposure can increase bronchial reactivity [2, 13, 19]. In addition, there is clear evidence that allergen avoidance in sanatoria [22, 54], in hospital rooms [34], by changing employment [10] and even in the home [30] can lead to reductions in nonspecific bronchial reactivity. Thus, there is little difficulty in proposing that allergens play a major role in the bronchial reactivity of allergic patients. However, the mechanism by which allergen exposure increases bronchial reactivity is not clear, and it is most unlikely that it is a simple correlation of immediate hypersensitivity responses [3, 4, 13, 19]. In avoidance studies, *reversal* of bronchial reactivity has always required weeks or months [10, 22, 34] while following experimental allergen exposure, increased reactivity correlated better with *late* reactions than with immediate reactions [13, 19]. These *late* and prolonged effects of allergens on the lung can involve several different mediators, including: prostaglandins, leukotrienes [25], platelet activating factor [18, 27], eosinophil major basic protein [17] and T-cell lymphokines [42]. Furthermore, the cumulative effect of these mediators on bronchial reactivity will presumably depend on both the degree of *inflammation* initially and the rate at which healing occurs. Thus, in a patient with IgE antibody, the relationship between allergen exposure and bronchial hyperreactivity probably involves several different steps which can be independently controlled, and we should not expect to find a simple relationship between the IgE antibody response and natural history of the disease. We do not understand why patients with negative skin tests (idiopathic or intrinsic asthma) develop bronchial hyperreactivity. The natural history of intrinsic asthma was vividly described by Rackemann in 1947 [39]. He noted that the patients were older, developed severe asthma within a period of a year or less and did not improve when they were admitted to the hospital. In 1947, intrinsic asthma was often rapidly fatal and this prognosis has only been significantly altered by the introduction of steroid treatment. At present, we only rarely see the *natural history* of intrinsic asthma and very often the history is dominated by the progressive side effects of high dose steroid therapy.

In this chapter, we will focus on allergic asthma because we know more about the etiology. We will also assume that most asthma is either extrinsic or idiopathic, implying that we do not believe that *mixed* asthma is an important entity. However, this position is rather dogmatic and will be discussed further when considering how much of bronchial reactivity is reversible.

2.1 How Close is the Relationship between Allergy and Asthma?

The percentage of asthmatic patients who are judged to have *allergic* or extrinsic asthma varies enormously from clinic to clinic. In a tertiary care pulmonary unit in which the assessment of allergy is based on histories, it would not be unusual to conclude that allergy was only an important factor in 30% of asthmatic patients. By contrast in a primary care setting, a community asthma clinic, or in school health surveys where skin testing is used, it is not unusual to find that ~85% of asthmatic patients are allergic [11, 33, 46]. These figures change even more if skin testing with a wider range of allergens, including foods, dermophytes and the wide range of house dust contributors is included. Probably the most important factor is whether the importance of allergy is judged by history or by the assessment of immediate hypersensitivity. Many authors imply that allergy is unlikely to be important if the patients are unaware of it [50]. On the other hand, it is well recognized that histories of house dust or dust mite sensitivity are very unreliable [20, 29]. Patients are usually aware if domestic or laboratory animal sensitivity is contributing to their asthma [12, 26, 31], while histories of seasonal hay fever correlating loosely with seasonal exacerbations of asthma may be clear. In view of the high incidence of positive skin tests to house dust in patients with asthma, we need to consider whether house dust is an important cause of bronchial reactivity. In particular, we need to ask why patients who are allergic to dust mite, cockroach or other house dust allergens do not know whether these allergens are an important cause of their disease.

2.2 The Relationship between Allergen Particle Size and Symptoms

Although allergic asthma is always classified as an immediate hypersensitivity disease and the relevance of allergens is usually assessed by immediate hypersensitivity skin tests, the majority of allergic asthmatic patients are not aware of an immediate or even a direct relationship between allergen exposure and most of their attacks [20, 29, 33, 50]. For some allergens, e.g., cats, horses or laboratory animals, allergic patients do report acute attacks of asthma developing within 20 min of increased exposure to the allergen. These responses appear to be very similar to the response to bronchial provocation with nebulized allergen extract. By contrast, patients allergic to pollens, dust mites and Alternaria, usually are not aware of acute attacks precipitated by increased exposure. In the past, bronchial provocation with nebulized allergen has often been taken as both a diagnostic test to establish that a particular allergen is a cause of asthma and also as a model of natural exposure. It is, therefore, important to ask whether bronchial provocation is comparable to natural exposure. It has been known for some years that the total quantity of ragweed allergen used for bronchial provocation was much higher than natural exposure. Bruce et al estimated that bronchial provocation with ragweed extract containing 0.1–1.0 μg antigen E represented nearly a season's exposure in 2 min [7]. It seems that provocation with either ragweed or mite antigen often represents a quantity equivalent to approximately 10 days of natural exposure. However, an equally important question is whether natural exposure is to particles of the same size as nebulized droplets. At a simple level, it is obvious that pollen grains, mite fecal particles and Alternaria spores (size range 10–40 μm) are much larger than the 2 μm diameter droplets used for bronchial provocation. However, since only a small proportion of these large particles will enter the lungs, it has been argued that the real contribution of these allergens to asthma comes from small particles. Two recent papers have argued that a significant proportion of ragweed allergen is airborne in

Table 2.1. Three different examples of inhaled allergens: relationship between particle size, allergen concentration and the number of particles

Size	Examples	Concentration/ qty of allergen	No. of particles	% entering the lung	Quantity of allergen
Large > 10 μm	Mite feces Pollen grains Large fungal spores	~0.2 ng/particle (~10 mg/ml)	~100	~5%	20 ng
Medium > 5–8 μm	Rat allergen	1 mg/ml[a]	~ 27,000	15–20%	20 ng
Small < 3 μm	Nebulized droplets Small fungal spores?	10 μg/ml[b]	~100 Million	15–25%	20 ng

[a] Concentration of rat allergen in male rat urine
[b] A concentration often used as the maximum in bronchial provocation

the form of particles smaller than 3 μm in diameter [1, 49]. However, these results are dependent on the fractionation of particles using a high volume Anderson sampler and there has to be some doubt about the technique. It seems most unlikely that 60% of ragweed allergen becomes airborne on small particles and one would like to see the results confirmed by other techniques.

We have analyzed airborne allergen exposure for two different allergens, dust mite antigen P_1 and the rat urinary allergen [35, 52]. Antigen P_1 from *D. pteronyssinus* only becomes airborne in houses during disturbance. Over 75% of the airborne allergen impacts on the first stage of a cascade impactor. 96% of the allergen that becomes airborne falls in 15 min, and finally, the particles carrying allergen that impact on the cascade impactor can be identified by electron microscopy as mite fecal particles. All these observations support the view that natural exposure to antigen P_1 is in the form of particles > 10 μm diameter (mean diameter 20 μm), and the maximum levels we have seen during disturbance in a house are ~ 20 ng collected in 20 min at 17 l/min which represents approximately 60 ng/m^3 or 300 fecal particles/m^3. The quantities of antigen P_1 associated with particles < 5 μm diameter were very low indeed, generally < 1 ng inhaled/hour. For the rat urinary allergen, airborne distribution was significantly different in that nearly half of the airborne allergen impacted on the second disc of the impactor and this allergen fell more slowly, i.e., only 80% in 15 min [35]. However, even the rat urinary allergen was airborne on particles significantly larger (7 μm diameter) than those produced by a nebulizer. It seems worth comparing the inhalation of 20 ng of allergen using these three forms: a) mite fecal particles which are very similar to pollen grains in their physical properties; b) 7 μm droplets of rat urine with a concentration of allergen approximately 1 mg/ml, i.e., the concentration of allergen in rat urine; and c) nebulized aqueous extract with a concentration of allergen of about 1 μg/ml (see Table 2.1). What is clear is that bronchial provocation and probably exposure to rat allergen would involve an even distribution of droplets throughout all the subsegments of the lung. Consequently, any response would involve all subsegments and would cause measurable increased airway resistance at the minimum dose necessary to cause a response. By contrast, occasional large particles entering the lung could cause a local inflammatory response in one small bronchus, including spasm without giving rise to measurable changes in airway resistance or to symptoms at that time (Fig. 2.1). The implication is that large particles could give rise to progressive inflammation of the lungs without any acute episodes of bronchospasm. Conversely, small particles might well cause acute diffuse bronchospasm without reaching sufficient concentration in any part of the lung to cause a prolonged inflammatory response. Obviously, most, if not all, natural allergens would represent a mixture of small and large particle exposure, but the fact that histories of dust mite (or pollen or

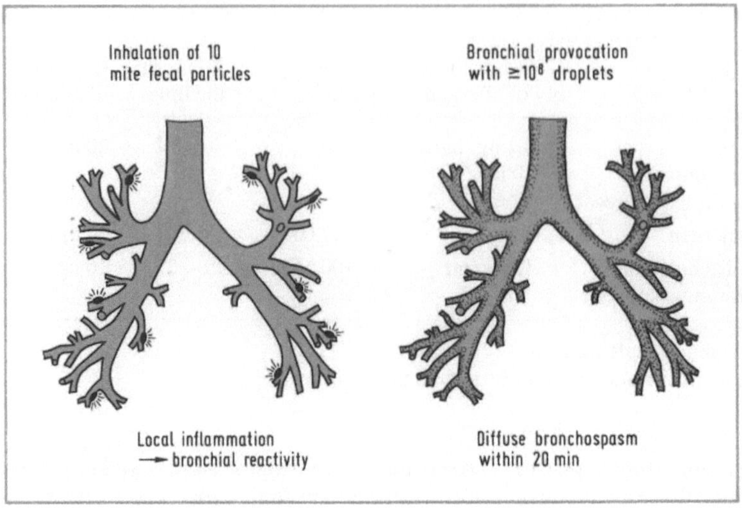

Fig. 2.1. A model of the effects of breathing either 100 mite fecal particles of which ≦ 10% enter the lung and cause a local inflammatory response, or 10^8 droplets of dilute allergen of which 25% enter the lungs and cause diffuse bronchospasm at the threshold dose. With droplets, late or prolonged inflammatory response would only be expected if the concentration used was greater than the threshold level for bronchospasm

fungal) allergy in asthma are so unreliable would be explained if the major role of these allergens was their contribution to bronchial reactivity mediated by a few large particles entering the lung each day. Similarly, as Hargreave and Dolovich and Cockcroft have shown, bronchial provocation only leads to prolonged increases in bronchial reactivity if the challenge is sufficient to cause not only an immediate response but also a late response [13, 19]. That is, the bronchial challenge dose usually has to be greater than the minimum quantity necessary to cause acute bronchospasm before any prolonged inflammatory effect occurs.

2.3 How Much of Bronchial Reactivity is Reversible?

If allergens play an important role in the maintenance of bronchial reactivity, the implication is that *complete* avoidance of allergens would lead to the reversal of bronchial reactivity. The effects of allergen *avoidance* can be observed in several different ways.

One way is by following patients, who are allergic to seasonal allergens, throughout the year. Several groups have now confirmed Altounyan's original observation that patients with *grass pollen asthma* lose their hyperreactivity during the autumn and winter, and it is obvious that reduction may not take place until several months after the end of the pollen season [2, 13, 19].

A second observation can be made by following workers, who have asthma associated with industrial exposure, after they leave that employment. The most elegant studies of this kind have been carried out by Dr. Chan-Yeung, in Canada [10]. Workers exposed to western red cedar who developed asthma generally improved after they stopped working with the wood dust and about two thirds lost their bronchial hyperreactivity over several months [10]. However, a few remained hyperreactive for years which suggests that in some cases bronchial hyperreactivity, even if induced by allergen exposure, may not always be reversible. Similarly, following workers with asthma apparently caused by toluene diisocyanate has given confusing results about whether prolonged avoidance can lead to full recovery or not [32].

Attempts to reduce house dust exposure by cleaning patients' houses have produced clinical improvement in some cases, but not others [8, 23, 30, 45]. However, where measurements of mites or mite allergens have been carried out, it appears that the failures have occurred because of the difficulty in reducing the number of mites in houses, rather than a failure of avoidance to reduce symptoms [8, 23]. One study has reported clinical improvement and a modest reduction in bronchial reactivity as a result of *cleaning* the bedrooms of mite-allergic asthmatic children [30]. However, changes in mite numbers or allergen levels were not documented in that study.

The biggest changes in bronchial reactivity have been reported in dust-allergic patients moved out of their houses into high altitude sanatoria or allergen-free rooms [22, 34, 54]. Kerrebijn reported in 1970 that a large proportion of the asthmatic children moved from Holland to Davos showed marked reductions in bronchial reactivity to histamine [22]. Indeed, many of the children showed progressive reductions in bronchial reactivity over a year and reached normal levels. At that time, most investigators considered that bronchial hyperreactivity was a physiological property of the asthmatic lung, and the authors did not really consider the possibility that allergen avoidance was responsible for the reduced reactivity. However, the children were known to be allergic to dust mites, and it is known, from the work of Dr. Spieksma, that mite numbers in Davos are much lower than those in Holland. In London (UK), 7 mite-allergic asthmatic adults spent long periods living in a hospital room; 5 of 7 showed > 8-fold increase in PD30 for histamine. For the group, this increase was highly significant [34]. The mite allergen levels in the room were approximately 2% of the levels in the patients' houses (mean level 240 ng/g in hospital versus 13,600 ng antigen P_1/g of dust at home). Strikingly, the time needed to observe noticeable changes were months. Typically, it took ~ 2–3 weeks before the patients were well enough to carry out bronchial provocation and 2–3 months to see an 8-fold change. Furthermore, the changes were not related to progressive relaxation of the lungs since FEV_1 and peak flow reached normal levels before changes in reactivity started. However, two of the seven patients who reached normal spirometry did not show any reduction in bronchial reactivity over 3 months.

Finally, it is worth remembering that the increased bronchial reactivity associated with viral infections or following bronchial provocation has been reported to return to normal after a few weeks [15, 19].

Taken together, these studies leave no doubt that allergen avoidance can lead to reduced levels of nonspecific bronchial reactivity. However, in all studies so far, the *allergen avoidance* has been nearly complete, and these changes have taken many weeks or months. In patients with pollen asthma, seasonal changes in reactivity have been clearly documented; whether similar changes occur in house dust-related asthma has not been established.

2.4 Is the Development and Cure of Asthma Related to the Time Course of Immune Responses to Allergens?

Studying the development of asthma in young children is very difficult because it is not easy to distinguish acute bronchiolitis or bronchitis with bronchospasm from asthma. Children typically have several ill-defined episodes of breathlessness or coughing before it becomes obvious that they are suffering from asthma. Many studies in children have attempted to relate specific viral infections to the onset of asthma. Those studies have suggested either that viral infection could be responsible for the initial lung damage or that viral infections could initiate the IgE Ab response to allergens [16, 37]. On the other hand, following a group of children who had bronchiolitis caused by RSV did not reveal an increased incidence of asthma [37]. An alternative approach is to follow high risk children prospectively and try to record the time sequence of viral infections, antibody responses to allergens and the development of asthma. In a study following 80 children in Poole (UK) for 5 years, Cogswell found that there were multiple episodes of respiratory disease in the first year with little clear pattern or relationship to asthma; however, in the fourth and fifth year, the children with repeated episodes of symptoms had a high incidence of sensitivity to dust mite allergens [44]. Although there appeared to be a correlation between the development of immediate hypersensitivity and the development of asthma, it was still very difficult to arrange the events in any strict time sequence.

In the Poole study, it was also clear that children developed antibodies to egg and milk proteins in the first year of life, while antibody responses to dust started in the second and third year. Only an occasional child had an antibody response to grass pollen allergen by the age of 5 years [44]. This sequential development of antibodies to different groups of allergens is in keeping with the much older views of Rackemann [40]. He observed that allergic patients often had food allergy, dust allergy and pollen allergy sequentially. In that study, it was observed that patients often lost sensitivity to one allergen while gaining sensitivity to another; however, at that time (1948), there were no antibody assays available suitable for documenting declining sensitivity. The spontaneous *cure* of allergic disease has been well documented in studies in Tecumseh, Michigan [6], but long-term follow-up studies on individual patients are very difficult. In order to study the changes in antibodies that occur over long periods, we have recently studied groups of patients diagnosed as having dust-allergic asthma in 1941, 1951, 1961, and 1971 [41]. The results showed that both IgE anti-antigen P_1 and IgE anti-*D. pteronyssinus* as measured by RAST were progressively lower the longer after diagnosis. In addition, approximately two thirds of the patients lost their symptoms over a 40-year period. However, the results suggested that on average patients lost their symptoms 10–15 years earlier than they lost their IgE antibodies. These results appeared to show that spontaneous cure was not a direct consequence of falling IgE antibody levels [41].

2.5 Possible Mechanisms Contributing to 'Cure' of Asthma

Marked reduction in symptoms of asthma often occurs without any clear explanation but may be related to changes in the patients' life-style or in response to treatment (Table 2.2). Both in *spontaneous cure* and following desensitization, improvement can occur with continued exposure to allergen and without a significant fall in IgE antibodies [41, 53]. A possible explanation of these spontaneous changes in *allergic* asthma could come from changes in sensitized T-cells. We know that many patients with asthma have T-cells sensitized to the same allergens against which they have IgE Ab [see 33 for refs., 42]. In addition, we know that the responses of T-cells *in vitro* alter during desensitization therapy [43]. However, no evidence is available about changes in T-cell function during prolonged follow-up or spontaneous cure. Examining T-cell proliferative responses of al-

Table 2.2. Remission or cure of asthma

Spontaneous cure over time:
- a) With loss of IgE antibodies
- b) With persistent IgE antibodies

Avoidance of an allergic cause:
- a) Moving (sanatorium, hospital room, changing houses)*
- b) Seasonal change in pollen allergen*
- c) Removing an animal from the house
- d) Change in employment*

Desensitization treatment:

a) Early (2–3 months)	= Loss of late reactions
	= Rise in IgG Ab
	= Altered *in vitro* T-cell response
b) Late (2–3 years)	= Progressive loss of IgE Ab

Pharmacological treatment:
- a) Cromolyn sodium*
- b) Steroids

* Demonstrated falls in bronchial reactivity

lergic patients with different symptoms (i.e., rhinitis, asthma and/or atopic dermatitis) did not reveal differences [42], so that it is unlikely that the *in vitro* proliferative response is a close reflection of the way in which T-cells contribute to lung damage. However, several studies have suggested that late reactions both in the skin and in the lung can be modified by desensitization treatment [38, 55]. This is particularly interesting since late reactions following bronchial provocation appear to correlate with increased bronchial reactivity [19]. At present, the mechanism of late reactions is still only partially resolved. It appears that some parts of a late response can be passively transferred with IgE antibody [14, 48]. On the other hand, the basophil infiltrate in a late reaction or in eczematous patch responses cannot be transferred with IgE antibody alone [28]. At present, it seems unlikely that changes in late reactions are simply a reflection of changes in IgE antibody levels and a regulatory role for T-cells or T-cell products in late reactions is by no means ruled out. Thus, the immunological mechanism of *cure,* either following desensitization or over long periods of time, is not clear but could include changes in T-cells or in mediator production and, in some cases, changes in IgE antibody. There is very little evidence that changes in IgG antibody are responsible for *cure* of inhalant allergy in any situation [41]. At present, it seems reasonable to conclude that, although skin tests and IgE antibody are excellent markers of an immune response to inhalant allergens, the response includes IgG Ab, IgA Ab and T-cells as well as IgE Ab [33]. The inflammatory effect of these allergens on the lung involves either a mechanism other than IgE Ab or involves a secondary consequence of IgE-triggered mediator release that can be modulated independently of IgE antibody.

2.6 Alternative Causes of Bronchial Reactivity

In all age groups, a significant proportion of asthmatic patients do not have positive skin tests to common inhalant allergens. The term *intrinsic* was first used by Robert Cook because he thought that most of these cases were caused by an internal allergen. However, Rackemann (1947) used the term *intrinsic* synonymously with idiopathic [39]. Rackemann's description of patients who had an onset of asthma after the age of 40, negative skin tests, who did not improve in hospital, and often died within a few years has dominated our vision of these patients since then. Certainly, some of these patients run a severe course and are persistently *steroid-dependent.* However, there appear to be some important subdivisions within this group. Firstly, there are the patients with only partially reversible obstruction. Using 20% reversal as the definition of asthma, there are many patients who have asthma but who never reach 50% of predicted FEV_1 (or particularly FEF_{25-75}) despite aggressive treatment. In our experience, most (but not all) of these patients are not allergic to common inhalant allergens and often require steroids for long periods. Secondly, there are occasional food-allergic patients whose allergy can be confirmed by skin testing and RAST and whose condition can be helped by specific diet. These patients should not be confused with the rather common phenomenon that patients with severe and largely fixed obstruction often report that *milk products* increase their mucus production, and they feel better on a diet. Thirdly, there are a group of patients who have intermittent very severe obstructive disease but who respond fully to steroids. Some of these patients have positive skin tests to surprising extracts, e.g. crude house dust without specific responses to any of the recognized components or epidermophytons, yeast or Aspergillus. The house dust sensitivity may be explained by cockroach, spiders, beetles, etc., and Aspergillus is recognized as an inhalant allergen as well as a cause of bronchopulmonary aspergillosis. However, there is no agreement about whether Trichophyton can contribute to lung inflammation and asthma. Bacterial allergy, which is often diagnosed in some European countries has been very difficult to prove as a cause of asthma, and in England and the United States, bacterial allergy is not generally accepted as a cause of asthma. At present, intrinsic asthma remains very unsatisfactory. No proof is forthcoming that the range of *intrinsic* allergens is really the cause of the disease but no alternative explanation for the steroid-responsive bronchial inflammation in these patients has been demonstrated.

2.7 Genetic Predisposition to Asthma

The Dutch hypothesis implied that patients with asthma had a genetically determined increased bronchial reactivity which was the real cause of asthma. In those patients various different trigger factors would be important, including exercise, allergens, etc. We would now interpret this information rather differently and suggest that individuals are either potentially asthmatic or normal and that both groups can become allergic. If potentially asthmatic patients become allergic and are exposed to sufficient allergen, they will get progressively increased bronchial hyperreactivity which will lead to symptoms or even severe symptoms.

In this model, the patients may have two separate controls, the control which makes them more likely to make immune responses to inhalant allergens, i.e. the atopic diathesis or atopy, and in addition, controls that decide whether their lungs are liable to develop increased bronchial reactivity. There are good reasons for believing that these two controls are at least in part hereditary and that they are largely independent. Genetic, or HLA, studies of asthma are not nearly as satisfactory as those of hay fever because, while it can be assumed that pollen exposure in a particular geographic area is reasonably similar, there are very large differences in the levels of house dust allergen exposure between houses. House dust from some houses contains > 100,000 ng antigen P_1/g, while in another house or apartment within 5 miles, dust may contain < 200 ng/g, i.e. < 1%. Nonetheless, there is good evidence from family studies that families can inherit inhalant allergy without a tendency to develop asthma while other families have a very high incidence of asthma which is only in part linked to atopy [see 33].

2.8 The Smoking Confusion

Smoking cigarettes probably does more harm than the whole hospital service does good, and there is no question that cigarette smoking is a very important cause of chronic bronchitis and emphysema. There is also evidence that smoking appears to cause mild increases in bronchial reactivity, increased IgE levels within the normal range, and small rises in eosinophils in nonallergic nonasthmatic patients [51]. In addition, many asthmatic patients are acutely sensitive to tobacco smoke and report not only discomfort but marked exacerbations of their bronchospasm on exposure to tobacco smoke. On the other hand, it is well-known that some asthmatic patients continue to smoke and maintain that they become worse if they stop smoking. Recently, a study from Australia reported that almost one third of asthmatic patients who stopped smoking suffered an exacerbation of their bronchospasm and about 10% felt they were unable to continue without smoking [21]. We have also seen this phenomenon in our clinical practice and now recommend that allergic asthmatic patients should carry out allergen avoidance measures and/or start desensitization before they stop smoking. The more interesting part of the smoking confusion, however, comes from a long-term follow-up of asthmatic patients and a large population study. In Phoenix, Arizona, Burrows found that smoking correlated with reduced lung function in all sections of the population *except* allergic asthmatic patients [9]. In South Wales, a retrospective survey by Rawle et al found that patients diagnosed as having house dust-allergic asthma 30 or 40 years earlier reported *less* symptoms of bronchospasm if they had continued to smoke [41]. While there are obviously many different interpretations of these results, it seems possible that smoking, while causing direct damage to the lung, can also reduce immunological inflammation caused by allergens. Certainly, there is evidence that smokers have a lower incidence of extrinsic allergic alveolitis which again suggests a direct immunosuppressive effect of smoking on the lung [5].

2.9 Conclusions

The symptoms of asthma often fluctuate dramatically from day to day. This variability results from a complicated interaction of trigger factors and the much slower changes in bronchial reactivity. The present discussion has been based on the premise that bronchial hyperreactivity is largely reversible, the onset of clinical asthma probably represents the onset of increased bronchial reactivity, and it is possible to identify factors causing alterations in reactivity. We are also assuming that most of the factors that trigger acute attacks of asthma are not causes of bronchial reactivity. Thus, we are assuming that most of the things that the patient recognizes as causes, e.g. emotion, cold air, changes in humidity, exercise, tobacco smoke, etc., are not the *causes* that we are interested in.

Two *causes* stand out, viral infections and allergens. However, in each case, their role in asthma is not simple. While viral infections can precipitate an acute attack in a patient with a preexisting reactivity, they can also increase reactivity without causing marked symptoms [15]. Many doctors believe that it is viral infections which cause the initial changes in the lung which develop into bronchial hyperreactivity. On the other hand, many episodes of increased nasal and sinus secretion which are accepted as viral infections by patients and doctors are not confirmed by viral cultures and may have some other basis. Similarly with allergens, it is clear that they can precipitate acute attacks of asthma in allergic patients, but they are also an important cause of bronchial reactivity. We believe that much of the confusion about the role of allergens comes because different forms of exposure can favor one response or another. That is, regular inhalation of a few large particles would cause progressive inflammation without any acute episodes of bronchospasm. By contrast, a large number of small particles can cause acute bronchospasm without any increase in inflammation. Thus, the patients may know which allergens cause acute attacks, but they would not be expected to recognize which allergens contribute to their bronchial reactivity.

Since only a few nanograms of allergen are inhaled, only individuals who have made an immune response would be expected to react, and it is common experience that there is an extremely good correlation between systemic IgE Ab response and lung response. Almost all patients whose lungs respond to ragweed or dust mite allergen have easily demonstrable IgE antibodies. However, there are many patients who have IgE Ab but not asthma, and there are good reasons for believing that the inflammatory response in the lung is not simply caused by mast cells releasing the mediators of *immediate* hypersensitivity. The implication is that we are looking at the time course of an immune response that includes IgE antibody but which also includes a delayed element.

Whether a given individual makes an immune response in the first place is decided by his genetic background, his reaction to viral infection, and the dose of exposure. Particles such as pollen grains or mite fecal pellets are the most effective way of carrying large quantities of a foreign protein into the nose. It is clear the pollen allergy is restricted to areas where the peak pollen count remains high, $>50/m^3$ for several weeks. Equally, it has now been recognized in several different parts of the world that dust mite counts $>100/g$ of fine dust are associated with symptoms of asthma [24]. This level translates to a value of 10,000 ng of antigen P_1 (or antigen P_1 equivalent)/g of fine dust [36]. Further similar levels may be associated with an increased incidence of antibody response in children [44]. Increasingly, the factors in a house that lead to high mite counts are being defined, and the early work of Spieksma showing that high relative humidity is the most important factor in a house has been amply confirmed [24, 47]. The combination of damp houses with fitted carpets and mild central heating, e.g. in England, Holland or New Zealand, is ideal for mite growth, and under these circumstances, it may be very difficult to reduce the quantity of mite allergen in a house.

Finally, the important conclusion is that, while asthma is a disease of rapidly reversible bronchospasm, it is also a disease in which bronchial hyperreactivity can increase or decrease over prolonged periods. Increasingly, the chronic management of asthma will be directed to encouraging the natural processes that can lead to reduced bronchial reactivity.

References

1. Agarwal MK, Swanson MC, Reed CE, Yunginger JW (1983) Airborne ragweed allergens: association with various particle sizes and short ragweed plant parts. J Allergy Clin Immunol 74:687–693
2. Altounyan REC (1970) Changes in histamine and atropine responsiveness as a guide to diagnosis and evaluation of therapy in obstructive airways disease. In: Pepys J, Frankland AW (eds) Disodium cromoglycate in allergic airways disease. Butterworth, London, pp 47–53
3. Askenase P (1977) Role of basophils, mast cells and vasoamines in hypersensitivity reactions with a delayed time course. Prog Allergy 23:199–320
4. Austen KF, Orange RP (1975) Bronchial asthma: the possible role of chemical mediators of immediate hypersensitivity on the pathogenesis of subacute chronic disease. Am Rev Respir Dis 112:423–436
5. Belin L (1980) Clinical and immunological data on 'wood trimmer's disease' in Sweden. Eur J Respir Dis [Suppl 107] 61:169–176
6. Broder I, Higgings MW, Mathews KP, Keller JB (1974) Epidemiology of asthma and allergic rhinitis in a total community, Tecumseh, Michigan. IV. Natural history. J Allergy Clin Immunol 54:100–110
7. Bruce CA, Rosenthal RR, Lichtenstein LM, Norman PS (1974) Diagnostic tests in ragweed-allergic asthma. A comparison of direct skin tests, leukocyte histamine release and quantitative bronchial challenge. J Allergy Clin Immunol 53:230–239
8. Burr ML, Dean BV, Merrett TG, Neale E, St. Leger AS, Verrier-Jones ER (1980) The effects of anti-mite measures on children with mite sensitive asthma. A controlled trial. Thorax 35:506
9. Burrows B, Halonen M, Lebowitz MD, Knudson RJ, Barbee RA (1982) The relationship of serum immunoglobulin E, allergy skin tests and smoking to respiratory disorders. J Allergy Clin Immunol 70:199–204
10. Chan-Yeung M (1977) Fate of occupational asthma. A follow-up study of patients with occupational asthma due to Western Red Cedar (*Thuja plicata*). Am Rev Respir Dis 116:1023–1029
11. Clarke CW, Aldons PM (1979) The nature of asthma in Brisbane. Clin Allergy 9:147–152
12. Cockcroft A, Edwards J, McCarthy P, Andersson N (1981) Allergy in laboratory animal workers. Lancet I:827–830
13. Cockcroft DW (1983) Mechanism of perennial allergic asthma. Lancet II:253–255
14. Dolovich J, Hargreave FE, Chalmers R, Shier KJ, Gauldie J, Bienenstock J (1973) Late cutaneous allergic responses in isolated IgE dependent reactions. J Allergy Clin Immunol 52:38
15. Empey DW, Laiteinen LA, Jacobs L, Gold WM, Nadel JA (1976) Mechanisms of bronchial hyper-reactivity in normal subjects after upper respiratory infection. Am Rev Respir Dis 113:131
16. Frick OL, German DF, Mills J (1979) Development of allergy in children. I. Association with virus infections. J Allergy Clin Immunol 63:228
17. Gleich GJ, Frigas E, Filley WV, Loegering DA (1984) Eosinophils and bronchial inflammation. In: Kay AB, Austen KF, Lichtenstein LM (eds) Asthma. Academic Press, London, pp 195–210
18. Hanahan DJ, Demopoulos CA, Liehr J, Pinkard RN (1980) Identification of platelet activating factor isolated from rabbit basophils as acetyl glyceryl ether phosphorylcholine. J Biol Chem 255:5514–5516
19. Hargreave FE, Dolovich J (1984) Bronchial responsiveness and late asthmatic response. In: Kay AB, Austen KF, Lichtenstein LM (eds) Asthma. Academic Press, London, pp 263–277
20. Hendrick DJ, Davies RJ, d'Souza MF, Pepys J (1975) An analysis of skin prick test reactions in 656 asthmatic patients. Thorax 30:2–8
21. Hillerdahl G, Rylander R (1984) Asthma and cessation of smoking. Clin Allergy 14:45–47
22. Kerrebijn KF (1970) Endogenous factors in childhood CNSLD. Methodological aspects in population studies. In: Orie NGM, van der Lende R (eds) Bronchitis III. Van Gorcum, Assen, pp 38–48
23. Korsgaard J (1982) Preventive measures in house-dust allergy. Am Rev Respir Dis 125: 80–84
24. Korsgaard J (1983) Mite asthma and residency: a case control study on the impact of exposure to house-dust mites in dwellings. Am Rev Respir Dis 128:231–235
25. Lewis RA, Mencia-Huerta JM, Lee CW, Austen KF (1984) Mast cell dependent synthesis of lipid mediators of immediate hypersensitivity. In: Kay AB, Austen KF, Lichtenstein LM (eds) Asthma. Academic Press, London, pp 63–83

26. Lutsky II, Kalbfleisch JH, Fink JN (1983) Occupational allergy to laboratory animals: employer practices. J Occup Med 25:372–376
27. Mencia-Huerta JM, Hadji L, Benveniste J (1981) Release of a slow-reacting substance from rabbit platelets. J Clin Invest 68: 1586–1591
28. Mitchell EB, Crow J, Rowntree S, Webster ADB, Platts-Mills TAE (1984) Cutaneous basophil hypersensitivity to inhalant allergens: local transfer of basophil accumulation with immune serum but not IgE antibody. J Invest Dermatol 83:290–295
29. Murray AB, Ferguson AC (1983) Diagnosis of house dust mite allergy in asthmatic children: what constitutes a positive history? J Allergy Clin Immunol 71:21–28
30. Murray AB, Ferguson AC (1983) Dust-free bedrooms in the treatment of asthmatic children with house dust or house dust mite allergy: a controlled trial. Pediatrics 71:418–422
31. Newman-Taylor A, Longbottom JL, Pepys J (1977) Respiratory allergy to urine proteins of rats and mice. Lancet II:847–849
32. Paggiaro PL, Loi AM, Rossi O, Ferrante B, Pardi F, Rosselli MG, Baschieri L (1984) Follow-up study of patients with respiratory disease due to toluene diisocyanate TDI. Clin Allergy 14:463–469
33. Platts-Mills TAE (1982) Type I or immediate hypersensitivity. In: Lachmann PJ, Peters DK (eds) Clinical aspects of immunology, 4th edn. Blackwell, London Oxford, pp 579–686
34. Platts-Mills TAE, Tovey ER, Mitchell EB, Mozarro H, Nock P, Wilkins SR (1982) Reversal of bronchial hyper-reactivity during prolonged allergen avoidance. Lancet II: 675–678
35. Platts-Mills TAE, Heymann PW, Longbottom J, Wilkins SR (1986) Airborne particles carrying dust mite and rat allergens. J Allergy Clin Immunol 77:850–857
36. Platts-Mills TAE, Heymann PW, Chapman MD, Hayden ML, Wilkins SR (1986) Cross-reacting and species specific determinants on the major allergen from *D. pteronyssinus* and *D. farinae*: development of a radioimmunoassay for 'Antigen P_1 Equivalent' in house dust. J Allergy Clin Immunol 78:398–407
36a. Platts-Mills TAE, Fiocco GP, Pollart S, Hayden ML, Jackson S, Wilkins SR (1986) Trichophyton allergy in a 24 year-old man with "intrinsic" asthma. Ann Allergy 56:454–455, 470–471
37. Polmer SH, Robinson LD, Minnefor AB (1972) Immunoglobulin E in bronchiolitis. Pediatrics 50:279
38. Price JF, Warner JO, Hey EN, Turner MW, Soothill JF (1984) A controlled trial of hyposensitization with adsorbed tyrosine *Dermatophagoides pteronyssinus* antigen in childhood asthma: in vivo aspects. Clin Allergy 14:209–219
39. Rackemann FM (1947) A working classification of asthma. Am J Med 3:601–606
40. Rackemann FM, Edwards RC (1952) Asthma in children: follow-up study of 688 patients after an interval of 20 years. N Engl J Med 246:815–823, 858–863
41. Rawle FC, Burr ML, Platts-Mills TAE (1983) Long-term falls in antibodies to dust mite and pollen allergens in patients with asthma or hay fever. Clin Allergy 13:409–417
42. Rawle FC, Mitchell EB, Platts-Mills TAE (1984) T cell responses to the major allergen from the house dust mite, *Dermatophagoides pteronyssinus*, Antigen P_1. J Immunol 133: 195–201
43. Rocklin RE, Sheffer AL, Greineder DK, Melmon KL (1980) Generation of antigen specific suppressor cells during allergy desensitization. N Engl J Med 302:1213–1216
44. Rowntree SR, Cogswell JJ, Mitchell EB, Platts-Mills TAE (1985) Development of antibodies to inhalant allergens during the first five years of life. Arch Dis Child 60:727–735
45. Sarsfield JK, Gowland G, Toy R, Norman AL (1974) Mite sensitive asthma of childhood trial of avoidance measures. Arch Dis Child 49:716–721
46. Smith MJ, Disney ME, Williams JD, Goels ZA (1969) Clinical significance of skin reactions to mite extracts in children with asthma. Br Med J 2:723–726
47. Smith TF, Kelly LB, Heymann PW, Wilkins SR, Platts-Mills TAE (1985) Exposure and antibody responses to house dust mite of mite allergic asthmatic children in Atlanta. J Allergy Clin Immunol 76:782–788
48. Solley GO, Gleich GJ, Jordan RE, Schoreter AL (1976) The late phase of the immediate wheal and flare skin reaction – its dependence on IgE antibodies. J Clin Invest 58:408–420
49. Solomon WR, Burge HA, Muilenberg ML (1983) Allergen carriage by atmospheric aerosol. 1. Ragweed pollen determinants in smaller micronic fractions. J Allergy Clin Immunol 72:443–447
50. Stevenson DD, Mathison DA, Tan EM, Vaughan JH (1975) Provoking factors in bronchial asthma. Arch Intern Med 135: 777–783
51. Taylor RG, Joyce H, Gross E, Holland F, Pride NB (1985) Bronchial reactivity to inhaled histamine and annual rate of decline

in FEV_1 in male smokers and ex-smokers. Thorax 40:9–16, 17–22
52. Tovey ER, Chapman MD, Wells CW, Platts-Mills TAE (1981) The distribution of dust mite allergen in the houses of patients with asthma. Am Rev Respir Dis 124:630–635
53. Turner MW, Yalcin I, Soothill JF, Price JF, Warner JO, Hey EN, Chapman MD, Platts-Mills TAE (1984) In vitro investigations in asthmatic children undergoing hyposensitization with tyrosine-adsorbed *Dermatophagoides pteronyssinus* antigen. Clin Allergy 14:221–231
54. Vervloet D, Penaud A, Razzouk H, Senft M, Arnaud A, Boutin C, Charpin J (1982) Altitude and dust mites. J Allergy Clin Immunol 69:290–296
55. Warner JO (1976) Significance of late reactions after bronchial challenge with house dust mite. Arch Dis Child 51:905–911

B. Epidemiology

3. Epidemiology of Bronchial Asthma

D. Charpin, J. Charpin

The epidemiological study of asthma includes:

Descriptive epidemiology, i.e., mortality and morbidity in relation to asthma and disease distribution according to some personal characteristics.

Analytic epidemiology in search of risk factors. Etiology being described in another chapter of this book, we will consider, among extrinsic risk factors, air pollution, allergens, meteorological conditions, and among intrinsic factors, atopy and hyperreactivity.

Experimental epidemiology, i.e., preventive and therapeutic interventions which are dealt with in another chapter of this book.

3.1 Asthma as a Public Health Problem

Mortality rate is a poor index because deaths from asthma are uncommon. Some deaths from wheezy bronchitis are probably misclassified as asthma deaths. A likely estimate for this mortality in France ranges from 0.5 to 1 death per year per 100,000 persons. However, from 1961 to 1967, especially in Great Britain, this rate reached 2 deaths per 100,000 persons. This increase in the death rate in 6 years amounted to 3,000 extra deaths. β-adrenergic sprays, marketed in Europe since 1960, have been charged with this increase in mortality [40]. In New Zealand, the same increase was noticed at the same time and is still going on [22]. This increase in mortality seems related to a therapeutic association of bronchodilators (β-agonists and theophylline), or to an unfortunate substitution of steroids with sprays of β-agonists, when these latter drugs were marketed, rather than to a β-agonist's proper toxicity.

Morbidity rate is evaluated in terms of the prevalence rate (proportion of patients in a given population, at a given time) rather than the incidence rate (number of new cases arising in a given population in a given time period) because it is often difficult to specify the beginning of the disease. There are large variations in morbidity rates in published studies. These variations are partly due to differences in defining the disease, partly due to variable characteristics of the population under study.

3.2 Prevalence Rates Depend on the Criteria for Diagnosis

In epidemiology, the diagnosis of asthma relies mainly on answers to standardized questionnaires; sometimes the questionnaire is supported with pulmonary function tests. The questionnaire includes either a diagnostic question: "Have you ever had asthma?", or questions about asthmatic symptoms. The diagnostic question is more direct but answers may be influenced by the medical knowledge conveyed from the physician to the patient and by the picture the population has of the disease. Questions about symptoms may be less biased but their sensitivity and specificity must be checked. The questionnaire set up by the British Medical Research Council (BMRC) in 1976 (can be obtained from the BMRC, 20 Park Crescent, London W1N 4A2, England) includes the following questions: "Does your chest ever sound wheezing or whistling?", "Have you ever had attacks of shortness of breath with wheezing?" and, in the "Past illnesses" section an inquiry about "bronchial asthma". In the 1978 American Thoracic Society questionnaire [13], the wording is slightly different. The first question is: "Does your chest ever sound wheezy or whistling?", the second: "Have you ever had an attack of wheezing

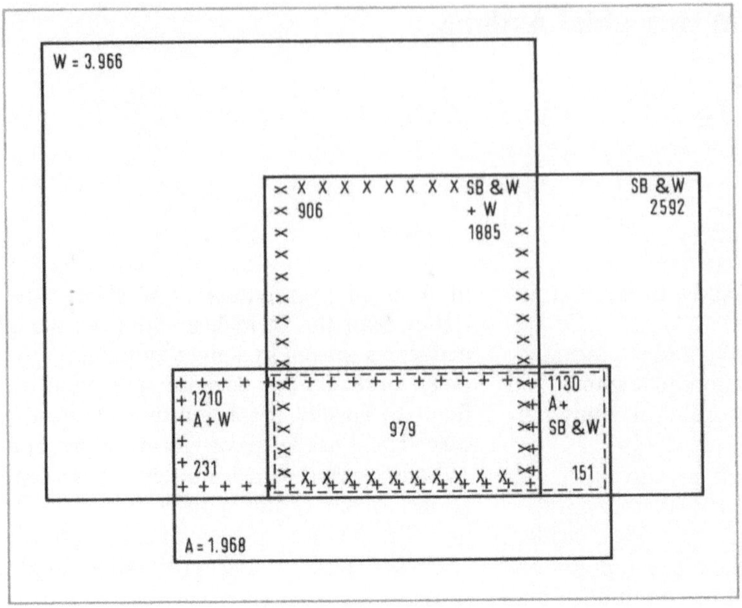

Fig. 3.1. Distribution of answers to questions about asthma in a survey made from 29,000 army recruits [10]. 979 subjects, i.e., 3.6% of the group, answered yes to all three questions. W = wheezing; SB & W = shortness of breath with wheezing; A = asthma

that has made you feel short of breath?" and the third, in the "Past illnesses" section: "Have you ever had asthma?". Helsing et al [17] compared these questionnaires as well as the American National Heart and Lung Institute questionnaire (NHLI) proposed in 1971. Lebowitz and Burrows evaluated the BMRC and NHLI respiratory questionnaires and a new self-completion questionnaire [26]. Because of subjectivity inherent to questionnaires, other tests have sometimes been included in epidemiological studies: measurement of the serum-immunoglobulin E (IgE) level; determination of serum or nasal eosinophilia; and, above all, pulmonary function tests. Between attacks, pulmonary function, appreciated by spirometry, is often normal in asthmatic subjects; thus bronchial provocation tests are useful although they are time consuming and may raise ethical issues.

In children, through the various studies performed around the world and reviewed by Gregg [14], 7 to 25% have had wheezing, but only 0.7 to 5% have had asthma, according to answers to questionnaires. Some epidemiological studies [27, 46] suggest that wheezy bronchitis is closely related to asthma because both are underlain by bronchial hyperreactivity and respond well to bronchodilators. This pooling does not apply to infants in whom any aggression can induce wheezing attacks without predictive value for subsequent asthma.

Similarly in adults, acute infection in chronic bronchitics often gives rise to wheezing. So, a diagnosis between asthma and wheezy bronchitis is often difficult. In London, 28% of men and 22% of women have had wheezing; in the Netherlands, 31% and 20% respectively. As in children, the prevalence rate ranges from 1.1 to 9.9% in published studies [14]. The broadness of this estimate lies partly in the questions used to identify asthma. In a recent epidemiological study performed in France, Dor [10] studied 29,000 army recruits. According to self-administered questionnaires, 9.7% answered positively to the question: "Have you ever had attacks of breathlessness, with wheezing?"; 7.4% to the question: "Have you ever had asthma?"; and 4.6% to both questions. Only 3.6% answered yes to questions about asthma attacks, attacks of breathlessness with wheezing, and about wheezing (Fig. 3.1). 1% answered yes to the question about asthma and attacks of breathlessness with wheezing, but denied having had wheezing.

Finally, prevalence figures depend on the consideration of period prevalence (past or present asthma) or point prevalence (present asthma only). In the former case, the figure is higher and the knowledge about the disease in a population is better, but the rate is underestimated because remote attacks may have been forgotten.

3.3 Prevalence Rates Depend on some Individual Characteristics such as Sex, Racial Group, Social Class and Month of Birth

In children the **male/female ratio** varies, in published studies, between 2 to 3. As occupational and smoking factors do not interfere at this age, males seem to be more susceptible to asthma. In contrast, in adults, the disease is equally distributed between both sexes. The clinical feeling of a predominance of late asthma in women arises, probably, from the fact that wheezing in smoking middle-aged males calls to mind the diagnosis of chronic bronchitis.

Prevalence rates are very dependent on **age**. Wheezy bronchitis is quite common in infants, but, as stated above, its predictive value for future asthma is poor, unless there is a history of familial atopy, atopic eczema or a high cordal IgE level. Youth is a strong predisposing factor, especially in children born into allergic families. In 1,106 clinical patients with marked skin reactions [32], the onset of asthmatic symptoms occurred under 10 years of age in over half of the cases, and under 20 years of age in over three quarters of the cases. One time out of three, the severity of asthma decreased at puberty, somewhat sooner and more often in girls than in boys. These data are derived from Rackemann's study [36]. This author followed up prospectively 459 persons during a period of 20 years; out of 459 children who had had asthma before 13 years of age, 30% had a quiescent asthma 20 years later. In a prospective study of asthma in the rural community of Lebanon (Connecticut), Schachter et al [38] counted 73 active asthmatics in 1972 (out of a population of 1,303 white residents). Six years later, in 1978, 50 (68%) were in remission. This improvement occurred in adults as well as in children. A second peak occurs around age fifty; these late asthmas are usually more severe. However, even in those cases long-term prognosis is unforeseeable. In women especially, once menopause is over, asthma attacks may diminish and even disappear.

According to published studies, asthma is unevenly distributed **around the world**. These discrepancies may be partly due to differences in methodology. In children (Table 3.1), prevalence rates are low in

Table 3.1. Intercountry variations of infantile asthma prevalence (according to Gregg [14])

Country	Class of age (years)	Authors	Year of publishing	Prevalence rate (%)
Scandinavia				
Sweden		Kraepelin	1954	0.7
Norway	7–14	Moeller	1955	2.0
Finland		Eriksson-Lihr	1955	0.7
Great Britain				
Birmingham	5–15	Morrison-Smith	1961	1.8
Aberdeen	10–15	Dawson et al	1969	4.8
London	5	Leeder et al	1975	3.2
United States				
Los Angeles	6–12	Harris and Shure	1956	2.0
Tecumseh	6–14	Broder et al	1962	4.1
Australia				
Queensland	5– 6	Patrick	1962	5.4
New Zealand	11–13	Milne	1959	7.1
Sydney	7–13	Leeder et al	1974	6.8

Table 3.2. Intercountry variations of asthma prevalence in adults (according to Gregg [14])

Country	Class of age (years)	Authors	Year of publishing	Prevalence rate (%)
Scandinavia				
Sweden	16–64	Juhlin and Wilhemsen	1967	2.0
Finland	40–64	Huhti	1965	1.1
Great Britain				
London	12	Fry	1961	2.0
United States				
Tecumseh	15	Broder et al	1962	4.1
Iowa	20	Smith and Knowler	1965	9.9
India				
Patna		Viswanathan et al	1965	5.0

Scandinavian countries (between 0.5 and 2%), medium in Great Britain and the United States of America (between 1.5 and 5.1%), and high in Australia (5.4 to 7.4%). Similarly, in adults, prevalence rates are very scattered (Table 3.2). The upper extreme figures are found in Tristan da Cunha island (South Atlantic). The proportion of active asthma was 22% in 1971, while the cumulative prevalence was 32% [6]. The lower figures were recorded in the New Guinea Highlands (0.2 to 0.3%) [47]. Hospital files from the Mackenzie Delta (Northwest Territories, Canada) include, in a 12-year period, 3 asthmatic cases only! Such differences in prevalence figures suggest the intervention of genetic factors which we will analyze later.

Social class may influence asthmatic risk through living conditions, occupational exposure or through health education or health care accessibility. Relationships between social class and the prevalence rate of asthma remain unclear. The Tecumseh (Michigan) study [3] concluded that asthma was more prevalent in high social classes; but Higgins et al [20], out of a sample of 4,699 men and women taken from this very community, did not find any correlation between asthma prevalence and occupation and education.

Morrison-Smith and Springett [34] evaluated the relationships between a **child's month of birth** and his/her subsequent risk for bronchial asthma. This risk seems to be higher when the birth occurs between May and October, and could be related to an allergy to house dust and Dermatophagoides pteronyssinus. Other authors have confirmed these data and concluded that atopic parents should be given a "Christmas pill"!

The study of **secular trends** suggests that, in western countries, asthma could be a more common disease than it used to be. Morrison-Smith [33] made, over a period of 20 years, three large prevalence studies in Birmingham, Great Britain. Using a similar definition of asthma and similar methods for gathering information, he showed a statistically significant progressive increase in prevalence from 1956–57 and 1974–75.

3.4 Risk Factors of Bronchial Asthma

The knowledge of these risk factors is important: *Extrinsic risk* factors can be modified; *intrinsic risk* factors make it possible to predict the individual risk of becoming asthmatic.

Extrinsic or Environmental Factors

These include domestic, occupational and general air pollution; meteorological and infectious factors.

As for **air pollution** we have only considered general air pollution; domestic and occupational aspects are dealt with in other chapters. Air pollution can, in some circumstances, induce bronchial asthma, but acts much more often as a triggering factor for asthma attacks.

Short-term repercussions of high peaks of air pollution on bronchial asthma were demonstrated in several instances in the past years: the Meuse Valley (1930), London (1952), and Donora, Pennsylvania (1958). During these episodes, asthmatics were not well. For example in Donora, 43% of the general population, but 88% of asthmatics felt chest discomfort. In contrast, many studies considered periods of several months or 1 or 2 years and looked for correlations between air pollutants and the number of home visits, or visits to the emergency room for asthma; these provided contradictory results (Table 3.3). These discrepancies may be linked to an uneven level of air pollutants in the various studies and the intervention of several pollutants in the induction of asthma attacks. In a specified area, the levels of these various pollutants may not vary in the same way; i.e., the part played by other bronchial aggressors, such as allergens or smoking could disguise the effect of air pollutants.

Is a **long-term exposure** to air pollutants able to induce bronchial asthma? A single study, performed on American soldiers stationed in Tokyo and Yokohama after World War II [21], demonstrated without a doubt that asthma could be created where there were no previous symptoms, by exposure to heavy air pollution, and disappear when the person was removed from this polluted area. Similar data have been reported by Maternowsky and Mathews [29] about immigrants; new cases of asthma may develop when people live in a more polluted area. However, in this latter situation, air pollution may be associated with allergen pollution, as well as with psychological factors, to create asthma.

Apart from those caricatural situations where exposure to air pollutants is drastically altered, *do people living in high pollution areas have more asthma?* In children, prevalence studies have shown a correlation between levels of air pollutants and the prevalence of upper airway infections and of chest wheezing. As for bronchial asthma, data are scanty. Peat et al [35], in Sydney, failed to find more asthmatic children in polluted areas. In adults, similarly, several studies did not find significant differences in prevalence rates of asthma between urban and rural areas [8], or in cities, between polluted and less polluted neighbourhoods [1]. However, a large scale French multicenter prevalence study [41] made in 1974–1975, did show a higher prevalence of asthma in the most polluted areas. In this study, the responsible pollutants were thought to be sulfur dioxide and dust. The above mentioned negative results may be due to relatively small sample sizes or to differential migration. Asthmatic subjects may choose to live in less polluted areas. Such a migration bias has been demonstrated in Tucson (Arizona)

Table 3.3. Correlations between air pollution and asthmatic symptoms. [From 24]

Data source	Place	Authors Year of publication	Conclusions
Visits of outpatient clinics for asthma	New York	Schoellin et al 1961	Correlation with ozone level
	Los Angeles	Greenburg et al 1964	No correlation
	Philadelphia	Girsh et al 1967	Overall association, but no specific pollutant responsible
	New York	Ribon et al 1972	No correlation
	Los Angeles	Kurata et al 1972	No correlation
Patient's diary	Nashville	Zeidberg et al 1961	Correlation with SO_2 level
	New Cumberland	Cohen et al 1972 [7]	Correlation with SO_2 and total suspended particles

by Lebowitz and Burrows [25]; ¾ of asthmatics found in their study already had asthma before moving to Arizona.

Tobacco smoke is a potent bronchial irritant. It can induce asthma attacks, but is it able to create bronchial asthma? As far as active tobacco smoking is concerned, the answer is negative: Before the onset of the disease, medical history does not include smoking in asthmatics more often than in a control population. In children, a study by Leeder et al [28] suggests that passive smoking is responsible for more upper respiratory tract infections and wheezing bronchitis, but does not induce an increase of asthma.

Role of inhaled allergens: A description of the various allergens and of the period of the year when they act ("Pollen calendars") is treated in another chapter. Epidemiology has contributed to the description of the role of allergens by studies involving geographic or temporal clustering of cases.

A geographic cluster means a spatial concentration of cases. In 1955–1956, several hundred new cases of asthma in relation to castor bean allergy appeared in the town of Marseille, France [5]. This allergy had developed because the process of extracting oil from grain had changed and become more drastic, leaving as residuum a volatile oil-cake (Fig. 3.2). Similarly, Bregevin [2] described asthma related to the inhalation of cereal dust in urban dwellings situated near grain storage units.

Temporal clustering studies make it possible to correlate two phenomena which occur simultaneously. For example, during spring, curves describing pollen counts in the air and symptoms of hay fever are parallel (Fig. 3.3).

Meteorologic conditions, apart from the cold which acts through a specific mechanism, operate through stagnancy of air pollutants over their original sources. Empiricially, most asthmatics feel the influence of meteorologic factors. Low wind, low barometric pressure, thermal inversions oppose pollutant dispersion, all the more in sunken valleys.

Rapid cooling of the weather seems to act as an independent triggering factor. Tromp [42] in the Netherlands, through diaries, showed that atmospheric cooling plays an important role. This cooling has also been studied by Salvaggio et al [37] in New Orleans and Cohen et al [7] in West Virginia. Actually, Mc Fadden and Ingram [30] demonstrated that, in those circumstances, air dryness is more important than air temperature.

Another variable included in climatic factors is **altitude**. Altitude generates a gradual decrease in one of the major allergens, Dermatophagoides pteronyssinus [44]. This can explain the clinical improvement and the drop in specific IgE to Dermatophagoides observed during a prolonged stay at a high altitude [43].

Intrinsic or Endogenous Factors

Psychological factors being studied elsewhere, we have concentrated on the one hand on atopy, on the other hand on hyperreactivity.

The role of **atopy** includes personal or family history of allergic disorders, skin testing to inhaled allergens and serum-IgE level.

The first problem when dealing with *allergic disorders* is to know what these words mean. Only atopic eczema, allergic rhinitis and hay fever should be included. Some authors include here drug allergies, headache and even food intolerance. Unfortunately this assimilation creates disorder. Several retrospective studies have shown that asthmatic subjects have, more often than a control group, a **personal history of allergic diseases**. However, how often this association is encountered depends on the type of asthma and on the institution which performed the study. Hendrick et al [18], in the Allergy and Clinical Immunology Department of the Brompton Hospital in London, found that ⅔ of asthmatics had a personal history of allergic disorders. This percentage was higher among extrinsic asthma (70%) than in intrinsic asthma (48%). In contrast, when the study considered a non-selected general population, as in the Tecumseh study [3], less than half of the asthmatics had such a personal history. Few prospective studies have considered the role of allergic diseases for future asthma. In pollinosis, many authors, working in a clinical setting, have stated that asthma

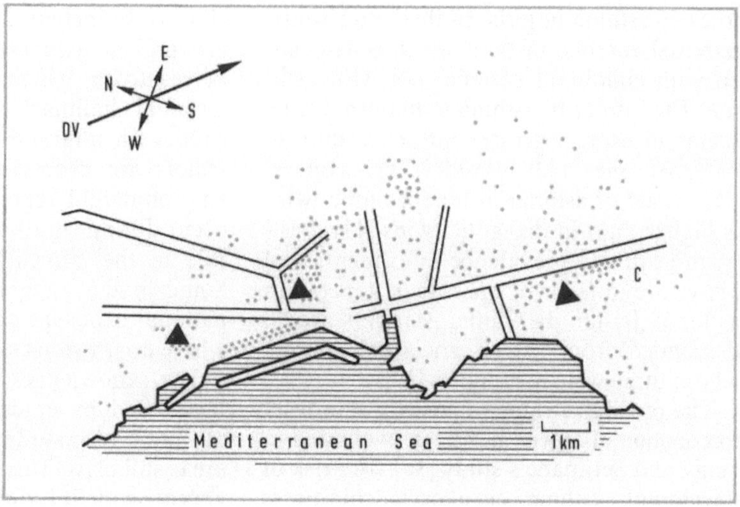

Fig. 3.2. Epidemic of asthma due to castor bean allergy [5]. Dots locate asthmatic patients. Note that they are situated down wind from an oil-mill (black triangles). The block of flats marked C concentrated many cases. Its ventilation system took in air on the northwest facade, which was down wind from an oil-mill

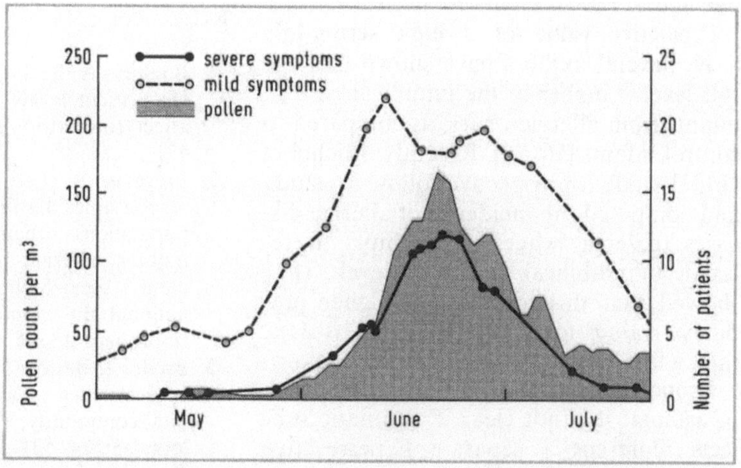

Fig. 3.3. Correlation between hay fever symptoms and pollen counts [9]

occurs in a range of 22 to 75% (mean, 43%) of persons having hay fever. However, allergists tend to see the more serious hay fever cases and may get a distorted picture of the natural history. The Tecumseh Community Health Study [3] showed not only that this bias actually occurred, but also indicated that the cumulative prevalence of asthma following hay fever is considerably lower (29%) than estimates made from clinical experience. Hagy and Settipane [15] followed up a group of 903 freshmen from Brown University, New York. They showed that subjects with a history of allergic rhinitis have, over a 7-year period, a 6% risk of developing bronchial asthma, while this risk is only equal to 1.3% in people without such a history.

The importance of a **family history of allergic diseases** is demonstrated in several types of epidemiological studies. Family studies have shown that the prevalence of asthma in asthmatics' parents is higher than in controls [4]. This association is encountered mainly in allergic (extrinsic) asthma [39]. Inversely, the risk of a child becoming asthmatic is greater when one of his/her parents, or a fortiori both, are themselves asthmatics [4]. In Fergusson's et al study [12], the risk of early childhood asthma is increased by nearly 2.5 times for boys, whereas parental asthma is unrelated to early asthma in girls. In this latter study, parental eczema, in both sexes, is associated with childhood eczema, not with asthma. The history of asthma in maternal issue seems to exert a greater influence than in paternal ones [32]. Besides, the concordance rate of asthma in monozygotic twins is higher than in dizygotic twins [11]. Lastly, the extreme prevalence rates mentioned above are in favor of the role of genetics in asthma: Tristan da Cunha islanders are all descended from fifteen ancestors, among whom three were asthmatics [19].

The predictive value of positive skin tests to common allergens has been evaluated in Hagy and Settipane's study [15]. The risk of developing asthma or allergic rhinitis is correlated with positive skin tests. For example the 7-year risk of asthma in this study was equal to 5% if the tests were positive and to 1.5% if they were negative.

Predictive value of a high serum-IgE level. Several authors have shown that the IgE level is higher in the umbilical cord in infants from allergic issues, as compared to control infants [16, 23]. Recently, Michel et al [31] made a prospective follow-up study and computed the incidence of allergic diseases (eczema, wheezy bronchitis) in relation to umbilical cord IgE level. They showed that this level has a higher predictive value, for future allergic diseases, than a family history of allergic diseases.

Bronchial hyperreactivity is the hallmark of asthma. It is not clear if asthmatic subjects represent a separate hyperreactive population uniquely different from normal individuals, or if they represent a hyperreactive extreme of a unimodal distribution. As pointed out by Mc Fadden [30], "until now, there have been no systematic measures made of the distribution of airway responsiveness, and these possibilities could not be tested". Recent studies in humans [45], as well as in animals, suggest that airway reactivity is a unimodal function, asthmatic subjects representing the most sensitive extreme of the population.

3.5 Conclusions

Suitable genetic background and environmental aggressors interact to produce clinical bronchial asthma. Genetic background is expressed by bronchial hyperreactivity, which is the permanent and essential hallmark of asthma. However, studies on migrants suggest that if genetic factors are necessary to produce asthma, environmental aggressors, especially if they occur during childhood, have a preeminent role in the clinical revelation of asthma. Some potent aggressors, such as occupational exposure can even induce asthma where no previous symptoms had existed.

The knowledge of asthma has been broadened by epidemiology. But, in spite of numerous studies, a lot of imprecise areas still exist. This comes from the lack of a precise definition of the disease. Bronchial hyperreactivity, as an objective tool, could fill this gap.

References

1. Bouhuys A, Beck GJ, Schoenberg JB (1978) Do present levels of air pollution outdoors affect respiratory health? Nature 276:466–471
2. Bregevin B (1976) Poussières de céréales responsables d'asthmes bronchiques dans les populations urbaines. In: Gervais P (ed) Asthme, allergie respiratoire et environnement socio-écologique. Congrès International du Mont-Dore, 29–31 Mai 1975. Imprimeca, Ussel, pp 151–158
3. Broder I, Barlow PP, Horton RJ (1962) The epidemiology of asthma and hay fever in a total community, Tecumseh, Michigan. J Allergy 33:524–531
4. Charpin J, Arnaud A (1971) Facteurs génétiques dans l' asthme et les maladies respiratoires. Poumon Cœur 27:111–119
5. Charpin J, Zafiropoulo A (1959) Allergie respiratoire au ricin dans la région de Marseille. Acta Allergologica 14:150
6. Citron KM, Pepys J (1964) An investigation of asthma amongst the Tristan da Cunha islanders. Br J Dis Chest 58:119–123
7. Cohen A, Bromberg S, Buechley RW, Heiderscheit LT, Shy CM (1972) Asthma and air pollution from a coal-fueled power plant. Am J Public Health 62:1181–1188
8. Comstock GW, Stone RW, Sakai Y, Matsuya T, Tonascia JA (1973) Respiratory findings and urban living. Arch Environ Health 27:143–150
9. Davies RJ (1973) Correlation between hay fever symptoms and pollen counts. Bull Ecol Res Comm 18:161–167

10. Dor PJ, Arnaud A, Barre A, Charpin J (1980) Prévalence des symptômes respiratoires en relation avec l'asthme dans une population d'adultes jeunes. Rev Fr Allergol 20:79–82
11. Edfors-Lubs ML (1971) Allergy in 7000 twin pairs. Acta Allergologica 26:249–285
12. Fergusson DM, Horwood LJ, Shannon FT (1983) Parental asthma, parental eczema and asthma and eczema in early childhood. J Chronic Dis 36:517–524
13. Ferris BG (1978) Epidemiology Standardization Project. Am Rev Respir Dis 118:1–120
14. Gregg I (1977) Epidemiology. In: Clark TJH, Godfrey S (eds) Asthma. Chapman and Hall, London
15. Hagy GW, Settipane GA (1976) Risk factors for developing asthma and allergic rhinitis. A 7-year follow-up study of college students. J Allergy Clin Immunol 58:330–336
16. Hamburger RN, Lenoir N, Groshong TE, Miller JR, Wallace W, Orgel HA (1973) Development of IgE and allergy during the first year of life: preliminary data. J Allergy Clin Immunol 51:129
17. Helsing KJ, Comstock GW, Speizer FE, Ferris BG, Lebowitz MD, Tockman MS, Burrows B (1979) Comparison for three standardized questionnaires on respiratory symptoms. Am Rev Respir Dis 120:1221–1231
18. Hendrick DJ, Davies RJ, d'Souza MF, Pepys J (1975) An analysis of skin prick test reactions in 656 asthmatic patients. Thorax 30:2–8
19. Henriksen SD, Oeding P (1946) Medical survey of Tristan da Cunha. In: Christophersen E (ed) Results of the Norwegian Expedition to Tristan Da Cunha 1937–38. Dybwad, Oslo, p 61
20. Higgins MW, Keller JB, Metzner HL (1977) Smoking, socio-economic status and chronic respiratory disease. Am Rev Respir Dis 116: 403–410
21. Huber TE, Joseph SW, Knoblock E, Redfearn PL, Karakawa JA (1954) New environmental respiratory disease (Yokohama asthma): preliminary report. Arch Industr Health 10:339–408
22. Jackson RT, Beaglehole R, Rea HH, Sutherland DC (1982) Mortality from asthma: a new epidemic in New Zealand. Br Med J 285:771–774
23. Kjellman NIM (1976) Predictive value of high IgE levels in children. Acta Paediatr Scand 65:465–471
24. Kurata JH, Glovsky MM, Newcomb RL, Easton JG (1976) A multifactorial study of patients with asthma. 2. Air pollution, animal dander and asthma symptoms. Ann Allergy 37:398–409
25. Lebowitz MD, Burrows B (1975) Tucson epidemiologic study of obstructive lung disease. II. Effects of in-migration factors on the prevalence of obstructive lung disease. Am J Epidemiol 102:153–163
26. Lebowitz MD, Burrows B (1976) Comparison of questionnaires: the BMRC and NHLI respiratory questionnaires and a new self-completion questionnaire. Am Rev Respir Dis 113:627–635
27. Lee DA, Winslow NR, Speight ANP, Hey EN (1983) Prevalence and spectrum of asthma in childhood. Br Med J 286:1256–1258
28. Leeder SR, Corkhill RT, Irwig LM, Holland WW, Colley JRT (1976) Influence of family factors on asthma and wheezing during the first five years of life. Br J Prev Med 30:213–218
29. Maternowski CJ, Mathews KP (1962) The prevalence of ragweed pollinosis in foreign and native students at a Midwestern University and its implications for determining the inheritance of atopy. J Allergy 33:130–140
30. McFadden ER, Ingram RH (1984) Pathogenesis of asthma. J Allergy Clin Immunol 73:413–424
31. Michel FB, Bousquet J, Greillier P, Robinet-Levy M, Coulomb Y (1980) Comparison of cord blood immunoglobulin E concentrations and maternal allergy for the prediction of atopic diseases in infancy. J Allergy Clin Immunol 65:422–430
32. Montgomery Smith J (1974) Incidence of atopic disease. Med Clin North Am 58:3–24
33. Morrison-Smith J (1976) The prevalence of asthma and wheezing in children. Br J Dis Chest 70:73–77
34. Morrison-Smith J, Springett VH (1979) Atopic disease and month of birth. Clin Allergy 9:153–157
35. Peat JK, Woolcock AJ, Leeder SR, Blackburn CR (1980) Asthma and bronchitis in Sydney schoolchildren. II. The effect of social factors and smoking on prevalence. Am J Epidemiol 111:728–735
36. Rackemann FM (1952) Asthma in children: a follow-up of 688 patients after an interval of twenty years. N Engl J Med 246:815–823
37. Salvaggio J, Hasselblad V, Seabury J, Heiderscheit LT (1970) New-Orleans asthma. II. Relationship of climatologic and seasonal factors to outbreaks. J Allergy 45:257–265
38. Schachter EN, Doyle CA, Beck GJ (1984) A prospective study of asthma in a rural community. Chest 85:623–630
39. Sibbald B, Turner-Warwick M (1979) Factors influencing the prevalence of asthma

among first degree relatives of extrinsic and intrinsic asthmatics. Thorax 34:332–337
40. Speizer FE, Doll R (1968) A century of asthma deaths in young people. Br Med J 285: 771–774
41. Teissier JF, Patois E, Lellouch J (1983) Pollution atmosphérique et affections pulmonaires. Résultats de l'Enquête Nationale Française. Communication présentée à la Conférence Internationale sur l'Environnement et les Maladies Respiratoires, Taormina, 22–27 Mars 1983
42. Tromp SW (1968) Influence of weather and climate on asthma and bronchitis. Rev Allergy 22:1027–1044
43. Vervloet D, Bongrand P, Arnaud A, Boutin C, Charpin J (1979) Données objectives cliniques et immunologiques observées au cours d'une cure d'altitude à Briançon chez des enfants asthmatiques allergiques à la poussière de maison et à Dermatophagoïdes. Rev Fr Mal Respir 7:19–27
44. Vervloet D, Penaud A, Razzouk H, Senft M, Arnaud A, Boutin C, Charpin J (1982) Altitude and house dust mites. J Allergy Clin Immunol 69:290–296
45. Weiss ST, Taeger IB, Weiss JW et al (1984) Am Rev Respir Dis 127:898–902
46. Williams H, McNicol KN (1969) Prevalence, natural history and relationship of wheezy bronchitis and asthma in children. Br Med J 4:321–325
47. Woolcock AJ, Blackburn CRB (1967) Chronic lung disease in the territory of Papua and New Guinea: An epidemiologic study. Aust Ann Med 16:11–28

4. Genetic Factors of Allergy

D. G. Marsh

In atopic allergy, as in other human diseases, knowledge of the epidemiology and genetics is fundamental to understanding the basic immunological, pharmacological and pathological mechanisms underlying the disease process, which should lead ultimately to its prevention and cure. The complexity of the disease presents a realistic challenge, because we now have the tools to unravel the reasonably well-defined immunological and pharmacological aspects. Furthermore, one can view allergy as a "model immunologic disease" since, unlike most other immunologically based diseases, a clear *causal* relationship has been established between specific immune responses and the expression of disease.

Since the pioneering work of Wyman [1] in 1872, and the more extensive classical study by Cooke and van der Veer in 1916 [2], it has been known that allergy "runs in families". By the 1950s and 1960s most researchers had realized that allergy is multifactorially determined; that is to say, the interaction of several genetic and nongenetic factors controls the expression of disease. This conclusion was augmented by two critical discoveries in the late 1960s: the importance of IgE in human atopy [3] and of major histocompatibility complex (*MHC*)-linked immune response (*Ir*) genes in laboratory animals [4]. Vaz and Levine [5] subsequently showed that, under highly limiting conditions of low dose immunization using complex protein allergens (chosen to simulate the induction of human allergy), mouse IgE antibody (Ab) responses normally parallelled IgG Ab responses, and the expression of both classes of specific response was linked to *H-2* (the mouse *MHC*). Later, they found that the induction of IgE Ab (as a class) was controlled by a gene(s) not linked to *H-2* [6]. These experiments suggested that two types of genetic control of IgE response should also exist in man, namely, *HLA*-linked control of *specific* responses and non-*HLA*-linked control of the overall production of IgE.

4.1 Basal IgE

Hamburger and associates estimated the proportions of the basal IgE due to *genetic* and *environmental* factors from studies of pairs of monozygotic and like-sexed dizygotic twins. Their initial findings in adults [7] suggested a remarkably high contribution of 84% for the genetic component. In a later study [8], they found that 59% of the variance of basal IgE in adult males and 79% for children was determined by genetic factors. Our preliminary studies on 28 families [9] suggested that a major gene (*R*/*r*) may be involved, with high IgE levels being recessive (low IgE being dominant). Gerrard and colleagues [10] subsequently analyzed data from a more comprehensive study of 173 Canadian families. Interestingly, they also found high IgE to be recessive and reported a frequency for the *r* allele of 0.49, a striking agreement with our earlier value of 0.52. These results have been neither negated nor confirmed in subsequent studies [11]. However, data from mouse experiments [12] show clear-cut evidence for recessive inheritance of high IgE production. Both human [11] and mouse [12] data show that the major genes regulating IgE levels are not linked to the *MHC* of the species.

Willcox and Marsh [13] have suggested that the dominant allele of the hypothesized human IgE-regulating gene *R*/*r* may be associated with increased suppressor T-cell activity, which greatly limits the number of IgE clones responding to an antigenic stimulus. Thus, individuals with the low genotypes *RR* and *Rr* hardly ever

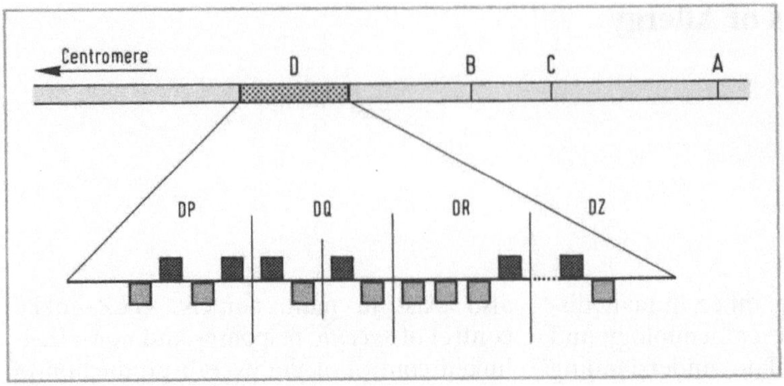

Fig. 4.1. A schematic diagram of the human major histocompatibility complex, *HLA*, emphasizing the *HLA-D* region (based on [14] and other sources). Each major subregion, *DP* (formerly *SB*), *DQ* (formerly *DC*) and *DR* contains α- and β-genes. (α-genes are shown by solid symbols and β-genes by shaded symbols.) Pairs of α- and β-genes code for the α- and β-chains of the corresponding D specificities. The *DZ* subregion contains one α- and one β-gene (*DO*) both of which are poorly expressed on the cell surface. This subregion has recently been mapped *DP* and *DQ*

make IgE Ab responses, and normally are clinically not allergic; if they are allergic, they make IgE Ab toward very few determinants and, consequently, are sensitive to very few allergens. Persons with high IgE levels (genotype *rr*) are seen as polyclonal responders with respect to IgE production and, therefore, are sensitive to many different allergenic determinants on many allergens.

4.2 The *HLA* Gene Complex

Before considering the genetics of allergy further, it is necessary to discuss briefly the *HLA* gene complex (Fig. 4.1). The *D* region contains important *Ir* genes that appear to be associated with at least three independent sets of specificities, DP, DQ and DR[1], each of which are coded by a pair of α- and β-genes which map in the respective region [14]. In Caucasian subjects, there is a very close (ca. 90%) correspondence between the "Dw"[1] specificities defined by mixed lymphocyte responses and DR specificities defined by serological typing. Most of the loci are extremely polymorphic, i.e., possess many different genetic variants (alleles). It is probable that this polymorphism is associated with important survival advantages for the human species, including an increased diversity of immune function.

4.3 *HLA*-associated Immune Hyperresponsiveness

Within defined ethnic groups, certain alleles of the loci of the *HLA* complex exhibit linkage disequilibrium, which is the tendency of specific alleles of the various loci to be found together on the same chromosome (as a *haplotype*) more frequently than expected by chance. For example, the frequencies of the two most common Euro-Caucasian *HLA* haplotypes, *A1,B8,Dw3* and *A3,B7,Dw2,* are about 35 times and 20 times higher than expected on the basis of chance association of the component alleles [15]. These associations appear to reflect selective advantages of particular combinations of alleles. However, an unfortunate by-product is the observed association of many autoimmune diseases with certain alleles of the two most common Caucasian *HLA* haplotypes, particularly *B8,D(R)3* and *B7,D(R)2* [15]. Especially since both allergy and autoimmunity are diseases of immune hyperresponsiveness, it has been of considerable interest to find that skin test responsiveness toward common environmental allergens is also associated

[1] These specificities are denoted by the revised nomenclature system of the 1984 Histocompatibility Testing Workshop [14]. The suffix "w" indicates a preliminary "workshop" designation.

Table 4.1. Summary of significant associations of specific IgE Ab responses to allergens with HLA and total IgE level in Euro-caucasian populations

Pollen allergen	Molecular weight (daltons)	HLA association		Association with total IgE
		Positive	Negative	
Ambrosiineae (ragweeds)				
Amb a V (AgE)	37,800	–	–	No effect
Amb a III (Ra3)	12,300	A2[a], A28[a]	A3[a], A11[a]	Strong effect
Amb a V (Ra5)	4,990	Dw2[c], B7[b]	–	No effect
Amb a VI (Ra6)	11,500	DR5[c]	–	No effect
Amb t V (Ra5G)	4,400	Dw2[b]	–	No effect
Gramineae (grasses)				
Lol p I (Rye I)	27,000	B8[c], Dw3[b], Al[b]	A9[a]	Weak effect
Lol p II (Rye II)	11,000	Dw3[c], B8[b]	–	Strong effect

Data were combined from two or more studies when available. Associations are listed in order of their significance. Significance of associations: [a] $0.05 \geqq p > 0.005$, [b] $0.005 \geqq p > 0.0001$, [c] $p \leqq 0.0001$

with these HLA specificities [15]. Comparison of the HLA frequencies in 157 people whose tests were positive to at least one of seven common allergens and in 191 people whose tests were negative to all of them, revealed significant associations with Dw3 ($p=0.002$), B8 ($p = 0.01$), and Dw2 ($p=0.02$). Examination of all the associations for all the various combinations of alleles, especially within *A3,B7,Dw2,* showed that the strongest associations were with phenotypic combinations of two or more HLA antigens rather than with the individual HLA specificities themselves. These and other data (currently being evaluated) suggest that alleles of the two most common Caucasian haplotypes are associated with immune hyperresponsiveness, which could well explain their selection.

4.4 Specific Immune Responses

In studying specific Ab responses, it is of course extremely important to use highly purified (≧ 97% pure) or, preferably, ultrapure (≧ 99.5% pure) preparations of allergens [16]. As seen in Table 4.1, several significant associations have been observed between particular HLA types and responses toward different highly purified allergen preparations. For certain allergens of *intermediate complexity,* such as *Amb a* III[2] (Ra3) and *Lol p* II[2] (Rye II), there appears to be an interaction between *HLA*-linked *Ir* and the IgE-regulating genes [13, 16, 18]. In such cases, individuals who are positive to the allergen in question, and who have low total IgE levels typical of nonallergic subjects, tend to show a much stronger association with the particular HLA type associated with response to the allergen.

The two cases to be discussed in detail here are the Ra5 homologues, *Amb a* V from short ragweed (*Ambrosia artemesiifolia*) and *Amb t* V from giant ragweed (*Ambrosia trifida*) pollens, which have mol. wts. of 5,000 and 4,400 daltons, respectively [19–21]. They also have similar structures, including the possession of 4 disulfide bonds, although the degree of homology of sequence (43%) leads only to extremely weak, or no, cross-reactivity [22].

In the *Amb a* V study, a total of 177 ragweed-allergic Caucasian subjects were HLA-D-typed [23]. Thirty-six out of 38 (95%) having serum-IgE Ab to *Amb a* V possessed Dw2, as compared with 22% of 139 *Amb a* V–subjects ($p<0.0001$) (Table 4.2). Analysis of IgG Ab responses to *Amb a* V following the immunotherapy of 61 patients with short ragweed antigens was, perhaps, even more interesting [24].

[2] These designations reflect a new nomenclature system for allergens [17].

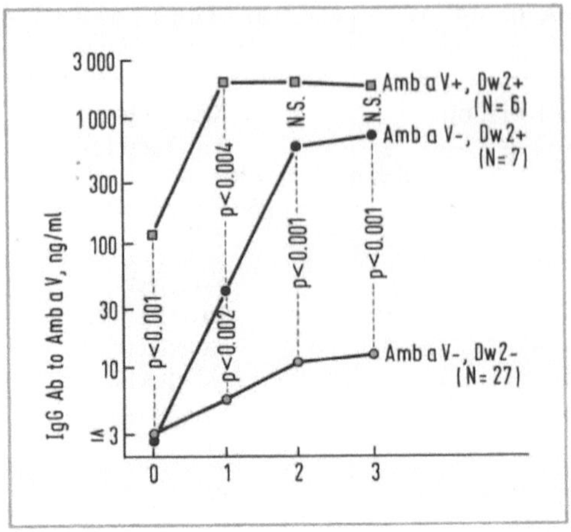

Fig. 4.2. Geometric mean IgG Ab responses to *Amb a* V (Ra5) in three subgroups of patients from a total of 40 subjects, who had been immunized with short ragweed for three successive years. The phenotypes of members of the subgroups are designated according to their pretreatment IgE Ab to *Amb a* V and whether or not they possess HLA-Dw2. The significance of differences between the groups before treatment (Year 0) and at each successive posttreatment year were calculated by t test. N.S. = not significant

Immunotherapy of 14 *Amb a* V IgE Ab+ subjects gave good IgG Ab responses to *Amb a* V (at least a 5-fold rise) in all cases; whereas injection of 47 *Amb a* V IgE Ab– (but ragweed-allergic) subjects gave good IgG Ab responses to *Amb a* V essentially only in the 9 subjects in this group who were Dw2+. Forty of the 61 subjects receiving therapy were followed for three successive years (Fig. 4.2). After two years, the IgG Ab responses in the *Amb a* V+, Dw2+ group were not significantly different from those of the *Amb a* V–, Dw2+ group. The responses of both of these two groups were, however, significantly higher than those of the *Amb a* V–, Dw2– group.

In the case of response toward *Amb t* V, IgG Ab levels have been studied in a limited number of people who were treated with giant ragweed extract. Since giant ragweed is much less prevalent than short ragweed in our area (Baltimore), we have not observed IgE Ab or IgG Ab responses to *Amb t* V as a result of natural exposure. In one group of 17 subjects who had previously received immunotherapy from their private physicians, 3/4 IgG Ab+ subjects were Dw2+, while 0/13 IgG Ab– were Dw2+ ($p = 0.01$). In a second group of 10 subjects, who were actively receiving therapy with giant ragweed, 3/3 high responders were Dw2+, while 1/7 low or negative responders were Dw2+ ($p = 0.03$). The overall p value for both groups was 0.0003.

These data, along with recent comparable results from Goodfriend et al [21], suggest that Dw2/DR2 itself may participate in the primary immune recognition of a common immunodeterminant on the two *Amb* V molecules.

4.5 Overall Conclusions

We postulate that the expression of atopic allergy is dependent on several genetic controls as well as a complex array of environmental influences. While the primary focus, here, has been on the immune response aspects of the disease, further controls may determine key steps in its pharmacological regulation and pathological

Table 4.2. Associations between HLA-Dw2 and immune responses to *Amb a* V (Ra5) in 177 ragweed-allergic Caucasian subjects

Response	No. of subjects		% with Dw2		p values
	Amb a V+	*Amb a* V–	*Amb a* V+	*Amb a* V–	
IgE Ab	38	139	95	22	≪0.0001
IgG Ab	46	131	85	21	≪0.0001

Analysis of the HLA association data has shown that the association with Dw2 (defined by MLR typing) is stronger than with DR2 (defined by serological typing) [23]

expression. Indeed, Marone et al [25] have recently obtained evidence that the ability of basophils to release mediators may be genetically determined. We hypothesize that genetic regulation of immune response includes at least one antigen-nonspecific control, namely the overall regulation of IgE responses, which is not *HLA*-linked. The major antigen-specific factors relate to *HLA*-linked *Ir* genes, which encode the HLA-D specificities themselves. In addition, one finds that immune hyperresponsiveness toward many different antigens is associated with alleles of the two most common Caucasian *HLA* haplotypes. This may imply the existence of additional genetic factors associated with these haplotypes and/or be a reflection of normal *Ir* gene action associated with D(R)3 and D(R)2.

Proof of the existence of human *Ir* and *Is* genes and their relation to *HLA* will require analysis of family data. Such analysis has, however, proved to be extremely difficult in view of the different degrees of expression of immune response in families that are determined by environment and by non-*HLA*-linked genetic factors [18].

References

1. Wyman M (1872) Autumnal Catarrh (Hay Fever). Hurd and Houghton, Cambridge, Mass., p 82
2. Cooke RA, van der Veer A (1916) Human sensitization. J Immunol 1:201
3. Ishizaka K, Ishizaka T (1968) Human reaginic antibodies and immunoglobulin E. J Allergy 42:330
4. Benacerraf B, McDevitt HO (1972) Histocompatibility-linked immune response genes. Science 175:273
5. Vaz NM, Levine BB (1970) Immune responses of inbred mice to repeated low doses of antigen: relationship to histocompatibility (H-2) type. Science 168:852
6. Levine BB, Vaz NM (1970) Two kinds of genetic control of reagin production in the mouse. J Clin Invest 49:58 a
7. Hamburger RN, Orgel HA, Bazaral M (1973) Genetics of human serum IgE levels. In: Goodfriend L, Sehon AH, Orange RP (eds) Mechanisms in Allergy. Reagin-mediated Hypersensitivity. Marcel Dekker, New York, p 131
8. Bazaral M, Orgel HA, Hamburger RN (1974) Genetics of IgE and allergy: serum IgE levels in twins. J Allergy Clin Immunol 54:288
9. Marsh DG, Bias WB, Ishizaka K (1974) Genetic control of basal serum immunoglobulin E level and its effect on specific reaginic sensitivity. Proc Natl Acad Sci USA 71:3588
10. Gerrard JW, Rao DC, Morton NE (1978) A genetic study of immunoglobulin E. Am J Hum Genet 30:46
11. Meyers DA, Marsh DG (1981) Report on an NIAID-sponsored workshop on the genetics of total IgE levels in man. J Allergy Clin Immunol 67:167
12. Watanabe N, Kojima S, Ovary Z (1976) Suppression of IgE antibody production in SJL mice. I. Non-specific suppressor T cells. J Exp Med 143:833
13. Willcox HNA, Marsh DG (1978) Genetic regulation of antibody heterogeneity: its possible significance in human allergy. Immunogenetics 6:209
14. Bodmer J, Bodmer W (1984) Histocompatibility 1984. Immunol Today 5:251
15. Marsh DG (1981) HLA and allergy. In: Steffen C, Ludwig H (eds) Clinical Immunology and Allergology. Proceedings of the XIth Congress of the European Academy of Allergology, Vienna. Elsevier, Amsterdam, p 157
16. Marsh DG, Hsu SH, Hussain R, Meyers DA, Freidhoff LR, Bias WB (1980) Genetics of human immune response to allergens. J Allergy Clin Immunol 65:322
17. Marsh DG, Goodfriend L, King TP, Løwenstein H, Platts-Mills TAE (1986) Allergen nomenclature. WHO Bulletin 64:767
18. Marsh DG, Meyers DA, Bias WB (1981) The epidemiology and genetics of atopic allergy. N Engl J Med 305:1551
19. Lapkoff CB, Goodfriend L (1974) Isolation of a low molecular weight ragweed pollen allergen; Ra5. Int Arch Allergy Appl Immunol 46:215
20. Mole LE, Goodfriend L, Lapkoff CB, Kehoe JM, Capra JD (1975) The amino acid sequence of allergen Ra5. Biochem 14:1216
21. Goodfriend L, Choudhury AM, Klapper DG, Coulter KM, Dorval G, Cartier M, delCarpio J, Osterland CK (1985) Ra5G, a homologue of Ra5 in giant ragweed pollen: isolation, HLA-DR-associated activity and amino acid sequence. Mol Immunol 22:899
22. Roebber M, Klapper DG, Goodfriend L, Bias WB, Hsu SH, Marsh DG (1985) Immunochemical and genetic studies of *Amb t* V (Ra5G), an Ra5 homologue. J Immunol 134:3062

23. Marsh DG, Hsu SH, Roebber M, Kautzky EE, Freidhoff LR, Meyers DA, Pollard MK, Bias WB (1982) HLA-Dw2: a genetic marker for human immune response to short ragweed pollen allergen Ra5. I. Response resulting primarily from natural antigenic exposure. J Exp Med 155:1439
24. Marsh DG, Meyers DA, Freidhoff LR, Kautzky EE, Roebber M, Norman PS, Hsu SH, Bias WB (1982) HLA-Dw2: a genetic marker for human immune response to short ragweed pollen allergen Ra5. II. Response after ragweed immunotherapy. J Exp Med 155:1452
25. Marone G, Poto S, Giugliano R, Celestino D, Bonini S (in press) International Symposium on Prevention of Allergic Diseases, Florence, June 24–27, 1984. O.I.C. Medical

5. Changing Prevalence of Asthma in Developing Countries

K. J. Turner

5.1 The Problem of Data Acquisition

Conflicting reports have emerged in literature regarding the prevalence and characteristics of asthma in developing countries, relative to those seen in people living in industrialized countries. Much of this conflict stems from: an inability to accurately define the term *developing countries*, variabilities in the social and racial characteristics and age of the study groups, unique features of the local environment, a satisfactory operational definition of asthma, and lack of uniformity in defining *prevalence*, e.g., whether the study describes point (current), period or cumulative prevalence.

Accurate diagnosis of asthma requires the use of different combinations of case history, clinical examination including studies of altered pulmonary physiology (particularly airways resonance), skin tests, *in vitro* tests, elimination and exposure tests and controlled challenge tests with allergen or by exercise [1]. Critical evaluation of the results from each test and from the sum of them provides a basis for the diagnosis of asthma. Prevalence figures for the disease based solely on answers to questionnaires may be exaggerated, yet this approach is still employed in many surveys. Stanhope and Prior [30] reported a prevalence rate of 11.3 per 100 for Tokelau adult females where asthma was defined by questions, only compared with a corresponding figure of 1.2 if the definition of the disease required that the subject should have clinical signs of asthma on examination or be currently undergoing treatment for asthma. Similarly, of the 1,817 residents in 8 villages of the South Fore linguistic group of the Eastern Highlands of Papua, New Guinea, 105 people gave a history of past or present episodes of breathlessness characteristic of asthma, yet of these only 54 could be classified as having asthma as a result of histamine inhalation test or bronchodilator test [41].

Much of the data reported in Table 5.1 was obtained from questionnaires which, in general, were followed by a detailed clinical examination including lung function studies. Asthma prevalence, which was not confirmed by clinical examination is identified by an asterisk.

5.2 Current Prevalence Rates

Numerous studies employing the narrow definition of asthma, clinical signs of asthma plus positive questionnaires have, over the past 15 years, established prevalence rates ranging from 0 (Gambia) [15] to 7.8 (Tanzania) [9] per 100 for developing countries all of which are located within the tropics or subtropics (Table 5.1). The upper range compares favorably with childhood prevalence rates established for the United States of America (2.6 to 9.0%), United Kingdom (1.2 to 9%), Australia (4.2 to 12%) and New Zealand (4.9 to 10%), while the lower range is comparable with childhood prevalence rates for the Scandinavian countries (Denmark, Sweden, Norway and Finland), Germany, Switzerland and Holland all of whom report asthma prevalence rates of less than 2% [27, 31].

Taken together, these studies suggest that the overall prevalence of asthma in the developing countries of the world is comparable with that reported for the industrialized countries where the disease is an important health problem causing considerable morbidity and appreciable mortality.

Table 5.1. Prevalence of asthma in developing countries

Continent/ country	Region	Rural (R)/ Urban (U)	Age (years)	Current prevalence (rate per 100 population)	References
Africa	Gambia	R	School children	0 (131)	[15]
			Adults	0.08 (1200)	
		U	All ages	NS (44/?)	
	Nigeria	NS	School children	2–4	[29]
	Nigeria (Ibidan)	NS	School children	(comparable with European rates)	[2]
	Nigeria (Zaria)	NS	Children	Very rare	[37]
			Adults	Relatively frequent	
	South Africa	R	Black school children	0.14 (671)	[33]
		U	Black school children	3.17 (694)	
	Sudan (Kalakla)	R	0– 4	2.0*	[15]
			5– 9	3.0*	
			10–14	4.0*	
			>30	>8.0	
			All ages	4.9 (5,261)*	
	Sudan (Umm-dawan-ban)	R	All ages	3.2 (2,634)*	
	Tanzania	R	School children	3.3 (240)	[8, 9]
		R	School children	7.8	
	Tanzania	NS	5–11	4.8 (2,511)	[10]
Barbados		NS	School children	1.1 (2,731)*	[23]
China		R	School children	1.3 (8,243)	[43]
		U	School children	1.9 (10,335)	
		R	All ages	1.3 } 142,035	
		U	All ages	0.69 } 142,035	
India		U	<9 M	0.16	[35]
			<9 F	0.19	
			>9 M	2.6	
			>9 F	2.1	
	Southern Maldives	R	Children	20.7 (2,903)	[39]
			Adults	3.3 (2,760)	
Indonesia	Bali (Banyuatis)	R	Children	3.7 (325)	[42]
Kuwait		NS	All ages	10	[14]
Mexico		NS	All ages	1.5	[7]

Table 5.1. (continued)

Continent/ country	Region	Rural (R)/ Urban (U)	Age (years)	Current prevalence (rate per 100 population)	References
Nepal		R	School children	6 (292)	[6]
Papua New Guinea	Highlands & coastal regions	R	All ages	0 (2,000)*	[34]
	Western Highlands	R	Adults	0.36 (2,500)	[40]
	Eastern Highlands	R	All ages	0.25 (2,000)	[3]
	Eastern Highlands	R	<20 >20	0.6 (1,081) 7.3 (736)	[13]
	Eastern Highlands	U	<20 >20	0.2 (489) 2.5 (404)	[12]
Polynesia	Tokelau		Adult M Adult F Adult F	12.4 (379)* 11.3 (478)* 1.2 (500)	[30]
	Tokelau	R	0–14 M 0–14 F	1.9 (373) 0.6 (333)	[36]
	Tokelau (resident in New Zealand)	U	0–14 M 0–14 F	8.3 (601) 5.4 (559)	
Puerto Rico			6 6–15	24.5 (534)* 5.4 (20,000)*	[26]
Singapore			4–6 8–12 13–17	2.9 (862)* 1.9 (10,549)* 1.1 (10,857)*	[22]
Tristan da Cunha		R	1–12 Adults	11.1 (288) 25	[19]
South America	Venezuela	R U	All ages All ages	1.8 (336) 5.8 (431)	[17]
	Venezuela (Amazon basin)	R	All ages	<1.0	[18]

NS = not stated; M = male; F = female; * data acquired by questionnaire only

5.3 Factors Influencing the Prevalence of Asthma

Closer examination of the data reported in Table 5.1, however, indicates that the above proposition may well be an over-simplification of the problem, as the prevalence of asthma is strongly dependent upon the unique features of the study group, including age, sex and life-style.

In general, in developing countries, the prevalence of asthma is lower in children than in adults with a mean age of onset in excess of 20 years. Warrell [37] reported that in his study group in Zaria, asthma among children was very rare though relatively frequent in adults. Similar age-dependent trends have been reported in Kenya [20, 38], India [35], Ibidan, Nigeria [2], Kalakla, Sudan [16] and the Eastern Highlands of Papua, New Guinea [13] although in the latter study the age effect extended to 20 years with an overall prevalence of 0.6%, compared with 7.3% for the over 20 years group. In contrast, Wolstenholme [39] reported a considerably higher prevalence of asthma in children (20.7%) than in adults (3.3%) in Addu Atoll in the Southern Maldives, and Sifontes and Maylo [26] established a fivefold difference in prevalence rates between 6-year old and 6–15-year old children in a Puerto Rico study group. It may be of relevance that the style of housing and furnishing of the Addu Atoll population reflected a higher level of material comfort than was present in other atolls in the Maldives [39]. The general trend for the majority of asthmatic individuals in developed countries is to exhibit symptoms before age 20 [27] and prevalence rates for children are higher than adult rates.

While asthma is less prevalent in rural than in urban areas of developed countries, this pattern is exaggerated in developing countries, particularly for rural communities living a traditional life-style [15, 17, 33, 36]. The epidemiological study of van Niekerk et al [33] employed the exercise tolerance test to identify the 23 (3.17%) asthmatics of 694 Xhosa children from a Cape Town African township and one (0.14%) asthmatic child among the 671 Xhosa children from a rural area in the Transkei. Lynch et al [17] examined two comparable but separate populations in Venezuela, both heavily parasitized, but one being purely rural and the other urban. The frequency of asthma, as defined by direct medical interrogation in those sex- and age-related groups was 1.8% for rural and 5.8% for urban, a difference which was also apparent in the frequency of skin test positivity to common inhalant allergens. These observations on relatively homogeneous populations suggest that the difference in prevalence rates for children from urban and rural areas is not genetic or racial in origin but likely to be related to the unique environmental characteristics of the study group, a concept developed by Smith et al [28] in his Birmingham study of emigrant West African and West Indian children. In some communities these environmental characteristics may range from traditional tribal patterns in the rural areas to a western urbanized society.

Possible exceptions to this general trend have been reported for China [43] and Papua, New Guinea [12, 13]. The study in the People's Republic of China [43] which involved sampling of 142,035 rural and urban inhabitants, demonstrated a different pattern for children than for adults as asthma prevalence was lower in rural children, but higher in rural adults than in the corresponding urban populations. Based on skin test reactions and histories in children, 70.1% of the urban cases and only 22.2% of the rural cases were attributed to extrinsic asthma. Of additional interest is the fact that solely breast feeding was practiced 4 to 5 times as frequently by rural than by urban mothers. Dowse et al [12, 13] reported comparable but low asthma prevalence rates for village children and young adults of the South Fore District of the Eastern Highlands of Papua, New Guinea and children living in Goroka, the administrative center for the Eastern Highlands. A subsequent study [32] did not distinguish any significant difference in the bronchial reactivity of asymptomatic rural and urban children but there was a significantly higher rate of skin test positivity to common allergens in the urban population. However, it is doubtful whether the urban population of Goroka can, in reality, be distinguished from the rural population in terms of life-styles and allergen exposures since most of the individuals in the study had been born in rural areas and frequently returned to their villages of origin. Moreover, there are no categorical differences in the way of life in these two areas.

5.4 Increasing Prevalence of Asthma

The possibility that asthma may be increasing in frequency and severity in Europe, Australia and the United States of America has been the subject of considerable discussion [3, 4, 11, 24, 25]. The current prevalence of 3–5% for Japanese children [21] also represents a considerable increase from the earlier figures of approximately 1% for male and 0.5% for female children [5]. Whether the actual prevalence and incidence of childhood asthma are increasing in these countries or whether the observations reflect improved diagnostic methods and recognition of these disorders, needs to be established.

Corresponding data from developed countries is difficult to obtain as, for reasons discussed earlier, prevalence of asthma only has relevance in relation to a clearly defined study group at a given space in time. Since most of the data in Table 5.1 has been derived from isolated studies, reports that asthma is increasing both in prevalence and severity in developing communities is largely anecdotal [14].

The studies in the Eastern Highlands of Papua, New Guinea, however, approximate closely to the requirements for defining shifts in prevalence of disease. Anderson [3] was unable to identify one asthmatic child or adolescent and only 3 asthmatic adults (0.28%) in the 1,076 people examined in a whole village community study undertaken in Lufa in the Eastern Highlands. A whole community study, employing criteria for definition of asthma comparable to that of Anderson's study [3], subsequently established a current prevalence of 0.6% for the 1,081 children and adolescents (< 20 years) and 7.3% for adults living in eight South Fore villages [13] of the Okapa District of the Eastern Highlands located approximately 50 miles from Lufa. This confirmed anecdotal reports by medical officers that inhabitants of villages in this area seemed to be manifesting the symptoms of asthma for the first time. Asthma in these sufferers is a severe disease which can now be provoked by a wide range of factors such as exertion, stress and antecedent respiratory tract infections. All of these have been common features of the South Fore way of life for generations yet, before the past decade, did not provoke asthma. Allergy to house dust mites appears to be a significant feature in the disease pathogenesis and it is likely that this is associated with modifications to traditional life-styles by the recent introduction of blankets and changes in sleeping habits which promote a more fertile environment for growth and multiplication of mites. These observations imply that some groups of highland people have the required genetic susceptibility for asthma, but that it is not expressed until the level of house dust mite in the environment (particularly in blankets) reaches the threshold for triggering asthma. In this context, it is significant that, while the village inhabitants of the Asaro Valley of the Eastern Highlands have not yet demonstrated this dramatic increase in asthma prevalence despite comparable modifications to their life-styles, their mite densities average 283/g blanket dust compared with 1,371/g blanket dust for the South Fore Group [Woolcock, unpublished].

The low childhood prevalence of asthma in the South Fore people may be attributed to endemic parasitism operating by suppressing production of IgE antibodies to ubiquitous allergens. This follows from the combined observations that serum-IgE antibody titers to *D. pteronyssinus* were significantly lower in children than in adults but increased positively ($p < 0.001$) with age, whereas helminth-specific IgE antibody and total IgE levels decreased with age to approach adult control levels at 20 years [32].

More longitudinal studies on populations such as this are needed to monitor the influence of modifications to traditional life-styles on prevalence of asthma in developing communities. The observation by Ellul-Micallef and Al-Ali [14] that the dramatic increase in bronchial asthma in Kuwait since the mid 1950s may be attributed to the importation in 1951 of *Prosopis* trees, the pollen of which is now suspected to be a major feature of asthma pathogenesis, further supports the proposition that the prevalence of asthma in these communities is not static.

5.5 Conclusions

While there are well-known problems in estimating the prevalence of asthma in industrialized countries, which enjoy a relatively affluent life-style, these problems are compounded in developing countries where age and environmental characteristics, which may range from traditional tribal patterns to a western urbanized society, significantly influence incidence of the disease. Since asthma is a disease whose prevalence in a population is determined by the interaction between potentially susceptible individuals and the adverse environmental factors present in the area of that population, any modification to traditional life-styles is likely to alter the pattern of asthma in these communities. It follows, therefore, that for developing countries the term *prevalence of asthma* can only be used in the context of describing the disease in a defined study group at a fixed period of time. Meaningful data relating to changes in prevalence can only be obtained by reexamination of that same study group. While isolated reports suggest that asthma is increasing in prevalence and severity in these communities, such reports are with limited exceptions largely anecdotal.

References

1. Aas K (1975) Diagnosis of immediate type respiratory allergy. Pediatr Clin North Am 22:33
2. Aderele WI (1979) Bronchial asthma in Nigerian children. Arch Dis Child 54:448–453
3. Anderson HR (1974) The epidemiological and allergic features of asthma in the New Guinea Highlands. Clin Allergy 4:171–183
4. Anderson HR (1978) Increase in hospitalisation for childhood asthma. Arch Dis Child 53:295
5. Baba M, Nakamura T, Mitsukawa M (1966) Clinical aspects of bronchial asthma in children in Tokyo: incidence, seasonal influence and results of skin tests. J Asthma Res 4:103–104
6. Bangham CRM, Hope RA (1981) Exercise-induced asthma in Nepalese children. Clin Allergy 11:273–280
7. Canseco C (1984) International Symposium on Prevention of Allergic Diseases, Florence, June 24–27, 1984, p 19 (abstract)
8. Carswell F, Meakins RH, Harland PSEG (1976) Parasites and asthma in Tanzanian children. Lancet 2:706–707
9. Carswell F, Merrett J, Merrett TG, Meakins RH, Harland PSEG (1977) IgE, parasites and asthma in Tanzanian children. Clin Allergy 7:445–453
10. Dawson B, Horobin G, Illsley R, Mitchell R (1969) Survey of childhood asthma in Aberdeen. Lancet 1:827–830
11. Derrick E (1973) Childhood asthma in Brisbane: epidemiological observations. Aust Paediatr J 9:135
12. Dowse GK, Turner KJ, Stewart GA, Alpers MP, Woolcock AJ (1985) The association between *Dermatophagoides* mites and the increasing prevalence of asthma in village communities within the Papua New Guinea highlands. J Allergy Clin Immunol 75:75–83
13. Dowse GK, Smith D, Turner KJ, Alpers MP (1985) The prevalence and features of asthma in a sample survey of urban Goroka, Papua New Guinea. Clin Allergy 15:429–438
14. Ellul-Micallef R, Al-Ali S (1984) The spectrum of bronchial asthma in Kuwait. Clin Allergy 14:509–517
15. Godfrey RC (1975) Asthma and IgE levels in rural and urban communities of the Gambia. Clin Allergy 5:201–207
16. Kay AB, MacLean Una CM, Wilkinson AH, Gad El Rab MO (1983) The prevalence of asthma and rhinitis in a Sudanese community seasonally exposed to a potent airborne allergen (the "green nimitti" midge *Cladotanytarsus lewisi*). J Allergy Clin Immunol 71:345–352
17. Lynch NR, Medouze L, di Prisco-Fuenmayor MC, Verde O, Lopez RI, Malave C (1984) Incidence of atopic disease in a tropical environment: Partial independence from intestinal helminths. J Allergy Clin Immunol 73:229–233
18. Lynch NR, Lopez R, Isturiz G, Tenias-Salazar E (1983) Allergic reactivity and helminthic infection in Amerindians of the Amazon basin. Int Arch Allergy Appl Immunol 72:369–372
19. Mantle J, Pepys J (1974) Asthma amongst Tristan da Cunha islanders. Clin Allergy 4:161–170
20. Mitchell HS (1970) Bronchial asthma in Kenya. East Afr Med J 47:142–145
21. Miyamoto T (1984) International Symposium on Prevention of Allergic Diseases, Florence, June 24–27, p 22 (abstract)

22. Mun CT (1972) Pattern of bronchial asthma in Singapore. Singapore Med J 13:154–160
23. Pearson RSB (1933) Asthma in Barbados. Clin Allergy 3:289–297
24. Richards W, Patrick J (1965) Death from asthma in children. Am J Dis Child 110:4
25. Schmerler A, Abramowicz M (1974) Childhood asthma in the Bronx. NY State J Med 2:166
26. Sifontes JE, Maylo PM (1976) Bronchial asthma in Puerto Rican children. Bol Assoc Med PR 68:336
27. Smith JM (1983) Epidemiology and natural history of asthma, allergic rhinitis and atopic dermatitis (eczema). In: Middleton E Jr, Reed CE, Ellis EF (eds) Allergy, Principles and Practice, vol 11, 2nd edn. Mosby, St. Louis, pp 771–803
28. Smith JM, Harding LK, Cumming G (1971) The changing prevalence of asthma in school children. Clin Allergy 1:57
29. Sofowara EO, Clarke B (1969) Cited in: Sofowara EO (1970) Bronchial asthma in the tropics: a study of 250 Nigerian patients. East Afr Med J 47:434–439
30. Stanhope JM, Prior IAM (1976) The Tokelau Island migrant study: prevalence of various conditions before migration. Int J Epidemiol 5:259–266
31. Turner KJ (1978) The conflicting role of parasitic infections in modulating the prevalence of asthma. Papua New Guinea Med J 21:86–104
32. Turner KJ, Dowse GK, Stewart GA, Alpers MP (1986) Studies on bronchial hyperreactivity, allergic responsiveness and asthma in rural and urban children of the highlands of Papua New Guinea. J Allergy Clin Immunol 77:558–566
33. van Niekerk CH, Weinberg EG, Shore SC, Heese H de V, van Schalkwyk DJ (1979) Prevalence of asthma: a comparative study of urban and rural Xhosa children. Clin Allergy 9:319–324
34. Vines AP (1970) An epidemiological sample survey of the Highland Mainland and Island regions of the Territory of Papua New Guinea. Department of Public Health, Port Moresby
35. Viswanathan R (1973) The problem of asthma. J Asthma Res 10:157
36. Waite DA, Eyles EF, Tonkin SL, O'Donnell TV (1980) Asthma prevalence in Tokelauan children in two environments. Clin Allergy 10:71–75
37. Warrell DA, Fawcett IW, Harrison BDW, Agamah AJ, Ibu JO, Pope HM, Maberly DJ (1975) Bronchial asthma in the Nigerian Savanna Region. Clinical and laboratory study of 106 patients with a review of the literature on asthma in the tropics. Q J Med 44:325–347
38. Wasunna AEO (1968) Asthma as seen at the casualty department, Kenyatta National Hospital, Nairobi. East Afr Med J 45:701–705
39. Wolstenholme RJ (1979) Bronchial asthma in the Southern Maldives. Clin Allergy 9:325–332
40. Woolcock AJ (1972) Asthma in the Highlands of New Guinea. Aust NZ J Med 2:310
41. Woolcock AJ, Dowse GK, Temple K, Stanley H, Alpers MP, Turner KJ (1983) The prevalence of asthma in the South Fore people of Papua New Guinea. A method for field studies of bronchial reactivity. Eur J Respir Dis 64:571–581
42. Woolcock AJ, Konthen PG, Sedgwick C (1984) Allergic status of children in an Indonesian village. Asian Pacific Allergy Immunol 2:7–12
43. Zhu JL, Chen XJ, Zhu HR (1981) Primary investigation of asthma in 142,035 inhabitants both in Shanghai urban and Jiashan rural areas. Chin J Tuberc Respir Dis 46:32

C. Etiology

6. Viruses

W. W. Busse

Upper respiratory tract infections precipitate wheezing in many asthma patients of all ages. Although epidemiologic studies have identified respiratory viruses and *Mycoplasma pneumoniae* as precipitants of these attacks, the mechanisms remain to be established. Identifying and understanding the mechanisms of these attacks is important both in terms of medical management and in providing insight into the pathogenesis of asthma itself. The following review will highlight some of the important contributions which have helped us to confirm the relationship between upper respiratory infections and asthma and to elucidate the mechanisms of these attacks.

6.1 The Epidemiology of Respiratory Infections and Asthma

Respiratory virus infections precipitate asthma: The relationship between respiratory tract infections and the exacerbation of asthma has long been a well-appreciated clinical observation. Between 1967 and 1969, McIntosh and co-workers [1] carefully and prospectively studied 32 young children with asthma. The children ranged in age from 1 to 5 years, had severe asthma, and were hospitalized at the National Jewish Hospital in Denver. The etiology of each acute upper respiratory infection (URI) was carefully evaluated by culturing for the presence of virus and bacteria along with serological testing for viral antibody titers. Each exacerbation of asthma was documented by physical examination and changes in bronchodilator medication. During the two-year study, the 32 children had 102 confirmed viral respiratory infections and 139 episodes of wheezing. Fifty-eight episodes of wheezing occurred in association with a viral respiratory infection. Of the viruses identified, respiratory syncytial virus (RSV) infection was the most prevalent and most likely to provoke asthma. RSV was recovered in 14 infections of which 13 were associated with wheezing. In contrast, the association of parainfluenza virus infections was quite variable; on 15 occasions parainfluenza viruses were found but wheezing was noted in only 3 patients. *H. influenzae,* pneumococcus, β-hemolytic streptococcus, and *staphylococcus aureus* were also recovered from the respiratory tract but their presence did not correlate with an attack of asthma.

Further confirmation of this relationship was found in a subsequent prospective outpatient study from our institution [2]. We enrolled 16 children, ages 3 to 11 years, and closely observed them from October 1971 to May 1972. These children formed a highly selective group as all had a history of four or more asthma attacks during the previous year which were associated with an apparent respiratory illness. Furthermore, to prevent confusion, a patient was excluded from the study if wintertime allergic reactions coexisted which might provoke asthma. Detailed clinical records were maintained along with biweekly examinations at which time the patients were cultured for virus and bacteria by a nurse. During an asthma exacerbation or an URI, the bacteria and virus cultures were obtained more frequently and the asthma symptoms were carefully quantitated.

During the 8 months, our 16 patients experienced 61 episodes of asthma. Forty-two of these episodes coincided with a symptomatic respiratory infection of which twenty-four were confirmed to be of viral etiology. Rhinovirus was the most frequently isolated virus during episodes of asthma. Interestingly, the probability of wheezing during the URI was directly related to the severity of URI symptoms. During periods of asymptomatic virus shedding, asthma was not precipitated. Only one episode of wheezing occurred with a bacterial respiratory infection.

Although epidemiological studies in adults have also shown a relationship between viral respiratory infections and the provocation of asthma, this is not nearly as striking as was found with children. We examined both children and adults in a subsequent study [3]. Eight adults participated in this investigation and on only three occasions were viruses isolated during times of increased wheezing. In contrast, respiratory viruses were more frequently identified during asthma attacks in the children less than 10 years old. Many factors may contribute to the difficulty of identifying respiratory viruses in adults. Perhaps the most important reason is that episodes of asthma in adults appear to be less sharply delineated and therefore the timing for virus cultures is not as accurate.

The difficulty of evaluating this relationship in adults is underscored by a study of Hudgel and co-workers [4]. They evaluated nineteen adult patients with chronic asthma over 15 months. Viral cultures and serum antibody titers detected a total of 8 separate viral infections during 243 routine clinical visits. In contrast, when the patients were evaluated during seventy-six exacerbations of asthma, 8 episodes (11%) were documented to be of viral etiology. Although respiratory viruses precipitate asthma in adults, the relative frequency of this event is less and more difficult to document than in children. But, as with children, wheezing is more likely when the respiratory infections are symptomatic.

Bacterial URIs do not exacerbate asthma: Bacterial respiratory infections do not cause attacks of asthma. To confirm this, Berman and co-workers [5] performed transtracheal aspirations to culture 27 adult asthma patients during a respiratory infection. They found the bacteria cultured from transtracheal aspirates was sparse and did not correlate with the clinical illness. More importantly, transtracheal isolates from normal subjects without respiratory infection yielded a similar degree of bacterial colonization. From this work and the other studies cited, there is little evidence that bacterial respiratory infections precipitate asthma.

A number of important conclusions can be drawn from these studies. First, symptomatic respiratory infections which provoke asthma in both children and adults are likely to be viral in origin, however, this association is more apparent in children less than 10 years old. Second, many viruses can provoke asthma and the most prevalent organism varies with the patient's age. In young children, respiratory syncytial virus is most common, whereas rhinovirus assumes prevalence in older subjects. Third, asymptomatic virus shedding or mild URIs are unlikely to provoke asthma. Finally, there is no evidence that bacterial respiratory infections cause wheezing.

Viral respiratory infections may cause asthma: Viral URIs may also cause asthma. This unique linkage is best illustrated in children recovering from bronchiolitis. Bronchiolitis is, in most cases, caused by viruses and particularly respiratory syncytial virus [6]. The majority of children with bronchiolitis recover without sequelae. Interestingly, in others, the initial bout of bronchiolitis is followed by recurrent episodes of wheezing which usually occur with subsequent viral respiratory infections.

Some investigations have found 40 to 50% of children will have recurrent wheezing following an acute episode of bronchiolitis [7]. The children most susceptible to recurrent episodes of wheezing are the offspring of allergic parents. Furthermore, the children with recurrent wheezing are also more likely to have strongly positive skin tests to allergens. The mechanism by which bronchiolitis ushers in recurrent virus-induced asthma, and possibly the atopic state as well, is largely unresolved but undoubtedly forms a critical link in the pathogenesis of asthma.

6.2 Respiratory Viruses Cause Airway Inflammation

Respiratory viral infections in normals cause airway obstruction: Our understanding of virus-induced asthma has been greatly advanced by evaluating lung function and airway reactivity in normal subjects during URIs. Studies in normals are important because subtle effects of a viral URI on airway function in asthma might easily be overlooked in the presence of advanced disease. Furthermore, the study of hyperreactivity in asthma is complicated by drug treatment, hypertrophy and hyperplasia of airway smooth muscle, and variable degrees of pulmonary obstruction, each of which makes it difficult to estimate virus-induced changes.

Hall et al [8] assessed airway function in 13 college-aged students with documented, uncomplicated influenza A infection. Measurements of large airway function remained unchanged throughout the illness. However, in tests of small airway mechanics, 10 of the 13 subjects evaluated had markedly abnormal frequency dependence measurements of airway resistance. Serial evaluations found these changes persisted in some patients for three to five weeks after the clinical illness. Furthermore, it was also found that the increase in pulmonary resistance was mild and confined principally to measurements of peripheral or small airway function.

Pathologic studies provide indirect evidence as to a mechanism for the mild airway obstruction. Biopsy specimens of bronchial epithelium in uncomplicated cases of influenza virus infection have documented extensive inflammation and even desquamation [9]. This process may directly cause peripheral airway obstruction noted in humans. In addition, influenza virus infections also cause a prolonged impairment in mechanisms of bronchial clearance [10]. This delayed clearance may further contribute to the airway dysfunction.

Viral respiratory infections cause airway hyperreactivity in normals: Viral URIs can also alter airway reactivity in normal individuals. Although respiratory syncytial virus (RSV) is a major pathogen of childhood bronchiolitis and, moreover, provokes asthma in youngsters, it is not a frequent cause of respiratory illnesses in adults except under unusual conditions. Hall et al [11] prospectively evaluated 10 adult employees of an infants' ward who were infected with RSV. Included in their evaluation were measurements of total airway resistance and the bronchial response to an aerosol of the cholinergic agonist carbachol. All 10 subjects were symptomatic during the RSV infection and had a cough which lasted at least one week. Four weeks later, almost all the patients were asymptomatic except for mild shortness of breath which also gradually resolved. Pulmonary function tests from these ten patients demonstrated increased airway resistance for at least 8 weeks after the onset of the RSV illness. Furthermore, all subjects had an exaggerated increase in airway resistance following an inhalation of carbachol. The airway hyperreactivity to carbachol was still present 8 weeks after the acute infection. The role of virus-induced airway inflammation is undoubtedly important to this enhanced cholinergic response.

There is a rather consistent pattern which emerges from the studies of normal subjects. Uncomplicated viral URIs produce pulmonary obstruction which is largely limited to the smaller airways. Moreover, the airway changes are subtle and transient but persist well beyond the clinical illness. Because airway hyperreactivity and obstruction already exists, the asthma patient appears more susceptible to the effects of a viral URI. In asthma, the URI consequences are not subtle but can produce severe wheezing.

6.3 Mechanisms of Virus-induced Airway Reactivity

Airway inflammation: Empey and coworkers [12] monitored airway reactivity in 12 young normal subjects with a clinical uncomplicated viral URI. Bronchial reactivity was measured by a change in the airway resistance to an aerosol of histamine and citric acid. The change in airway resistance to histamine was measured in the URI patients and compared to 11 matched controls without a cold. The subjects with a cold had a significantly greater increase in airway resistance to aerosol histamine ($218 \pm 54.6\%$) than did the controls ($30.5 \pm 5.5\%$). Furthermore, it was also found that the threshold for citric acid to

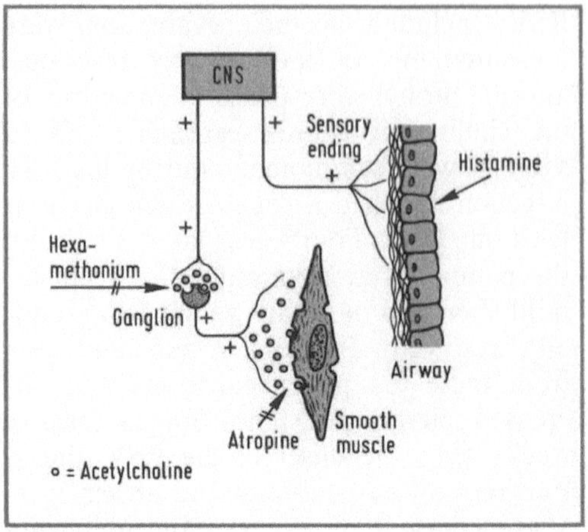

Fig. 6.1. The normal airway epithelium is supplied by afferent sensory fibers from the vagus. When the bronchial epithelium is stimulated by histamine, these sensory fibers are activated to cause a reflex increase in airway tone (+). In the normal subject, histamine does not cause a significant increase in airway tone. The reflex response is blocked by hexamethonium at the ganglion and by atropine at the neuromuscular junction

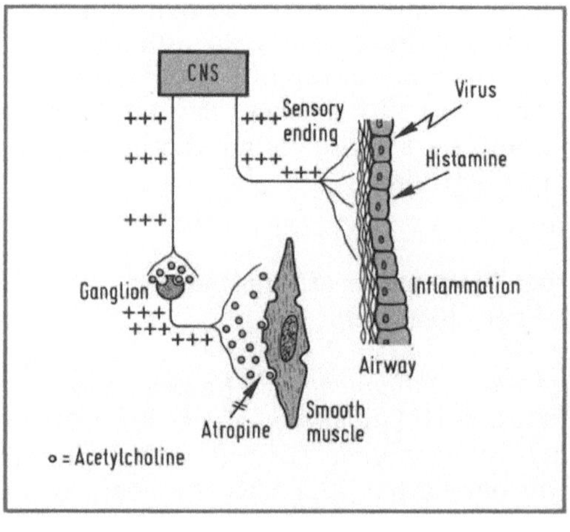

Fig. 6.2. During a respiratory viral infection, inflammation of the bronchial epithelium develops. As a consequence, the rapidly adapting sensory fibers of the afferent vagus nerve are sensitized. The sensitized afferent fibers become more responsive to stimulation, e.g., histamine (+ + +). As a consequence, the reflex airway reactivity to histamine is also enhanced during the viral infection (+ + +). Atropine blockage of this enhanced response is evidence for participation of the vagus reflex

stimulate cough was lowered during the URI. Although the URI symptoms disappeared within a week, the airway hyperreactivity persisted for up to 6 weeks in some subjects.

The investigators speculated that virus-induced inflammation of the airway epithelium increased the sensitivity of the rapidly adapting sensory airway receptors to a variety of stimuli including histamine and citric acid. Stimulation of these sensitized receptors activates vagus-mediated reflex bronchospasm. When the URI patients were pretreated with aerosolized atropine and then given an aerosol of either histamine or citric acid, the airway resistance was not enhanced nor was the cough response as great. Atropine protection is strong presumptive evidence that the virus-associated airway reactivity was mediated by a vagus reflex.

To explain their observations, the authors postulated that respiratory viruses damage bronchial epithelium to sensitize rapidly adapting sensory vagus fibers found in the airways. These afferent sensory receptors are located principally in the subepithelium of larger airways. A wide variety of stimuli, e.g., citric acid or histamine, are able to activate the sensitized afferent receptors to elicit vagus-mediated reflex bronchoconstriction (Figs. 6.1, 6.2). The airway damage from respiratory viruses requires weeks to heal as does the recovery of airway hyperreactivity. Interestingly, the length of time required for epithelial healing to occur corresponds to the persistence of airway irritability.

We have developed an animal model to study mechanisms of virus-induced asthma. The guinea pig is infected by nasal insufflation with parainfluenza 3. Four days later the animals are evaluated for virus effects on airway reactivity and compared to control animals insufflated only with a culture medium [13]. Specifically, we have evaluated the bronchial response to histamine with measurements of airway overflow pressure [Buckner, Songsiridej, Dick, and Busse, unpublished observations]. The pulmonary overflow pressure produced by histamine was significantly greater in the guinea pigs infected with parainfluenza virus. This enhanced airway response to histamine is similar to the observations of Empey et al [12] in humans. When the animal's vagus is severed, the enhanced airway response to histamine does not occur. Pretreatment with hexamethonium diminished the enhanced overflow pressure to histamine in the virus-treated animals. Furthermore, when large doses of atropine were given, airway sensitivity to histamine was diminished in the infected animal.

Interestingly, when the severed vagus nerve was electrically stimulated, there was also a substantial increase in the magnitude of overflow pressure in the virus-infected animals. This suggests that the efferent arm of the vagus is also altered by the virus infection (Fig. 6.3). In addition, tissue from infected and control animals was isolated and suspended in a water bath to measure contractile activity. The contractile response of isolated airway smooth muscle to acetylcholine and histamine is normal.

A number of conclusions can be drawn from the studies in humans and parainfluenza 3-infected guinea pigs. First, viral respiratory infections enhanced vagus-mediated reflex bronchospasm. This appears to occur because airway inflammation sensitizes the afferent vagus sensory fibers to a wide variety of stimuli. Second, data from our animal model also showed that the efferent vagus response was enhanced by the virus infection. Finally, we had no evidence from studies with airway smooth muscle-isolated parainfluenza 3-infected guinea pig, that the intrinsic contractile activity of the airway was altered by virus (Fig. 6.3).

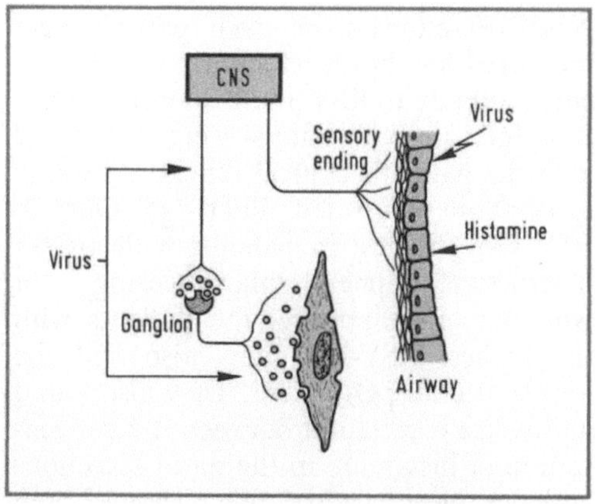

Fig. 6.3. The parainfluenza 3-infected guinea pig has increased airway reactivity to histamine. This has been postulated to occur because airway inflammation sensitizes afferent vagus sensory fibers to enhance the reflex bronchospastic response to histamine. In the guinea pig, we have also found that stimulation of the efferent vagus nerve causes enhanced airway contraction. Thus, in the parainfluenza 3-infected guinea pig, there is participation of both the afferent and efferent limb of vagus nerve to produce an enhanced airway reactive response

IgE antibody production: The IgE-dependent release of mast cell mediators is an important factor in the pathogenesis and precipitation of asthma. If viruses stimulated production of specific antibodies, this could contribute to increases in airway reactivity and asthma. In a study of 42 infants with respiratory syncytial virus infection, Welliver and co-workers [14] found IgE attached to exfoliated nasopharyngeal epithelial cells. Cell-bound IgE appeared in 70 to 80% of all patients during the first 10 days of illness. When the investigators examined the relationship of the particular clinical illness pattern to the frequency and persistence of cell-bound IgE, an interesting pattern emerged. All the patients with bronchiolitis or asthma had cell-bound IgE in their nasal secretions when tested 7 to 20 days into the illness. In contrast, only 33% of patients with pneumonia or upper respiratory tract illness had detectable cell-bound IgE at the same time. The persistence of cell-bound IgE, but not its early appearance, correlated with the presence of airway obstruction. Moreover, patients with higher levels of cell-bound IgE were more likely to have a family history of wheezing.

In a subsequent study, Welliver et al [15] evaluated an additional 79 children, all less than 12 months of age, with documented RSV infection. The clinical pattern of illness in these children could be divided into four types:

- upper respiratory tract illness,
- pneumonia without wheezing,
- pneumonia and wheezing, and
- wheezing (bronchiolitis).

Nasal secretions from each patient were measured for the development of IgE-specific antibody to RSV and histamine. When RSV-IgE antibody titers were compared with the patient's clinical illness, a striking association was noted. First, IgE titers to RSV were highest in patients with airway obstruction, pneumonia/wheezing or wheezing. Furthermore, the patients with the highest RSV-IgE titers also had the lowest arterial pO_2 values. They also found an inverse correlation between the concentration of histamine in the nasal secretions and the lowest arterial pO_2. That is, high nasal histamine concentrations were more likely to be found in patients with a low arterial pO_2.

At present, the interpretation of these exciting findings and their relevance to the pathogenesis of virus-induced asthma is speculative (Fig. 6.4). Clearly, Welliver and co-workers have documented that RSV elicits the production of a specific IgE antibody. It is possible that the newly formed IgE antibody attaches to mast cells and then interacts with the RSV antigen. An IgE-RSV interaction could activate mast cell and basophil mediator release to produce airway obstruction. At present, it is only conjecture that the identified IgE-specific antibody reacts with RSV to cause both histamine release and airway obstruction. In the interpretation of these data, it is important to emphasize that mediator release by itself does not usually cause asthma. However, the coexistence of bronchial inflammation may enhance airway sensitivity to the vasoactive hormones. Welliver's studies are important in that they clearly demonstrate that IgE antibodies can develop to respiratory viruses, respiratory syncytial [14, 15] and parainfluenza [16], during a respiratory illness.

Respiratory viral infections can also be important in the development of IgE antibodies to other environmental antigens. Frick and colleagues [17] prospectively followed 13 children, who had a biparental allergic background, for the onset of IgE-mediated hypersensitivity. All but 2 of the 13 children developed significant allergic symptoms and immunological evidence of allergic sensitization during the first year of life. Interestingly, the development of allergic sensitization was associated with the child having had a recent virus infection. The type of viruses associated with the onset of symptoms included parainfluenza and respiratory syncytial virus; the same viruses associated with the precipitation of asthma.

Although a number of mechanisms have been postulated to explain how viruses can lead to the development of allergic sensitization, recent work by Sakamota, Ida, and Takishima [18] is most provocative. They found that IgE antibody sensitization to an inhaled antigen occurred in mice who were infected with influenza A virus, but not in mice without the viral infection. Because influenza virus infections are associated with acute airway inflammation and exfoli-

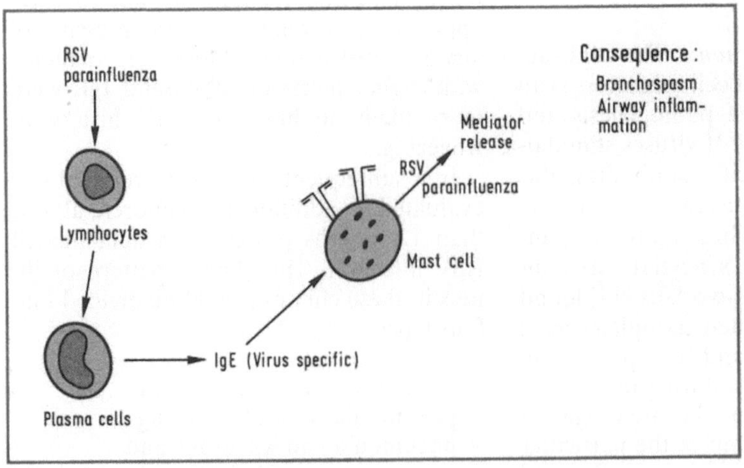

Fig. 6.4. Respiratory syncytial virus (RSV) and parainfluenza virus infections stimulate IgE production. The RSV and parainfluenza virus initiate IgE antibody production by interaction with lymphocyte. The newly produced IgE antibody becomes attached to mast cells. When IgE antibody interacts with RSV or parainfluenza virus, mediator release can occur to cause airway obstruction

ation of epithelial cells, the investigators speculated that permeability of the mucosal barrier is increased to antigen and with this the increased potential for sensitization. Possibly the same sequence of events occurs in humans.

Diminished β-adrenergic function: Szentivanyi [19] proposed that a major factor contributing to the pathogenesis of asthma may be an imbalance in the autonomic nervous system control of airway smooth muscle, specifically diminished β-adrenergic responsiveness. Decreased β-adrenergic response of the airway smooth muscle would favor bronchoconstriction. In some patients with asthma, β-adrenergic activity is defective. The importance of the adrenergic system to asthma is further emphasized by knowing that an asthma attack follows the administration of β-adrenergic antagonists like propranolol. Therefore, if respiratory viruses also compromised β-adrenergic function in the asthmatic airways, increased wheezing would be a likely consequence.

We have used leukocytes isolated from asthma patients as a model to evaluate β-adrenergic function in this disease. Specifically, we have examined the granulocyte response to isoproterenol, which inhibits lysosomal enzyme release via the cyclic adenosine monophosphate system, as a measurement of β-adrenergic function in asthma [20]. In asthma, this granulocyte isoproterenol response is diminished and further impaired during a viral URI which provokes asthma. Although unproven, we have speculated that respiratory viruses would increase wheezing if they diminished β-adrenergic function of airway smooth muscle.

To further evaluate and establish this relationship, isolated human granulocytes were incubated with live respiratory viruses. Influenza A virus- and rhinovirus-treated granulocytes were less responsive to isoproterenol [21, 22]. Because both rhinovirus and influenza virus altered leukocyte β-adrenergic function and also were associated with clinical episodes of asthma, our observations may have direct clinical application to attacks of wheezing.

Airway inflammation is a major contribution to obstruction in severe asthma of any cause and neutrophils undoubtedly play a role in this function. Like respiratory viruses, ozone exposure will produce airway hyperreactivity. In dogs, ozone produces an increase in airway reactivity which is associated with neutrophil infiltration of bronchial epithelium and the presence of neutrophils in the bronchial lavage [23]. Because catecholamines can reduce neutrophil-provoked inflammation by inhibiting lysosomal enzyme release, a virus impairment in this β-adrenergic function means lysosomal release increases and with it tissue inflammation, airway hyperreactivity and asthma (Fig. 6.5).

Enhanced basophil mediator release and movement: Mediator release and its modulation are undoubtedly pivotal to the pathogenesis of asthma and airway reactivity. Although the pulmonary mast cell is biologically the most relevant cell in this secretory process, basophil histamine release has proven to be a reliable and instructive model to study immediate hypersensitivity reactions. To evaluate the effects of respiratory viruses on basophil histamine release, Ida et al [24] conducted the following experiments. Isolated human leukocytes which were incubated with herpes simplex virus, influenza A, and adenovirus had enhanced IgE-dependent basophil histamine release. The degree of enhanced release correlated to the degree of virus infectivity.

Basophil histamine release also occurred with inactivated viruses. Further, Ida et al [24] found that the enhanced basophil histamine release paralleled interferon production which occurred during the virus incubation. In addition, leukocyte histamine release was also enhanced when exogenous interferon was substituted for virus in the incubation mixture. We have found similar enhancement in leukocyte histamine release to ragweed antigen E following an incubation with influenza A virus or interferon [25]. These observations suggest that not only can respiratory viruses directly increase asthma by causing airway inflammation, they can also generate and release factors from virus-infected cells to enhance this process (Fig. 6.6).

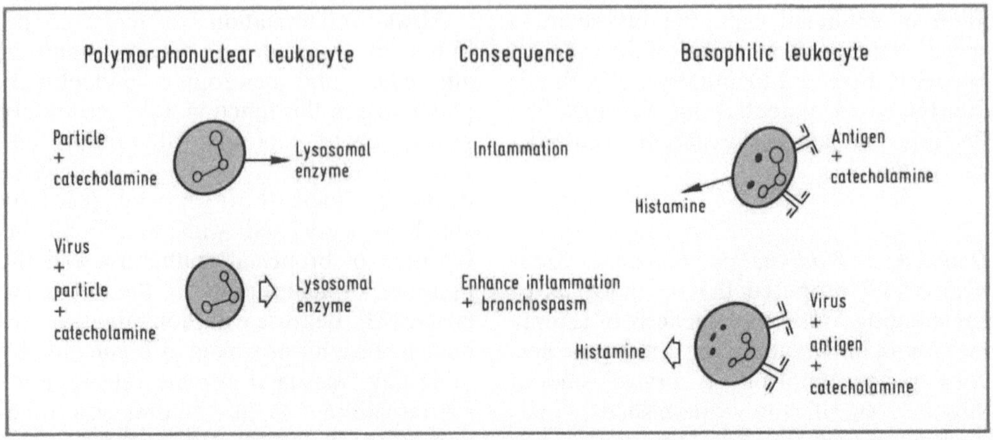

Fig. 6.5. Respiratory viruses can diminish the β-adrenergic response in the human polymorphonuclear (PMN) leukocyte and basophil. When the PMN is stimulated by particles like zymosan, lysosomal enzyme occurs. This secretory process is decreased by catecholamines which increase cellular levels of CAMP. In the presence of respiratory viruses, the PMN response to catecholamines is diminished and lysosomal enzyme release enhanced. A similar chain of events occurs where the human basophil histamine release to antigen is modulated by catecholamines. This negative modulation is diminished by respiratory viruses. The consequence of this virus action on both the PMN and basophil is to enhance the secretion of inflammatory and bronchoconstrictory factors

Circulating basophils increase during episodes of asthma. If more basophils are recruited to airways during a viral URI, the release of bronchospasm mediators would also enhance airway inflammation and obstruction. Lett-Brown and co-workers [26] incubated leukocytes with a parainfluenza virus. Following the virus incubation, leukocyte chemotaxis was measured to a C5 peptide of complement or a lymphocyte-derived chemotactic factor. Interestingly, the only leukocyte which had enhanced chemotaxis was the basophil. When interferon was substituted for virus, basophil migration was also enhanced. If respiratory viruses promote basophil accumulation in airways, stimulation of spasmogenic mediator release is likely to result in greater airway contraction. Therefore, respiratory viruses have a multiplicity of ef-

Fig. 6.6 Respiratory viruses enhance human basophil histamine release. When human basophil histamine release is performed in the presence of respiratory viruses, this response is enhanced. Furthermore, it has been shown that this enhanced activity is also caused by interferon which is generated during the virus incubation. The consequence of this enhanced response can be increased airway inflammation and asthma

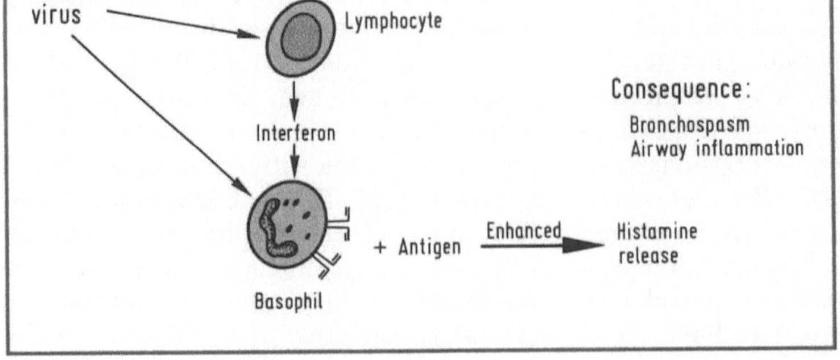

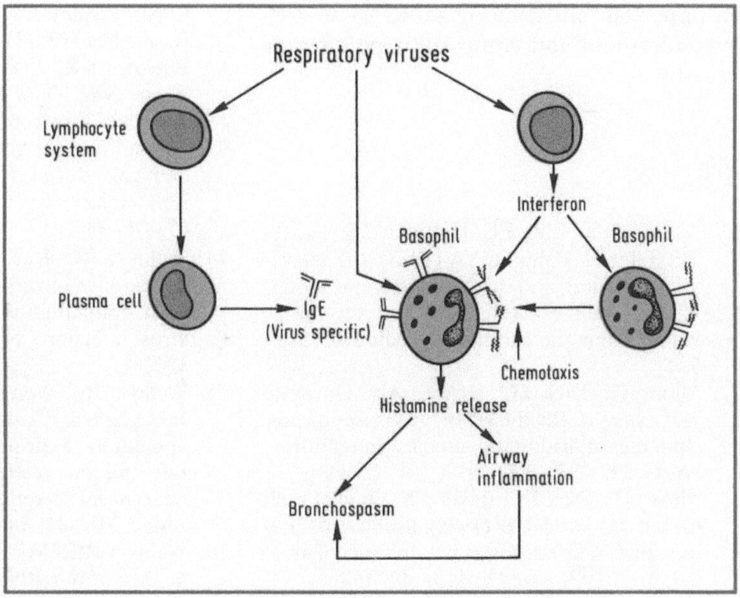

Fig. 6.7. Respiratory viruses can interact with the lymphocyte system to produce virus-specific IgE antibody. Theoretically, the virus-specific IgE will sensitize basophils and mast cells. A subsequent interaction of cell-bound IgE with the respiratory virus causes mediator release. This response can be compounded as either virus, or the product of virus-infected cells, interferon, enhances mediator release. Histamine release can produce airway obstruction directly or increase bronchial hypersensitivity by producing airway inflammation

fects on basophil function all of which could enhance the severity of airway reactivity and asthma (Fig. 6.7).

An animal model for virus-induced asthma: The parainfluenza 3-infected guinea pig provides an animal model in which virus-associated changes can be systemically examined. Guinea pigs actively sensitized with ovalbumin were inoculated with parainfluenza 3 virus four days before performing in vitro pharmacological studies on tracheal and bronchial smooth muscle [13]. The isolated airway segments were contracted with cumulative doses of ovalbumin in the presence and absence of a β-adrenergic receptor agonist, which reduced the contractile response to ovalbumin. Although the virus infection did not alter the dose response contractions with ovalbumin, the magnitude of β-adrenergic inhibition was smaller in airway segments from virus-infected animals. Our studies also showed that in the respiratory infection, β-agonist did not alter the airway smooth muscle contractile response to histamine or carbachol. The infection of the guinea pig with parainfluenza 3 caused a selective blockade of the β-adrenergic-mediated inhibition of antigen-induced contraction of airway smooth muscle. One plausible explanation is that the respiratory virus alters the airway mast cell's inhibitory response to a β-agonist thus ablating normal catecholamine suppression of mediator secretion.

6.4 Conclusions

A number of important mechanisms have been identified by which viruses can provoke asthma. From the available data a single mechanism does not appear able to explain virus-induced asthma. Rather, the relationship between viral URIs and asthma is complex and involves many organ systems: airway epithelium, autonomic nervous system control, and the immediate hypersensitivity system. A common factor associated with respiratory viruses is their ability to enhance leukocyte inflammatory activity. If this enhanced inflammation is directed toward the airway, a vicious cycle occurs with increased airway reactivity and asthma. Identifying the effects of respiratory viruses on airway function remains an important undertaking as we try to better understand and control this precipitant of asthma.

References

1. McIntosh K, Ellis EF, Hoffman LS, Lybass TG, Eller JJ, Fulginiti VA (1973) The association of viral and bacterial respiratory infections with exacerbations of wheezing in young asthmatic children. J Pediatr 82:578–590
2. Minor TE, Dick EC, DeMeo AN, Ouellette JJ, Cohen M, Reed CE (1974) Viruses as precipitants of asthmatic attacks in children. JAMA 227:292–298
3. Minor TE, Dick EC, Baker JW, Ouellette JJ, Cohen M, Reed CE (1976) Rhinovirus and influenza A infections as precipitants of asthma. Am Rev Respir Dis 113:149–153
4. Hudgel DW, Langston E Jr, Selner JC, McIntosh K (1979) Viral and bacterial infections in adults with chronic asthma. Am Rev Respir Dis 120:393–397
5. Berman SZ, Mathison DA, Stevenson DD, Tan EM, Vaughan JH (1975) Transtracheal aspiration studies in asthmatic patients in relapse with "infective" asthma and in subjects without respiratory disease. J Allergy Clin Immunol 56:206–214
6. McIntosh K (1976) Bronchiolitis and asthma: possible common pathogenetic pathways. J Allergy Clin Immunol 57:595–604
7. Zweiman B, Schoenwetter WF, Pappano JE, Tempest B, Hildreth EA (1971) Patterns of allergic respiratory disease in children with a past history of bronchiolitis. J Allergy 48: 283–289
8. Hall WJ, Douglas RG Jr, Hyde RW, Roth FK, Cross AS, Speers DM (1976) Pulmonary mechanics after uncomplicated influenza A infection. Am Rev Respir Dis 113:141–147
9. Walsh JJ, Dietlein LF, Low FN, Burch GE, Mogabgab WJ (1961) Tracheobronchial response in human influenza. Arch Intern Med 108:376
10. Camner P, Jarstrand C, Philipson K (1973) Tracheobronchial Clearance in patients with influenza. Am Rev Respir Dis 108:131–135
11. Hall WJ, Hall CB, Speers DM (1978) Respiratory syncytial virus infection in adults. Clinical, virologic, and serial pulmonary function studies. Ann Intern Med 88:203–205
12. Empey DW, Laitinen LA, Jacobs L, Gold WM, Nadel JA (1976) Mechanisms of bronchial hyperreactivity in normal subjects after upper respiratory tract infection. Am Rev Respir Dis 113:131–139
13. Buckner CK, Clayton DE, Ain-Shoka AA, Busse WW, Dick EC, Shult P (1981) Parainfluenza 3 infection blocks the ability of a beta-adrenergic receptor agonist to inhibit antigen-induced contraction of guinea pig isolated airway smooth muscle. J Clin Invest 67:376–384
14. Welliver RC, Kaul TN, Ogra PL (1980) The appearance of cell-bound IgE in respiratory-tract epithelium after respiratory syncytial virus infection. N Engl J Med 303:1198–1202
15. Welliver RC, Wong DT, Sun M, Middleton E Jr, Vaughan RS, Ogra PL (1981) The development of respiratory syncytial virus specific IgE and the release of histamine in nasopharyngeal secretions after infection. N Engl J Med 305:841–846
16. Welliver RC, Wong DT, Middleton E Jr, Sun M, McCarthy RN, Ogra PL (1982) Role of parainfluenza virus-specific IgE in pathogenesis of croup and wheezing subsequent to infection. J Pediatr 101:889–896
17. Frick OL, German DF, Mills J (1979) Development of allergy in children. 1. Association with virus infections. J Allergy Clin Immunol 63:228–241
18. Sakamoto M, Ida S, Takishima T (1984) Effect of influenza virus infection on allergic sensitization to aerosolized ovalbumin in mice. J Immunol 132:2614–2617
19. Szentivanyi A (1968) The beta-adrenergic theory of atopic abnormality in asthma. J Allergy 42:203–232
20. Busse WW (1977) Decreased granulocyte response to isoproterenol in asthma during upper respiratory infections. Am Rev Respir Dis 115:783–789
21. Busse WW, Cooper W, Warshauer DM, Dick EC, Wallow IHC, Albrecht R (1979) Impairment of isoproterenol, H2 histamine, and prostaglandin E_1 response of human granulocytes after incubation *in vitro* with live influenza vaccines. Am Rev Respir Dis 119: 561–569
22. Busse WW, Anderson CL, Dick EC, Warshauer D (1980) Reduced granulocyte response to isoproterenol, histamine, and prostaglandin E, after *in vitro* incubation with rhinovirus 16. Am Rev Respir Dis 122:641–646
23. Fabbri LM, Aizawa H, Alpert SE, Walters EH, O'Byrne PM, Gold BD, Nadel JA, Holtzman MJ (1984) Airway hyperresponsiveness and changes in cell counts in bronchoalveolar lavage after ozone exposure in dogs. Am Rev Respir Dis 129:288–291

24. Ida S, Hooks JJ, Siraganian RP, Notkins AL (1977) Enhancement of IgE-mediated histamine release from human basophil by viruses: role of interferon. J Exp Med 145:892–906
25. Busse WW, Swenson CA, Borden EC, Treuhaft MW, Dick EC (1983) The effect of influenza A virus on leukocyte histamine release. J Allergy Clin Immunol 71:382–388
26. Lett-Brown MA, Aelvoet M, Hooks JJ, Georgiades JA, Thueson DO, Grant JA (1981) Enhancement of basophil chemotaxis in vitro by virus-induced interferon. J Clin Invest 67:547–552

7. Allergic Bronchopulmonary Aspergillosis

A. B. Tonnel, Ph. Gosset, B. Wallaert

The ubiquitous presence of *Aspergillus* in decaying vegetation, soil, air and also, in households makes human pulmonary exposure inevitable. Moreover, *Aspergillus* spores can develop at body temperature in the bronchial lumen and form mycelia, conferring on it special status among inhaled allergens. This endoluminal growth of the fungus induces a continuous allergen release which probably explains the clinical and biological particularities of this disease.

7.1 Incidence

Among the different species of Aspergillus, *Aspergillus fumigatus* is the most frequently observed in allergic bronchopulmonary aspergillosis (ABPA), but other species (i.e., *A. niger, flavus, terreus*) may be implicated. The actual incidence of the disease is not easy to ascertain. Incidence seems to be more elevated in Great Britain and northern European countries than in the United States. However, a recent study conducted both in London and in Cleveland (Ohio), involving two groups of asthmatics [1] showed that sensitization to *Aspergillus* antigens occurred with similar frequency in both cities (28% in Cleveland vs 23% in London). It appears also that the incidence as well as the frequency of symptoms are increased during autumn and winter when *Aspergillus* spore counts are up to 100 times

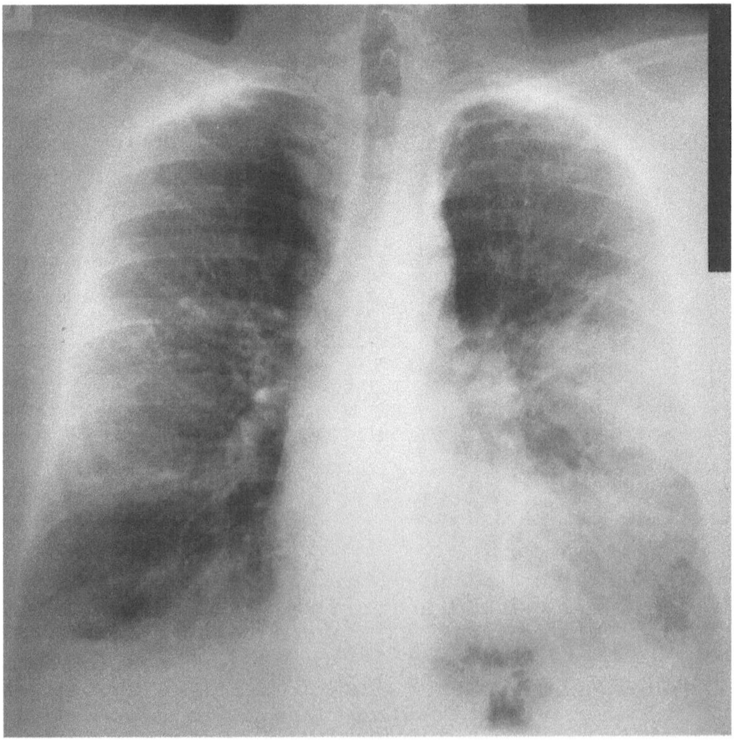

Fig. 7.1. Massive homogenous consolidation of the lingular segment

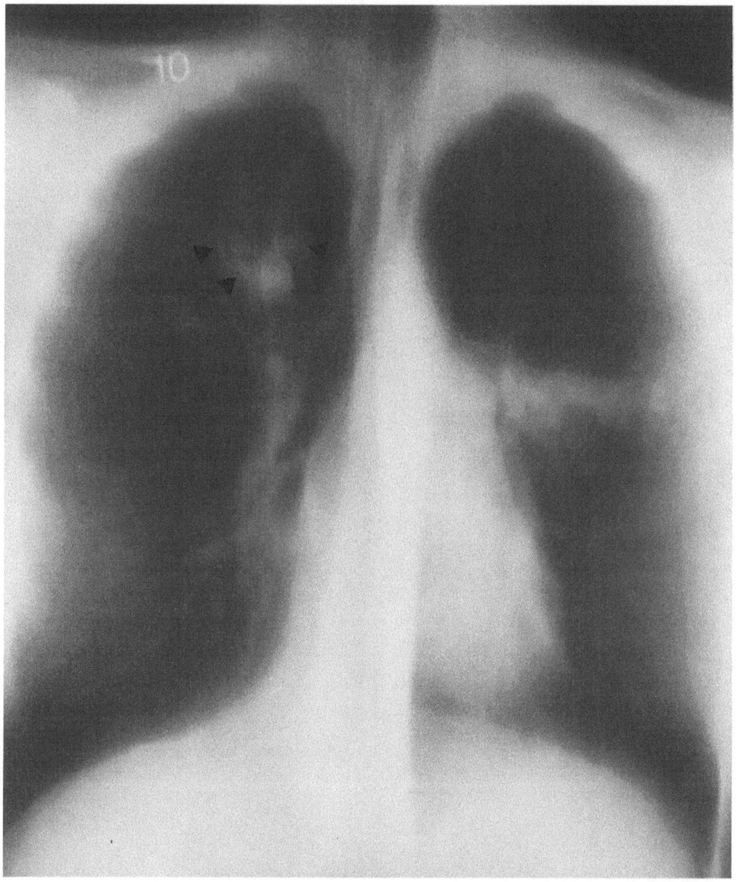

Fig. 7.2. Anteroposterior tomogram showing mucoid impaction with gloved-finger shadows (arrowheads)

more numerous in the atmosphere. It is likely that massive occupational exposure explains the higher incidence in agricultural areas, but many cases reported in urban dwellers support the view that host susceptibility also plays a role in the pathogenesis of ABPA [2].

7.2 Clinical and Radiological Features

Patients with ABPA are usually atopic with a long history of recurrent bronchospastic episodes, the duration of asthma before the diagnosis of ABPA being often longer than 15 or 20 years (29 years in our experience [3]). The asthma is severe, sometimes corticosteroid-dependent. During acute exacerbations, productive cough is common and golden-brown plugs of viscous material are found in the sputum. Hemoptysis can occur but usually remains minimal. Pleuritic chest pain is noted in 50% of ABPA patients, often localized in front of the radiological abnormalities. Sometimes ABPA is identified only at the stage of chronic respiratory failure, demonstrating the major delays in identification of the disease.

Radiological abnormalities often aid in the diagnosis of ABPA. Chest film findings include transient and/or permanent abnormalities [4].

The *transient shadows* are described as:

- parenchymal infiltrates with homogeneous opacities without shrinkage, or nonhomogeneous patchy clouding (Fig. 7.1). They were bilateral in 72 of 111 cases reported by MacCarthy and Pepys [2] with a predilection for the upper lobes;

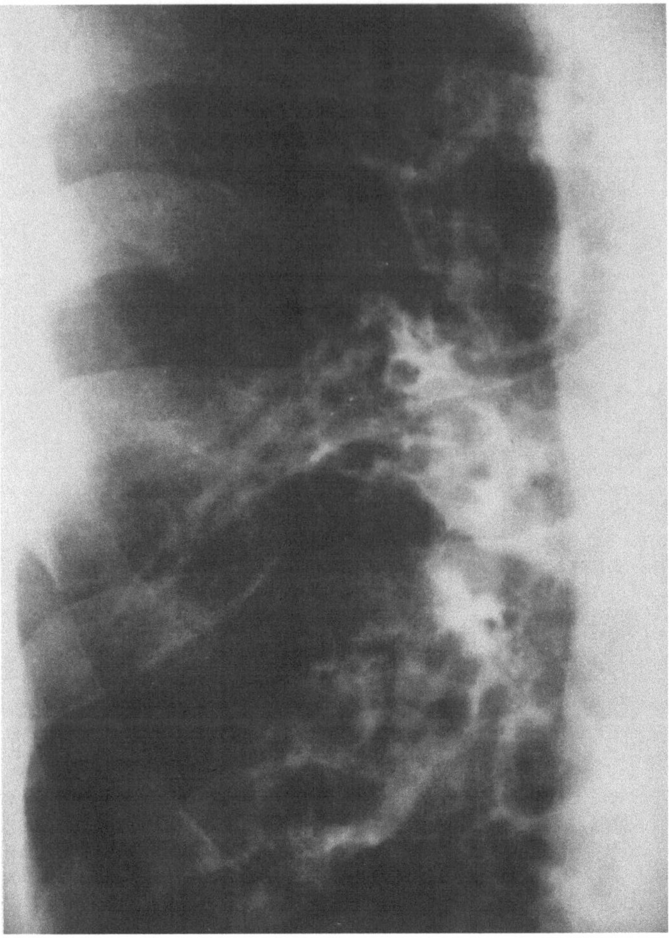

a

Fig. 7.3. Right upper lobe proximal bronchiectasis on chest roentgenogram (**a**) and lateral tomogram (**b**)

- atelectasis of a lung or a lobe;
- mucoid impaction with *toothpaste* or *gloved finger* shadows (Fig. 7.2).

The *permanent abnormalities* include:

- tubular and ring shadows related to the development of central bronchiectasis which represent one of the most characteristic features of ABPA (Fig. 7.3);
- less often, persistent shrunken but aerated segment or lobe;
- in addition to these classical features, Mintzer et al [5] described in some patients perihilar infiltrates simulating adenopathy, and air fluid levels secondary to dilated and partially obstructed bronchi. Occurrence of spontaneous pneumothorax and development of aspergillomas terminating in disseminated aspergillosis has been recently reported [6].
- It must be emphasized that 20% of chest x-ray abnormalities are asymptomatic but on the other hand, ABPA may exist despite normal chest roentgenogram [17]. Malo et al [4] have demonstrated a statistical correlation between the number of transient radiological changes through a long period of follow-up and the extent of bronchiectasis.

7.3 Laboratory Findings

Sputum examination: As a widespread microorganism, *Aspergillus* can be cultured from the sputum of controls and allergic

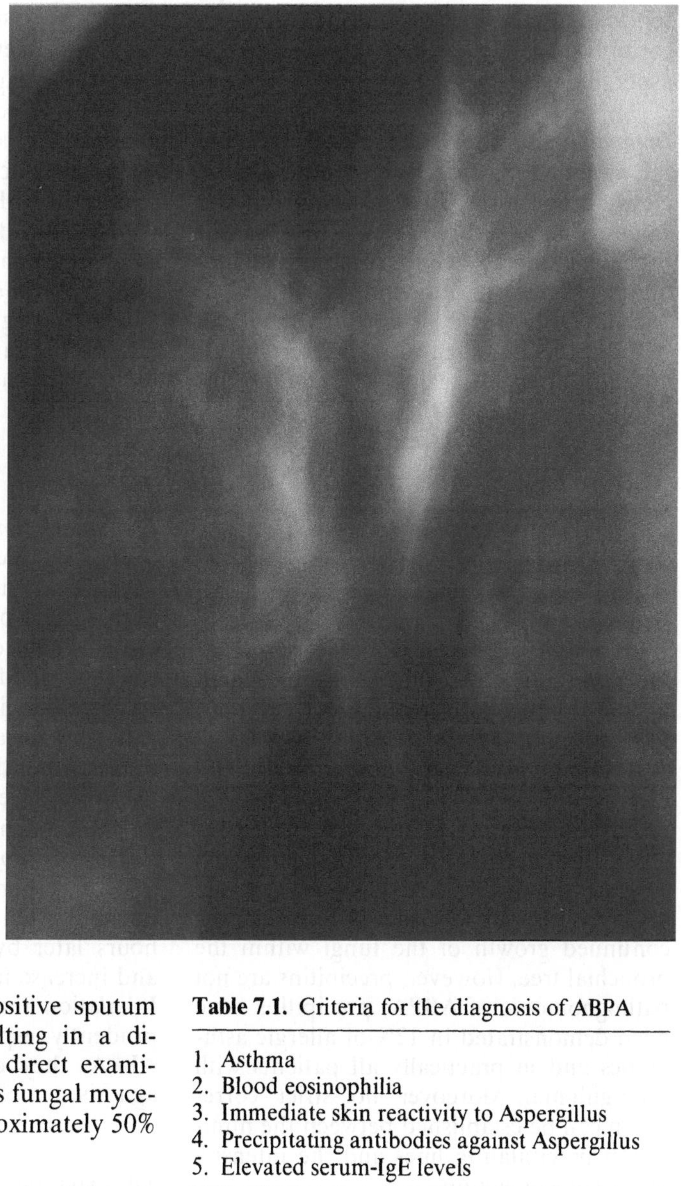

Fig. 7.3b

asthmatic subjects with a positive sputum culture not necessarily resulting in a diagnosis of ABPA. However, direct examination of sputum plugs shows fungal mycelium and eosinophils in approximately 50% of the patients [2].

Peripheral blood eosinophilia: An absolute eosinophil count higher than 600/mm³ is recognized as a typical feature in ABPA. Eosinophilia over 2,000/mm³ occurs in 20% of ABPA patients, particularly during the acute phase of the disease, often associated to the presence of eosinophils in sputum (Table 7.1).

Skin tests: All patients develop an immediate wheal and flare response to skin tests and a majority demonstrate a late cutaneous reaction after 6 to 8 hours. Mac Carthy and Pepys [2] found the dual reaction in almost all of the 111 patients tested. Although other studies have noted a late reaction in a more restricted number of ABPA patients (35–80%), most of those not demonstrating the late reaction were taking prednisone. Of course, an immediate positive test is not specific of ABPA; among 656 allergic asthmatics Hendrick et al [8] found

Table 7.1. Criteria for the diagnosis of ABPA

1. Asthma
2. Blood eosinophilia
3. Immediate skin reactivity to Aspergillus
4. Precipitating antibodies against Aspergillus
5. Elevated serum-IgE levels

16% skin prick tests positive to *Aspergillus fumigatus.* Likewise, Hoehne et al [9] reported dual positive skin reactions in controls, allergic asthma and even in aspergillomas.

Immunological tests: Both **total IgE and IgE specific** for *Aspergillus* are found to be elevated in most ABPA patients but the values of total serum-IgE in ABPA and in extrinsic asthma overlap, limiting the usefulness of this test in the individual patient. Specific IgE are also significantly higher in ABPA patients but most of the serum-IgE are not directed against *Aspergillus,* indicating that the marked IgE increase results partly from nonspecific stimulation of IgE-producing plasma cells. Nevertheless IgE levels correlate with disease activity and total serum-IgE can be considered as a sensitive marker of ABPA, rising prior to clinical exacerbations and decreasing with remission [10].

Precipitins: Specific precipitins measured by the double diffusion method or counterelectrophoresis are present in 70–80% of ABPA patients. When the serum is concentrated 3- or 4-fold, the percentage of positive precipitins increases to well over 90%. The precipitating antibodies to *Aspergillus fumigatus* are generally of the IgG-type and are considered to reflect the continued growth of the fungi within the bronchial tree. However, precipitins are not pathognomonic of ABPA; precipitins have been demonstrated in 12% of allergic asthmatics and in practically all patients with aspergilloma. Moreover no strict correlation can be established between the number of precipitating lines and the intensity of the clinical picture.

Other tests: These difficulties explain the interest of many investigators in additional laboratory tests: quantitative evaluation of IgE and IgG antibodies by radioimmunoassay [11] or enzyme assay [12], measurement of IgG subclasses [13], specific IgA detection [14] which seems unfortunately unable to discriminate all ABPA patients from asthmatics positive to *Aspergillus* skin tests. Recently Ghory et al [15] studied also the in vitro IgE formation by peripheral blood lymphocytes from ABPA patients, and demonstrated a high in vitro IgE synthesis, either spontaneously or after stimulation by pokeweed mitogen. In our experience, the comparison between in vitro IgE synthesis in patients with ABPA, mite hypersensitivity and controls, showed a much higher production than in the other two groups. In ABPA large differences were observed depending on the patients, and on an identical patient during the course of the disease. In one case, the IgE increased up to 258,100 pcg/ml, while in the 3 previous tests on the same patient, in vitro IgE synthesis was successively 1,980, 1,040 and 1,000 pcg/ml. This sudden increase was contemporary of an acute phase of the disease.

Pulmonary function tests: Results differ according to the stage of the disease; from pure obstructive pattern at an early stage of disease to predominant restrictive profile in cases of irreversible damage with bronchiectasis and fibrosis. The diffusing capacity is decreased in some patients, correlated with the duration of the disease, which suggests that this parameter can be used to measure the severity of involvement [16]. As for the bronchial challenge, inhalation with *Aspergillus fumigatus* extracts usually causes a dual response with an immediate and transitory fall in FEV_1, followed 4 to 6 hours later by a late response with fever and increase in white blood cells (Fig. 7.4). Inhalation tests must be carried out very prudently, especially in advanced stages of ABPA; they do help to establish the diagnosis.

7.4 Evolution

The prognosis of ABPA is severe but the evolution is difficult to anticipate. It may begin in childhood, remain latent for years and result, because of its insidious nature, in severe fibrotic lung disease [17]. Delay in recognition of ABPA is frequent and usually related to the lack of typical symptoms during acute exacerbation. Patterson et al [18] identified five stages of ABPA: acute stage; remission; exacerbation; corticosteroid-dependent asthma; and fibrosis. In the

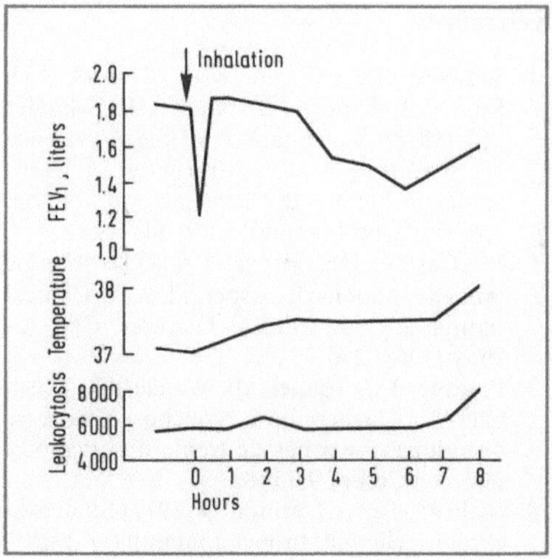

Fig. 7.4. Bronchial provocation test in allergic bronchopulmonary aspergillosis: early and late changes of FEV_1, temperature and leukocytosis

Table 7.2. Different stages in the evolution of ABPA

I	*Acute stage*
II	*Remission*
III	*Exacerbation* usual characteristics of the acute phase may be asymptomatic (asymptomatic pulmonary infiltrates and/or increasing IgE level)
IV	*Corticosteroid-dependent asthma* most patients with identified ABPA
V	*Fibrosis* usual criteria for ABPA extensive fibrosis obstructive lung disease (irreversible with high dose prednisone therapy)

last two stages, the major problem is that the dose of corticosteroids needed to control asthma may not be sufficient to prevent repeated exacerbations and further lung damage (Table 7.2).

Besides late sequelae of ABPA, other complications have to be considered: occurrence of mycetoma; bronchocentric granulomatosis; and dissemination of aspergillosis, possibly related to systemic and/or aerosolized corticosteroids.

ABPA is also associated with cystic fibrosis (CF). First described by Mearns et al [19], the actual incidence of ABPA in CF is not clearly established (10% for Laufer et al [20]). Indeed the classical findings of ABPA including centrally located bronchiectasis, high frequency of positive skin tests, sputum cultures and precipitins to *Aspergillus* can be seen in CF without ABPA.

7.5 Pathophysiology

The exact pathogenesis of ABPA remains poorly understood, but two main processes have been implicated: local proliferation of the fungus in the bronchial tree; and hypersensitivity to fungal allergens. A particular feature of ABPA compared to other allergies to inhaled antigens is the growth of the antigen source within the bronchial tree. While the growth of most molds is inhibited at body temperature, *Aspergillus* spores germinate, form mycelia and continuously shed antigen in the surrounding tissue. In response to the local high concentration of antigens, a double-type immunological reaction develops. **IgE antibodies** interact with mast cells, leading to bronchospasm and increased permeability of bronchial mucosa. Ricketti and co-workers [21] recently demonstrated a hyperreactivity of mediator releasing cells in ABPA, compared to patients with mold-sensitive asthma. **Specific IgG** react with absorbed antigen, leading to the formation of antigen-antibody complexes and complement fixation. The weak titer of precipitin provides a condition of moderate antigen excess which leads to the formation of toxic immune complexes and subsequently to bronchial and parenchymal alterations.

Other mechanisms can also be implicated in ABPA. Marx and Flaherty [22] suggest that *Aspergillus* extracts may activate the complement sequence through the alternate pathway.

7.6 Treatment

Prophylaxis: Attempts to prevent ABPA exacerbation by decreasing exposure to materials known to harbor high levels of *Aspergillus* are ineffective. Moreover, many ABPA patients are urban dwellers without special exposure to materials containing high concentrations of spores.

Antifungal therapy: In order to reduce the growth of fungi in the bronchial tree, systemic antifungal drugs including amphotericin B, clotrimazole, and more recently ketoconazole have been proposed but with poor results. A variety of regimens using aerosols (nystatin or amphotericin) seems able to reduce the number of acute exacerbations. However, inhalation of the antifungal drug is often followed by a bronchospastic reaction and it is not known whether the drug given by aerosol may effectively penetrate the viscid secretions in which the fungus is lodged.

Corticosteroid therapy: In fact, prednisone is currently considered the therapeutic agent of choice although not without risk: Long-term corticosteroid treatment in asthmatics might facilitate the development of ABPA as demonstrated by Clayton and Busse [23] and Basich et al [24].

However, corticosteroids are currently considered the best therapeutic approach for ABPA, resulting in a rapid clinical improvement with a resolution of pulmonary infiltrates and reduction of late skin and bronchial reactions [25]. Rosenberg et al [26] reported a rapid improvement with one week of prednisone (0.5 mg/kg/day) and MacCarthy and Pepys [2] noted that an effective dose was 7.5 mg prednisone per day. After the resolution of the acute phase, the daily dose corticotherapy is followed by alternate day prednisone as maintenance therapy over a sufficient period of time (2 or 3 months). To guide the evaluation of corticosteroid treatment, it appears useful to survey IgE levels the rise or decrease of which correlates with clinical and radiographic recurrences. The effects of prednisone may result in a variety of reactions [26]: reduction in acute inflammation in the lung, but also the mucus hypersecretion, thus eliminating the culture medium for *Aspergillus.* Another reaction may be the decrease of both total IgE and specific IgE, perhaps by a suppressive action on IgE T helper cells.

References

1. Schwartz HJ, Citron KM, Chester EH, Kaimal J, Barlow PB, Baum GL, Schuyler MR (1978) A comparison of the prevalence of sensitization to *Aspergillus* antigens among asthmatics in Cleveland and London. J Allergy Clin Immunol 62:9–14
2. MacCarthy DS, Pepys J (1971) Allergic bronchopulmonary aspergillosis. Clinical Immunology 1. Clinical Features. Clin Allergy 1:261–286
3. Fournier EC, Tonnel AB, Wallaert B, Voisin C (1983) L'aspergillose broncho-pulmonaire allergique. A propos de trente observations. Poumon Cœur 39:75–82
4. Malo JL, Pepys J, Simon G (1977) Studies in chronic allergic bronchopulmonary aspergillosis. II. Radiological findings. Thorax 32:262–268
5. Mintzer RA, Rogers LF, Kruglik GD, Rosenberg M, Neiman HL, Patterson R (1978) The spectrum of radiologic findings in allergic bronchopulmonary aspergillosis. Radiology 127:301–307
6. Anderson CJ, Craig S, Bardana EJ (1980) Allergic bronchopulmonary aspergillosis and bilateral fungal balls terminating in disseminated aspergillosis. J Allergy Clin Immunol 65:140–144
7. Rosenberg M, Mintzer R, Aaronson DW, Patterson R (1977) Allergic bronchopulmonary aspergillosis in three patients with normal chest x-ray films. Chest 72:597–600
8. Hendrick DJ, Davies RJ, d'Souza MF, Pepys J (1975) An analysis of skin prick test reactions in 656 asthmatic patients. Thorax 30:2–7
9. Hoehne JH, Reed CE, Dickie HA (1973) Allergic bronchopulmonary aspergillosis is not rare. Chest 63:177–181
10. Ricketti AJ, Greenberger PA, Patterson R (1984) Serum IgE as an important aid in management of ABPA. J Allergy Clin Immunol 74:68–81
11. Patterson R, Wang JLF, Roberts M, Zeiss CR (1978) Comparison of radioimmunoassay techniques in the detectives of IgE and IgG antibody activity against Aspergillus fumigatus antigens. J Immunol 120:66–74
12. van der Heide S, Kauffman HF, de Vries K (1984) Measurement of specific IgE and IgG antibodies against Aspergillus fumigatus antigen in patient sera by use of enzyme immunoassays: influence of different procedures of antigen immobilization. J Allergy Clin Immunol 73:813–818
13. Stokes TC, Turton CWG, Turner-Warwick M (1981) A study of immunoglobulin G subclasses in patients with allergic bron-

chopulmonary aspergillosis. Clin Allergy 11:209–215
14. Patterson R, Roberts M, Ghory A, Greenberger PA (1982) IgA antibody against Aspergillus fumigatus antigen in patients with ABPA. Clin Exp Immunol 42:395–398
15. Ghory AC, Patterson R, Roberts M, Suszko I (1980) In vitro IgE formation by peripheral blood lymphocytes from normal individuals and patients with ABPA. Clin Exp Immunol 40:581–585
16. Safirstein BH, d'Souza M, Simon G, Tai EH, Pepys J (1973) Five year follow up of ABPA. Am Rev Respir Dis 108:450–459
17. Greenberger PA, Patterson R, Ghory A, Arkins JA, Walsh T, Graves T, Saker J (1980) Late sequelae of allergic bronchopulmonary aspergillosis. J Allergy Clin Immunol 66: 327–335
18. Patterson R, Greenberger PA, Radin RC, Roberts M (1982) Allergic bronchopulmonary aspergillosis: staging as an aid to management. Ann Intern Med 96:286–291
19. Mearns M, Young W, Batten J (1965) Transient pulmonary infiltrates in cystic fibrosis due to allergic aspergillosis. Thorax 20:385–392
20. Laufer P, Fink JN, Bruns T, Unger GF, Kalbfleisch JH, Greenberger PA, Patterson R (1984) Allergic bronchopulmonary aspergillosis in cystic fibrosis. J Allergy Clin Immunol 73:44–48
21. Ricketti AJ, Greenberger PA, Pruzansky JJ, Patterson R (1983) Hyperreactivity of mediator-releasing cells from patients with allergic bronchopulmonary aspergillosis evidenced by basophil histamine release. J Allergy Clin Immunol 72:386–392
22. Marx JJ, Flaherty DK (1976) Activation of the complement sequence by extracts of bacteria and fungi associated with hypersensitivity pneumonitis. J Allergy Clin Immunol 57:328–334
23. Clayton DE, Busse WW (1981) Development of allergic bronchopulmonary aspergillosis during treatment of severe asthma with systemic corticosteroids. J Allergy Clin Immunol 67:243–246
24. Basich JE, Graves TS, Baz MN, Scanlon G, Hoffmann RG, Patterson R, Fink JN (1981) Allergic bronchopulmonary aspergillosis in corticosteroid-dependent asthmatics. J Allergy Clin Immunol 68:98–102
25. Imbeau SA, Nichols D, Flaherty D, Dickie H, Reed C (1978) Relationships between prednisone therapy, disease activity and the total serum IgE levels in allergic bronchopulmonary aspergillosis. J Allergy Clin Immunol 62:91–95
26. Rosenberg M, Patterson R, Roberts M, Wang J (1978) The assessment of immunologic and clinical changes occurring during corticosteroid therapy for allergic bronchopulmonary aspergillosis. Am J Med 64: 599–605

8. Bacterial Asthma

J. Pepys

There is considerable controversy, no general agreement and inadequate evidence for definitive conclusions regarding the role of *bacterial allergy* in asthma and even the role of infection per se. From the therapeutic point of view the main object of establishing bacterial allergy has been the use of vaccines of mixed respiratory tract and potentially pathogenic common commensal bacteria for immunotherapy. This approach is hallowed more by time, with its long usage, than by acceptably proven findings and will be dealt with first. Theoretical possibilities of bacterial allergy in asthma will then be discussed together with the problems which need to be considered and require resolution for results of practical value to be obtained.

The use of bacterial vaccines for asthma was subjected to a searching and critical survey by the Food and Drug Administration of the USA (1977) who appointed a highly representative and knowledgeable panel of experts. They examined "Bacterial vaccines and bacterial antigens with no U.S. standards of potency" in an "Implementation of Efficacy Review".

Three categories were used: Category I, biological products determined to be safe and effective and not misbranded; Category II, biological products determined to be unsafe, ineffective or misbranded; and Category III, biological products not falling within I or II above, on the basis of the Panel's conclusion that the available data were insufficient for their classification and that further testing was required. For Category III A it was recommended that the product licence should be retained while adequate data of safety and effectiveness were generated under controlled conditions and revoked for Category III B.

In relation to allergic disease, symptomatic allergy, the *requirements* were: identification of the suspected antigen; proof of causal relationship of the antigen to the signs and symptoms under consideration; and identification of the immunological mechanism involved and its causal relationship to the signs and symptoms. For each product the questions were: Does the final product, as given to the patient, contain the active ingredients stated to be present? Has the active substance been clearly shown to be safe in a defined population? Has it been clearly demonstrated that the active agent is effective for the specific indications under defined conditions?

The panel recommended that the assessment of these factors needed to be determined as follows: "Effectiveness and safety of treatment with a product for a given disease can be judged properly by adequate and well-controlled studies in populations of patients having the most well-defined states and carefully selected to be as homogeneous as possible."

The panel's conclusions regarding mixed respiratory bacterial vaccines were: There were no acceptable standards of potency or adequately detailed methods of production; the various products appeared to be safe as judged by their long continued use and lack of reported side effects; and the reports on efficacy came from unconfirmed and uncontrolled studies based on clinical impressions. None of the vaccines qualified in Category I; most fell into Category II and were regarded as unsatisfactory for production.

8.1 Bacterial Vaccine Immunotherapy

Among the possible effects of injections of bacterial vaccine are a decrease in hypersensitivity or an increased resistance to infection, or both. Table 8.1 cites a series of reports of double-blind trials showing no

Table 8.1. Studies of aqueous hyposensitization with bacterial vaccine. (From Weiss EB, Segal MS (eds) (1976) Bronchial Asthma. Little, Brown & Co. Boston, p 630)

Author Year reported	Antigen(s) used	Technique	Disease(s) treated	Type of study	Treated patients	Controls	Results
Aas et al 1963 [2]	Stock bacterial vaccine	Perennial	Infectious bronchial asthma	Double-blind	15 children	10 children	Treatment not better than placebo
Frankland et al 1955 [18]	Autogenous bacterial vaccine	Perennial	Intrinsic bronchial asthma	Double-blind	100 children and adults	84 children and adults	Treatment not better than placebo
Johnstone 1959 [26]	Stock and autogenous bacterial vaccine	Perennial	Mixed bronchial asthma	Double-blind	60 children	58 children	Treatment not better than placebo
Fontana et al 1965 [16]	Stock bacterial vaccine	Perennial	Infectious bronchial asthma	Double-blind	15 children	15 children	Placebo superior to treatment
Barr et al 1965 [4]	Stock bacterial vaccine	Perennial	Mixed bronchial asthma	Double-blind	22 children and adults	22 children and adults	Inconclusive; treated group somewhat better than controls
Helander 1959 [22]	Stock bacterial vaccine	Perennial	Infectious bronchial asthma	Double-blind	77 adults	79 adults	Treatment not better than placebo

beneficial effect of the vaccine treatment as has been the case with later studies [28]. All of these are subject to questions concerning the nature of the bacterial allergens and the dosages and duration of treatment, very much as is the case, with few exceptions, with the more familiar common environmental allergens. Improvement in both vaccine- and control-treated groups was attributed to better general care, a possible source of erroneous assessments [26].

Mueller and Lanz [33] in a selected group of children with *infective* asthma found that with vaccine treatment there were fewer and milder episodes of asthma with infection, though no difference in the number of infections. The possibility has also been raised that without careful selection of patients, some with asthma not due to infection may have been included in the studies giving negative results.

In a series of reports Oehling et al [35, 36] and Martin-Gil et al [30] claim very favorable results in asthmatic children, classified as bacterial allergy on the basis of negative skin tests to inhalant allergens, a "clear history" and skin test reactions [34] to *bacterial antigens* giving both immediate and delayed reactions. Injections of a mixed lyophilized bacterial vaccine of common respiratory tract bacteria were given over a period of 3 years [35]. Emphasis is laid upon: the duration of treatment, longer than in other negative reports; higher dosages of vaccine; and the use of effective antibiotic treatment of recurrent infections. Further studies were then made with bacterial ribosomal antigen preparations given by injection at weekly intervals for 4 weeks followed by monthly injections, together with, after the second month, aerosol administration of the preparation in 9 doses per day for 15-day periods with 15-day rest periods in between. The use of ribosomal preparations was based on the extensive work of Youmans and Youmans [51] on the protective immunizing effect of such material from *M. tuberculosis.* Martin-Gil et al [30] reported almost 100% improvement in *catarrhal* episodes after 2 years. Good results to such treatment were claimed in both children and adults [36]. The mechanisms claimed for such responses are not clear, possibly an influence on T-lymphocyte function and/or increased synthesis of IgA. It is also not evident whether clinical responses could be related to specific or nonspecific mechanisms. These studies suffer, however, from the fact that they were not made under the stringent requirements of double-blind controls. The findings could also have been influenced by the duration of the treatment and may allow for changes in asthma with time, particularly in children. Closer attention, with the effective use of antibiotics, in their studies could have played a part in the control of recurrent infections. There is no indication of relationships between the skin test reactions to the bacterial antigens and the clinical conditions, which may have served as a guide.

8.2 Bacterial Allergy

Allergy to bacteria is often a prerequisite for the production of disease characteristic of the particular organism. In asthma, however, the clinical manifestations are characteristic of the type or types of allergy involved whatever the nature of the causal agent, and against which antibodies and allergic reactions are present mainly in clinically affected subjects. As far as common commensal respiratory tract bacteria are concerned, antibodies and allergic reactions to them are commonly present. It is necessary to establish whether these are clinically relevant or simply epiphenomena resulting from episodes of infection. Whereas with the common extrinsic allergens exposure occurs mainly following inhalation or ingestion, the bacterial allergens are presumably produced in the upper and/or lower respiratory tract, except for certain occupational inhalant exposures. Thus, while a number of the objective findings taken to support a causal role for extrinsic allergens, can also be shown with bacterial allergens, the differences in mode of exposure dictate caution in drawing the same conclusions. The well-known problems of standardization of even the common allergens and the paucity of objective evidence for assessing clinical efficacy of immunotherapy with them imply that the absence of unequivocal evidence of a response to bacterial vaccines cannot be taken to preclude the possibility of bacterial allergy in asthma.

8.3 Definitive Terms

Classification of clinical asthma: A commonly used classification is: **extrinsic**, where exogenous causal agents can be identified and where atopic, nonatopic, or combined mechanisms may be present; **cryptogenic** (*intrinsic*) where exogenous causal agents are not identified. In this group it has been assumed that bacterial allergy may be present; **infectious** or **infective asthma** where the attacks appear to be related to the infection itself, with or without participation of bacterial allergy. A preferable term for such a group would be *infection asthma,* because the terms infectious or infective, taken literally, mean disease transmissible by the infective agent. It is desirable to try and avoid confusion between the concepts of bacterial allergy and infection asthma by the use of strict criteria, since there are suggestions that infection asthma may benefit from vaccine or other treatment.

Criteria laid down by Mueller and Lanz [33] for symptomatic respiratory tract infection in relation to asthma in a selected group of children were: onset of asthma from infancy up to 5 years and rarely after 8 years of age; asthma with every respiratory tract infection and symptom-free in between; skin tests negative or if positive of no clinical significance; attempts at elimination or avoidance of possible allergens without effect; bronchodilator less effective with successive attacks; attacks decreasing rapidly as the infection decreases, i.e., antibiotic treatment; and acute attacks associated with an increase in the neutrophil count and a low eosinophil count, the latter rising in between attacks. The diagnosis of the respiratory infection is made in the presence of malaise, fever, cough, nasal discharge and inflamed nasal mucosa, raised white cell count and a positive culture. It is supported by the presence of similar symptoms in others in the household.

8.4 Patterns of Asthmatic Reaction

The elicitation of immediate, nonimmediate and combined patterns of asthmatic reaction to provocation tests with common environmental allergens and occupational allergens has its clinical counterparts [41]. The absence of immediate asthmatic reactions and of atopy has in the past been taken on the basis of negative evidence to suggest bacterial allergy. However, should bacterial allergy be relevant to asthma, similar patterns of asthmatic reaction might occur, as suggested indeed by provocation tests [42].

8.5 Bronchial Infection and Asthma

Intensive studies of possible associations between respiratory tract infections and asthma have shown a close relationship to viral infections and only a limited number to bacterial infections [6, 11, 19, 23, 31–33]. Hudgel et al [23] conclude that "respiratory tract infections can occur without necessarily worsening the asthma" and that "in some asthmatic patients the respiratory tract may be chronically colonized with pathogenic bacteria without increased frequency of asthmatic exacerbations". However a study of prophylaxis with sulfamethoxazole, penicillin and placebo, given continuously for 6 winter months to children in a low socioeconomic group with severe asthma showed reductions in upper respiratory tract infections, patient visits, emergency room visits and hospital admissions and in the severity of the asthma [46]. In a study of selected patients conforming to the above criteria for infection asthma, Aas [1] found that injections of minute doses of vaccine were followed in some patients by eosinophilia of the nasal secretions, suggestive of an allergic reaction. Elimination of infection was found by Aas et al [2] to result in marked improvement in allergic symptoms.

As far as sputum culture is concerned, in addition to the diagnostic problems of distinguishing between exacerbations of chronic bronchitis and episodes of cryptogenic asthma in middle-aged patients, there is the need to exclude bacterial contamination from the pharynx. Far fewer positive cultures are obtained in asthma from bronchoscopic or transtracheal specimens than from expectorated sputum. No differences were found between asthmatics and healthy controls [5, 8]. Examination of sinus secretions, taken with care to prevent contamination, gave positive cultures in about 20% of the cases [7].

Emphasis is laid upon the presence of eosinophils as an argument against infection. If allergy to bacteria does indeed occur in this context, eosinophils could be present on that account. The fact that there is little or no difference in the culture findings in asthmatics and normals is also not an argument against an allergy role for those that are present. In the case of atopy, for example, 30 to 40% of the population have evidence of IgE antibody to common allergens without symptoms. Nevertheless in affected subjects this can be shown to be relevant.

8.6 Sinus Infection and Asthma

There are reports of rare patients whose asthma is improved by treatment of bacterial sinus infections. It is not known whether the relationship to asthma is due to reflex bronchoconstriction or to allergy to bacterial allergens from the infected sinuses. Focal reactions in the sinuses to injection of bacterial vaccines have been regarded as evidence of bacterial allergy.

Intensive medical treatment with heat, decongestants and antibiotics, supplemented, if ineffective, by surgical intervention have been reported beneficial [12, 44]. Patients may however become asymptomatic in spite of the persistence in the sinuses of purulent material with a high concentration of bacteria, suggesting that allergy to these bacteria is not involved.

8.7 Bacterial Agents Mediating Reactions

Bacteria contain a mixture of protein, polysaccharide and lipid containing agents potentially capable of causing reactions by immunological, nonimmunological and combined mechanisms.

Bacterial allergens: The different classes of antibody can be found against protein and polysaccharide components. Conditions may therefore be present for the elicitation of the different types of allergic reaction by appropriate tests. It is difficult to equate such reactions with those elicited by exogenous common environmental allergens because of the endogenous origin of the bacterial allergens. Where bacterial allergens are met by exogenous exposure, as with the enzymes of *B. subtilis* used in biological detergents, they act in the same way as the common inhalant allergens, inducing IgE antibody and also antibodies in the other immunoglobulin classes [15, 39, 40].

A variety of bacterial preparations, ranging from suspensions of whole killed or disrupted bacteria to protein and polysaccharide components are commonly used. The proteins give Type I, III and IV reactions whereas the polysaccharides give Type I and III reactions only. These materials have been used arbitrarily and empirically. More studies are needed with well-defined, reproducible and standardized materials for the correlation with immunological and possibly clinical findings.

Skin tests with bacterial agents: Protein extracts of common commensal bacteria were used by Walker [50] for scratch tests. Positive reactions were given in asthmatics to *S. aureus* in 18%, *S. albus* in 6%, and to other bacterial proteins in 1 to 2%. Stevens and Jordani [47] used nucleoproteins for intradermal tests in asthmatics. Positive reactions were given to *S. aureus,* both immediate and late, in 28%. There was no difference between atopic and nonatopic subjects.

Extensive intradermal tests by Swineford and Holman [48] with 34 crude polysaccharide and nucleoprotein fractions of 14 bacteria gave more positive immediate reactions to the polysaccharides and delayed reactions to the proteins.

Tests with purified type-specific proteins of 10 strains of *S. aureus* from nasal cultures and with the crude residue containing the polysaccharide fraction were made by Kahn et al [27]. Comparable numbers of allergic and control subjects gave delayed reactions to the proteins. Immediate but not delayed reactions were given to the polysaccharide fraction in 72% of the allergics and 32% of the controls.

Tests with fragmented bacteria by Kraft et al [29] gave more immediate reactions in asthmatics than in the general population, but there appeared to be little correlation with what was regarded as clinical evidence of bacterial allergy.

Immediate reactions were given to prick tests with α-teichoic acid of *S. aureus* in 77 to 84% of controls and asthmatics [11]. While these and other skin test investigations show the common presence of allergy to bacterial components, there is little evidence from them in favor of clinically relevant bacterial allergy in asthmatics. Cooke [10], a leading proponent of bacterial allergy in sinusitis and asthma, emphasized the point that the skin test reactions, in themselves, had little diagnostic or prognostic value.

As far as the types of allergic reaction elicited, roles for Type I allergy, in particular, and possible for Type III allergy in asthma are established. No definitive role has been found for Type IV allergy. In this respect more attention needs to be given to the polysaccharide fractions, though not to the exclusion of the proteins. This applies equally, if not more so, to fungal and bacterial polysaccharides in relation to their possible clinical roles and the effects of injection for immunotherapeutic purposes. Finland and Dowling [14] found that injections of pneumococcal polysaccharide could induce immediate-type allergy in normals together with an increase in antibodies. Similar findings resulted from intradermal injection of mannan from *C. albicans,* with elicitation of Type I and III reactions in previously skin test-negative subjects, together with increased amounts of precipitins [38]. The observations with *C. albicans* resemble the situation with the respiratory tract bacteria, in that skin test evidence of allergy and antibodies are common. The question is to decide whether these can be clinically relevant.

Skin tests/immunotherapy/local and focal reactions: Local reactions, as in skin tests, can be regarded, if specific, as evidence of allergy, though their diagnostic relevance is not definitely established. More weight has been placed on focal reactions, namely rhinitis and/or asthma. Cooke [10] regarded such reactions to small doses appearing after 12 to 48 hours as evidence of clinically relevant bacterial allergy. But here too, it is not clear whether an expected allergic reaction was being elicited by a route of exposure different from that which might have occurred naturally.

Nonspecific effects of bacterial agents: There are a number of bacterial properties which need to be distinguished from allergy and which might, in themselves, elicit tissue and clinical reactions or may contribute to allergic reactions. These also need an answer to the question of how their effects could arise from endogenous exposure in such a way as to cause or influence asthma.

Among these factors are bacterial endotoxins capable of causing the release of histamine and other mediators. Lectins from a number of common respiratory bacteria have been shown to liberate histamine from human leukocytes and rat mast cells by both immunological IgE-mediated and nonimmunological mechanisms [24, 25].

The ability of protein A from *S. aureus* to fix nonspecifically to the Fc piece of the IgG molecule may be responsible for the release of histamine [17]. Complexes of IgG and protein A have also elicited Arthus reactions in the rabbit [20].

8.8 Antibodies to Common Respiratory Bacteria

IgE antibodies: The development of a RAST (radioallergosorbent test) for IgE antibodies to intact organisms, *S. aureus* [23, 37, 43–45, 49, 50] and to *Strep. pneumoniae* and *H. influenzae* [50] was a useful development for the study of bacterial allergy in asthma. Comparisons of well-defined clinical groups showed the highest RASTs for all three of the above bacteria in patients with allergic bronchopulmonary aspergillosis. In chronic bronchitis and cystic fibrosis raised RASTs were present to *H. influenzae.* A positive correlation was found between immediate skin prick test reactions to extracts from ultrasonically disrupted *S. aureus* and the supernatant of a *Strep. pneumoniae* culture and the RAST to these bacteria and to the total serum-IgE levels [50]. The RAST results were confirmed by specific inhibition tests. Such findings make the interpretation in immunological terms of the skin test reactions more meaningful.

Using the ELISA, IgE antibodies to noncapsular antigens of *Strep. pneumoniae* were found in patients with middle ear effusion and confirmed by Prausnitz-Küstner tests [46]. IgE antibodies to pneumococcal antigens have also been reported in cigarette smokers [9]. The report by Jensen et al [25] of a role for IgE antibody in histamine release from mast cells by bacterial lectins is further evidence for IgE antibodies to bacterial antigens. The availability of specific antibiotics or chemotherapeutic agents against different bacteria makes it possible to monitor their effects on IgE antibody levels. In an unreported study of the effect of miconazole in patients with allergic bronchopulmonary aspergillosis [Pepys et al] falls in specific IgE levels were observed not only to *C. albicans,* for which this agent was intended, but also to *S. aureus* against which miconazole is also effective. Clinical studies incorporating such objective findings could contribute materially to the assessment of whether particular bacteria had a role in asthma.

Tests have not yet been made for short-term sensitizing IgG (IgG-S-TS) antibodies to bacteria in asthma and these too need to be pursued.

Bacterial precipitins: Precipitins against bacteria are commonly present. Precipitins against the α-teichoic acid of *S. aureus* were found in comparable proportions of atopic asthmatics (64%) and controls (78%). Similar percentages of atopic patients (28%) and nonatopics (32%) had precipitins to *Strep. pneumoniae* as compared with controls (36%). No significant differences were found in precipitins to *H. influenzae* in patients and controls. In patients with chronic bronchitis, as would be expected, more than one-half had specific precipitins to *H. influenzae* as compared with 6 to 8% in controls and asthmatics [11].

The above precipitins were mainly in the IgG class. Precipitins to the α-teichoic acid of *S. aureus* were found in 70% of sera tested and the same antigen was found in a variety of organic dusts [13]. Such dusts could be a source of exposure to this antigen by inhalation and in view of its capacity to elicit immediate reactions, should be considered as a possible cause of asthmatic symptoms.

Bronchial provocation tests with bacterial antigens: The asthmatic reactions elicited by provocation tests could be due to nonspecific or specific mechanisms. In patients with asthma and bronchial hyperreactivity nonspecific agents would be more likely to provoke reactions. It is necessary therefore in assessing such reactions to have information on nonspecific bronchial reactivity before the test. It is also to be expected that in the presence of specific IgE antibody positive reactions to the allergen would be elicited. Such a response would have to be regarded, in the first place, as the result of an immunological experiment and not necessarily as evidence of clinical allergy. Clinical confirmation would have to be sought from direct observation of the effects of clinical exposure, supported if possible by the effects of elimination of the particular bacteria.

Hampton et al [21] elicited asthmatic reactions after the inhalation of *N. catarrhalis* in 14 out of 16 patients. Fever and malaise occurred both in asthmatics and controls. Ricci et al [42] used suspensions of bacteria for inhalation tests and elicited asthmatic reactions in 17 out of 39 patients to autogenous α-hemolytic streptococci. Positive reactions were elicited in 39% of *infective* asthma cases and 29% of those regarded as combined infective and exogenous allergic cases (Tables 8.2, 8.3). The reactions were either immediate, delayed or combined. Reactions occurring between the 1st and 16th hour were regarded as *delayed.* They would probably be regarded at present as *late* reactions, with delayed reactions occurring after 24 hours. No precipitins were found in these cases, a surprising find in view of the report by Davies et al [11]. No asthmatic reactions were elicited in patients with chronic bronchitis.

Table 8.2. Table of case material (number of cases: 113). [From 42]

Type of asthma	No. of cases	Positive to bronchial tests		Chronology of asthmatic reactions		
		No. of cases	%	Immediate only	Immediate and delayed	Delayed only
Infective	69	24	39	3	13	8
Infective and exogenous allergic	44	13	29	3	4	6

Table 8.3. Bacteriological results of an examination of the sputum and bronchoscopic aspirates of 113 patients suffering from infective asthma. [From 42]

Bacterial strain	Incidence resulting from cultural examination of the bronchial secretion (113 cases)	Positive results of bronchial tests induced by the various strains (37 cases)
α-hemolytic streptococcus	77	17
Neisseria	69	9
Hemolytic staphylococcus aureus (coagulase +)	26	5
Candida albicans	12	–
Nonhemolytic staphylococcus albus (coagulase –)	11	–
Escherichia coli	11	3
Nonhemolytic streptococcus	7	–
Klebsiella	8	3
Enterococcus	4	–
Hemolytic staphylococcus aureus (coagulase +)	3	1
Proteus mirabilis	2	1
Nonhemolytic staphylococcus albus (coagulase +)	1	–
Alkaligenes	1	1
Pseudomonas aeruginosa	1	–

NB. In three cases, the tests yielded positive results with two different strains

Inhalation of suspensions of killed *H. influenzae* [52], not tested by Ricci et al [42], elicited immediate plus late (dual or biphasic) asthmatic reactions with fever and malaise in patients with specific precipitins, but only late reactions in the controls. Immediate and late skin test reactions were elicited in the patients, the controls giving delayed (? late) reactions only. As possible mechanisms for the late asthmatic reactions, endotoxin activity or precipitin-mediated reactions were postulated. The bronchial reactivity to histamine showed a lowered threshold lasting for several days in the reacting patients. The patients were described as having chronic nonspecific lung disease. It is difficult to know what this term covers and whether these had cryptogenic (intrinsic) asthma or chronic bronchitis or a combination of both.

Provocation tests with *S. aureus, K. pneumoniae* and *D. pneumoniae* by Bacigaluppi [3] in patients with *bacterial* rhinitis and asthma showed a good correlation between exacerbation of rhinitis or asthma and a positive MIF test and positive delayed skin test reactions. These findings, as with the others, show that reactions specific and/or nonspecific can be elicited by bacterial antigens and are evidence, if specific, of the presence of bacterial allergy.

8.9 Conclusions

There are formidable theoretical and practical problems in trying to reach unequivocal conclusions about *bacterial allergy* in asthma. These concern both diagnostic problems, i.e., demonstration of a specific causal relationship to the asthma, and therapeutic aspects, mainly concerning vaccine immunotherapy. Past studies have not been helped by arbitrary selection of bacteria and dosages for diagnostic and therapeutic purposes. Most bacterial respiratory vaccines have been mixtures of strains of streptococci and staphylococci, pneumococci, Klebsiella, Pseudomonas, *E. coli,* Neisseria, *Hemophilus influenzae* and sometimes others. These represent a complexity of antigens and other reactive substances without objective evidence of their possible relevance.

The questions arising from the above analysis of the literature are: 1) Is there any evidence favoring the possibility of bacterial allergy which might be relevant to clinical asthma? 2) What steps could and should be taken to establish this?

The items favoring a possible role for bacterial allergy in asthma are: the presence of immediate skin test reactivity to some of the bacteria; the presence of specific IgE antibodies; immediate asthmatic reactions to provocation tests, and nonimmediate reactions as well; and focal reactions, rhinitis/asthma to injection of low dosages of bacterial antigens. These findings show that bacterial allergic reactions can provoke asthma, but they do not establish that this can happen when the source of the antigens is endogenous. Similar problems apply with regard to the generally accepted role of atopy and asthma. For example, between 30 and 40% of the asymptomatic population gives immediate reactions to prick tests with extracts of common environmental allergens. There is also often no evidence in many asthmatic subjects, with evidence of atopy, that the allergens to which they give positive reactions are related to their asthma. Bronchial provocation tests serve to confirm that the allergen could cause an asthmatic reaction, as would be expected if specific IgE antibody is present, but not necessarily that it is the cause of the clinical asthma. This applies equally to common and bacterial allergens.

Etiological diagnostic tests for possible causally related bacteria require the use of standardized, purified protein and polysaccharide antigens, together with specific antibody immunoglobulin and lymphocyte profiles. The influence of specific antibiotic or chemotherapeutic agents capable of reducing or eliminating the particular bacteria, together with profiles of specific antibodies needs to be studied, where possible, and matched with the clinical findings. Positive findings could provide strong support for the role of the bacteria and for an allergic mechanism.

Immunotherapy with bacterial antigens may be intended to serve two purposes, namely increased resistance to infection or decreased bacterial allergy. The latter should be based on selected bacterial antigens guided by objective criteria. Caution is needed with polysaccharide antigens which may and can increase allergic sensitivity. This is an indication of the problems of using mixed vaccines containing all the bacterial components. The trials of immunotherapy should be on a controlled basis, with clear definitive criteria, which is lacking in many of the existing reports. The final conclusion, in this respect, is that there is no substantive evidence for efficacy of the bacterial vaccines in use, and that the information for clinical guidance lies in the future.

References

1. Aas K (1961) Nasal eosinophilia in so-called bacterial hypersensitivity in asthmatic children. Acta Paediatr Scand 50:1
2. Aas K, Berdal P, Henricksen SD, Gardberg O (1963) "Bacterial Allergy" in childhood asthma and the effect of vaccine treatment. Acta Paediatr Scand 52:338–344
3. Bacigaluppi JE (1977) Human bacterial allergy. In: Mathov E, Sindo T, Naranjo P (eds) Allergy and Clinical Immunology. Proceedings of the IXth International Congress of Allergy and Clinical Immunology. Excerpta Medica, Amsterdam, pp 429–433
4. Barr SE, Brown H, Fuchs M, Orvis H, Connor A, Murray FJ, Seltzer A (1965) A double-blind study of the effects of bacterial vaccine on infective asthma. J Allergy 36:47
5. Bergman S, Colldahl H, Nilsson E (1955) Bronchial infection and B.S.R. in asthma with a description of a method for sterile removal of bronchial secretion. Acta Allergologica 8:163
6. Berkovich S, Millian SJ, Snyder RD (1970) The association of viral and mycoplasma infections with recurrence of wheezing in the asthmatic child. Ann Allergy 28:43–49
7. Berman SZ, Mathison DA, Stevenson DD, Usselman JA, Shore S, Tan EM (1974) Maxillary sinusitis and bronchial asthma. Correlation of roentgenograms, cultures and thermograms. J Allergy Clin Immunol 53:311
8. Berman SZ, Mathison DA, Stevenson DD, Tan EM, Vaughan JH (1975) Transtracheal aspiration studies in asthmatic patients in relapse with "infective" asthma and in subjects without respiratory disease. J Allergy Clin Immunol 56:206
9. Bloom JW, Farland AM, Halonen M, Burrows B (1984) Pneumococcus-specific IgE in cigarette smokers. Am Rev Respir Dis 129:A191 (abstract)
10. Cooke RA (1947) Allergy in theory and practice. Saunders, Philadelphia
11. Davies RJ, Holford-Stevens VC, Wells ID, Pepys J (1976) Bacterial precipitins and their immunoglobulin class in atopic asthma, nonatopic asthma, and chronic bronchitis. Thorax 31:419–424
12. Eisen AH (1969) The role of infection in allergic disease. Pediatr Clin North Am 16:67
13. Faux JA, Holford-Stevens V, Wells ID, Pepys J (1970) False positive precipitation reactions to extracts of organic dusts due to a teichoic acid from *S. aureus*. Clin Exp Immunol 7:897
14. Finland M, Dowling HF (1935) Cutaneous reactivity and antibody response to intracutaneous injections of pneumococcus polysaccharides. J Immunol 29:285
15. Flindt ML-H (1969) Pulmonary disease due to the inhalation of derivatives of *Bacillus subtilis* containing proteolytic enzyme. Lancet 1:1177
16. Fontana VJ, Salanitro AS, Wolfe HI, Moreno F (1965) Bacterial vaccine and infectious asthma. JAMA 193:895–900
17. Forsgren A, Sjoquist J (1966) "Protein A" from *S. aureus*. I. Pseudo-immune reaction with human γ-globulin. J Immunol 97:822
18. Frankland AW, Hughes MW, Gorrill RH (1955) Autogenous "bacterial vaccine" in the treatment of asthma. Br Med J 2:941–944
19. Graham VAL, Knowles GK, Milton AF, Davies RJ (1982) Routine antibiotics in hospital management of acute asthma. Lancet 1:419
20. Gustafson GT, Sjoquist J, Stalènheim G (1967) "Protein A" from *Staphylococcus aureus*. II. Arthus-like reaction produced in rabbits by interaction of "Protein A" and human γ-globulin. J Immunol 98:1178
21. Hampton SF, Johnson MC, Galaktos E (1963) Studies of bacterial hypersensitivity in asthma. I. The preparation of antigens of *Neisseria catarrhalis*, the induction of asthma by aerosols, the performance of skin in passive transfer tests. J Allergy 34:63–95
22. Helander E (1959) Bacterial vaccines in the treatment of bronchial asthma. Acta Allergologica 13:47–66
23. Hudgel DW, Langston L Jr, Selner JC, McIntosh K (1979) Viral and bacterial infection in adults with chronic asthma. Am Rev Respir Dis 120:393–397
24. Jensen C, Norn S, Skov PS, Espersen F, Koch C, Permin H (1984) Bacterial histamine release by immunological and non-immunological lectin-mediated reactions. Allergy 39:371–377
25. Jensen C, Skov PS, Norn S, Espersen F, Borg-Hansen TC, Lihme A (1984) Complexity of lectin-mediated reactions in bacteria-induced histamine release. Allergy 39:451–456
26. Johnstone DE (1959) Study of the value of bacterial vaccine in the treatment of bronchial asthma associated with respiratory infections. Paediatrician 24:427–433
27. Kahn MC, Baldwin HS, Zeitlin BR, Smart M (1951) Cutaneous reactions to staphylococcus polysaccharide, protein and an unfractionated extract in hypersensitive and normal individuals. J Allergy 22:237–248
28. Koivikko A (1973) Bacterial vaccine in childhood asthma: a double-blind study. Acta Allergologica 28:202

29. Kraft B, Mothersill MH, Nestman RH (1949) Immediate urticarial reactions to intradermal injections of bacterial antigens. Ann Allergy 7:162–164
30. Martin-Gil D, Diéquez I, Oehling A, Subira M-L (1981) Immunotherapy with bacterial ribosomal antigen. I. Clinical study. Allergol Immunopathol 9:509
31. McIntosh K, Ellis EE, Hoffman LS, Lybass TG, Eller JJ, Fulgitini VA (1973) The association of viral and bacterial respiratory infections with exacerbations of wheezing in young asthmatic children. J Pediatr 82:578–590
32. Minor TE, Dick EC, de Meo AN, Ouelette JJ, Cohen M, Reed CE (1974) Viruses as precipitants of asthmatic attacks in children. JAMA 227:292–298
33. Mueller HL, Lanz M (1969) Hyposensitisation with bacterial vaccine in infectious asthma. JAMA 208:1379–1383
34. Oehling A (1965) Hyposensibilisierungsbehandlung des Asthma bronchiale und der sinobronchopulmonalen Erkrankungen in bezug auf die bakterielle Allergie. Allergie und Asthma II:3–109
35. Oehling A, Baena-Cagnani CE, Neffen H (1980) Bacterial immunotherapy of childhood bronchial asthma. Allergol Immunopathol 8:177–184
36. Oehling A, Subira M-L, Diéquez I, Martin-Gil D (1981) Immunotherapy with bacterial ribosomal antigens. In: Steffen C, Ludwig H (eds) Clinical Immunology and Allergology. Elsevier, Amsterdam, p 399
37. Pauwels R, Verschraegen G, van der Straeten M (1980) IgE antibodies to bacteria in patients with bronchial asthma. Allergy 157:665–669
38. Pepys J, Faux JA, Longbottom JL, McCarthy DS, Hargreave FE (1968) Candida precipitins in respiratory disease. J Allergy 41:305
39. Pepys J, Hargreave FE, Longbottom JL, Faux J (1969) Allergic reactions of the lungs to enzymes of *Bacillus subtilis.* Lancet I:1181
40. Pepys J, Wells ID, d'Souza MF, Greenberg M (1973) Clinical and immunological responses to enzymes of *Bacillus subtilis* in factory workers and consumers. Clin Allergy 3:143
41. Pepys J, Hutchcroft BJ (1975) Bronchial provocation tests in etiologic diagnosis and analysis of asthma. Am Rev Respir Dis 112:829
42. Ricci M, Fishlewitz J, Ricca M, Passalera A (1967) A study on bacterial sensitisation in the infective asthma. Acta Allergologica 22:47–56
43. Schopfer K, Baerlocher K, Price P, Krech U, Quiè PG, Douglas D (1979) Staphylococcal IgE antibodies, hyperimmunoglobulinemia E and *Staphylococcus aureus* infections. N Engl J Med 15:835–838
44. Slavin RG (1982) Relationship of nasal disease and sinusitis to bronchial asthma. Ann Allergy 49:76
45. Sloyer JL, Ploussard JH, Karr LJ (1980) Otitis media in the young infant: an IgE mediated disease? Ann Otol Rhinol Laryngol 89 [Suppl 68]:133
46. Snyder RD, Stiefel FH (1970) Prophylactic antibiotics in asthmatic children. Ann Allergy 28:307
47. Stevens FA, Jordani L (1936) Reactions to intracutaneous injections of nucleoproteins of the upper respiratory pathogenic bacteria in asthmatic patients. J Allergy 7:443
48. Swineford O, Holman J (1949) Studies in bacterial allergy: results of 3,860 cutaneous tests with 34 crude polysaccharide and nucleoprotein fractions of 14 different bacteria. J Allergy 20:420–427
49. Tee RD, Pepys J (1982) Specific serum IgE antibodies to bacterial antigens in allergic lung disease. Clin Allergy 12:439
50. Walker IC (1916) Studies on the sensitisation of patients with bronchial asthma to bacterial proteins as demonstrated by the skin reaction and the methods employed in the preparation of these proteins. J Med Res 35:487
51. Youmans GP, Youmans AS (1971) "Mycobacterium tuberculosis" immunogens. Ann Sclavo 13:706
52. van der Zwan JC, Orie NGM, de Vries K (1975) Biphasic reaction after inhalation of *Haemophilus influenzae* in patients with chronic non-specific lung disease. Clin Allergy 5:225

9. Exercise-induced Asthma: Clinical Aspects

S. D. Anderson

Exercise-induced asthma (EIA) is the name which describes the transitory increase in airways resistance which occurs after 6–8 min of strenuous exercise. It is defined as a reduction in peak expiratory flow rate (PEFR) or forced expiratory volume in one second (FEV_1) of 10% or more from the preexercise level [1, 2]. If specific conductance (SGaw) or the flow rates in the middle half of the vital capacity (FEF_{25-75}) are measured, a reduction of 35% or more from the preexercise level is characteristic of EIA [3, 4]. The values used to define an abnormal response are based on the changes in lung function recorded after exercise in normal subjects [5, 6]. Under laboratory conditions 70–80% of asthmatics exhibit EIA [7, 8].

Fig. 9.1 illustrates typical changes in PEFR and FEV_1 recorded during and after exercise of an asthmatic with mild airways obstruction at rest. During the first few minutes of exercise, bronchodilation occurred and this was reflected as an increase in PEFR and FEV_1. When this change in PEFR or FEV_1 is expressed as a percentage of the preexercise value it is called the % Rise. There is an inverse relationship between the % Rise in PEFR and FEV_1 and the degree of airways obstruction which is present at rest [9]. A rise greater than 22% of the preexercise value is abnormal and is characteristic of asthma although it can also occur in smokers and in patients with cystic fibrosis and hay fever [10]. This bronchodilation lasts only for a few minutes and is thought to be due to a withdrawal of parasympathetic tone and the release of catecholamines. After 6 min of exercising at between 70–85% of predicted maximal oxygen uptake, the flow rates begin to fall. After 8 min of exercise the flow rates are usually lower than the preexercise value. The lowest PEFR or FEV_1 recorded after exercise is the value used to calculate the % Fall which is the index used to express the severity of EIA (Fig. 9.1). The reduction in flow rates in children reaches a maximum around 5–7 min after exercise. In adults the maximum fall occurs between 7–12 min. The severity of EIA cannot be predicted from the preexercise level of lung function [11]. For example, a patient may have normal lung function at rest but a reduction of 50% or more in FEV_1 after exercise. However the preexercise lung function of the 20–30% of patients who do not exhibit EIA is likely to be normal.

Exercise is distinguished from other tests of bronchial hyperresponsiveness by the potential to document overall bronchial lability in response to a single stimulus. To assess this, the exercise lability index (also called the top-bottom index) was introduced by Silverman and Anderson [7]. It is

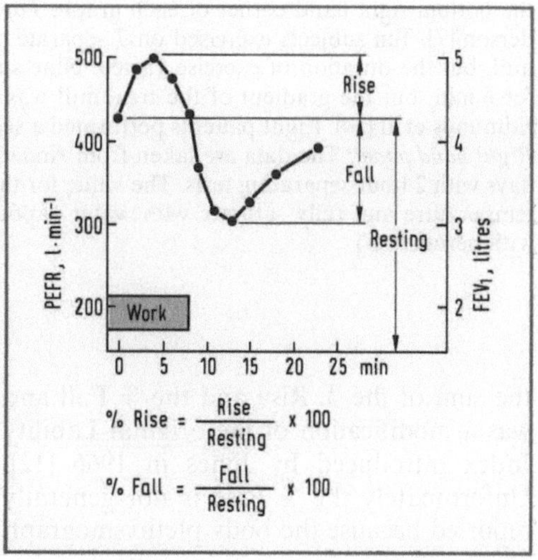

Fig. 9.1. Changes in peak expiratory flow rate (PEFR) and forced expiratory volume recorded during and after 8 min of treadmill running in an asthmatic patient. (Reproduced from [69], with permission)

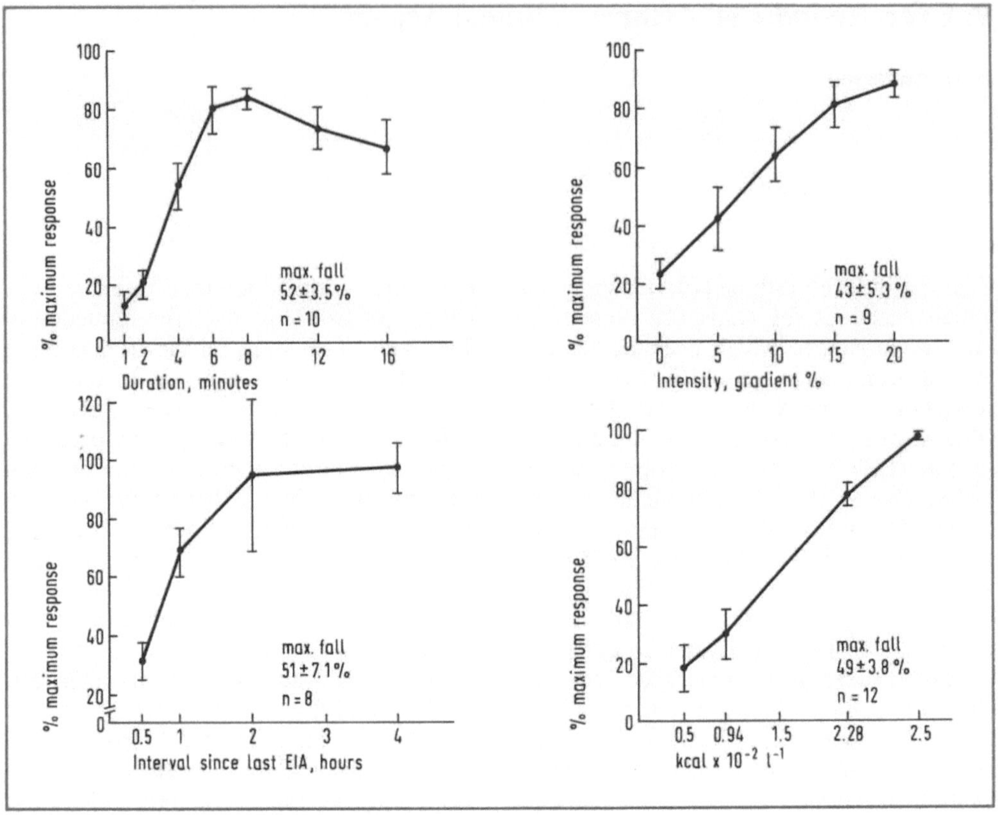

Fig. 9.2. The percent fall in peak expiratory flow rates (PEFR) expressed as a percentage of the maximum percent fall in PEFR. The group mean maximum fall in PEFR ± 1 SEM recorded is shown in the bottom right hand corner of each graph. *Top panel:* The data are taken from Silverman and Anderson [7]. Ten subjects exercised on 7 separate occasions at the same speed and slope on the treadmill, but the duration of exercise varied. Nine subjects exercised 5 separate times at the same speed for 6 min, but the gradient of the treadmill was varied. *Bottom left panel:* The data are taken from Edmunds et al [54]. Eight patients performed a second running test after the specified interval of time. *Right hand panel:* The data are taken from Anderson et al [27]. Twelve subjects exercised 4 times on 2 days with 2-hour separating tests. The value for the heat required to condition the inspired air to body temperature and fully saturate with water vapour is expressed in kcal L^{-1}. (Reproduced from [75], with permission)

the sum of the % Rise and the % Fall and was a modification of the original Lability Index introduced by Jones in 1966 [12]. Unfortunately the % Rise is not generally reported because the body plethysmograph has been used to measure lung function before and after, but not during exercise.

It is not easy to assess the changes in lung function to exercise as a dose response relationship. Investigators have aimed for the maximum airway response by adjusting the duration and intensity of exercise and the conditions of the inspired air (Fig. 9.2). The workload or *dose* of exercise relates to the size and sex of the patient and is limited by the subject's ability to perform external work. For this reason isocapnic hyperventilation (ISH) is now frequently used instead of exercise to provoke asthma. The use of ISH overcomes the problem of physical fitness and the response can be related to the level of ventilation (i.e., the *dose*) [13].

Table 9.1. Mean ± 1 SEM for peak expiratory flow rate (PEFR) expressed as a percentage of predicted value, arterial blood gas tensions (PaO_2, $PaCO_2$), pH, heart rate (HR), and change in base excess (BE); at rest, during, and after exercise in 14 adult asthmatic males and 5 normal males who exercised for 8 min by running on a treadmill. [From 16]

	Asthmatics		Normals		Significance	
	P	A	P	A	P	A
Rest						
PEFR % predicted	73±4	92±2	89±3	93±5	<0.05	NS
PaO_2 mm Hg	85±3	94±3	96±1	96±4	<0.05	NS
$PaCO_2$ mm Hg	39±1	37±1	40±1	41±2	NS	<0.02
pH[a]	7.43	7.42	7.43	7.42	NS	NS
During exercise						
PEFR % predicted[b]	84±4	98±3	98±4	100±5	NS	NS
PaO_2 mm Hg[a]	100±2	105±2	103±3	105±4	NS	NS
$PaCO_2$ mm Hg	39±1	37±1	41±2	39±2	NS	NS
pH[a]	7.35	7.37	7.35	7.37	NS	NS
HR beats min^{-1}	175±4	179±3	177±5	193±4	NS	<0.05
After exercise						
PEFR % predicted[b]	41±4	82±4	89±3	94±5	<0.001	NS
PaO_2 mm Hg[c]	71±3	91±2	91±4	88±2	<0.005	NS
$PaCO_2$ mm Hg[b]	39±1	35±1	40±1	42±2	NS	<0.005
pH[a, c]	7.30	7.34	7.34	7.35	NS	NS
BE	-8±1	-7±1	-7±1	-6±1	NS	NS

[a] All standard errors less than 0.02; [b] highest values measured; [c] lowest values measured; A = terbutaline sulfate aerosol given 15 min before exercise; P = placebo; NS = not significant

9.1 Arterial Blood Gas Tensions and pH

Mild arterial hypoxemia is commonly observed at rest in asthmatic patients who have airways obstruction (Table 9.1). During exercise, as bronchodilation occurs, there is an increase in arterial oxygen tension (PaO_2). At this time there is no significant difference recorded for blood gas tensions and pH between asthmatics and normal subjects [14]. After exercise, however, there are marked differences and where exercise has induced asthma, the PaO_2 falls to about 60–70 mmHg. The reduction in PaO_2 occurs as a result of the mismatching of ventilation and perfusion [15]. When EIA is prevented, hypoxemia does not occur and the responses of the asthmatic to exercise are normal [14, 16] (Table 9.1).

9.2 Lung Volumes

As exercise induces an attack of asthma there is an increase in functional residual capacity and, in some patients, an increase in total lung capacity [17, 18]. In this situation the work of breathing may be increased leading to a further reduction in oxygen tension and, ultimately, to the retention of carbon dioxide. It is these physiological changes which make it difficult and potentially dangerous for many asthmatics to resume exercising once they have EIA. Many asthmatics lack confidence in their ability to perform exercise without being stressed and this has often led to poor physical fitness and in some patients, a lack of social development.

9.3 Initiating Stimuli

In 1977 Chen and Horton proposed that EIA was due to the cooling or drying of the airways as a result of conditioning the inspired air [19]. Their hypothesis came from their observation that EIA was inhibited when air at body temperature and fully saturated with water vapour was inspired during exercise. Strauss and co-workers confirmed these observations and also demonstrated that the inhalation of cold dry air during exercise enhanced the airway response [20, 21]. Direct evidence that cooling occurred came from the measurement of the airway temperature during ISH. This was recorded as abnormally low when air at ambient and subfreezing temperatures was inhaled at 60 l min^{-1} [22]. It was proposed that the colder and drier the air, the greater the number of airways involved in conditioning the air and the greater the predicted reduction in lung function [23]. Originally the airway cooling theory seemed to account very well for the variation that was recorded for the prevalence and reproducibility of EIA. The importance of intensity and duration of exercise in EIA could be explained by the differences in airway cooling resulting from an increased requirement for ventilation. It was later demonstrated that exercise *per se* was not necessary to induce asthma and that it was possible to provoke the response simply by increasing the ventilation in response to inhaling CO_2 [24–26].

In 1982 a study from this laboratory reported the effect of varying the temperature and water content of the air inspired during exercise. It concluded that a stimulus, other than cooling of the airways, was acting to induce asthma [27]. It was later proposed that the abnormally high rate of water loss from the airways during exercise led to a transient hyperosmolarity of the epithelial fluid which induced asthma by an unknown mechanism [28]. The rate of water loss under resting conditions of ventilation is normally 0.15–0.4 ml min^{-1}. During exercise, when ventilation can increase by a factor of 10–20, the loss can be as high as 3 ml min^{-1} in an adult male. Most conditioning of the inspired air occurs in the first 6–7 generations where the surface area is approximately 250–375 cm^2 [29]. At high rates of ventilation there is very little epithelial fluid available to humidify the air. Even if the depth of periciliary fluid is exaggerated to 20 microns there is still only 0.75 ml surface water available and this would need to be replaced approximately every 15 s if the osmolarity were to remain constant.

There is now evidence to support the proposal that hypertonicity of the airways is more important than airway cooling as the stimulus to EIA. Exercise-induced asthma has been recorded when hot dry air is inspired during exercise and expired air temperature is higher than normally observed under resting conditions [30, 31]. The potential to reduce mucosal temperature by evaporative heat loss is overcome under these conditions. Thus, when sufficient heat is delivered to the airways to prevent abnormal airway cooling, EIA will still occur. Furthermore there are now several studies which report that a reduction in the temperature of the inspired air (Ti) is not as critical to the response as was originally thought. When the inspired water content is constant, enhancement of EIA with a reduction in Ti is not a universal finding [32, 33]. For an individual there is a good relationship between the total amount of water lost during an 8 min exercise test and the severity of EIA (Fig. 9.3). Asthmatics are known to be very sensitive to the changes in osmolarity induced by the inhalation of ultrasonically nebulized aerosols of hypertonic solutions [34, 35]. In fact the airway response to the loss of water induced by exercising and ISH is similar to the response induced by the inhalation of hypertonic saline [36]. These observations suggest that there is a similar mechanism for the asthma provoked by exercise, ISH and the inhalation of hypertonic aerosols.

The precise mechanisms by which hypertonicity of the airway mucosa leads to contraction of bronchial smooth muscle is still not known. There is evidence that hypertonicity can act as a stimulus to induce a release of mediators from lung mast cells [37] and also to increase vagal activity [38]. Some of the differences observed, however, between exercise and ISH asthma, [39] have made it difficult to be certain about

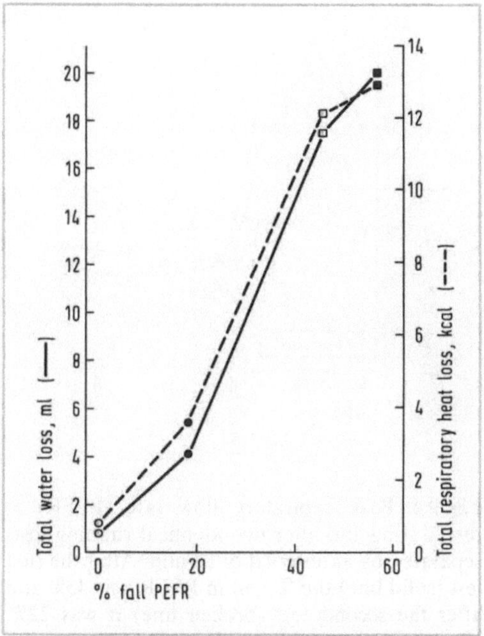

Fig. 9.3. Total water loss and total respiratory heat loss during exercise in relation to the percent fall in peak expiratory flow rate (PEFR) after exercise in a 17-year-old boy who performed cycling exercise at 73% of his maximum working capacity for 8 min at four different inspired air conditions (1 kcal = 4.2 kJ). (Reproduced from [3], with permission)

the mechanisms even though the initiating stimulus appears to be the same for both these forms of induced asthma.

9.4 The Role of Circulating Substances in EIA

There are many studies which report measurements of plasma concentration of noradrenaline (NAD), adrenaline (AD), cyclic adenosine monophosphate (CAMP), and histamine in response to exercise [9, 15, 40–44]. These circulating substances have been considered to be important for their potential to modulate airway smooth muscle function during and after exercise. For example it was originally thought that AD and NAD may mediate bronchoconstriction through stimulation of α-receptors [45]. The increase in plasma catecholamines is reported as normal in adult asthmatics [40–42]. The levels are highest at the end of exercise and return rapidly to preexercise levels. There is some evidence, however, that the response is blunted in asthmatic children [46]. As similar changes in lung function occur after ISH, a challenge which is not associated with an increase in catecholamines [46], it would appear these substances are more likely to modulate bronchodilatation than EIA.

An increase of between 7–14 pmole ml^{-1} in plasma concentration of histamine has been measured after exercise in some, but not all, patients with EIA [42–44]. The significance of these relatively small changes in histamine is unknown but may reflect disproportionately larger changes in the lung as a result of mast cell degranulation [47]. An increase in the number of circulating basophils is the explanation given by several investigators for the increase in histamine [48, 49]. This argument is supported by the observation that plasma histamine levels do not increase with ISH when basophil numbers remain unchanged. In addition to an increase in number, the fragility of basophils has also been thought to be a contributing factor to the increase in plasma histamine levels [50]. Differences in the ability to release histamine could explain why only some asthmatics have increases in plasma levels. Technically histamine is difficult to measure [51] and there is little published information on the results of multiple measurements of the same samples [34].

During exercise there is an increase in the concentration of CAMP which is related to the increase in numbers of circulating white cells. The changes occurring in asthmatics are normal in response to exercise and also after the inhalation of β-sympathomimetic agents [14]. The bronchodilatation which occurs during exercise probably reflects an increase in intracellular CAMP. The circulating levels of CAMP remain high for at least 30 min after exercise and thus do not protect the patient from EIA.

An increase in neutrophil chemotactic activity (NCA) in serum has been reported after EIA in 75% of asthmatics studied [52]. The increase in NCA is due to the release of a high molecular weight neutrophil chemotactic factor (NCF). The release of NCF is blocked by sodium cromoglycate (SCG) and by inspiring hot humid air during exercise. The release of NCF is not due to bronchoconstriction *per se* as NCA does not increase after challenge with histamine or methacholine. Furthermore NCF is not released as a consequence of exercise as normal subjects performing the same task do not inhibit changes in NCA. NCF is not released during ISH and this has made it difficult to interpret its role in EIA [53]. NCF is thought to be derived from mast cells but, as yet, this has not been confirmed.

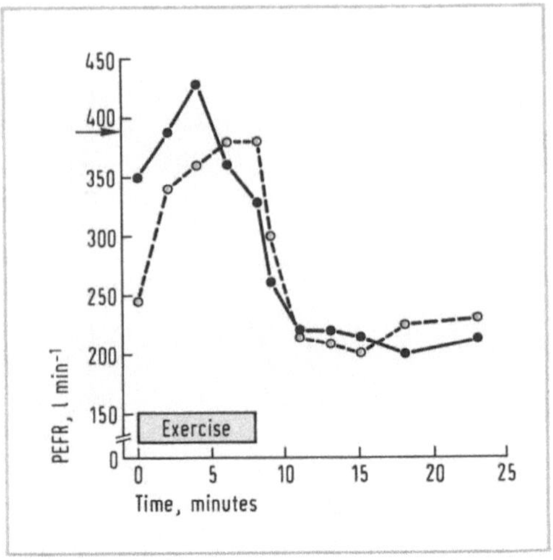

Fig. 9.4. Peak expiratory flow rate (PEFR) at rest, during and after two identical running tests separated by an interval of 32 min. After the first test (solid line) the % Fall in PEFR was 43% and after the second test (broken line) it was 22%. (Reproduced from [75], with permission)

9.5 Refractory Period

The refractory period after EIA is the time during which a second challenge with exercise will induce less asthma [54, 55]. If the % Fall after the second test is less than half of that recorded on the first test the patient is said to be refractory [55]. A refractory period can only be identified in patients who recover to initial lung function before a second challenge. When prechallenge lung function is similar, approximately 50% of patients will be refractory to an identical exercise task [56]. Even when these strict criteria are used care should be taken when interpretating the refractory index. For example, a patient may be defined as being refractory when EIA persists (Fall 1st test 79%, 30% on repeated challenge) or not refractory when EIA does not occur (Fall 1st test 17%, 9% on repeated challenge).

Bundgaard and Anderson [57] used the ELI to assess the response to exercise and found no significant change when six challenges were performed at hourly intervals. The response was not analyzed in terms of % Fall but any reduction in preexercise lung function was probably compensated by the bronchodilation induced by exercise. An example of this is illustrated in Fig. 9.4 of a patient who, on the basis of the % Fall Index, could be described as refractory. Assessed in terms of the ELI or Jones Lability Index there is little change. It is perhaps important to comment that the bronchoconstriction induced by the initial test was almost completely reversed during the first few minutes of the second exercise test.

On the basis of differences in the response to repeated exercise challenge and the inhibitory action of drugs such as SCG and ipratropium bromide (IPB; see later) it appears that there is more than one mechanism for EIA. In the context that the initiating stimulus to EIA is hypertonicity of the respiratory tract [28] it is possible to suggest that contraction of airway smooth muscle will result from mediator release and/or increase in vagal activity. In those patients who are refractory, mediators may be depleted and take some time to replenish. Bronchoconstriction arising from increased vagal stimulation is unlikely to be diminished by repetition, as patients respond repeatedly to inhalation of methacholine. In support of the argument for different mechanisms in EIA, IPB has been shown to be ineffective in blocking the response in patients who are refractory, but effective in those who are not [58]. Furthermore some patients refractory to exercise may respond to allergen inhalation [59].

There are a number of clinical questions to be asked regarding these observations.

Firstly, is the bronchodilatation induced by exercise a useful adjunct to aerosol therapy? Secondly, can a patient benefit from the identification of a refractory period? Finally, is EIA necessary to induce refractoriness or will exercise itself induce a diminished airway response to repeated challenge? There is evidence that recovery from EIA is faster if 1–2 min of exercise are performed before the aerosol bronchodilator is given [60]. There is no formal study to answer the second question although many asthmatics claim to have more endurance when refractory. There is certainly some evidence that exercise itself may induce a refractory state but the issue remains controversial. Schnall and his colleagues have shown that multiple sprints of 30 s duration can render a patient refractory [61] while others [62] have failed to show any benefits from warm-up before formal exercise testing. Ben-Dov and colleagues [63] have reported that patients are refractory to EIA when hot humid air is inspired during exercise and throughout recovery. These observations have not been supported by others [64, 65]. More studies are required to resolve these discrepant findings.

9.6 Drugs in the Treatment and Prevention of EIA

EIA can be treated when it occurs, or prevented with prophylactic therapy. In most patients EIA is rapidly reversed by giving a bronchodilator as an aerosol from a metered dose inhaler. EIA may be partially reversed before the aerosol is given by having the patient exercise for 1–2 min.

In approximately 10% of patients who exercise in the laboratory EIA is severe and not readily reversed by 2–3 inhalations of bronchodilator aerosol. In these patients it is frequently required to give a bronchodilator through a nebulizer driven by oxygen. The failure of the metered dose aerosol to work under these conditions may be due to inadequate delivery of the aerosol when a patient has severe airways obstruction.

During the last 15 years drugs used in the treatment of asthma have been investigated and their effects have been previously reviewed [1, 11]. Most studies have clearly shown that β-sympathomimetics and sodium cromoglycate, delivered as wet aerosols, inhibit or totally prevent EIA when given in the clinically recommended dose immediately before exercise [66, 67]. The protective effect, however, is usually less than 2 hours [68]. As the β-sympathomimetic aerosols induce bronchodilation, in addition to their preventative action in EIA, they are the drug of choice by patients who have airways obstruction before exercise. Sodium cromoglycate is recommended for use in patients who have normal lung function at rest and who may wish to take therapy prophylactically many times a day. Agents administered orally are less effective in preventing EIA probably due to lower concentrations of the drug being available locally in the airway mucosa.

When EIA is not prevented by either of these two aerosols then the dose is doubled. If this fails a combination of the two agents is used and if necessary the dose of each aerosol is doubled. If EIA still occurs IPB in a dose of 80 μg is added [69]. In patients with chronic symptoms of asthma the daily use of aerosol steroids may enable normal doses of β-sympathomimetics to be effective in preventing EIA [70].

9.7 Recommendation for the Assessment of Exercise-induced Asthma

The intensity and duration of exercise have long been recognized as important determinants of the magnitude of the airway response [7, 71]. This is understandable as the rate and amount of ventilation and consequent loss of water and heat from the airways increases in response to these factors. Reducing the water content and temperature of the inspired air will also enhance the airway response although the water content of the air is more important than is temperature [30, 32, 33] (Fig. 9.5).

The measurement of PEFR or FEV_1 is adequate to diagnose EIA in most patients. The measurements should be made immediately before exercise, after 2 min of exercise, at the end of exercise, and preferably 1, 3, 5, 7, 10, and 15 min after exercise. Changes in lung function assessed by more

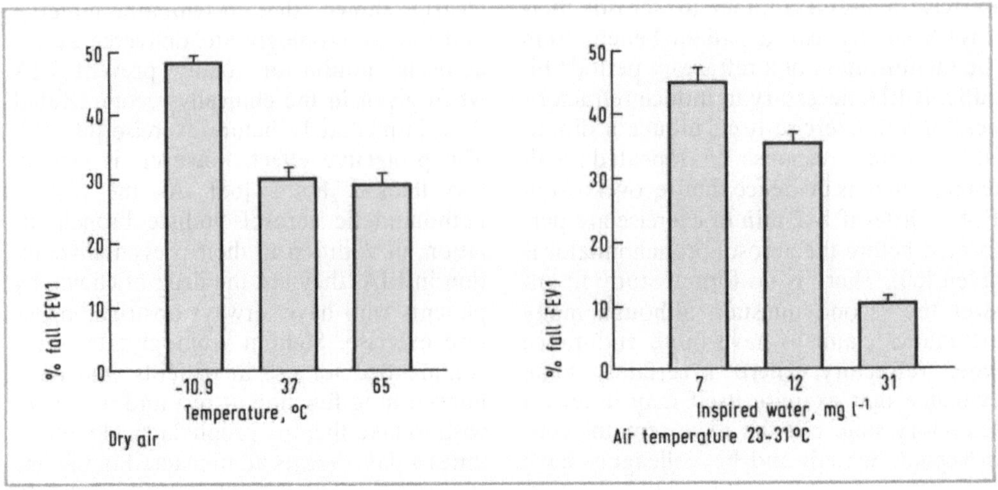

Fig. 9.5. *Left hand panel:* The fall in FEV_1 expressed as a percentage of the prechallenge level in 8 asthmatics who performed 3–4 min of exhausting cycling exercise while inspiring dry air at various temperatures. The data have been redrawn from Deal et al [30]. *Right hand panel:* The fall in 12 asthmatics who performed 6–8 min of exercise while inspiring air of different water contents. The time of exercise remained constant for each subject. The data are redrawn from Anderson et al [27]. (Reproduced from [75], with permission)

sensitive techniques, in the absence of changes in FEV_1, are unlikely to be of clinical significance. They may be useful however in the assessment of the site of drug action. Reproducible airway responses can be obtained when exercise is performed with the same prechallenge lung function at the same ventilation for the same time and with identical conditions of inspired air [1].

There are a number of recommendations for optimising the airway response: The air inspired should be dry but not necessarily cold; the exercise performed for 6–8 min at the highest possible workload; the subject should breathe only by mouth and a nose clip should be used; at least 3 hours should have elapsed since exercise last induced an attack of asthma; and the time since last medication should be greater than 4 hours, preferably 6 hours for aerosols and 24 hours for drugs given orally. Heart rate is a useful measurement of stress because asthmatics differ in their level of fitness. Suitable and safe adjustments to the work load can be made by monitoring it [72].

The amount of water and heat lost from the airways is measured by recording the ventilation and the temperature and water content of the inspired and expired air. Because this involves the use of expensive equipment, the documentation of ventilation alone, while keeping the inspired air condition constant may be all that is required. When the inspired air is dry and between 26–42 °C the concentration of water in the expired air is approximately 33 mg l^{-1} [73] and there is no difference between asthmatic and normal subjects [74]. When dry air is inhaled at these temperatures water loss (ml) may be simply assessed at ($\dot{V}E$ L BTPS $\times 33 \times 10^{-3}$). To investigate the effects of airway drying as distinct from airway cooling, the inspired air may be heated so that the expired air temperature is higher than the value recorded at rest, breathing ambient air. Under these conditions the heat lost due to the vaporization of water seems insufficient to induce abnormal cooling of the airways [31].

For the assessment of drug efficacy, it is probably best to aim for optimal conditions to obtain the maximum airway response with the placebo and match these conditions for assessment of the active drug. This technique is recommended for clinical

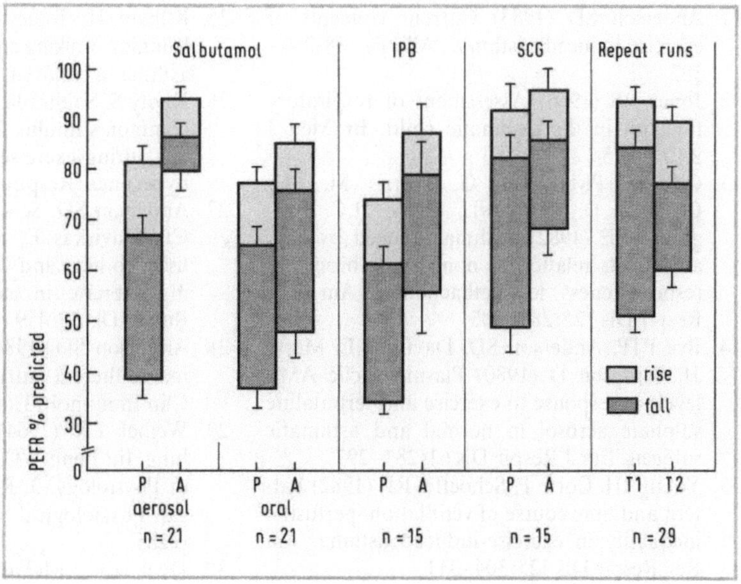

Fig. 9.6. The mean ± 1 SEM values for PEFR expressed as a percentage of the predicted value at rest , during , and after exercise. The resting levels are taken after administration of the placebo or active drug and using the lowest value recorded after exercise. (Reproduced from [11], with permission)

investigation because it is important to aim for normal lung function and the inhibition of EIA with the appropriate dose of one or more aerosol medications. Measurements of lung function should be documented before and at the appropriate time after the active drug and its placebo. The % Falls should be calculated and compared, and the preexercise lung function expressed as a percentage of predicted normal values [11, 74] (Fig. 9.6).

Exercise must still be considered the provocation test of choice in the patient who complains of breathlessness during or after exertion. It is only by documenting the changes in lung function in response to exercise, that the diagnosis of EIA can be made and the appropriate prophylactic drug treatment prescribed and assessed.

References

1. Anderson SD, Seale JP, Ferris L, Schoeffel RE, Lindsay DA (1979) An evaluation of pharmacotherapy for exercise-induced asthma. J Allergy Clin Immunol 64:612–624
2. Mellis CM, Kattan M, Keens TG, Levison H (1978) Comparative study of histamine and exercise challenges in asthmatic children. Am Rev Respir Dis 117:911–915
3. Anderson SD, Schoeffel RE (1983) The importance of standardising exercise tests in the evaluation of asthmatic children. In: Oseid S, Edwards A (eds) The asthmatic child in play and sport. Pitman, London, pp 145–158
4. Chatham M, Bleecker ER, Smith PL, Rosenthal RR, Mason P, Norman PS (1982) A comparison of histamine, methacholine and exercise airway reactivity in normal and asthmatic subjects. Am Rev Respir Dis 126:235–240
5. Anderson SD (1972) Physiological aspects of exercise-induced bronchoconstriction. PhD Thesis, University of London
6. Burr ML, Eldridge BA, Borysiewicz LK (1974) Peak expiratory flow-rates before and after exercise in school-children. Arch Dis Child 49(12):923–926
7. Silverman M, Anderson SD (1972) Standardization of exercise tests in asthmatic children. Arch Dis Child 47:882–889
8. Kattan M, Thomas CM, Keens TG, Mellis CM, Levison H (1978) The response to exercise in normal and asthmatic children. J Pediatr 92(5):718–721
9. Anderson SD, Schoeffel RE, Bye PTP (1983) Physiological aspects of exercise-induced asthma. In: Oseid S, Edwards A (eds) The asthmatic child in play and sport. Pitman, London, pp 21–35
10. Anderson SD, Silverman M, Konig P, Godfrey S (1975) Exercise-induced asthma. Br J Dis Chest 69:1–39

11. Anderson SD (1983) Current concepts of exercise-induced asthma. Allergy 38:289–302
12. Jones RS (1966) Assessment of respiratory function in the asthmatic child. Br Med J 2:972–975
13. O'Byrne PM, Ryan G, Morris M, McCormack D, Jones NL, Morse JLC, Hargreave FE (1982) Asthma induced by cold air and its relation to nonspecific bronchial responsiveness to methacholine. Am Rev Respir Dis 125:281–285
14. Bye PTP, Anderson SD, Daviskas E, Marty JJ, Sampson D (1980) Plasma cyclic AMP levels in response to exercise and terbutaline sulphate aerosol in normal and asthmatic subjects. Eur J Respir Dis 61:287–297
15. Young IH, Corte P, Schoeffel RE (1982) Pattern and time course of ventilation–perfusion inequality in exercise-induced asthma. Am Rev Respir Dis 125:304–311
16. Anderson SD (1982) Changes in airways resistance and arterial blood gas tensions in response to exercise in patients with asthma. In: Billimoria AR, Anand MP (eds) Heart and Lung Diseases Update. Bombay, pp 285–293
17. Anderson SD, McEvoy JDS, Bianco S (1972) Changes in lung volumes and airway resistance after exercise in asthmatic subjects. Am Rev Respir Dis 106:30–37
18. Freedman S, Tattersfield AE, Pride NB (1975) Changes in lung mechanics during asthma induced by exercise. J Appl Physiol 38(6):974–982
19. Chen WY, Horton DJ (1977) Heat and water loss from the airways and exercise-induced asthma. Respiration 34:305–313
20. Strauss RH, McFadden ER, Ingram RH, Jaeger JJ (1977) Enhancement of exercise-induced asthma by cold air. N Engl J Med 297:743–747
21. Strauss RH, McFadden ER, Ingram RH, Deal EC, Jaeger JJ (1978) Influence of heat and humidity on the airway obstruction induced by exercise in asthma. J Clin Invest 61:433–440
22. McFadden ER, Denison DM, Waller JF, Assoufi B, Peacock A, Sopwith T (1982) Direct recordings of the temperatures in the tracheobronchial tree in normal man. J Clin Invest 69:700–705
23. McFadden ER (1983) Respiratory heat and water exchange: physiological and clinical implications. J Appl Physiol 54:331–336
24. Deal EC, McFadden ER, Ingram RH, Jaeger JJ (1979) Hyperpnea and heat flux: initial reaction sequence in exercise-induced asthma. J Appl Physiol 46:476–483
25. Kilham H, Tooley M, Silverman M (1979) Running, walking and hyperventilation causing asthma in children. Thorax 34(5):582–586
26. Kivity S, Souhrada JF (1980) Hypernea: The common stimulus for bronchospasm in asthma during exercise and voluntary isocapnic hyperpnea. Respiration 40:169–177
27. Anderson SD, Schoeffel RE, Follet R, Perry CP, Daviskas E, Kendall M (1982) Sensitivity to heat and water loss at rest and during exercise in asthmatic patients. Eur J Respir Dis 63:459–471
28. Anderson SD (1984) Exercise-induced asthma. Is there a unifying hypothesis? J Allergy Clin Immunol 73:660–665
29. Weibel ER (1964) Morphometrics of the lung. In: Fenn WO, Rahn H (eds) Handbook of Physiology. 3. Respiration, vol. 1. American Physiological Society, Washington D.C., p 285
30. Deal EC, McFadden ER, Ingram RH, Strauss RH, Jaeger JJ (1979) Role of respiratory heat exchange in production of exercise-induced asthma. J Appl Physiol 46:467–475
31. Anderson SD, Schoeffel RE, Black JL, Daviskas E (1985) Airway cooling as the stimulus to exercise-induced asthma; A Re-evaluation. Eur J Respir Dis 67:20–30
32. Hahn A, Anderson SD, Morton AR, Black JL, Fitch KD (1984) A re-interpretation of the effect of temperature and water content of the inspired air in exercise-induced asthma. Am Rev Respir Dis 130:575–579
33. Eschenbacher WL, Shepphard D (1985) Respiratory heat loss is not the sole stimulus for bronchoconstriction induced by isocapnic hyperpnea with dry air. Am Rev Respir Dis 131:894–901
34. Schoeffel RE, Anderson SD, Altounyan REC (1981) Bronchial hyperreactivity in response to inhalation of ultrasonically nebulised solutions of distilled water and saline. Br Med J 283:1285–1287
35. Anderson SD, Schoeffel RE, Finney M (1983) An evaluation of ultrasonically nebulized solutions as a provocation in patients with asthma. Thorax 38:284–291
36. Smith CM, Anderson SD (1986) Hyperosmolarity as the stimulus to asthma induced by hyperventilation. J Allergy Clin Immunol 77:729–736 (abstract)
37. Eggleston PA, Sobotka AK, Schleimer R, Lichtenstein LM (1984) Interaction between hyperosmolar and IgE-mediated histamine release from basophils and mast cells. Am Rev Respir Dis 130:86–91
38. Colebatch HJH, Halmagyi DJF (1962) Reflex airway reaction to fluid aspiration. J Appl Physiol 17(5):787–794

39. Ingram RH, McFadden ER (1983) Are exercise and isocapnic voluntary hyperventilation identical bronchial provocations? Eur J Respir Dis 64:242–245
40. Chryssanthopoulos MD, Barboriak JJ, Fink JN, Stekiel WJ, Mksud MG (1978) Adrenergic responses of asthmatic and normal subjects to submaximal and maximal work levels. J Allergy Clin Immunol 61:17–22
41. Zielinski J, Chodosowska E, Radomyski A, Araszkiewicz Z, Kozlowski S (1980) Plasma catecholamines during exercise-induced asthma. Thorax 35:823–827
42. Anderson SD, Bye PTP, Schoeffel RE, Seale JP, Taylor KM, Ferris L (1981) Arterial plasma histamine levels at rest, during and after exercise in patients with asthma: Effects of terbutaline aerosol. Thorax 36:259–267
43. Hartley JPR, Charles TJ, Monie RDH, Seaton A, Taylor WH, Westwood A, Williams JD (1981) Arterial plasma histamine after exercise in normal individuals and in patients with exercise-induced asthma. Clin Sci 61:151–157
44. Barnes PJ, Brown MJ (1981) Venous plasma histamine in exercise- and hyperventilation-induced asthma in man. Clin Sci 61:159–162
45. Griffiths J, Leung FY, Grzybowski S, Chan-Yeung MMW (1972) Sequential estimation of plasma catecholamines in exercise-induced asthma. Chest 62(5):527–533
46. Barnes PJ, Brown MJ, Silverman M, Dollery CT (1981) Circulating catecholamines in exercise and hyperventilation induced asthma. Thorax 36:435–440
47. Anderson SD (1983) Recent advances in the understanding of exercise-induced asthma. Eur J Respir Dis 64:225–236
48. Howarth PH, Pao GJK, Church MK, Holgate ST (1984) Exercise and isocapnic hyperventilation-induced bronchoconstriction in asthma: Relevance of circulating basophils to measurement of plasma histamine. J Allergy Clin Immunol 73:391–399
49. Morgan DJR, Moodley I, Phillips MJ, Davies RJ (1983) Plasma histamine in asthmatic and control subjects following exercise: influence of circulating basophils and different assay techniques. Thorax 38:771–777
50. Neijens HJ, Dengenhart HJ, Raatgeep R, Kerrebijn KF (1980) The correlation between increased reactivity of the bronchi and of mediator releasing cells in asthma. Clin Allergy 10:535–539
51. Gleich GJ, Hall WM (1980) Measurement of histamine: a quality control study. J Allergy Clin Immunol 66:295–298
52. Kay AB, Lee TH (1982) Neutrophil chemotactic factor of anaphylaxis. J Allergy Clin Immunol 70:317
53. Lee TH, Nagakura T, Papageorgiou N, Cromwell O, Iikura Y, Kay AB (1984) Mediators in exercise-induced asthma. J Allergy Clin Immunol 73:634–639
54. Edmunds AT, Tooley M, Godfrey S (1978) The refractory period after exercise-induced asthma: Its duration and relation to the severity of exercise. Am Rev Respir Dis 117:247–254
55. Schoeffel RE, Anderson SD, Gillam I, Lindsay DA (1980) Multiple exercise and histamine challenge in asthmatic patients. Thorax 35:164–170
56. Anderson SD (1985) Exercise-induced asthma. The state of the Art. Chest 875: 1915–1955
57. Bungaard A, Anderson KK (1983) Diurnal variation in exercise-induced asthma. Eur J Respir Dis 64(128):424–426
58. Wilson NM, Barnes PJ, Vickers H, Silverman M (1982) Hyperventilation-induced asthma: Evidence for two mechanisms. Thorax 37:657–662
59. Weiler-Ravell D, Godfrey S (1981) Do exercise- and antigen-induced asthma utilize the same pathways? J Allergy Clin Immunol 67: 391–397
60. Joseph J, Bandler L, Anderson SD (1976) Exercise as a bronchodilator. Aust J Physiother XXII:47–50
61. Schnall R, Landau LI, Phelan PD (1983) The use of short periods of exercise in the prevention and reversal of exercise-induced asthma. Oseid S, Edwards A (eds) The asthmatic child in play and sport. Pitman, London, pp 107–115
62. Morton AR, Hahn AG, Fitch KD (1982) Continuous and intermittent running in the provocation of asthma. Ann Allergy 48:123–129
63. Ben-Dov I, Bar-Yishay E, Godfrey S (1982) Refractory period after exercise-induced asthma unexplained by respiratory heat loss. Am Rev Respir Dis 125:530–534
64. Anderson SD, Daviskas E, Schoeffel RE, Unger SF (1979) Prevention of severe exercise-induced asthma with hot humid air. Lancet 2:629
65. Hahn AG, Nogrady SG, Burton GR, Morton AR (1985) Absence of refractoriness in asthmatic subjects after exercise with warm humid inspirate. Thorax 40:418–421
66. Schoeffel RE, Anderson SD, Lindsay DA (1983) Sodium cromoglycate as a pressurized aerosol (Vicrom) in exercise-induced asthma. Aust NZ J Med 13:157–161

67. Tullet WM, Tan KM, Wall RT, Patel KR (1985) Dose-response effect of sodium cromoglycate pressurised aerosol in exercise-induced asthma. Thorax 40:41–44
68. Schoeffel RE, Anderson SD, Seale JP (1981) The protective effect and duration of action of metaproterenol aerosol on exercise-induced asthma. Ann Allergy 46:273–275
69. Anderson SD (1981) Exercise-induced asthma; Current views. Patient Management 6:43–55
70. Henriksen JM, Dahl R (1983) Effects of inhaled budesonide alone and in combination with low-dose terbutaline in children with exercise-induced asthma. Am Rev Respir Dis 128:993–997
71. Wilson BA, Evans JN (1981) Standardization of work intensity for evaluation of exercise-induced bronchoconstriction. Eur J Appl Physiol 47:289–294
72. Eggelston PA, Rosenthal RR, Anderson SD et al (1979) Guidelines for the methodology of exercise challenge testing of asthmatics. J Allergy Clin Immunol 64:642–645
73. Mitchell JW, Nadel ER, Stolwijk JAJ (1972) Respiratory weight losses during exercise. J Appl Physiol 32:474
74. Anderson SD, Schoeffel RE, Gonda I, Daviskas E (1984) Water concentration in the expired air of humans during exercise under aired conditions. Am Rev Respir Dis 129:A260
75. Anderson SD, Schoeffel RE (1985) Standardization of exercise testing in the asthmatic patient: A challenge in itself. In: Hargreave FE, Woolcock AJ (eds) Airway Responsiveness: measurement and interpretation. Astra Pharmaceuticals, Ontario, pp 51–59

10. Asthma and Gastroesophageal Reflux

M. Perrin-Fayolle

For many years authors have reported the existence of an abnormal frequency of gastrointestinal reflux in asthma and have discussed the possibility of connections between these two diseases. A better knowledge of this problem is a result of clinical observations of many experimental data in animals, accurate diagnostic methods and therapeutic results.

10.1 Physiological Reminders

The reflux of gastric contents into the esophagus is normally prevented by three mechanisms.

The lower esophageal sphincter (LES): It is not a distinct muscle but rather an area of increased intraluminal pressure about 3 cm long [1]. The role of lower esophageal sphincter pressure (LESP) is considered the crucial factor in the prevention of reflux.

Efficient esophageal clearing: Usually the esophagus is efficiently cleared by the peristaltic pressure wave. This activity is able to clear the esophagus from a gastric reflux in only one direction.

Glottis shutting reflex: It prevents any false passage in case of deficiency of either of these two mechanisms.

10.2 Reflux Disease

Many factors can trigger off, perpetuate or increase the pathological reflux. Some of them are particularly interesting for our purpose.

The pressure fall of the lower esophageal sphincter: It appears to be the main cause of the pathological gastroesophageal reflux (GER). This abnormality may be permanent or transient, explaining some of the discrepancies between the recording of an isolated sphincter pressure and clinical evidence of a reflux [2, 3]. This fact has been well demonstrated in recent studies by Dent and colleagues [4]. These authors, using simultaneous prolonged intraesophageal monitorings of pH and pressure, showed that gastroesophageal reflux was critically related to low sphincter pressure (LSP) and that reflux disease (RD) might be produced by a permanent fall of pressure or only by a transient relaxation of the sphincter.

Anatomical abnormalities: The existence of a cardiotuberositar malformation or a hiatal hernia is inconstant in reflux disease, although a high percentage of patients with reflux symptoms have a hiatal hernia. Cohen and Harris [5] in 1971, compared patients with chronic persistent reflux symptoms to asymptomatic persons, and found an equal incidence of hiatal hernia in both groups.

Mechanical factors: Any action producing either a violent or a progressive and prolonged stretching of the gastroesophageal junction can trigger off a reflux: a traumatism with a violent and acute compression of the thoracoabdominal region, or a prolonged and important pulling down of the diaphragm (by pulmonary distension for instance). In the same way, short-term monitoring shows that reflux can occur with increases in abdominal pressure or gastric volume [6, 7].

Decrease of the esophageal peristalsis: In some patients, acid refluxed into the distal esophagus has been shown to initiate a series of segmented contractions [8]. This effect results in a delay of acid-clearing although the lower esophageal sphincter remains relaxed, setting the stage for further reflux injury.

Role of esophagitis: The popular concept of reflux disease is that an incompetent lower esophageal sphincter causes GER which produces esophagitis. Recent animal studies showed, both in cats and baboons, that esophagitis could result in significant decreases of LESP [9, 10]. These experiments suggest that in human reflux disease a cyclic mechanism may occur which perpetuates this process once it is finished.

Life-style and iatrogenic factors: These may play an important role. Cigarette smoking [11, 12] and alcohol consumption [13] significantly reduce LESP. Many drugs can produce a fall in LESP inducing a reflux: caffeine [14], PGE, PGE_2, PGA_2 [14, 15], morphine [14] and progesterone [14, 15]. The similar action of theophylline, on the one hand [15–18], and salbutamol and other β-mimetics, on the other hand, is more interesting in asthma [19–21].

Other factors may be important in the development of reflux and esophagitis such as the gastric contents (pH, peptin, bile) and the resistance of the esophageal mucosa to injury [22, 23].

10.3 Frequency of the Esophageal Reflux in Asthma

It is impossible to assess the precise incidence of GER in asthma. In fact, no study has yet been made of all the varieties of asthma, including a sufficient number of patients, to be statistically significant. Many studies, however, have been carried out regarding this problem, including, almost exclusively, chronic and severe asthma patients.

Among *children* with severe asthma, a GER could exist in 43 to 63% of the cases [2, 24–30]. In cases of chronic *asthma in adults,* similar results are found (between 30 and 45%) [30–34].

10.4 Pathogenicity

Three mechanisms have been proposed to account for the respiratory symptoms related to gastroesophageal reflux.

Aspiration of gastric contents: It has long been assumed that the precipitation of asthma is due to this phenomenon [29, 31, 33, 35, 36]: Small amounts of the refluxed acid juice are aspirated into the tracheobronchial tree, thereby inducing a chemical tracheobronchitis [37, 38]. This aspiration of the gastric juice occurs only in decubitus. It could explain the predominance of night attacks among asthmatic patients with GER. But proof of aspiration in these patients has yet to be found and in some studies evidence of aspiration of gastric contents has been especially sought during a barium study or by isotope monitoring [30, 39].

Esophagobronchial vagal reflex: The existence of such a reflex was first mentioned in 1935 by Bray [40]. The knowledge of locoregional vagal reflexes uniting the different parts of the esophagus and the respiratory apparatus [41, 42] leads one to think that such reflexes might exist between organs with vagal innervation. After observing esophagitis induced by hydrochloric acid in a dog model, Mansfield and Stein [43, 44], using an infusion of acid in the esophagus, obtained a small, but significant, deterioration of pulmonary functions in 15 asthmatic patients with GER, while digestive signs of reflux appeared. Other more recent studies confirmed these results [45, 46]. They particularly demonstrated the simultaneous apparition of bronchoconstriction and reflux symptoms during the esophageal acid perfusion [45].

Abnormal production of reagins from food: Several authors [24, 47] suggested that esophagitis could facilitate the contact between regurgitated food antigens and immune cells with abnormal production of IgE. In fact this hypothesis remains to be proven.

Role of asthma in the reflux: The worsening of GER by asthmatic disease is a possibility which has been discussed by many authors. Clemencon and Osterman [48] suggested that intrathoracic intraabdominal pressure changes, as such, occurring in asthma, may induce reflux. Pellegrini et al [42] showed that an asthmatic attack may precede episodes of reflux. Thus, a potential self-propagating situation can be envisaged where reflux can aggravate asthma, which can itself induce further reflux [30].

10.5 Diagnostic Methods of Gastroesophageal Reflux

Clinical digestive criteria: They are very well-known, but their search in asthma patients requires great care and a conducted inquiry; patients often forget to mention them spontaneously because they are anxious about their pulmonary disturbances (pyrosis, heartburn, retrosternal pains are the more common signs). Clinical symptoms may be atypical: belching, angina-like chest pain, and postprandial sensation of repletion. In each case, it is very important to determine whether the signs are posture-dependent or not. One must remember that sometimes digestive signs are absent or discreet because the reflux is limited to the lower esophagus. Its probable action upon the tracheobronchial apparatus is then possible by means of the reflex mechanism.

Radiological criteria: A barium esophagogram can give prominence to two types of abnormalities: on the one hand, a barium reflux on the Trendelenburg posture and, on the other hand, the existence of an anatomical malformation such as a cardiotuberositar malformation or a hiatal hernia. In children, the presence of a hiatal hernia correlates closely with evidence of clinical GER [1]. In adults, the situation is debatable; some authors suggest that most of the pathological reflux could be associated with a hiatal hernia [49], while others think there is no correlation between hernia and reflux [50]; the reflux could exist without any radiological abnormality [5, 8, 34].

Esophageal fibroscopy: The double interest of this exam is to allow the direct visualization of a reflux, and to evaluate the possible consequences on the mucosa (esophagitis).

Manometry: It is theoretically the most interesting test since it objectively shows the most constant abnormality, i.e., the lower sphincter hypotonia, while it explores the esophageal peristalsis tonicity and quality. About 25% of patients with GER have pressure within the normal range when manometry is performed [51].

pH-metry: It permits a precise and direct measurement of acid regurgitation. Several methods are usable: either measurements of the esophageal pH variations in several postures, after an acid instillation in the stomach cavity, or similar measurements after a meal test with prolonged pH and reflux measures. About 20% of healthy controls have a positive test during short pH-metry. So the test should include prolonged measurements to be reliable.

Acid perfusion test: This cannot be performed in children. It was first proposed by Kjellen et al [46], and makes it possible to determine whether thoracic symptoms originate in the esophagus or not. It may also identify those asthmatic patients whose asthma is exacerbated by esophageal reflux through a reflex mechanism. This test is very reliable, with very few false positive and rarely false negative results [8, 27].

Prolonged pH monitoring: First described by Spencer [52] in 1969 and popularized by Johnson and de Meester [53] it permits a precise study of the radiological signs during the reflux, particularly during sleep. This test is usable both in children and adults [53–55]. It appears more interesting than the acid perfusion test and tends to supplant it.

Scintiscanning: This is a promising technique [56] but, thus far, insufficient studies have been reported to determine its appropriate place in the diagnosis of GER.

In conclusion, since none of these diagnostic criteria are sufficiently specific or sensitive, one must resort to the concordant positivity of them before admitting the reality of the reflux [2, 27, 29]. In our daily practice, we require four positive tests [34].

10.6 Meaning of Gastroesophageal Reflux in Asthma

The discovery of a GER in asthmatic patients can have two significations: a fortuitous association, or a pathological situation with an interdependence between these two abnormalities.

Fortuitous association: This situation is still arguable for it has been established that GER regularly occurs in both normal children and adults coming from a transient inappropriate LES relaxation. These regurgitations occur mainly after a food intake and when healthy subjects are upright [58]. Normally refluxed material is rapidly cleared from the esophagus by swallowing. However, symptoms of heartburn are common; in one survey of hospital employees, 70% had heartburn every day and 30% had it at least once a month. 4 to 5% of healthy controls are estimated to have an asymptomatic reflux.

Unlike these data, GER appears to be particularly frequent in asthma. This fact cannot be a coincidence. However, this notion has only been well-established in severe chronic, often cortico-dependent, asthma. The literature data exposed in the annexed table refer to these kinds of asthma (Table 10.1).

Table 10.1. Compared frequency of GER in asthmatic patients and controls

Healthy controls	
asymptomatic reflux	4 to 5%
occasional heartburn	7 to 36%
Asthmatic children (pathological reflux)	
Berquist et al [16]	51%
Shapiro and Christie [28]	43%
Friedland et al [24]	48%
Asthmatic adults (pathological reflux)	
Overholdt and Woorhees [31]	30% (n=497)
Mays [33]	46% (n= 28)
Perrin-Fayolle et al [34]	65% (n=150)

To eliminate the eventuality of a fortuitous association, some authors insist on the acid perfusion test and the isotopic exploration; the former can establish the proof (without any risk of error) of the gastric content passage into the respiratory apparatus.

Interdependence: The demonstration of an interdependence between asthma and GER encounters various difficulties.

Clinical criteria of the GER role in asthma: Besides the specific tests mentioned above, we insist on the possibility of identifying clinical criteria of a GER intervention in asthma: The postural trigger of the crises, their nocturnal predominance and particularly the preexistence of coughing fits, especially abundant bronchorrhea (during crises or not), and retrosternal pains are several signs of some diagnostic value, when associated, even though they are, of course, not specific of the reflux [34, 42, 54].

When one is quite sure of the existence of a GER and suspects connections with asthma, the exact nature of these connections remains to be ascertained. Asthma can be dependent exclusively on the digestive disease, or it may be induced by the bronchial disease, which in turn can aggravate the digestive disease.

Asthma induced by GER: This situation is quite exceptional, but knowing that it exists is of great interest because the surgical treatment of GER can cure the asthma. Three facts of unequal value make it possible to identify this situation [5].

Etiological data: The GER is sometimes the consequence of a thoracoabdominal traumatism, followed by the first dyspnea crisis of a so-called intrinsic asthma.

Clinical data: These types of asthma are severe, with little response to usual therapeutics. And none of the classical triggering factors of the attacks can usually be found (except ancient asthma). Above all, the precise study of the chronology of the symptoms brings to the forefront the fact that the digestive signs have preceded the respiratory symptoms (sometimes by several years). The predominance of coughing fits during the night is constant; their appearance after a copious meal is frequent.

Gastrodigestive data: It is a rule that all the GER tests should be positive; the existence of cardiotuberositar malformation or especially hiatal hernia is very frequent.

Asthma complicated with GER: Most of the reflux discovered in asthma comes under this heading. This situation raises several questions [57]. *The GER is a consequence of asthma* when the respiratory symptoms precede the digestive ones (sometimes by several years). This fact is of great diagnostic value. The results of the tests are rarely all positive; the existence of a hiatal hernia is uncommon in adults [34] while it is relatively frequent in children [24]. *We do not know very well the mechanisms* that could explain the great frequency of GER in asthma, although several factors could provoke a reflux in such conditions; the most common explanation is the lung overdistension and the diaphragm lowering which induces a stretching of the gastroesophageal junction with a widening of the His angle. The fall in LESP of these patients [26–29, 34] is otherwise favored by the different etiological factors described above. Goyal and Staish [59] showed that theophylline and isoproterenol decrease LESP in opossums, presumably by enhancing CAMP which relaxes smooth muscle [27]. Stein et al [17] confirmed this work in man. They reported a drop in LESP with therapeutic levels of aminophylline in both normal and asthmatic volunteers. *GER can have an aggravating role in asthma.* The determination of this fact is another main question which has already been mentioned. It is not always possible to give an answer because undoubtedly some asthmatic patients can have a secondary reflux without any worsening of their asthma. Its noxious role can, however, be suspected. Reflux could appear in cases of ancient, chronic and severe asthma (with or without an allergic component), and criteria which allow us to establish the proof of their aggravating role in asthma can then be found. Besides the criteria mentioned at the beginning of this chapter, one must be careful of asthma becoming aggravated for no apparent reason, particularly if there is an increase in nocturnal signs or a decrease in the efficacy of usually active treatments. A medical treatment test of the reflux must be started when it is quite sure that the reflux exists or even if it is only suspected.

10.7 Therapeutic Deductions

The aim of the treatment is to reduce gastric acidity, to avoid an increase in intragastric pressure, to maintain or restore LES tonus and to speed up the esophageal clearance. Two types of treatment can be used.

Medical treatment: It includes hygienic and dietetic rules (raising of the head of the bed, banning of copious evening meals, suppression of food and drugs capable of lowering the LESP) and a drug association: antacids which act by increasing LESP and reducing the acid content of refluxed fluids; cimetidine whose benefit action on the reflux symptoms and the nocturnal asthmatic attacks has been proven by several studies; alginic acid (Gaviscon®), which reacts with saliva to form a highly viscous solution that floats on the surface of the gastric pool during the night, acting as a mechanical barrier; and metoclopramide hydrochloride, a dopamine agonist, which increases LESP and speeds esophageal and gastric emptying.

Antireflux surgery: Different techniques aim to improve the competence of the lower esophageal sphincter. The most used are the Nissen transabdominal gastropexy and the Belsey transthoracic fundoplication.

Indications and Therapeutic Results

Medical treatment: It must be undertaken in the presence of every severe asthma whose symptomatology evokes the aggravating role of reflux.

In *children,* the various published statistics show poor results of medical antireflux treatment on the respiratory symptom [19, 26, 28, 61].

In *adults,* results vary greatly depending on the severity of the reflux, the quality of the treatment, and the duration of follow-up. Overall, the results seem better than in children. Some authors report 88% [62] and even 95% [63] good results (Table 10.2). Ac-

Table 10.2. Effect of conservative treatment* of esophageal dysfunction on bronchial asthma [62]

	Treatment group n=31	Control group n=31	
Improvement of esophageal symptoms	20	2	$p<0.001$
Improvement of bronchial symptoms			
dyspnea	15	3	$p<0.01$
wheezing	11	1	
coughing	14	1	$p<0.05$
expectoration	14	5	$p<0.001$

* Treatment required a special regimen and an alginate/antacid compound. Patients were asked to elevate the head of their bed, to end all meals with a glass of luke-warm water, to eat no later than 3 hours before bed-time and to refrain from aspirin and anticholinergic drugs

cording to our experience, medical treatment can remove completely the digestive signs; its favorable action on asthma is very often noted. However, we have never observed a perfect control of asthma by the medical antireflux treatment alone.

Surgical treatment: In children, numerous statistics show improvements in, or recoveries from asthma after surgical therapy in a high number of cases [26, 29, 53, 58, 60, 64–66]. It is interesting to note that medical treatment results do not make it possible to forecast the surgical ones. Jolley et al surgically controlled 12/27 times a reflux which had not been improved by medical treatment [54], while Christie et al obtained the same results 5/15 times [26].

In adults, the surgical indications must be considered.

In reflux-induced asthma (exceptional situation) surgical therapy must be applied. This completely cures the asthma when the intervention is early enough. In 1980 we reported 13 recoveries from these conditions [67].

When the GER is the consequence of asthma, the surgical treatment of reflux cannot cure the respiratory disease. It can, however, improve it considerably. We obtained an improvement in 18/37 cases [68] and numerous authors have also noted similar results [30–32, 58]. We must, however, realize that the reappearance of reflux in the following years is not exceptional, in children as well as in adults.

In practice, surgical treatment should be proposed only in the presence of severe, possibly cortico-dependent asthma, complicated with neat reflux and severe esophagitis, which represents in itself a surgical indication owing to the risk of secondary peptic ulcer.

10.8 Conclusions

The study of the relationship between asthma and gastroesophageal reflux produces two situations in which the recognition of reflux can be of great interest. The first, exceptional in fact, concerns asthma caused by more or less ancient reflux, and which can be surgically cured. The second, occurring more frequently, concerns severe chronic and readily cortico-dependent asthma which are later complicated with a reflux, which in turn aggravates the respiratory disease. The discovery of the gastroesophageal reflux can lead to precise therapeutic prescriptions capable of really improving the asthma.

References

1. Herbst JJ (1981) Gastroesophageal reflux. J Pediatr 98:59–62
2. Behar J, Biancani P, Sheahan DG (1976) Evaluation of esophageal tests in the diagnosis of reflux esophagitis. Gastroenterology 71:9–15
3. de Meester TR, Wang CI, Wernly JA et al (1980) Technique, indications and clinical use of 24 hours esophageal pH monitoring. J Thorac Cardiovasc Surg 79:656–670
4. Dent J, Doods WJ, Friedman RH et al (1980) Mechanism of gastroesophageal reflux in recumbent asymptomatic human subjects. J Clin Invest 65:256–267
5. Cohen S, Harris LD (1971) Does hiatus hernia affect competence of the gastroesophageal sphincter? N Engl J Med 284: 1053–1056
6. McCallum RW, Berkowitz DM, Lerver E (1981) Gastric emptying in patients with gas-

troesophageal reflux. Gastroenterology 86: 285–291

7. Ahtaridis G, Snape WJ, Cohen S (1981) Lower esophageal sphincter pressure as an index of gastroesophageal acid reflux. Dig Dis Sci 26:993–998
8. Nelson HS (1984) Gastroesophageal reflux and pulmonary disease. J Allergy Clin Immunol 73:547–556
9. Eastwood GL, Castell DO, Higgs RH (1975) Experimental esophagitis in cats impairs lower esophageal sphincter pressure. Gastroenterology 69:146–153
10. Sinar DR, Fletcher JR, Cordova CC, Eastwood GL, Castell DO (1981) Acute acid-induced esophagitis impairs esophageal peristalsis in baboons. Gastroenterology 80:1286 (abstract)
11. Stanci C, Bennett JR (1972) Smoking and gastro-esophageal reflux. Br Med J 10:793–795
12. Dennish GW, Castell DO (1971) Inhibitory effect of smoking on the lower esophageal sphincter. N Engl J Med 284:1136–1137
13. Hogan WJ, Viegas de Andrade SR, Winship DH (1972) Ethanol-induced acute esophageal motor dysfunction. J Appl Physiol 32:755–760
14. Castell DO (1978) Medical measures that influence the gastro-esophageal junction. South Med J 71 [Suppl 1]:26
15. Richter JE, Castell DO (1982) Gastroesophageal reflux. Pathogenesis, diagnosis and therapy. Ann Intern Med 97:93–103
16. Berquist WE, Rachelefsky GS, Kadden M et al (1981) Effect of theophylline on gastroesophageal reflux in normal adults. J Allergy Clin Immunol 67:407–411
17. Stein MR, Weber RW, Towner TG (1978) The effect of theophylline on the lower esophageal sphincter pressure (LESP). J Allergy Clin Immunol 61:135 (abstract)
18. Goyal PK, Rattan S (1973) Mechanism of the lower esophageal sphincter relaxation. Action of prostaglandin E_1 and the theophylline. J Clin Invest 52:337–341
19. Cohen S, Snape WJ (1978) The pathophysiology and treatment of gastroesophageal reflux disease. Arch Intern Med 138:1398–1401
20. di Marino AJ, Cohen S (1974) Characteristics of lower esophageal function in symptomatic diffuse esophageal spasm. Gastroenterology 66:1–6
21. Christensen J (1976) Effects of drugs on esophageal motricity. Arch Intern Med 136:532–537
22. Dodds WJ, Hogan WJ, Helm JF, Dent J (1981) Pathogenesis of reflux esophagitis. Gastroenterology 61:376–394
23. Harmon JW, Johnson LF, Maydonovitch LL (1981) Effects on acid and bile salts on the rabbit esophageal mucosa. Dig Dis Sci 26:65–72
24. Friedland GW, Yamate M, Marinkovich VA (1973) Hiatal hernia and chronic unremitting asthma. Pediatr Radiol 1:156–160
25. Danus O, Casar C, Larrain A (1976) Esophageal reflux – an unrecognized cause of recurrent obstructive bronchitis in children. J Pediatr 89:220–224
26. Christie DL, O'Grady LR, Mack DV (1978) Imcompetent lower esophageal sphincter and gastroesophageal reflux in recurrent acute pulmonary disease of infancy and childhood. J Pediatr 93:23–27
27. Euler AR, Byrne WJ, Ament ME (1979) Recurrent pulmonary disease in children: a complication of gastroesophageal reflux. Pediatrics 63:47–51
28. Shapiro GG, Christie DL (1979) Gastroesophageal reflux in steroid-dependant asthmatic youths. Pediatrics 63:207–212
29. Berquist WE, Rachelefsky GS, Kadden M, Siegel SC, Katz RM, Fonkalsrud EW, Ament ME (1981) Gastroesophageal chronic asthma in children. Pediatrics 68:29–35
30. Goodall RJR, Earis JE, Cooper DN, Bernstein A, Temple JG (1981) Relationship between asthma and gastroesophageal reflux. Thorax 36:116–121
31. Overholt RH, Woorhees RI (1966) Esophageal reflux as trigger in asthma. Dis Chest 49:464–466
32. Urschell HC, Paulson DL (1967) Gastroesophageal reflux and hiatal hernia. J Thorac Cardiovasc Surg 53:21–29
33. Mays EE (1976) Intrinsic asthma in adults. Association with gastroesophageal reflux. JAMA 236:2626–2628
34. Perrin-Fayolle M, Bel A, Kofman J, Harf R, Montagnon B, Pacheco Y, Daudet J, Nesmoz J, Perpoint B (1980) Asthme et reflux gastro-oesophagien (résultats d'une enquête portant sur 150 cas). Poumon Coeur 36:225–230
35. Babb RR, Notarangelo J, Smith VM (1970) Wheezing: A clue to gastroesophageal reflux. Am J Gastroenterol 53:230–232
36. Huxley EJ, Viroslav J, Gray WR, Pierre AK (1978) Pharyngeal aspiration in normal adults with depressed consciousness. Am J Med 64:564–568
37. Wolfe JE, Bone RC, Ruth WE (1976) Diagnosis of gastric aspiration by fiberoptic bronchoscopy. Chest 70:458–459
38. Wynne JW, Ramphal R, Hood C (1984) Tracheal mucosal damage after aspiration: a scanning electron microscope study. Am Rev Respir Dis 124:728–732

39. Ghaej N, Stein MR (1979) Assessment of a technique for scintigraphic monitoring of pulmonary aspirations of gastric contents in asthmatics with gastroesophageal reflux. Ann Allergy 43:306–309
40. Bray GW (1935) The treatment of asthma. Br Med J 1:118–123
41. Hunt PS, Colnnell AM, Smiley TB (1970) The crico-pharyngeal sphincter in gastric reflux. Gut 11:303–306
42. Pellegrini CA, de Meester TR, Johnson IF, Skinner DB (1979) Gastroesophageal reflux and pulmonary aspiration: incidence, functional abnormality and results of surgical therapy. Surgery 86:110–118
43. Mansfield LE, Hameister HH, Spaulding HS, Smith NJ, Glab N (1981) The role of the vagus nerve in airway narrowing caused by intraesophageal hydrochloric acid provocation and esophageal distension. Ann Allergy 47:431–434
44. Mansfield LE, Stein MR (1978) Gastroesophageal reflux and asthma. A possible reflex mechanism. Ann Allergy 41:224–226
45. Spaulding HS, Mansfield LE, Stein MR, Sellner JC, Gremillion DE (1982) Further investigations of the associations between gastroesophageal reflux and bronchoconstriction. J Allergy Clin Immunol 69:516–519
46. Kjellen G, Tibbling L, Wranne B (1981) Bronchial obstructions after esophageal acid perfusion in asthmatics. Clin Physiol 1:285–287
47. Sandmark S (1970) Hiatal incompetence. Mechanical studies and principles of examination for hiatus hernia and gastroesophageal reflux. Ann Surg 170:627–637
48. Clemencon GH, Osterman PO (1961) Hiatal hernia in bronchial asthma. The importance of concomitant pulmonary emphysema. Gastroenterologia 95:110–120
49. Lichter I (1974) Measurement of gastro-esophageal acid reflux: its significance in hiatus hernia. Br J Surg 61:253–258
50. Pope CE (1976) Pathophysiology and diagnosis of reflux esophagitis. Gastroenterology 70:445–454
51. Denis P, Le Bihan M, Galmiche JP, Hecker TS, Weiler P, Colin R, Pasquis P (1980) Syndrome de reflux gastro-oesophagien. Exploration fonctionnelle de l'eosophage chez 55 malades. Nouv Presse Méd 9:2125–2127
52. Spencer J (1969) Prolonged pH recording in the study of gastroesophageal reflux. Br J Surg 56:912–914
53. Johnson LF, de Meester TR (1974) Twenty-four hour pH monitoring of the distal esophagus: a quantitative measure of gastroesophageal reflux. Am J Gastroenterol 62:325–332
54. Jolley SG, Gerbst JJ, Johnson DG, Matlak ME, Book LS (1981) Esophageal pH monitoring during sleep identifies children with respiratory symptoms from gastroesophageal reflux. Gastroenterology 80:1501–1506
55. Branicki FJ, Evans DF, Ogilvie AL, Atkinson M, Hardcastle JD (1983) Ambulatory monitoring of esophageal pH in reflux oesophagitis using a portable readiotelemetry system. Gut 23:992–998
56. Guillet J, Basse-Cathalinat B, Soubiran G, Blanquet P, Saudubray F, Battin J (1982) Asthme provoqué ou aggravé par reflux gastro-oesophagien. Preuve directe par la cinéoesogastroscintigraphie. Nouv Presse Méd 11:529
57. de Meester TR, Johnson LF, Joseph GJ, Toscano MS, Hall AW, Skinner DB (1976) Patterns of gastroesophageal reflux in health and disease. Ann Surg 184:459–469
58. Perrin-Fayolle M (1981) Asthme et reflux gastro-oesophagien. Nouv Presse Méd 10:1503–1505
59. Goyal RK, Staish R (1973) Mechanism of the lower esophageal sphincter relaxation. J Clin Invest 52:337–341
60. Behar J, Sheahan DG, Bianconi P (1975) Medical and surgical management of reflux esophagitis. N Engl J Med 293:263–268
61. Roufail WM (1978) Medical management of patients with reflux esophagitis. South Med J 43 [Suppl]: 12
62. Kjellen G, Tibbling L, Wranne B (1981) Effect of conservative treatment of esophageal dysfunction on bronchial asthma. Eur J Respir Dis 62:190–193
63. Carcassonne M, Bensoussan A, Aubert S (1973) The management of gastroesophageal reflux in infants. J Pediatr Surg 8:575–586
64. Randolph JG, Willy JR, Anderson KD (1974) Surgical treatment of gastroesophageal reflux in infants. Ann Surg 180:479–486
65. Funkalsrud EW, Ament ME, Bryne WJ (1978) Gastroesophageal fundoplication for management of reflux in infants and children. J Thorac Cardiovasc Surg 76:655–664
66. Perrin-Fayolle M, Bel A, Braillon G, Lombard-Platet R, Kofman J, Harf R, Montagnon B, Pacheco Y, Perpoint B (1980) Asthme et reflux gastro-oesophagien. Résultats de la cure chirurgicale chez 50 malades. Poumon Coeur 36:231–237
67. Pearson JEG, Wilson RSE (1971) Diffuse pulmonary fibrosis and hiatus hernia. Thorax 20:300–306
68. Klotz SD, Moeller RK (1971) Hiatal hernia and intractable bronchial asthma. Ann Allergy 29:325–328

D. Immunology

11. The IgE Receptors (Introduction)

It is well-known that stimulation of the receptor, with high affinity for IgE on mast cells and basophils, initiates an allergic reaction. This has been extensively studied during the past 20 years. There is no doubt that this receptor is of major importance in the understanding of allergic diseases. But more recently, a *second* IgE receptor, of low affinity, was revealed on other cells such as eosinophils, macrophages, platelets and lymphocytes. This receptor appears to be involved in helminth expulsion and also in allergy. Although this *second receptor* was recognized latter, its importance seems to be identical with the first receptor in the understanding and eventual treatment of allergic patients. Antireceptor molecules, or drugs blocking the early steps of the cascade of events initiated by receptor activation, may represent an alternative to specific immunotherapy with allergens.

11.1 IgE Receptors in Bronchial Asthma

A. Kulczycki

The pathogenesis of asthma can be examined from many different perspectives. Clinically, one often distinguishes asthma which is initiated by antigen, IgE, and mast cell mediators (where pathogenetic mechanisms are relatively clear) from asthma which is termed *idiopathic*. In this review, a more complex view of some of the known (and potential) mechanisms involved in asthma is explored using the cell surface receptors for IgE as reference points.

11.1.1 IgE

IgE was discovered in 1966 after its isolation from sera of ragweed-allergic individuals [28]. The unique properties of IgE corresponded to known properties of *reaginic antibody,* including the ability to transfer the immediate hypersensitivity response [29]. Like other immunoglobulins, IgE is synthesized by plasma cells and consists of two light and two heavy chains covalently linked by disulfide bonds [2]. Unlike other immunoglobulin classes, IgE is present in extremely low concentrations in normal individuals (e.g., 180 to 350 ng/ml) [34], it has the ability to bind with high affinity to receptors on mast cells and basophils, and it functions as a cell surface antibody.

One characteristic of IgE is that a heating at 56 °C for several hours or mild reduction destroys its ability to bind to IgE receptors [30]. Studies on the rate of sequential digestion of IgE by trypsin in the presence and absence of an IgE receptor suggest that the $C_\varepsilon 3/C_\varepsilon 2$ interdomain region of IgE is bound to the high affinity IgE receptor [51].

11.1.2 High Affinity IgE Receptors of Mast Cells and Basophils

The specificity of the high affinity IgE receptors was first demonstrated in studies using human IgE and human basophils from peripheral blood [32, 57]. In studies with rat IgE and IgE receptors derived from rat basophilic leukemia (RBL) cell cultures [42, 44] it was found that IgE-binding to cell surface receptor is a temperature-dependent and reversible reaction, consistent with the simple biomolecular forward reaction and the first-order reverse reaction:

$$[\text{IgE}]+[\text{receptor}] \underset{k_{-1}}{\overset{k_1}{\rightleftarrows}} [\text{IgE receptor complex}]$$

Although the forward rate constant (k_1) of approximately 1×10^5 l/mole-sec at 37 °C [44] is not unusual for biological reactions, the extremely low concentration of IgE in serum explains why IgE-binding to high affinity receptors requires long *latent* periods *in vivo* in the passive cutaneous anaphylaxis (PCA) reaction. The reverse rate constant (k_{-1}) of $< 10^{-5}$/s explains why *sensitization* with IgE may persist for weeks. The affinity constant, K_a ($=k_1/k_{-1}$), is at least 10^{10} l/mole in the rat system [44], and is similar in the human system [33].

The high affinity IgE receptor appears to be composed of multiple subunits (Fig. 11.1). The surface-exposed glycoprotein α-component was the first component recognized. It was purified from ^{125}I-labeled rat mast cells and RBL cells by immunoprecipitation and was characterized as an ~50,000 M_r glycoprotein in SDS-polyacrylamide gels [11, 43]. A similar ^{125}I-labeled α-component has been isolated from human basophils [12, 20]. The α-component appears as a broad band in SDS-polyacrylamide gels and in isoelectric focusing gels because of microheterogeneity of attached N-linked oligosaccharides [21]. The rat IgE receptor α-component contains about 30% carbohydrate and only a modest proportion of hydrophobic amino acids [36]. The α-component can be enzymatically cleaved into two similar-sized fragments [18].

In the isolation of an IgE receptor from RBL cells biosynthetically labeled with ^3H-labeled amino acids, an $\sim 33{,}000\ M_r$ macromolecule was discovered which copurified with the α-component, but was not a glycoprotein [21, 45]. Since a $\sim 33{,}000\ M_r$ macromolecule could be chemically cross-linked to the α-component [22], it has been termed the "β-component" [23]. Associated with each α- and β-chain are two $\sim 9{,}000\ M_r$ "γ-chains", linked to each other by disulfide bonding [52].

Mast cells and basophils express large numbers of IgE receptors on their surfaces. It is estimated that there are 300,000 high affinity IgE receptors per mast cell [10], 300,000 to 1,400,000 per RBL cell [44], and approximately 40,000 to 100,000 receptors per human basophil [33]. In studies with RBL cells it has been shown that receptor density varies according to the cell cycle, with the receptor density highest when cells are in the G_1 phase of the cell cycle [24]. It also appears that the α-component of the IgE receptor must be glycosylated before it can be expressed on the cell surface [21].

Membrane proteins have been classified into two groups: *migrant* proteins (e.g., LDL receptors), which recycle from one membrane containing organelle to another via *coated pits,* and *resident* proteins (e.g., histocompatibility antigens), which do not recycle [4]. Even though IgE together with IgE receptors can be internalized after antigen-induced cross-linking, the receptor is neither recycled nor replaced by active synthesis [25], so it should be classified as a *resident* membrane protein. Nevertheless, the internalization of a multivalent antigen bound to IgE molecules (bound in turn to IgE receptors) does serve to remove both antigen and IgE antibody from the cell surface. This may account, at least in part, for the *antigen-specific desensitization* phenomenon observed when low concentrations of a specific antigen render a mast cell or basophil unresponsive to further challenge

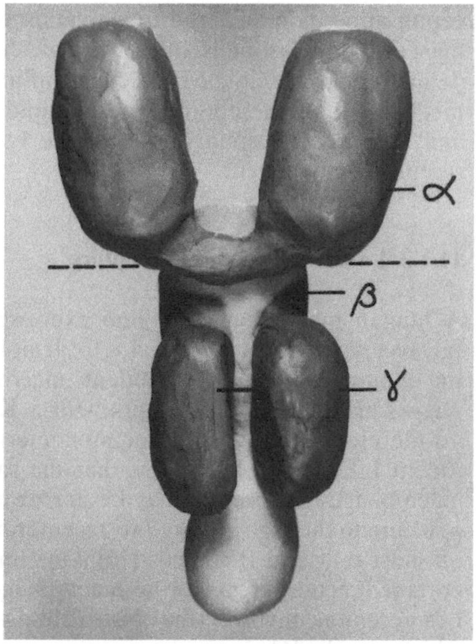

Fig. 11.1. Artist's model of the high affinity receptor for IgE of the mast cell/basophil. Components from top to bottom (outside of cell membrane to inside) consist of: 1 α- ($\sim 50{,}000\ M_r$), 1 β- ($\sim 33{,}000\ M_r$), and 2 γ- ($\sim 9{,}000\ M_r$) chains [52]. Appropriate weights of modeling clay were shaped in ovoid masses, except for narrow segments which represent postulated enzymatic cleavage sites. The α-component is a glycoprotein exposed to the outer cell surface, proposed to be a U-shaped molecule of two domains [18]. The nonglycosylated β-component seems to have two enzymatically separable domains [23], the larger associating with the α-component [18] and with two disulfide-linked γ-components [52]. The approximate position of the cell membrane is indicated by dashed lines

with that antigen yet responsive to a different antigen.

It is the cross-linking of the IgE receptors (brought into apposition by the binding of a multivalent antigen to several receptor-bound IgE molecules) which appears to be the critical cellular event which triggers mediator release and production [41]. This was established definitively by demonstrations that rabbit antibodies to rat IgE receptor induced histamine release from rat mast cells and RBL cells [26, 27]. The biochemical mechanisms which follow IgE receptor apposition and lead to activation of mast cells and basophils are not completely defined but may involve calcium influx, methylation of membrane phospholipids, and increased phosphorylation of the IgE receptor α-component.

11.1.3 Lower Affinity IgE Receptors

A human macrophage cell line expresses IgE receptors with a K_a of $\sim 4 \times 10^7$ l/mole for monomeric IgE [1]. Rodent macrophages also have IgE receptors with a K_a on the order of 10^7 l/mole for monomeric rodent IgE [3, 15]. It appears that the rat macrophage IgE receptor may be similar in structure to the high affinity IgE receptor of rat mast cells and RBL cells [16]. One important function of monocyte-macrophage IgE receptors involves the destruction of schistosomules [6].

B- and T-lymphocytes in humans and rats have also been shown to express IgE receptors [19, 59]. Lymphocyte receptors for IgE appear similar to monocyte receptors in affinity for IgE (K_a $\sim 6 \times 10^7$ l/mole), in size (both contain $\sim$ 47,000 M_r molecules), and in antigenic determinants [47]. Since infection of rats with *N. brasiliensis* and exposure of patients to appropriate allergens both induce increases in Fc_ε receptor-bearing lymphocyte populations, it is presumed that such populations are involved in regulating IgE synthesis [55, 59]. Fc_ε-bearing T-lymphocytes are capable of releasing IgE-binding factors which appear to regulate IgE responses *in vitro*. The factor which potentiates IgE synthesis is glycosylated (by another soluble T-cell factor), whereas the factor which suppresses IgE production is not glycosylated [reviewed in 31]. Lymphocyte Fc_ε receptors themselves can be induced *in vitro* by incubation with IgE [60] and, in humans, with cross-linked IgE [50].

Rat and human eosinophils also express receptors for IgE. Since they are demonstrated by using IgE-coated erythrocytes [7], it is presumed that they have a low affinity (compared with basophils) for monomeric IgE. Eosinophil Fc_ε receptors appear to have an important role in mediating eosinophil cytotoxicity against parasites [8].

11.1.4 Involvement of IgE Receptors in Asthma

In the etiology of an individual's asthma, IgE receptors may have a known role, a potential role, or no role at all (Fig. 11.2). The classical pathway of extrinsic asthma, in which high affinity IgE receptors are clearly involved in the pathogenesis of the disease, is emphasized in the center of Fig. 11.2. Allergens bind to receptor-bound IgE antibodies, which brings high affinity IgE receptors into apposition and activates mast cells to produce a variety of mediators – some of which lead directly to asthma. Several surveys indicate that *extrinsic* allergens play an important etiologic role in the majority of patients with asthma [5, 17, 58]. (Although numerous antigens are well-known causes of asthma, the antigen most commonly implicated is derived from the house dust mite *Dermatophagoides*, e.g., in one study 85% of unselected asthmatic children appeared to be allergic to *Dermatophagoides* [48].) It also follows that the lower affinity IgE receptors of lymphocytes (Fc_ε receptors) can play an important role in the etiology of asthma because they regulate the synthesis of IgE [31].

There are a variety of potential roles of IgE receptors in the pathogenesis of asthma. First, it is very likely that additional antigens, presently unrecognized, will in the future be implicated in the etiology of asthma, just as the importance of antigens from cockroaches [37], rodents [46], relatively unusual molds [40], grain storage mites [13], and pepsin [9] has been appreciated in the past decade.

Second, it had been suggested that spontaneous autoantibodies against IgE or IgE receptors could conceivably be involved in idiopathic asthma [41] because several groups have found a high frequency of various autoantibodies in patients with idiopathic asthma and because antibodies deliberately produced against IgE or IgE receptors can induce mediator release. Recently, anti-IgE autoantibodies of the IgG class were found in 93% of atopic asthmatics and 72% of nonatopic asthmatic (compared to 7% (1 of 15) of normal individuals [49]. The anti-IgE antibody levels were correlated with the total IgE levels in the sera

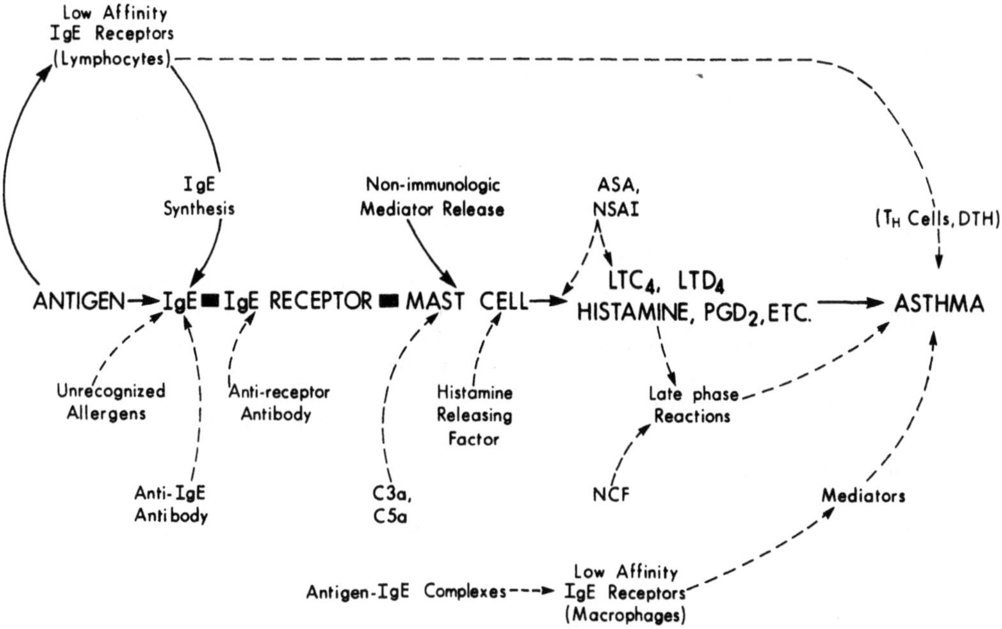

Fig. 11.2. Sequence of pathogenetic events involved in asthma, emphasizing known and potential roles of IgE receptors. The *classical extrinsic* pathway leading to asthma is represented with capital letters. Solid lines represent the well-defined mechanisms of clinical importance

of 76 individuals studied. Gel filtration studies suggested that the anti-IgE autoantibodies were present in the immune complex form (bound to IgE) in asthmatic patients' sera. The autoantibodies appeared to mediate reversed-type immediate hypersensitivity reactions in the skin of normal individuals, which suggests that anti-IgE autoantibody might play a pathogenetic role in asthma [49].

Third, IgE immune complexes might also be involved in the pathogenesis of asthma. It has been shown that allergic patient populations frequently have elevated levels of IgE containing immune complexes [56]. It is known that aggregates containing IgE can induce mediator release *in vitro* from macrophages [14]; it is presumed that complexes bind to lower affinity IgE receptors and that they might be involved in asthma pathogenesis. Another cell type potentially involved with IgE complexes and asthma pathogenesis is the sensitized T-cell. Most dust-allergic patients (but not controls) have T-lymphocytes which are sensitized to the antigen P_1 of house dust [53]. The sensitized cells (apparently T helper cells) are probably involved in the production of antibody but may also be involved in the delayed manifestations of asthma.

Not all paths culminating in asthma involve IgE receptors (Fig. 11.2). Aspirin sensitivity occurs in 8–14% of all asthmatics and does not involve IgE or IgE receptors. It is known that aspirin and nonsteroidal anti-inflammatory drugs inhibit the cyclooxygenase pathway of arachidonic acid metabolism, but their precise site(s) and mechanism(s) of producing asthma are not known [54]. Certain other drugs are known to cause nonimmunologic release of mediators from mast cells *in vitro* (e.g., opiates, polymyxin, radiocontrast dyes, mannitol, etc.) and are sometimes clinically important. The anaphylatoxins, C3a and C5a, are known to cause mediator release from mast cells *in vitro,* and recently a 20,000 M_r histamine releasing factor has been isolated from human mononuclear cells [38]. However, the clinical significance of these latter substances is not clear.

It is known that mast cell-derived mediators and neutrophil chemotactic factor (NCF) [39] may produce late phase allergic reactions (which may involve eosinophils, neutrophils, monocytes, and lymphocytes). Late phase reactions also seem to have a potentially important role in the pathogenesis of asthma [35].

The diagram on Fig. 11.2 is not meant to be comprehensive. For example, it is widely recognized that viral respiratory infections can initiate or exacerbate symptoms in a subset of asthmatic patients, but the pathogenetic mechanisms involved are not clear. Likewise, exposure to metabisulfites, to toluene diisocyanate, and to Cuprophane hemodialysis membranes are known to induce asthma, yet the responsible mechanisms have not been defined.

References

1. Anderson CL, Spiegelberg HL (1981) Macrophage receptors for IgE: Binding of IgE to specific IgE Fc receptors on a human macrophage cell line, U937. J Immunol 126: 2470–2473
2. Bennich H, von Bahr-Lindstrom H (1974) Structure of immunoglobulin E (IgE). In: Brent L, Holborow J (eds) Progress in Immunology, II, vol. I. North Holland Publishing, Amsterdam
3. Boltz-Nitulescu G, Plummer JM, Spiegelberg HL (1982) Fc receptors for IgE on mouse macrophages and macrophage-like cell lines. J Immunol 128:2265–2268
4. Brown MS, Anderson RGW, Goldstein JL (1983) Recycling receptors: the round-trip itinerary of migrant membrane proteins. Cell 32:663–667
5. Burrows B, Lebowitz MD, Barbee RA (1976) Respiratory disorders and allergy skin-test reactions. Ann Intern Med 84:134–139
6. Capron A, Dessaint J-P, Capron M, Bazin H (1975) Specific IgE antibodies in immune adherence of normal macrophages to Schistosoma mansoni schistosomules. Nature 253:474–475
7. Capron M, Capron A, Dessaint J-P, Torpier G, Johansson SGO, Prin L (1981) Fc receptors for IgE on human and rat eosinophils. J Immunol 126:2087–2092
8. Capron M, Bazin H, Joseph M, Capron A (1981) Evidence for IgE-dependent cytotoxicity by rat eosinophils. J Immunol 126:1764–1768
9. Cartier A, Malo JL, Pineau RT, Dolovich J (1984) Occupational asthma due to pepsin. J Allergy Clin Immunol 73:574–577
10. Conrad DH, Bazin H, Sehon AH, Froese A (1975) Binding parameters of the interaction between rat IgE and rat mast cell receptors. J Immunol 114:1688–1691
11. Conrad DH, Froese A (1976) Characterization of the target cell receptor for IgE. II. Polyacrylamide gel analysis of the surface IgE receptor from normal rat mast cells and from rat basophilic leukemia cells. J Immunol 116:319–326
12. Conrad DH, Wingard JR, Ishizaka T (1983) The interaction of human and rodent IgE with the human basophil IgE receptor. J Immunol 130:327–333
13. Cuthbert OD, Brostoff J, Wraith DG, Brighton WD (1979) "Barn allergy": asthma and rhinitis due to storage mites. Clin Allergy 9:229–236
14. Dessaint J-P, Waksman BH, Metzger H, Capron A (1980) Cytophilic binding of IgE to the macrophage. Cellular Immunology 51:280–292
15. Finbloom DS, Metzger H (1982) Binding of immunoglobulin E to receptor on rat peritoneal macrophages. J Immunol 129:2004–2008
16. Finbloom DS, Metzger H (1983) Isolation of cross-linked IgE-receptor complexes from rat macrophages. J Immunol 130:1489–1491
17. Ford RM (1969) Aetiology of asthma: a review of 11,551 cases (1958 to 1968). Med J Aust 1:628–631
18. Goetze A, Kanellopoulos J, Rice D, Metzger H (1981) Enzymatic cleavage products of the α subunit of the receptor for immunoglobulin E. Biochemistry 20:6341–6349
19. Gonzalez-Molina A, Spiegelberg HL (1977) A subpopulation of normal human peripheral B lymphocytes that bind IgE. J Clin Invest 59:616–624
20. Hempstead BL, Parker CW, Kulczycki A Jr (1979) Characterization of the IgE receptor isolated from human basophils. J Immunol 123:2283–2291
21. Hempstead BL, Parker CW, Kulczycki A Jr (1981) The cell surface receptor for IgE. Effect of tunicamycin on molecular properties of receptor from rat basophilic leukemia cells. J Biol Chem 256:10717–10723
22. Holowka D, Hartman H, Kanellopoulos J, Metzger H (1980) Association of the receptor for IgE with an endogenous polypeptide on rat basophilic leukemia cells. J Recept Res 1:41–68
23. Holowka D, Metzger H (1982) Further characterization of the β-component of the receptor for immunoglobulin E. Mol Immunol 19:219–227

24. Isersky C, Metzger H, Buell DN (1975) Cell cycle-associated changes in receptors for IgE during growth and differentiation of a rat basophilic leukemia cell line. J Exp Med 141:1147–1162
25. Isersky C, Rivera J, Segal DM, Triche T (1983) The fate of IgE bound to rat basophilic leukemia cells. II. Endocytosis of IgE oligomers and effect on receptor turnover. J Immunol 131:388–396
26. Isersky C, Taurog JD, Poy G, Metzger H (1978) Triggering of cultured neoplastic mast cells by antibodies to the receptor for IgE. J Immunol 121:549–558
27. Ishizaka T, Ishizaka K, Conrad DH, Froese A (1981) A new concept of triggering mechanisms of IgE-mediated histamine release. J Allergy Clin Immunol 61:320–330
28. Ishizaka K, Ishizaka T, Hornbrook MM (1966) Physiochemical properties of human reaginic antibody. IV. Presence of a unique immunoglobulin as a carrier of reaginic activity. J Immunol 97:75–85
29. Ishizaka K, Ishizaka T, Hornbrook MM (1966) Physiochemical properties of human reaginic antibody. V. Correlation of reaginic activity with γE-globulin antibody. J Immunol 97:840–853
30. Ishizaka K, Ishizaka T, Menzel AEO (1967) Physiochemical properties of human reaginic antibody. VI. Effect of heat on γE-, γG-, and γA-antibodies in the sera of ragweed sensitive patients. J Immunol 99: 610–618
31. Ishizaka K (1984) Regulation of IgE synthesis. In: Paul WE, Fathman CG, Metzger H (eds) Annual Review of Immunology 2:159–182. Annual Reviews, California
32. Ishizaka K, Tomioka H, Ishizaka T (1970) Mechanisms of passive sensitization. I. Presence of IgE and IgG molecules of human leukocytes. J Immunol 105:1459–1467
33. Ishizaka T, Soto C, Ishizaka K (1973) Mechanisms of passive sensitization. III. Number of IgE molecules and its receptor sites on human basophil granulocytes. J Immunol 111: 500–511
34. Johansson SGO, Bennich HH, Berg T (1972) The clinical significance of IgE. Prog Clin Immunol 1:165–171
35. Kaliner M (1984) Hypothesis on the contribution of late-phase allergic responses to the understanding and treatment of allergic diseases. J Allergy Clin Immunol 73:311–315
36. Kanellopoulos JM, Liu T-Y, Poy G, Metzger H (1980) Composition and subunit structure of the cell receptor for IgE. J Biol Chem 255:9060–9066
37. Kang B, Sulit N (1978) A comparative study of prevalence of skin hypersensitivity to cockroach and house dust antigens. Ann Allergy 41:333–336
38. Kaplan AP, Halbert E, Fauci A, Dinarello C (1984) A histamine releasing factor from human mononuclear cells. J Allergy Clin Immunol 73:120 (abstract)
39. Kay AB, Lee TH (1982) Neutrophil chemotactic factor of anaphylaxis. J Allergy Clin Immunol 70:317–320
40. Kozak PP, Gallup J, Cummins LH, Gillman SA (1980) Currently available methods for home mold surveys. II. Examples of problem homes surveyed. Ann Allergy 45:167–176
41. Kulczycki A Jr (1981) Role of immunoglobulin E and immunoglobulin E receptors in bronchial asthma. J Allergy Clin Immunol 68:5–14
42. Kulczycki A, Isersky C, Metzger H (1974) The interaction of IgE with rat basophilic leukemia cells. I. Evidence for specific binding of IgE. J Exp Med 139:600–616
43. Kulczycki A, McNearney TA, Parker CW (1976) The rat basophilic leukemia cell receptor for IgE. I. Characterization as a glycoprotein. J Immunol 117:661–665
44. Kulczycki A, Metzger H (1974) The interaction of IgE with rat basophilic leukemia cells. II. Quantitative aspects of the binding reaction. J Exp Med 140:1676–1695
45. Kulczycki A, Parker CW (1979) The cell-surface receptor for IgE. I. The use of repetitive affinity chromatography for the purification of a mammalian receptor. J Biol Chem 254: 3187–3193
46. Lim DT, Ganju A (1980) Reaginic sensitivity to mus musculus extract in a group of Chicago urban asthmatics. Ann Allergy 44:267–272
47. Melewicz FM, Plummer JM, Spiegelberg HL (1982) Comparison of the Fc receptors for IgE on human lymphocytes and monocytes. J Immunol 129:563–569
48. Morrison Smith J, Disney ME, Williams JD, Goels ZA (1969) Clinical significance of skin reaction to mite extracts in children with asthma. Br Med J 2:723–726
49. Nawata Y, Koike T, Yanagisawa T, Iwamoto I, Itaya T, Yoshida S, Tomioka H (1984) Anti-IgE autoantibody in patients with bronchial asthma. Clin Exp Immunol 58: 348–356
50. Parker CW, Schechtel L, Falkenhein S, Huber M (1983) Induction of IgE receptors on human lymphocytes. Immunol Commun 12:1–10
51. Perez-Montfort R, Metzger H (1982) Proteolysis of soluble IgE receptor complexes: localization of sites on IgE which interact with the Fc receptor. Mol Immunol 19:1113–1125

52. Perez-Montfort R, Kinet J-P, Metzger H (1983) A previously unrecognized subunit of the receptor for immunoglobulin E. Biochemistry 22:5722–5728
53. Rawle FC, Mitchell EB, Platts-Mills TAE (1984) T cell responses to the major allergen from the house dust mite dermatophagoides pteronyssinus, antigen P: Comparison of patients with asthma, atopic dermatitis, and perennial rhinitis. J Immunol 133:195–201
54. Simon RA, Pleskow WW, Stevenson DD, Mathison DA (1984) Aspirin sensitivity. In: Korenblat PE, Wedner HJ (eds) Allergy: Theory and Practice. Grune and Stratton, San Diego, pp 435–452
55. Spiegelberg HL, Simon RA (1981) Increase of lymphocytes with Fc receptors for IgE in patients with allergic rhinitis during the grass pollen season. J Clin Invest 68:845–852
56. Stevens WJ, Bridts CH (1984) IgG-containing and IgE-containing circulating immune complexes in patients with asthma and rhinitis. J Allergy Clin Immunol 73:276–282
57. Sullivan AL, Grimley PM, Metzger H (1971) Electron microscopic localization of IgE on the surface membrane of human basophils. J Exp Med 134:1403–1416
58. van Asperen PP, Mellis CM, South RT, Simpson SJ (1980) Allergen skin-prick testing in asthmatic children. Med J Aust 2:266–268
59. Yodoi J, Ishizaka K (1979) Lymphocytes bearing Fc receptors for IgE. I. Presence of human rat T lymphocytes with Fc_ϵ receptors. J Immunol 122:2577–2583
60. Yodoi J, Ishizaka T, Ishizaka K (1979) Lymphocytes bearing Fc receptors for IgE. II. Induction of Fc_ϵ-receptor bearing rat lymphocytes by IgE. J Immunol 123:455–462

11.2 IgE Receptors on Inflammatory Cells

A. Capron, J.-P. Dessaint, A. B. Tonnel

Formerly restricted to high affinity, monovalent binding to mast cells or basophils, the cellular interactions of IgE have been extended, now, to an array of cells. These include subpopulations of lymphocytes, the function of which might be to regulate the production of IgE itself [33, 42, 68] and many of the cells known to participate in inflammatory responses. Even if the production of many of the mediators of anaphylaxis were already attributed to inflammatory cells, the recent identification of IgE receptors on their surface leads one to reconsider the function of these cells in IgE-dependent reactions.

Interestingly, a dualistic role of IgE has emerged in addition with the demonstration that IgE antibodies can participate not only in hypersensitivity states, but also in immune defense, especially against helminth parasites.

It is beyond the scope of this review to analyze in detail all the experimental work which led to the identification of IgE receptors on inflammatory cells in rodents and in man. We shall concentrate instead on the essential characteristics of the Fc_ε receptors and on the possible consequences of IgE-dependent cell activation in inflammatory reactions.

11.2.1 Characteristics of IgE Receptors on Inflammatory Cells

The study of IgE receptors on inflammatory cells came from convergent observations made in our laboratory during the investigation of immunity in human schistosomiasis and in experimental *Schistosoma mansoni* infection of the rat. These parasitic models are characterized, as in many other helminthic infections, by a massive production of antiparasite IgE [20, 65], part of which is complexed with circulating schistosome antigens [68, 72].

The study of immunity to schistosomes pointed to antibody-dependent, cell-mediated cytotoxicity (ADCC) systems as prominent effector mechanisms, at least *in vitro* [8]. At variance with the tumor or allograft situation, however, ADCC against helminths did not involve lymphoid K-cells. Depending on the stage of immunity, macrophages, eosinophils and platelets were indeed identified as the effector cells responsible for parasite killing.

The essential role of IgE antibody in these ADCC systems was indicated by several experimental evidences:

- Selective absorption of IgE resulted in the abrogation of schistosome killing by macrophages, eosinophils or platelets;
- conversely, the addition of aggregated myeloma IgE protein induced a significant inhibition of the ADCC by immune serum in both rats and humans; and
- finally, schistosome targets could be killed by macrophages, eosinophils or platelets in the presence of an anti-schistosome monoclonal antibody of the IgE class in the rat model (Fig. 11.3) [9, 12, 14, 19, 36, 37].

These observations, made in experimental or human schistosomiasis, were confirmed in other helminthic infections [reviewed in 11], and the *in vivo* relevance of IgE-dependent cell-mediated cytotoxicity was shown in rat schistosomiasis by the passive transfer of immunity by each of the three cell types participating in ADCC [18, 36].

However suggestive of interactions between IgE and inflammatory cells, these observations in immune defense against helminths do not rule out the participation of IgE and mast cell interactions. At least in cytotoxicity by rat eosinophils, mast cells were indeed found to potentiate killing and, among their mediators, ECF-A tetrapeptides were found to enhance IgE-

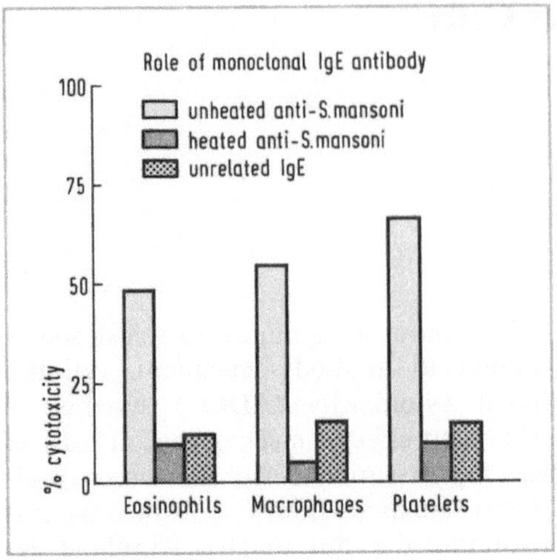

Fig. 11.3. Killing of *S. mansoni* schistosomula *in vitro* by rat eosinophils, macrophages and platelets incubated with a (rat) monclonal IgE antibody to *S. mansoni*

dependent, eosinophil-mediated cytotoxicity [15, 19].

Fc$_\varepsilon$ Receptors on Mononuclear Phagocytes

IgE receptors on mononuclear phagocytes were characterized by using several techniques. With peroxidase-labeled myeloma IgE protein, the specific binding of IgE to the surface of rat peritoneal macrophages could be demonstrated [23]. A rosette assay using fixed erythrocytes coated with either rat or human myeloma IgE protein showed that mononuclear phagocytes or macrophage/monocyte cell lines formed IgE rosettes in rats, mice and humans. The rosetting was specific for IgE since heated or reduced and alkylated IgE did not bind and IgG did not inhibit the rosetting [3, 5, 39, 49–51, 69].

The percentages of Fc$_\varepsilon$ receptor-positive cells varied in cells from different anatomical locations, monocytes showing lower percentages than peritoneal or alveolar macrophages. Interestingly, monocytes or alveolar macrophages from healthy donors formed a lower percentage of IgE rosettes than cells from patients with severe allergic disorders [39, 41, 52]. Likewise in the rat, infection by helminth parasites was associated with elevated percentages of Fc$_\varepsilon$ receptor-positive macrophages and the role of IgE in inducing this increase was demonstrated *in vitro* as well as *in vivo* [4, 60, 70]. Interferon γ was also shown to increase IgE receptor expression on the monocytic cell line U937 [54].

Saturable binding of radiolabeled monomeric IgE to human, rat or mouse mononuclear phagocytes can be demonstrated and the fixation is specifically inhibited by native IgE or its Fc$_\varepsilon$ fragment, but not by IgG [2, 23]. About 40,000–500,000 receptors per cell were detected and this number was increased in *Nippostrongylus brasiliensis*-infected rats, in rats bearing an IgE-producing myeloma or in rats injected with 5 mg IgE [70]. An average association constant of $0.8–6 \times 10^7$ M^{-1} for unaggregated IgE was measured, and monomeric IgE dissociated rapidly from the cells ($t_{1/2} \sim 2–3$ min) [2, 3, 26].

Dimeric IgE binds to rat macrophages with a higher association constant (2.3×10^8 M^{-1}) than monomers, and IgE dimers have a much slower rate of dissociation ($t_{1/2}$ 94 min) [26]. When the Fc$_\varepsilon$ receptor-positive human monocytic cell line U937 is incubated with radiolabeled IgE monomers or dimers, the binding of each label is competitively inhibited by a moderate ($\times 50$) excess of unlabeled dimers, when monomers do not inhibit significantly in these conditions [21].

An antiserum prepared against lymphocyte Fc$_\varepsilon$ receptors was shown to inhibit the binding of IgE to human monocytes or to U937 macrophage-like cells. This antiserum precipitated two surface components from U937 cells of approximately 47 and 23 kDa [50]. A chain with similarities with the β-chain of the receptor of rat basophilic leukemia cells has been identified in the Fc$_\varepsilon$ receptor of rat peritoneal macrophages [27].

Fc$_\varepsilon$ Receptors on Eosinophils

By using homologous IgE-coated erythrocytes, the rosetting of a significant proportion of rat or human eosinophils was obtained and the specificity of the binding was shown by inhibition with aggregated IgE, but not with IgG [15]. The binding of

IgE by eosinophils was also shown by ultrastructural studies [13, 31], by fixation of ^{125}I-labeled IgE [15, 19] and by time-course studies in experimental rat schistosomiasis, where surface-IgE could be detected on eosinophils from 5 weeks of infection onward by using anti-IgE-coated indicator cells [16, 18].

Both in hypereosinophilic patients and in *S. mansoni*-infected rats, an increase in the proportion of Fc_ε receptor-positive eosinophils was observed, an indication of a possible *in vivo* modulation of the expression by eosinophils of their receptor for IgE. Incubation of normal rat eosinophils with either purified myeloma IgE protein or with the reaginic antibodies in schistosome-infected rat serum indeed led to a dose-dependent increase in the proportion of Fc_ε receptor-positive eosinophils [16].

Besides IgE itself, other factors seem to participate in the modulation of eosinophil receptors for IgE. ECF-A tetrapeptides, in particular, were shown to induce *in vitro* a significant increase in the proportion of eosinophils forming IgE rosettes [16]. Another factor accounting for variations in the expression of Fc_ε receptors by eosinophils is related to the heterogeneity of these cells mainly in hypereosinophilic patients. In such patients, and particularly in those with the hypereosinophilic syndrome, blood eosinophils were mainly formed of abnormal light density cells with few granules (*hypodense* eosinophils), which bear an increased number of Fc_ε receptors [19], and exhibit a higher cytotoxic capacity than eosinophils with normal density [62].

The antiserum against the Fc_ε receptor of human lymphocytes was recently shown to inhibit also the formation of IgE rosettes by eosinophils from hypereosinophilic patients at the same dilution that previously reported to block IgE-dependent rosetting by lymphocytes, monocytes or macrophage-like cell lines [19].

Fc_ε Receptors on Platelets

The binding of IgE to platelets was shown by flow cytofluorometry with a monoclonal anti-IgE antibody and by using ^{125}I-labeled IgE myeloma protein, with approximately 6,000 sites on platelets and an average affinity constant of about 1.5×10^7 M^{-1}.

The binding of IgE was restricted to a fraction of rat or human platelets, ranging from 10–20% in controls and up to 50% in schistosome-infected rats or allergic patients [35].

Interestingly, the binding of IgE to platelets was inhibited also by the antiserum against the Fc_ε receptor of lymphocytes [10].

The Case of Neutrophils

No clear-cut evidence has yet been provided, that neutrophils could bind IgE. By using IgE-coated erythrocytes, no significant rosetting was observed with neutrophils [19], although it has been reported that in the mouse, neutrophils could interact with IgE-coated particles [46].

In the case of filarial parasites, complex cell-antibody interactions were identified, and a synergistic effect of IgG and IgE antibodies with complement and neutrophils has been suggested [1, 48].

Common Characteristics of Fc_ε Receptors on Inflammatory Cells

From these observations, several properties appear to be shared by IgE receptors on inflammatory cells:

- the binding of IgE with lower affinity than the Fc_ε receptor of mast cells or basophils;
- preferential interaction with aggregated or complexed IgE;
- presence on subpopulations of inflammatory cells, the percentage of Fc_ε receptor-bearing cells being directly or indirectly modulated by IgE itself; and
- common antigenicity distinct from the basophil receptor, as shown by the use of the antiserum against the anti-Fc_ε receptor. Confirming the observations made in immunity to schistosomes, this antiserum was shown to inhibit IgE antibody-dependent killing of the parasites by macrophages, eosinophils or platelets (Fig. 11.4) [10].

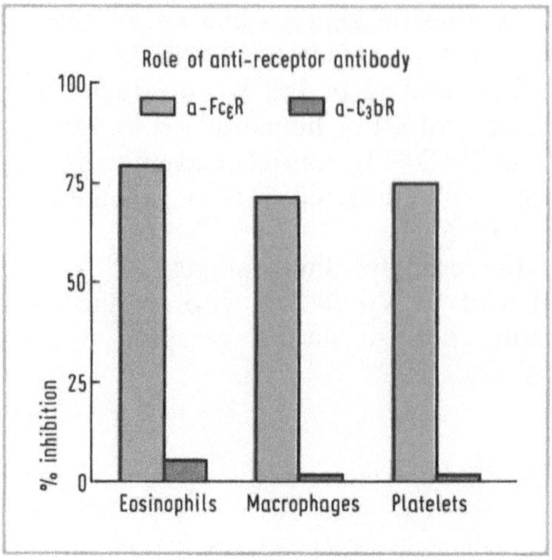

Fig. 11.4. Inhibition of IgE antibody-dependent cytotoxicity to *S. mansoni* schistosomula by an anti-receptor antibody against the Fc_ε receptor (a Fc_ε R) (a-C3b R = anti-C3b receptor (CR1) antibody)

11.2.2 Activation of Inflammatory Cells by IgE

The use of different molecular forms of myeloma IgE protein, from purified monomers to various sizes of polymers, together with IgE-anti-IgE reactions, has led to the study of some biochemical events associated with the activation of inflammatory cells. These can be summarized as follows:

- The binding of monomeric IgE does not induce any activating signal, the minimal degree of aggregation required being IgE dimers [24];
- the binding of IgE to macrophage receptors is followed by a rapid increase (10–15 min) of intracellular cyclic GMP in a calcium-dependent process. It is noticeable that these IgE-dependent changes are much faster than the IgG-dependent ones, which only appear to be optimal after 6 hours. It should also be stressed that the successive triggering of macrophages by IgG and IgE leads to a sustained activation while IgG added in a second step does not modify a previous triggering by IgE [24, 59]; and
- this activation process is also evidenced by many changes depending on the inflammatory cell considered, which ultimately can lead to cytotoxicity against targets corresponding to the specificity of the receptor-bound IgE.

Consequences of Macrophage Activation by IgE

Upon IgE-dependent triggering, mononuclear phagocytes were shown both in humans and rats: to secrete lysosomal enzymes or neutral proteases [22, 40, 41]; to release oxygen metabolites [40, 41]; and to produce arachidonic acid metabolites, including prostaglandins, prostacyclins, leukotriene C [58, 63, 64, 66, 67, 70] and PAF [41].

Interestingly, human alveolar macrophages successively incubated with the serum from allergic patients and with anti-human IgE, specifically released β-glucuronidase, excreted neutral proteases and produced the superoxide anion O_2^-. The release was dependent on IgE antibody in patients' sera, as shown by the disappearance of the anti-IgE-induced exocytosis after heating at 56 °C or after the depletion of IgE of the sensitizing serum. Alveolar macrophages collected from allergic patients or cultured with the serum from patients allergic to house mites or to grass pollen released lysosomal enzymes selectively with the addition of the specific allergen (+ 830% increase), and the depletion of IgE but not of IgG prevented enzyme release by the corresponding allergen [40, 41].

Eosinophil Activation by IgE

Since markers of eosinophil activation are poorly defined, most of the information on the consequences of their interaction with anaphylactic antibodies or complexes are drawn from cytotoxicity systems. The triggering of eosinophils by IgE immune complexes can also account for their preferential phagocytosis by the cell [29, 32, 74].

By measuring the extracellular release of rat eosinophil peroxidase, it was shown that IgE-anti-IgE induced the release of up to 26% of the cellular content of the enzymes. Accordingly, eosinophil peroxidase was released by eosinophils from schistosome-infected rats collected at the period when IgE antibody-dependent cytotoxicity could be demonstrated, upon the addition of anti-rat IgE or schistosome antigens [43].

Platelet Activation by IgE

Oxygen metabolite generation was found to be stimulated by successive incubation of normal platelets with IgE and anti-IgE or with serum from allergic patients and anti-IgE. In the latter situation, previous absorption of IgE from allergic serum prevented platelet triggering by anti-IgE. Furthermore, platelets collected from allergic donors were triggered to release oxygen metabolites by the addition of the corresponding allergen or anti-IgE antibody, but not by unrelated antigens or anti-IgG [35].

In conclusion, both in ADCC to schistosomes and by assaying appropriate biochemical markers of activation, it was found that inflammatory cells exposed to IgE molecules could be selectively activated when IgE was specifically complexed or nonspecifically aggregated. Although it is clear that the massive production of IgE and immune IgE complexes in helminthic disease is favorable to the *in vivo* expression of IgE-dependent immune reaction, the direct participation via their IgE receptors of inflammatory cells in adverse reactions may also be questioned.

11.2.3 Participation of IgE Receptor-bearing Inflammatory Cells in Human Pathology

Role of IgE immune complexes: As far as ADCC reactions against helminths are considered, the involvement of antiparasite IgE antibody, as complexed with parasite antigen, was indicated by several experimental evidences:

- Inhibition experiments using rat myeloma IgE added to the immune rat serum during the incubation with the macrophages showed that disaggregated IgE protein exerted little inhibitory activity contrary to chemically cross-linked IgE, which prevented schistosomula killing [38];
- the inducing factor in the immune rat serum was absorbed out not only by *S. mansoni* antigen but also by anti-*S. mansoni* immunosorbent [12];
- immune complexes containing both antiparasite IgE antibody and schistosome antigen were characterized in the immune rat serum [68];
- ultracentrifugation of the immune serum and separate testing of the supernatant and the pellet showed that only the latter induced macrophage killing. Almost all antiparasite IgE antibody and 69% of the total circulating *S. mansoni* antigen were characterized in this pellet, and the role of IgE to induce macrophage killing was confirmed by demonstrating that heating the pellet at 56 °C abolished the cytotoxic reaction. Thus, IgE antibody triggers normal cells to kill the homologous target predominantly when complexed with circulating parasite antigen, in the form of IgE antibody-excess immune complexes [12].

These observations have to be related with the demonstration of circulating immune IgE complexes in allergic patients. Such IgE complexes have indeed been characterized, especially after oral allergen challenge [7]. The frequency of circulating IgE complexes appears significantly elevated in patients with allergic asthma or rhinitis [71]. Furthermore, anti-IgE autoantibody can be detected in 95.5% of patients with allergic asthma, which can form circulating complexes with self-IgE [55]. That raises the question of the participation of IgE complexes in the pathogenesis of allergic reactions, all the more as local formation of such complexes may be assumed, resulting from local exposure to the allergen when (free) anaphylactic antibodies circulate.

Presence of IgE on inflammatory cells in human diseases: Surface-bound IgE can indeed be characterized on inflammatory cells in various diseases. In the case of eosinophils for instance, cytophilic IgE could be detected by flow microfluorometry with anti-IgE on about 75% of the cells from patients with hypereosinophilia. A significant increase in the percentage of IgE-bearing cells was found in those patients with elevated serum-IgE levels (>240 kU/l). In patients with the PIE syndrome, eosinophils collected by bronchoalveolar lavage showed higher percentages of surface-bound IgE than blood cells [17]. Similarly, IgE could be detected on a fraction of nasal eosinophils [29]. Interestingly, a very low percentage of blood, nasal or lung eosinophils was found to bear cytophilic IgG [17, 29].

Similar observations were made with bronchoalveolar macrophages from asthmatic patients [41] and with platelets from allergic asthmatics [35].

IgE-dependent activation of inflammatory cells in vivo: The recent reports that macrophages, after their interaction with IgE immune complexes, can release leukotriene C and other arachidonic acid metabolites [63, 64, 66, 67, 70] and PAF-acether [41] suggest that the release of many mediators of immediate-type hypersensitivity can in fact be the result of interactions between mononuclear phagocytes and IgE. Another study showed that human monocytes had an enhanced phagocytic activity and displayed specific *in vitro* cytotoxicity for IgE-coated erythrocytes, this cytotoxicity being highly correlated to the percentage of monocytes bearing Fc_ε receptors [51]. This IgE-dependent cytotoxicity of blood monocytes was increased in patients with severe atopic disease, whose monocytes bear more IgE receptors [53].

The demonstration that alveolar macrophages from asthmatic patients bear surface-IgE but can also be triggered specifically via their surface-IgE is also strongly suggestive [39, 41]. For instance, after incubation with anti-IgE or the specific allergen, macrophages from allergic asthmatics, collected by bronchoalveolar lavage, could release a chemotactic factor for neutrophils and eosinophils [30].

Interestingly, the IgE-dependent release of β-glucuronidase by macrophages from allergic patients was inhibited by a 15 min treatment of the cells with anti-inflammatory drugs, such as disodium cromoglycate, methylprednisolone, or β_2-mimetics each at a concentration of 100 ng/ml *in vitro.* The inhibition was more effective for allergen-induced exocytosis, which probably involves a smaller number of Fc_ε receptors, than for anti-IgE-induced release which concerns the whole of IgE molecules on the macrophage surface [39].

Finally, supportive evidence of the participation of alveolar macrophages in allergic reactions has been brought about by the decrease in macrophage concentrations of lysosomal enzymes found after a local provocation test, while the enzyme levels in bronchoalveolar lavage fluids were significantly higher than in the control lung [75].

Although the exact role of eosinophils in allergic reactions through their activation by anaphylactic antibodies remains to be evaluated, it should be pointed out that the same eosinophil subpopulation, (i.e., hypodense cells), is identified in the tissue lesions of the hypereosinophilic syndrome and demonstrates higher cytotoxic capability in the presence of IgE. The cross-linking of IgE antibody molecules by the antigens may lead to the release of very active mediators, among which the cationic proteins showing toxic properties against tracheal epithelium [28], heart cells [73] or nervous cells [25] and also the peroxidase system shown to be tumoricidal [34] are especially interesting in the context of human pathology associated to eosinophils. In this respect, a previous study has clearly shown the presence of ruptured eosinophils and free eosinophil granules on lung biopsy specimens obtained in the acute phase of eosinophilic pneumonia, and their association with high levels of IgE, leading the authors to postulate a role of eosinophil degranulation in the pathogenesis of this disease [47]. Coming back to the possibility of eosinophils to participate in allergic reactions, it should be noted that the granule components were found to potentiate histamine release by basophils or mast cells [56] and to release smooth muscle-active mediators like PAF or leukotriene C_4 [6, 45].

Finally, platelet accumulation within the pulmonary vessels and platelet activation have been reported to be associated with bronchospasm in humans or in experimental models [44, 57, 61, 76]. In this respect, the release of platelet activating factor by macrophages activated by IgE [41] should be kept in mind, all the more since the results mentioned above indicate the possibility of direct activation of platelets by IgE.

11.2.4 Conclusions

The characterization of IgE receptors on inflammatory cells has enlarged our knowledge of the cellular interactions of IgE molecules. There is now much evidence that IgE not only can bind to inflammatory cells like mononuclear phagocytes, eosinophils or platelets, but also specifically trigger these cells. The presence of IgE immune complexes, either circulating or formed locally, facilitates the fixation of aggregated IgE to its Fc_{ε} receptors on inflammatory cells, when free IgE will dissociate rapidly. The circumstantial evidence gained in the study of allergic patients or individuals with hypereosinophilia opens fascinating views on an alternative pathway in immediate-type hypersensitivity, in addition to the classical activation of mast cells or basophils by IgE. These observations will undoubtedly have, in the near future, an important input into our understanding of many areas of human pathology, and especially in hypereosinophilic syndromes and allergic diseases.

References

1. Aime N, Haque A, Bonnel B, Torpier G, Capron A (1984) Neutrophil-mediated killing of *Dipetalonema viteae* microfilariae: simultaneous presence of IgE, IgG antibodies and complement is required. Immunology 51:585–594
2. Anderson CL, Spiegelberg HL (1981) Macrophage receptors for IgE: binding of IgE to specific IgE Fc receptors on a human macrophage cell line, U937. J Immunol 116: 2470–2473
3. Boltz-Nitulescu G, Plummer JM, Spiegelberg HL (1982) Fc receptors for IgE on mouse macrophages and macrophage-like cell lines. J Immunol 128:2265–2268
4. Boltz-Nitulescu G, Plummer JM, Spiegelberg HL (1984) Increased expression of the IgE-Fc receptors on rat macrophages induced by elevated IgE levels. Immunology 53:9–16
5. Boltz-Nitulescu G, Spiegelberg HL (1981) Receptors specific for IgE on rat alveolar and peritoneal macrophages. Cell Immunol 59:106–114
6. Borgeat P, Fruteau de Laclos B, Rabinovitch H, Picard S, Braquet P, Hebert J, Laviolette P (1984) Eosinophil-rich human polymorphonuclear leukocyte preparations characteristically release leukotriene C_4 on ionophore A23187 challenge. J Allergy Clin Immunol 74:310–315
7. Brostoff J, Stanworth DR, Johns P (1977) Immune complexes in atopy. Lancet I:741–744
8. Capron A, Capron M, Dessaint JP (1980) ADCC as primary mechanisms of defence against metazoan parasites. In: Fougereau M, Dausset J (eds) Immunology 80, Progress in Immunology IV. Academic Press, London, pp 782–793
9. Capron A, Dessaint JP, Capron M, Bazin H (1975) Specific IgE antibodies in immune adherence of normal macrophages to *Schistosoma mansoni* schistosomules. Nature 253:474–475
10. Capron A, Dessaint JP, Capron M, Joseph M (1983) Effector mechanisms against schistosomes. In: Yamamura Y, Tada T (eds) Progress in Immunology V. Academic Press, New York, pp 1305–1316
11. Capron A, Dessaint JP, Haque A, Capron M (1982) Antibody-dependent cell-mediated cytotoxicity against parasites. Prog Allergy 31:234–267
12. Capron A, Dessaint JP, Joseph M, Rousseaux R, Capron M, Bazin H (1977) Interaction between IgE complexes and macrophages in the rat: a new mechanism of macrophage activation. Eur J Immunol 7:315–322
13. Capron A, Dessaint JP, Joseph M, Torpier G, Capron M, Rousseaux R, Santoro F, Bazin H (1977) IgE and cells in schistosomiasis. Am J Trop Med Hyg 26:39–46
14. Capron M, Bazin H, Joseph M, Capron A (1981) Evidence for IgE-dependent cytotoxicity by rat eosinophils. J Immunol 126:1764–1768
15. Capron M, Capron A, Dessaint JP, Johansson SGO, Prin L (1981) Fc receptors for IgE on human and rat eosinophils. J Immunol 126:2087–2092
16. Capron M, Capron A, Joseph M, Verwaerde C (1983) IgE receptors on phagocytic cells and immune response to schistosoma infection. Monogr Allergy 18:33–44
17. Capron M, Kusnierz JP, Prin L, Spiegelberg HL, Khalife J, Tonnel AB, Capron A (1985)

Cytophilic IgE on human blood and tissue eosinophils. In: 15th Symposium, Collegium Internationale Allergologium. Int Arch Allergy Appl Immunol 77:246–248
18. Capron M, Nogueira-Queiroz JA, Papin JP, Capron A (1984) Interaction between eosinophils and antibodies. *In vivo* protective role against rat schistosomes. Cell Immunol 83:60–72
19. Capron M, Spiegelberg HL, Prin L, Bennich H, Butterworth AE, Pierce RJ, Ouaissi MA, Capron A (1984) Role of IgE receptors in effector function of human eosinophils. J Immunol 132:462–468
20. Dessaint JP, Capron M, Bout D, Capron A (1975) Quantitative determination of specific IgE antibodies to schistosome antigens and serum IgE levels in patients with schistosomiasis (*S. mansoni,* or *S. haematobium*). Clin Exp Immunol 20:427–436
21. Dessaint JP, Capron A, Joseph M, Auriault C, Pestel J (1983) Macrophage-mediated IgE ADCC to helminth parasites and IgE-dependent macrophage activation. In: Koren HS (ed) Macrophage Mediated Antibody. Marcel Dekker, New York, pp 315–338
22. Dessaint JP, Capron A, Joseph M, Bazin H (1979) Cytophilic binding of IgE to the macrophage. II. Immunologic release of lysosomal enzyme from macrophages by IgE and IgE in the rat: a new mechanism of macrophage activation. Cell Immunol 46:24–34
23. Dessaint JP, Torpier G, Capron M, Bazin H, Capron A (1979) Cytophilic binding of IgE to the macrophage. I. Binding characteristics of IgE on the surface of macrophages in the rat. Cell Immunol 46:12–23
24. Dessaint JP, Waksman BH, Metzger H, Capron A (1980) Cytophilic binding of IgE to the macrophage. III. Involvement of cyclic GMP and calcium in macrophage activation by dimeric or aggreated rat myeloma IgE. Cell Immunol 51:280–292
25. Durack DT, Ackerman SJ, Loegering DA, Gleich GJ (1981) Purification of human eosinophil-derived neurotoxin. Proc Natl Acad Sci USA 78:5165–5169
26. Finbloom DS, Metzger H (1982) Binding of immunoglobulin E to the receptor on rat peritoneal macrophages. J Immunol 129: 2004–2008
27. Finbloom DS, Metzger H (1983) Isolation of cross-linked IgE-receptor complexes from rat macrophages. J Immunol 30:1489–1491
28. Frigas E, Loegering DA, Gleich GJ (1980) Cytotoxic effects of the guinea pig eosinophil major basic protein on tracheal epithelium. Lab Invest 42:35–43
29. Fujita Y, Rubinstein E, Greco DB, Reisman RE, Arbesman CE (1975) Antigen-antibody complexes in or on eosinophils in nasal secretions. Int Arch Allergy 48:577–583
30. Gosset P, Tonnel AB, Joseph M, Prin L, Mallart A, Charon J, Capron A (1984) Secretion of a chemotactic factor for neutrophils and eosinophils by alveolar macrophages from asthmatic patients. J Allergy Clin Immunol 74:827–834
31. Hubscher T (1975) Role of the eosinophil in the allergic reactions. I. EDI An eosinophil derived inhibitor of histamine release. J Immunol 114:1379–1388
32. Ishikawa T, Wicher K, Arbesman CE (1974) *In vitro* and *in vivo* studies on uptake of antigen-antibody complexes by eosinophils. Int Arch Allergy Appl Immunol 46:230–248
33. Ishizaka K (1984) Isotype-specific regulation of the IgE response. In: Yamamura Y, Tada T (eds) Progress in Immunology V. Academic Press, New York, pp 455–464
34. Jong EC, Klebanoff SJ (1980) Eosinophil-mediated mammalian tumor cell cytotoxicity: role of the peroxidase system. J Immunol 124:1948–1953
35. Joseph M, Ameisen JC, Kusnierz JP, Pancre V, Capron M, Capron A (1984) Participation du récepteur pour l'IgE à la toxicité des plaquettes sanguines contre les schistosomes. CR Acad Sci Paris 298:55–60
36. Joseph M, Auriault C, Capron A, Vorng H, Viens P (1983) A role for platelets in IgE-dependent killing of schistosomes. Nature 303:810–811
37. Joseph M, Capron A, Butterworth AE, Sturrock RF, Houba V (1978) Cytotoxicity of human and baboon mononuclear phagocytes against schistosomula *in vitro:* induction by immune complexes containing IgE and Schistosoma mansoni antigens. Clin Exp Immunol 33:45–56
38. Joseph M, Dessaint JP, Capron A (1977) Characteristics of macrophage cytotoxicity induced by IgE immune complexes. Cell Immunol 34:247–258
39. Joseph M, Tonnel AB, Capron A, Dessaint JP (1981) The interaction of IgE antibody with human alveolar macrophages and its participation in the inflammatory processes of lung allergy. Agents Action 11:619–622
40. Joseph M, Tonnel A, Capron A, Voisin C (1980) Enzyme release and superoxide anion production by human alveolar macrophages stimulated with immunoglobulin E. Clin Exp Immunol 40:416–422
41. Joseph M, Tonnel AB, Torpier G, Capron A, Arnoux A, Benveniste J (1983) Involvement of immunoglobulin E in the secretory processes of alveolar macrophages from asthmatic patients. J Clin Invest 71:221–230

42. Katz DH, Marcelletti JF (1984) Regulation of the IgE antibody system in humans and experimental animals. In: Yamamura Y, Tada T (eds) Progress in Immunology V. Academic Press, New York, pp 465–482
43. Khalife J, Capron M, Grzych JM, Bazin H, Capron A (1985) Extracellular release of rat eosinophil peroxidase (EPO). I. Role of Anaphylactic Immunoglobulins. J Immunol 134:1968–1974
44. Knauer LA, Lichtenstein LM, Adkinson NF, Fish JE (1981) Platelet activation during antigen-induced airway reactions in asthmatic subjects. N Engl J Med 304:1404–1407
45. Lee TC, Lenihan DJ, Malone B, Roddy LL, Wasserman SI (1984) Increased biosynthesis of Platelet-activating factor in activated human eosinophils. J Biol Chem 259:5526–5530
46. Lopez AF, Strath M, Sanderson CJ (1983) Mouse immunoglobulin isotypes mediatory cytotoxicity of target cells by eosinophils and neutrophils. Immunology 48:503–509
47. McEvoy JDS, Donald KJ, Edwards PL (1978) Immunoglobulin level and electron microscopy in eosinophil pneumonia. Am J Med 64:529–536
48. Mehta K, Sindhu RK, Subrahmanyam D, Nelson DS (1980) IgE-dependent adherence and cytotoxicity of rat spleen and peritoneal cells to *Litomosoides carinii* microfilaria. Clin Exp Immunol 41:107–114
49. Melewicz FM, Kline LE, Cohen AB, Spiegelberg HL (1982) Characterization of Fc receptors for IgE on human alveolar macrophages. Clin Exp Immunol 49:364–370
50. Melewicz FM, Plummer JM, Spiegelberg HL (1982) Comparison of the Fc receptors for IgE on human lymphocytes and monocytes. J Immunol 129:563–569
51. Melewicz FM, Spiegelberg HL (1980) Fc receptors for IgE on a subpopulation of human peripheral blood monocytes. J Immunol 125:1026–1031
52. Melewicz FM, Zeiger RS, Mellon MH, O'Connor RD, Spiegelberg HL (1981) Increased peripheral blood monocytes with Fc receptors for IgE in patients with severe allergic disorders. J Immunol 126:1592–1595
53. Melewicz FM, Zeiger RS, Mellon MH, O'Connor RD, Spiegelberg HL (1981) Increased IgE-dependent cytotoxicity by blood mononuclear cells of allergic patients. Clin Exp Immunol 43:526–533
54. Náray-Fejes-Tóth A, Guyre PM (1984) Recombinant human immune interferon induces increased IgE receptor expression on the human monocyte cell line U-937. J Immunol 133:1914–1919
55. Nawata Y, Koike T, Yanagisawa T, Iwamoto I, Itaya T, Yoshida S, Tomioka H (1984) Anti-IgE autoantibody in patients with bronchial asthma. Clin Exp Immun 58:348–356
56. O'Donnell MC, Ackerman SJ, Gleich GJ, Thomas LL (1983) Activation of basophil and mast cell histamine release by eosinophil granule major basic protein. J Exp Med 157:1981–1991
57. Page CP, Paul W, Morley J (1984) Platelets and bronchospasm. Int Arch Allergy 74:347–350
58. Passwell JH, Geiger B, Levanon M, Davidsohn J, Cohen BE, Ramot B (1984) IgE induces secretion of prostaglandin E_2 by human monocytes. Clin Exp Immunol 58:566–572
59. Pestel J, Dessaint JP, Joseph M, Bazin H, Capron A (1984) Macrophage triggering by aggregated immunoglobulins. II. Comparison of IgE and IgG aggregates or immune complexes. Clin Exp Immunol 57:404–412
60. Pestel J, Joseph M, Dessaint JP, Capron A (1986) Variation in the expression of macrophage Fc_ε receptors in relation to schistosome infection. Clin Exp Immunol (in press)
61. Pinckard RN, Halonen M, Palmer JD, Botler C, Shaw JP, Henson PM (1977) Intravascular aggregation and pulmonary sequestration of platelets during IgE-induced systemic anaphylaxis in the rabbit: abrogation of lethal anaphylactic shock by platelet depletion. J Immunol 119:2185–2193
62. Prin L, Capron M, Tonnel AB, Bletry O, Capron A (1983) Heterogeneity of human peripheral blood eosinophils: variability in cell density and cytotoxic ability in relation to the level and origin of hypereosinophilia. Int Arch Allergy Appl Immunol 72:336–346
63. Rankin JA, Hitchcock M, Merrill WW, Bach MK, Brashler JR, Askenase PW (1982) IgE-dependent release of leukotriene C_4 from alveolar macrophages. Nature 297:329–331
64. Rankin JA, Hitchock M, Merrill WW, Huang SS, Brashler JR, Bach MK, Askenase PW (1984) IgE immune complexes induce immediate and prolonged release of leukotriene C_4 (LTC_4) from rat alveolar macrophages. J Immunol 132:1993–1999
65. Rousseaux-Prévost R, Capron M, Bazin H, Capron A (1978) IgE in experimental schistosomiasis. II. Quantitative determination of specific IgE antibodies against *S. mansoni:* a follow-up study of two strains of infected rats. Correlation with protective immunity. Immunology 35:33–39
66. Rouzer CA, Scott WA, Hamill AL, Liu FT, Katz DH, Cohn ZA (1982) IgE immune complexes stimulate arachidonic acid release by mouse peritoneal macrophages. Proc Natl Acad Sci USA 79:5656–5660

67. Rouzer CA, Scott WA, Hamill AL, Liu FT, Katz DH, Cohn ZA (1982) Secretion of leukotriene C and other arachidonic acid metabolites by macrophages challenged with immunoglobulin E immune complexes. J Exp Med 156:1077–1086
68. Santoro F, Capron M, Joseph M, Rousseaux-Prévost R, Capron A (1978) Circulating antigens and immune complexes in *Schistosoma mansoni*-infected rats. Characterization by radioimmunoprecipitation-PEG assay (RIPEGA). Clin Exp Immunol 32:435–442
69. Spiegelberg HL (1984) Structure and function of Fc receptors for IgE on lymphocytes, monocytes and macrophages. Adv Immunol 35:61–88
70. Spiegelberg HL, Boltz-Nitulescu B, Plummer JM, Melewicz FM (1983) Characterization of the IgE Fc receptors on monocytes and macrophages. Fed Proc 42:124–128
71. Stevens WJ, Bridts CH (1984) IgG-containing and IgE-containing circulating immune complexes in patients with asthma and rhinitis. J Allergy Clin Immunol 73:276–282
72. Stevens WJ, Feldmeier H, Bridts CH, Daffalla AA (1983) IgG and IgE circulating immune complexes, total serum IgE and parasite related IgE in patients with mono- or mixed infection with *Schistosoma mansoni* and/or *S. haematobium*. Influence of therapy. Clin Exp Immunol 52:142–152
73. Tai PC, Hayes DJ, Clark JB, Spry CJF (1982) Toxic effects of human eosinophil secretion products on isolated rat heart cells *in vitro*. Biochem J 204:75–80
74. Takenaka T, Okuda M, Kawabori S, Kubo K (1977) Extracellular release of peroxidase from eosinophils by interaction with immune complexes. Clin Exp Immunol 28:56–60
75. Tonnel AB, Joseph M, Gosset P, Fournier E (1983) Stimulation of alveolar macrophages in asthmatic patients after local provocation test. Lancet 8339:1406–1408
76. Vargaftig BB, Lefort J, Chignard M, Benveniste J (1980) Platelet-activating factor induces a platelet-dependent bronchoconstriction unrelated to the formation of prostaglandin derivatives. Eur J Pharmacol 65:185–192

12. Immunological Mechanisms

C. W. Parker

In view of the central role of IgE antibodies in the immunology of allergic asthma, much research effort has been directed toward defining the basis for the increased IgE antibody levels in susceptible individuals. While there is little doubt that IgE biosynthesis is increased in familial respiratory allergy the basis for the increase is uncertain. IgE-producing B-lymphocytes appear to be derived from a pool of precursor cells which initially produce only cytoplasmic IgM but later express both IgM and IgD on their surfaces. Eventually a commitment is made to produce a single class of immunoglobulin but even though this immunoglobulin may be secreted in large quantities other types of immunoglobulins may still be present on the cell surface [1]. The percentage of cells which ultimately become IgE-producing cells is ordinarily well below 10% even in respiratory organs but under conditions of markedly increased IgE biosynthesis (as in certain parasitic infections) the proportion is considerably increased, particularly in regional nodes near sites of active infection [2]. The capacity to markedly increase IgE biosynthesis in response to an appropriate stimulus indicates that B-cells are subject to regulatory influences which markedly affect IgE production. While a variety of mechanisms for the control of IgE synthesis are possible, current emphasis is centering on the possible role of helper or suppressor T-cells that have selectivity for the IgE system. Evidence based primarily on animal studies is accumulating that soluble factors released by T-cells may directly affect the biosynthesis of various immunoglobulin classes including IgE [3–5]. While evidence exists for the presence of isotype specific regulation of overall IgE synthesis there is also data indicating the existence of antigen-specific factors affecting IgE biosynthesis which may help control IgE responses at the individual antigen level [6]. The physicochemical properties of the various regulatory factors and their importance in immune regulation *in vivo* is only beginning to be elucidated. While a number of laboratories have described such factors, considerable disagreement exists in regard to their chemical characteristics [3–5]. One attractive mechanism for regulation might involve T-cells or B-cells with IgE receptors on their surfaces. IgE receptors have recently been demonstrated on T-cells, B-cells, macrophages and eosinophils in addition to their long recognized presence on basophils and mast cells [7]. The existence of IgE receptor molecules at these locations may permit the cells to respond selectively to IgE, particularly when the IgE is bound to antigen in the form of a multimeric complex [8]. Cross-linking by IgE and antigen may stimulate the release of IgE receptor-bearing molecules or other products into the cell supernatants where they may then act as soluble mediators to control further IgE biosynthesis [3, 4]. The possible role of direct cell-cell interactions involving IgE molecules bound to several different cell types simultaneously also deserves attention. Control may also be produced by mediators released in IgE-dependent reactions. Mediators of immediate hypersensitivity such as histamine have been shown to alter specific T-cell functions and under appropriate circumstances antibody production by B-cells *in vitro* may be suppressed [9, 10].

Any attempts to understand the role of IgE in allergy must deal with local as well as systemic IgE biosynthesis. The best data available would indicate that most of the IgE in secretions in the respiratory tract is synthesized locally rather than systemically in plasma cells within and below the respiratory mucosa [11]. The extent to which B-lymphocytes which are producing or have the potential to produce IgE antibodies are selectively localized in the respiratory mucosa and whether or not they are subject to regional rather than systemic control at this location remains to be clarified.

While it has been argued that the proteins in pollens which are the most effective allergens tend to show similarities in structure, it is nonetheless clear that airborne allergens can include a broad range of molecules with differing physicochemical properties and may even include small molecular weight chemicals such as penicillin which have to combine with endogenous proteins in order to elicit a hypersensitivity response [12]. Another level of immunologic control in allergic asthma relates to the presence of marked differences in the patterns of allergic reactivity between different allergic individuals. One individual with allergic rhinitis or asthma may be primarily sensitive to trees, another to grasses or ragweed and a third responds to perennial allergens. Some individuals exhibit a broad spectrum of allergies with reactions to essentially every allergen that is tested, but in others an apparently isolated allergy is present. Since the dose of airborne allergens encountered by allergic and nonallergic individuals is low allergic responsiveness may in part be a threshold phenomenon where individuals who are best able to respond to low concentrations of allergen are selected. Certainly there is no convincing evidence that mucosal permeability to antigen, per se, is an important controlling feature.

Because of the well-recognized relationship between major histocompatibility (MHC) antigens and immune responsiveness, linkage studies have been performed in allergic families with large numbers of surviving members. Seven families with allergic rhinitis produced by ragweed were studied by Levine et al [13]. In 20 of 26 individuals apparent linkage was observed between skin reactivity to ragweed allergen and inheritance of a particular parental HLA haplotype (which, however, differed from one family to another). In 20 individuals with other haplotypes, very little or no allergic reactivity was observed. Similar conclusions were drawn by Blumenthal et al [14] in a single large family with 57 members where the presence of IgE antibodies to ragweed appeared to be correlated with the HLA-A 12 haplotype. However, later studies by this group suggested a closer relationship to the HLA-D locus. Marsh et al [15] concluded that with the exception of relatively simple allergens such as ragweed Ra-5, linkage of IgE antibody formation to the MHC was no more marked for ragweed antigen than for other purified pollen antigens. Other studies have suggested a possible linkage of HLA-A or HLA-B antigens to the presence or absence of idiopathic asthma or to the particular combination of target organs (nasal passages, bronchi or skin) affected by IgE allergy in a given individual [1]. Genetic influences on allergy are also possible at the level of tissue receptors for allergic mediators or IgE, mast cell number, reactivity or mediator content, mediator catabolism or end organ reactivity. So regardless of the basis for the increased IgE-forming capacity in allergic individuals a variety of other factors are undoubtedly of importance in determining the distribution and magnitude of allergic symptoms.

In considering the immunology of allergic asthma it is also important to keep in mind that IgE is produced in the presence of antibodies in other immunoglobulin classes of the same specificity which may, by competing for antigen or other mechanisms help regulate IgE biosynthesis. Moreover, there may be suppressor cells which affect the overall response to an antigen rather than its distribution in particular immunoglobulin classes such as IgE. Non-IgE-antibodies may also compete with IgE antibodies for antigen in the allergic target tissue tending to dampen the allergic response. The possibility that some immediate hypersensitivity reactions may not be IgE-dependent also must be born in mind. There is convincing evidence that IgG_4 can also produce immediate hypersensitivity responses although the time of maximal sensitization differs from that for IgE [12] under appropriate circumstances. Even IgG or IgM antibodies can release mediators from mast cells. This may occur when the complement is activated and polypeptide fragments with direct mediator releasing properties derived primarily from C5 and C3 (anaphylatoxins) are produced [10]. Secretion from mast cells may also be produced by the 2-acetyl-1-alkyl phosphorocholines (platelet activating factors) and various kinins which have the property of stimulating secretion from mast cells and leukocytes whereas adenosine, acetylcholine and several polypeptides of importance in the nervous system may markedly enhance the response. Additional factors which may be of importance include histamine releasing lymphokines produced by T-lymphocytes which alone or in the presence of other modulatory agents such as the interferons may directly affect mast cell or basophil secretion. Another T-cell product which may affect mast cells although the nature of the effect is very different is the lymphokine interleukin 3 [16], IL-3, which stimulates mast cell replication. IL-3 is produced by T-lymphocytes under conditions of mitogenic stimulation providing a mechanism through which T-cells undergoing antigen-dependent reactions might expand the number of mast cells in their local environment. Taken together these various observations indicate that the humoral and cellular immune responses are tightly linked to one another and cannot be considered as isolated systems. Interrelations between these two systems may ultimately be of critical importance in determining both the level of IgE antibodies and their effectiveness in producing allergic inflammation.

References

1. Teale JM, Klinman NR (1984) Control of the production of different classes of antibody. In: Paul WE (ed) Fundamental Immunology. Raven Press, New York, pp 519–535
2. Sedgewick JD, Holt PG (1983) Kinetics and distribution of antigen-specific IgE-secreting cells during the primary antibody response in the rat. J Exp Med 157:2178
3. Ishizaka K (1983) IgE-binding factors from rat T lymphocytes. Lymphokines 8:41–80
4. Kishimoto T, Suemura M, Sugimura K, Okada M, Nakanishi K, Yamamura Y (1982) Characterizations of T cell-derived immunoregulatory molecules from murine or human T hybridomas. Lymphokines 5:129–160
5. Katz D (1982) IgE antibody responses in vitro: from rodents to man. Prog Allergy 32:105–160
6. Tada T (1975) Regulation of reaginic antibody formation in animals. Prog Allergy 19:122–126
7. Spiegelberg HL (1981) Lymphocytes bearing Fc receptors for IgE. Immunol Rev 56:199–218
8. Parker CW, Schechtel T, Falkenhein S, Huber M (1983) Induction of IgE receptors on human lymphocytes. Immunol Commun 12:1–10
9. Rocklin RE (1976) Modulation of cellular immune responses *in vivo* and *in vitro* by histamine receptor bearing lymphocytes. J Clin Invest 57:1051–1058
10. Parker CW (1984) Mediators: release and function. In: Paul WE (ed) Fundamental Immunology. Raven Press, New York, pp 697–747
11. Platts-Mills TAE (1979) Local production of IgG, IgA, and IgE antibodies in grass pollen hay fever. J Immunol 122:2218–2518
12. Parker CW (1984) Asthma and Rhinitis. In: Parker CW (ed) Clinical Immunology. Saunders, Philadelphia, p 1372
13. Levine FB, Stember RH, Fotino M (1972) Ragweed hay fever: Genetic control and linkage to HL-A haplotypes. Science 178:1201
14. Blumenthal MN, Amos DB, Noreen H, Mendell NR, Yunis EJ (1974) Genetic mapping of Ir locus in man: Linkage to second locus of HL-A. Science 184:1301–1303
15. Marsh DG, Bias WB, Ishizaka K (1975) Allergens and the genetics of allergy. In: Sela M (ed) The Antigens, vol. III. Academic Press, New York, pp 271–350
16. Ihle JW, Lee JC, Hapel AJ (1982) Interleukin 3: Biochemical and biologic properties and possible roles in the regulation of immune responses. Lymphokines 6:239–262

13. Mechanisms of IgE-mediated Immediate Reactions

A. L. de Weck

The association of immediate allergic reactions with a peculiar category of antibodies denominated *reagins* became apparent with the experiments of Prausnitz and Küstner [1], passively transferring immediate skin reactions to allergens with serum antibodies, which at the time gave none of the usual serological reactions in vitro, such as precipitation, hemagglutination, etc. Even when the main immunoglobulin classes such as IgG, IgA and IgM were identified at the beginning of the 1960s, the quest for the elusive *reagins* continued. Only in 1967 could Ishizaka et al [2] and Johannson and Bennich [3] independently attribute the property of causing immediate-type skin reactions to a new class of immunoglobulins, denominated then IgE.

The IgE differ from other immunoglobulin classes essentially by their ability to bind strongly to homologous tissue mast cells and blood basophils, their very low concentration in serum of normal individuals (usually less than 250 μg/ml or 100 IU) and their thermolability at 56 °C. Later structural analyses have also revealed that the Fc portion of IgE is somewhat larger than that of other Ig classes, possessing a fourth (C4) domain.

However, even before the structural identity of antibodies responsible for immediate allergic reactions became known, their relationship with tissue mast cells and blood basophils, as well as the molecular events leading to triggering of the reaction by bridging of the antibody molecules on the cell surface [4, 5], had been extensively investigated. Many factors affecting the production of IgE had been identified, including the strong genetic components which influence this type of allergic hypersensitivity. Later, experiments with purified allergen-specific IgE and/or anti-IgE antibodies often merely permitted to confirm, at the molecular level in a direct manner, what had been inferred before, on the basis of assessment of reaginic activity by passive transfer experiments.

In this chapter, I shall briefly review our current concepts about the factors influencing the production of IgE antibodies and the regulation of IgE formation, either in a nonspecific manner (isotypic regulation) or in relationship to allergens (specific regulation). The molecular mechanisms by which IgE antibodies may trigger reactions on tissue mast cells and blood basophils will be discussed, as well as recent data indicating that IgE-mediated mechanisms may also play a role in the activation of macrophages/monocytes and of platelets.

13.1 Factors Affecting the Production of IgE

In experimental animals: The first recorded experimental immunization leading to an IgE-mediated immediate reaction is probably the ill-fated experiment by Richet and Portier [7], who involuntarily produced an immediate hypersensitivity to sea star extracts in a dog, leading them to the discovery of anaphylaxis. Since then, numerous authors investigated the mechanisms of such reactions in animals, using mostly passive serum transfer techniques (PCA: passive cutaneous anaphylaxis) [8, 9]. However, the interpretation of such experiments is complicated by the fact that rodents apparently produce two kinds of anaphylactic antibodies: on the one hand, some which appear to be *IgE-like* in term of strong prolonged binding to homologous tissue mast cells and blood basophils and thermolability. On the other hand, another subclass of IgG antibodies, thermostable at 56° and less strongly bound to cells (sometimes denominated *short-sensitizing* antibodies), can also cause passively transferrable immediate allergic reactions.

Despite this difficulty, several basic facts and principles have emerged over the years. Many factors may foster or prevent the formation of IgE antibodies, some of them related to the antigen and its mode of presentation, others related to the host mounting an immune response.

From the side of the **antigen**, the following points should be made: Some antigens appear more prone to cause the formation of IgE than others (e.g., pollens, parasites), although precise rules defining molecular characteristics common to IgE-producing allergens have not been identified. It has been claimed also that IgE are preferentially produced against some specific epitopes (antigenic determinant) of a given pollen allergen, while IgG would be directed against some other epitopes on the same allergen.

IgE is preferentially formed upon administration of low doses of antigen, a fact which was systematically established by Levine [10] in mice and which has been confirmed in several other species, such as guinea pigs [11] and dogs. While IgE production is usually fostered by injection of protein antigens in the nanogram range, administration of micrograms or milligrams of protein antigens leads to the preferential production of IgG antibodies.

The frequency of administration of antigen also seems to play a role: Infrequent administration at long intervals fosters the establishment of a long-lasting IgE response. In guinea pigs the optimal regimen for establishing a long-lasting sustained IgE response has been 5–8 injections every 3rd week. More frequent injections lead to diminished and transient IgE responses [de Weck and Toffler, unpublished results].

The route of administration also appears of importance. Mucosal application (by inhalation or nasal drops) as well as intradermal injection are more conducive to IgE formation than the intraperitoneal or subcutaneous injection.

Of great significance appears to be the adjuvant(s) in which the antigen is presented. While IgE may also be produced by allergen/antigen in aqueous solution, the adjunction of some adjuvant such as aluminum hydroxide or *B. pertussis* greatly enhances IgE formation [12]. On the other hand, adjuvants containing mycobacteria or mycobacterial products (e.g., Freund's complete adjuvant) markedly depress the IgE response, while fostering the production of IgG antibodies.

From the side of the **host undergoing an IgE immune response**, the following factors have been identified: Like for most antigen-specific responses, immune response genes (Ir genes) are at play and will decide whether a strong or weak immune response can be mounted by a given animal strain towards a defined antigen. Such immune response genes have been identified in relationship to the IgE response in mice [13], guinea pigs [14] and rats [15]. There is no indication, however, that different Ir genes influence the specific IgE or the IgG response to a given antigen. Provided the appropriate form of immunization is chosen, high IgG responders for a given antigen also appear to be high IgE responders. Ir genes have been linked in several species to class II histocompatibility antigens [16] and appear to be involved in antigen recognition.

Besides Ir genes, there appear to be other genes governing the IgE response in a non allergen-specific manner, namely by influencing the general propensity to form IgE-like antibodies towards any allergen (isotypic IgE regulation). This type of regulation has been observed extensively in mice [17] and to some extent in rats [18] and dogs [19]. SJL mice, for example, appear to be universally poor IgE responders towards a variety of antigens, while they are perfectly capable of intense IgG response to the same antigens. By the same token, some strains of rats (Lister, Brown Norway) appear to be high IgE responders and families of *atopic* dogs, producing IgE antibodies in large amounts to inhaled [19] or injected [17] antigens have been described. Although the quality of being a high IgE responder seems to correspond to one of the main features of the atopic predisposition in man, there is not yet a clear identification of the gene(s) governing this predisposition in experimental animals and of their level of operation.

The regulation of antigen-specific immune responses appears to be dependent upon an elaborate idiotype/anti-idiotype network, implying recognition and interactions between immunocompetent cells even in the absence of antigen. There is evidence that this regulatory network affects IgE responses, as well as other types of response. As discussed below, there are even some indications that the IgE response may be particularly sensitive to this type of regulation [20].

One of the major discoveries in experimental studies on the IgE response has been the observation by Tada and his colleagues [21] that various immunosuppressive measures such as thymectomy, anti-T-lymphocyte serum or irradiation, favor in rats the development and persistence of a sustained IgE response. In normal animals, on the other hand, the IgE response is transient and obviously suppressed. It was later confirmed in mice [22] and further established that immunological manipulations primarily affecting T suppressor cells have a profound and, in operational terms, preferential influence on the IgE response. When T suppressor cells are preferentially rendered inoperative (e.g., by mild irradiation or cyclophosphamide treatment), IgE responses are much enhanced while IgG responses may remain unaffected. This confirms the genetic observations reported above, according to which regulation of the IgE response appears to function independently from the regulation of IgG responses. Appropriate immunological manipulations affecting T suppressor cells may convert low IgE responder SJL mice into high IgE responders [23]. Conversely, it is possible to suppress the IgE response of high responders with T suppressor cells from low responder strains.

Despite the importance of T suppression deficiency in the regulation of IgE responses, it would be too one-sided to attribute high IgE responses solely to the relative absence of suppression. Indeed, evidence has been obtained, mostly in rats, by Ishizaka and his colleagues [24] that isotypic enhancing factors are also involved in high IgE responses. Such factors appear to be produced by T-cells and to promote the differentiation of IgE-bearing B-cells into IgE-secreting cells.

In man: Although for obvious reasons, the experimental study of IgE responses in man is limited by ethical considerations, numerous observations, such as experiments of nature, and immunological experiments on IgE biosynthesis in vitro suggest that the same rules established for IgE-like responses in rodents also apply to man.

In terms of antigen administration, it also appears in a general way that low doses of antigen favor IgE responses over IgG responses. It appears that the amount of pollen allergens inhaled and producing an IgE response in potentially high IgE responders (*atopic*) is extremely small (1 μg in an entire season!) [25]. In patients repeatedly injected with protein antigens (e.g., stung by bees, and bee keepers), it is evident that the ratio of IgE versus IgG antibodies formed is in an inverse relationship to the number and frequency of stings. A bee sting corresponds to the injection of 50–100 μg of foreign peptides and proteins; apparently the antigen dose favoring IgE formation is of the same order of magnitude as in rodents. Similar observations have been made in the development of IgE antibodies and immediate-type skin reactions to insulin in treated diabetics: An initial rise in IgE antibodies is followed by a decrease and a corresponding rise in IgG antibodies, as total dose and number of injections increase [J. Gutersohn, A. L. de Weck, unpublished observations]. In penicillin allergy, it has also been observed in prospective studies [26] that high dose penicillin therapy regularly induces an immune response in terms of specific IgG and lymphocyte reactivity, but practically never induces detectable anti-penicillin IgE antibodies. In breast fed infants, traces of milk or egg proteins in the milk of mothers not complying with an egg- and milk-free diet appear to be potent IgE sensitizers [27]. On the other hand, massive administration of antigenic foods markedly increases IgG responses [27]. All these observations point to the same conclusion: Low amounts of allergen administered infrequently mostly favor IgE production.

There are, for obvious ethical reasons, almost no systematic experimental studies comparing various routes of administration of potentially allergenic substances in man.

However, it is remarkable that the large majority of IgE-mediated allergic diseases are due to inhaled or ingested allergens. Whether this is merely a matter of allergen dose, of local availability of IgE-producing cells and/or of local concentration of IgE-bearing effector cells cannot be decided.

There are few data pertaining to the role of adjuvants for IgE formation in man, in part because a number of adjuvants experimentally used in rodents (e.g., Freund's complete adjuvant) are unsuitable for human use. It may appear paradoxical that aluminum hydroxide has been so widely used in allergen formulations for hyposensitization therapy; in how far the rise in IgE following the beginning of hyposensitization therapy may be related to such adjuvant effects is not clear. In one instance at least, it is documented that penicillin therapy in aluminum monostearate more frequently produces anti-penicillin IgE than penicillin treatment without such additions.

From the side of the host himself the following considerations may apply: There is evidence that the propensity to develop IgE response to specific allergens is also inherited and under the influence of Ir genes. This has been demonstrated for various allergens of ragweed [28] and possibly others [29]. In analogy to mice, class II histocompatibility antigens appear here to play a substantial role.

There is no doubt that the propensity to form high levels of IgE upon exposure to a variety of ubiquitous allergens (pollens, house dust mites, molds, food allergens, etc.) is a genetically inherited trait, as well shown by studies in twins and in atopic families. Although this type of inheritance most likely involves two genes not linked to the histocompatibility system, little is known about the mode of inheritance. The obvious high IgE response capacity is a main characteristic of *atopic* patients, although this seems to apply essentially to inhaled and ingested allergens. For allergens which are injected (e.g., insulin, drugs, bee venoms), the atopic state does not appear to offer a particular predisposition to IgE responses. The difference, however, may merely be a matter of intensity of exposure; atopic patients may be especially prone to form IgE upon exposure to minute amounts of allergens. This question could only be answered by establishing IgE dose response curves to some synthetic allergen in normal and atopic individuals.

Evidence for regulation of IgE levels by idiotype/anti-idiotype network interactions in man is still scarce, since the appropriate reagents to identify idiotypes and anti-idiotypes in human IgE-mediated allergy are mostly not available. Some preliminary attempts in IgE responses to phospholipase A (in bee venom allergy) and to grass allergens have been made. It has been speculated that the effect of IgG responses in hyposensitization therapy as well as some effects of combined antigen administration with passive transfer of specific IgG antibodies might be due to an idiotypic suppression of IgE responses. There is evidence for the presence of cross-reactive idiotypes to phospholipase A between IgG and IgE antibodies [A. Wetterwald, K. Blaser, personal communication].

Concerning the importance of T suppressor cells for the regulation of IgE in man, several lines of evidence are currently available. In a number of experiments of nature, increases in IgE levels occur concomitantly with a congenital or acquired deficiency in T suppressor cells. Among primary T-cell immunodeficiencies accompanied by high serum-IgE levels figure the Wiskott-Aldrich syndrome and ataxia-telangiectasia. In some secondary immunodeficiencies, such as transient hypo-γ-globulinemia in children [30] and some forms of lymphoid cancer (e.g., Hodgkin) elevated IgE levels have been reported. Diminished T suppressor activity, either in terms of diminished T8-lymphocyte levels or diminished activity in functional lymphocyte tests have been reported in hyper-IgE syndromes and in atopic patients [31]. The brisk elevation of IgE levels following viral infections (e.g., influenza) affecting T suppressor activity points in the same direction. Recently we have observed an increase in specific IgE production to drugs in patients concomitantly undergoing radiation therapy or *Amanita* poisoning, a T-cell immunosuppressant [M. Wälti, A. de Weck, unpublished]. Therefore, an accumulation of evidence, mostly indirect, points to the fact that a breakdown in T-cell suppressive activity favors IgE responses. This has been qualified as *allergic breakthrough* [32], suggesting that impairment in the normal damping (suppressing) mechanism of control will lead to IgE-mediated allergy.

Experimentally, some confirmatory evidence for the concept of T-cell-mediated suppression and its breakdown in IgE-mediated allergic conditions is available. T-cells from normal nonallergic individuals have a depressing effect on IgE biosynthesis in vitro, when using spontaneously IgE-producing cells from atopic or hyper-IgE patients in culture [33]. Furthermore, the serum from normal nonallergic patients appears to contain factors depressing the IgE biosynthesis in vitro from leukocytes of the same patients [34]. However, it is probably erroneous to consider the production of IgE and the emergence of IgE-mediated allergic hypersensitivity merely as the consequence of a breakdown in T-cell suppression. There is evidence that enhancing factors are promoting IgE response, even in the presence of an intact T suppressor mechanism. For example, a transient but marked IgE increase has been reported in acute graft-versus-host disease, at a time where no decrease in T suppressor activity may be noticed [35]. Furthermore, supernatants of stimulated T-cells or serum from hyper-IgE or atopic patients may increase IgE biosynthesis in vitro, using either normal or atopic leukocytes [36]. It is striking that allogeneic stimulation by normal T-cells or T-cell clones seems peculiarly efficient in promoting IgE biosynthesis in vitro.

13.2 Mechanisms of IgE-mediated Allergic Reactions

For several decades, it has been considered that the main (and possibly only) effector cells involved in the initiation of IgE-mediated allergic reactions have been tissue mast cells and blood basophils, which possess high affinity receptors for IgE. In recent years, however, it has been realized that IgE may also bind, albeit to receptors of lower affinity, to other types of cells, such as monocytes/macrophages, eosinophils, lymphocytes and platelets [37]. This, together with the increasing awareness that the triggering of mast cells and basophils by an IgE-mediated mechanism initiates a chain reaction involving numerous mediators and inflammatory cells such as eosinophils, neutrophils, macrophages, lymphocytes and platelets, has enormously complicated the relatively simple immunopathological scheme put forward over 20 years ago by Gell and Coombs [67] to describe type I, alias anaphylactic reactions. Several of the interactions between mediators and inflammatory cells of various types are described in this book at various places and many of the mechanisms demonstrated and studied in vitro probably also exist and play a role in vivo. However, the presentation of a balanced and integrated picture of the IgE-mediated reaction in tissues and of its secondary consequences is still difficult, because the dynamic analysis of pathological events at the various sites of allergic reactions in man is still incomplete and because IgE-mediated reactions seldom occur alone in a sensitized individual, other elements such as specific IgG, IgM and IgA antibodies, or sensitized effector T-lymphocytes, concomitantly intervene in the overall scene.

The following is an attempt to summarize the various elements building up the overall immunopathological picture of the IgE-mediated allergic reactions and their modulation by various factors. Several elements of this overall picture are described in more detail in other chapters of this volume.

Triggering of IgE-mediated reactions in blood basophils and tissue mast cells: IgE binds to specific receptors on blood basophils and tissue mast cells. These receptors are of high affinity (see Chapter 11) and are composed of 3 polypeptide chains. In studies already performed in the early 60s by Ovary [38] and Eisen and colleagues [39], it had been indirectly established that bridging of adjacent antibody molecules on the surface of the effector cells was the decisive element for eliciting wheal-and-erythema reactions in human skin as well as passive cutaneous anaphylactic reactions in rodents. An essential condition for achieving such a bridging was the use of antigens which are at least bivalent, i.e., which carry at least two identical antigenic determinants per molecule. Subsequent studies with synthetic allergens have shown that: a) trivalent to hexavalent antigens are optimally efficient in inducing bridging and triggering [40]; b) the distance between antigenic determinants available for bridging is not indifferent and that sterical considerations obviously influence bridging efficiency [41]. A logical consequence of the bridging concept is that monovalent antigens should function as inhibitors of IgE-mediated allergic reaction [35, 42], a prediction which was soon confirmed experimentally [42] and which has found its clinical applications in the field of allergy to drugs, such as penicillin [43, 44] or dextran. Once IgE was identified as the immunoglobulin molecule binding to effector cells, it became possible to induce bridging with anti-IgE antibodies [45], with chemically prepared IgE dimers or polymers [46] or with molecules interacting and bridging nonspecifically IgE molecules, such as concanavalin A. Thus, the requirement for bridging was confirmed in several ways. At a later date, it was established that bridging through IgE molecules is in fact not the required event but that bridging of IgE receptors themselves, as brought about by anti-receptor antibodies [47] yields the signal required for triggering. The bridging of IgE receptors apparently brings about the activation of some membrane proteolytic enzyme (serine esterase?) and gives the required activating signals both to the adenylate cyclase pathway and to the arachidonic acid metabolization pathways. However, the precise molecular mechanisms by which the corresponding signals are transmitted from the IgE receptors to these various intramembrane activation systems is not yet known.

In practical terms, the requirement of bridging by antigen in IgE-mediated allergic reactions provides some constraints on the molecular characteristics and properties of natural antigens susceptible to elicit such reactions. If the patient is sensitized to a single epitope (or antigenic determinant), the antigen will be eliciting only when carrying the same epitope in a repetitive manner. This may be the reason why polysaccharides with repetitive polymeric structures are relatively efficient anaphylactogens. On the other hand, proteins will only function as anaphylactogens if the same epitope is present more than once or if the patient is sensitized to various epitopes on the same molecules, enabling the formation of antigen-IgE bridges of mixed specificities on the cell surface. These immunochemical considerations may explain, at least in part, why some antigens are much better anaphylactogens than others. Drug polymers and chemicals with *mirror* structures (e.g., myorelaxants) functioning as bivalent antigens may elicit allergic reactions directly, without prior conjugation to a protein, as required for sensitization. This is indeed the mechanism of anaphylactic reactions to penicillins [48].

According to the bridging mechanism elucidated for IgE-mediated reactions, it becomes possible that, under exceptional circumstances, such reactions could be triggered also in the absence of antigen-specific IgE. As already indicated, concanavalin A triggers such reactions by binding nonspecifically to IgE [49]; a similar mechanism has been reported for protein A from Staphylococcus aureus and for other bacterial products [50]. Indeed, it becomes then possible that bacterial infections would trigger *pseudoallergic* reactions based on mast cell triggering via nonspecific bridges with IgE or IgE receptors. In how far some of the pseudoallergic reactions based on mast cell triggering and observed with various drugs or peptides may be based on such nonspecific bridging interactions remains to be elucidated. A special case appears to be the triggering of IgE-mediated allergic reactions by monovalent antigens, where a single epitope reacts with specific IgE. Although in most instances, such a reaction would block antibody combining sites and prevent bridging [42], there are reported instances where apparently monovalent compounds react solely with one IgE combining site and nevertheless trigger the cell. In that case, detailed analysis of the molecular characteristic of such triggering antigens, using a series of analogs, has indicated that bridging occurs through some additional nonspecific binding of the antigen molecule, either to an adjacent IgE molecule, to an IgE receptor, or even to some other *anchoring* membrane protein.

An understanding of the immunochemical requirements for IgE-mediated mast cell triggering makes it easier to visualize why many potent anaphylactogens are relatively small molecules (between 10,000 and 50,000 daltons), since diffusability and permeability considerations are probably important for effectively bridging molecules.

Releasability of mediators by IgE-triggered tissue mast cells and blood basophils: Studies on the bridging of IgE by multivalent antigens or anti-IgE antibodies have clearly shown that triggering and mediator release only require a limited amount of such bridges on the cell surface; mediator release will be achieved long before bridging of IgE becomes apparent in fluorescence microscopy in the form of visible capping [51]. It has become obvious that, in addition to the triggering effect of an IgE antigen bridge, other factors ultimately affect the release of mediators. These factors have been collectively considered under the concept of *releasability,* meaning the relative ease with which the mast cells or blood basophils of a given individual may be triggered to mediator release. As demonstrated several years ago by Conroy et al [52], using anti-IgE antibodies as a standard bridging reagent, histamine release from blood basophils is in no way correlated with the amount of IgE bound to blood basophils and to the density of IgE bridges brought about by anti-IgE. Various individuals triggered by anti-IgE may be classified as *high* or *low releasers,* independently from the formation of IgE-anti-IgE bridges on their basophils' membranes. The releasability characteristics seem to remain rather constant with time and are quite reproducible for a given individual [52], although no good correlation exists between IgE serum levels and releasability, atopic individuals seem to possess a higher releasability with anti-IgE than normal subjects. This is especially the case for spontaneous mediator release, without the addition of anti-IgE but in the presence of deuterium oxide [53]. Releasability may be influenced by drugs, such as prostaglandin synthesis inhibitors; indomethacin increases releasability triggered by anti-IgE [54] while some local anesthetics depress it. The study of other factors influencing releasability such as hormones, lymphokines [55] or neuropeptides [56] is only beginning. There is little doubt that the basic capacity of the cells to react and the factors influencing this parameter may turn out to be as, if not more, important for the ultimate clinical outcome of the reaction than the presence of allergen-specific IgE itself.

It is of interest that the releasability parameter, in contrast to what might have been expected, is not constant for all forms of triggers in basophils or mast cells. There is no apparent correlation between histamine release elicited by anti-IgE antibodies, anaphylatoxins or various histamine releasing peptides. This underlines the fact that despite common features and intracellular phenomena following cell triggering (e.g., calcium mobilization and influx), different pathways of activation may lead to mediator release. Since mediator release brought about by various triggering agents obviously plays an important role in the development of bronchial hyperreactivity and bronchial inflammation, it is likely that the information gained from in vitro experiments with blood basophils may also be relevant for asthmatic patients. Tissue and bronchial mast cells, however, may be influenced somewhat differently than blood basophils by the various factors affecting releasability.

Elicitation of IgE-mediated reactions by monocytes/macrophages: It has long been quasi a dogma that IgE molecules are only able to bind to blood basophils and monocytes. However, the group of A. and M. Capron [57] has produced in recent years a string of compelling evidence indicating that macrophages/monocytes, eosinophils and platelets possess receptors of somewhat lower affinity for IgE and become loaded with IgE in appropriately immunized individuals. These authors demonstrated also that the cells loaded with IgE do not play merely a passive role, but may become active in immune reactions. Indeed, the interaction of antigen with IgE stimulates the cells to become cytotoxic and to release some of their mediators [58]. The same can be achieved with anti-IgE antibodies [58]. Although most of these observations were made with an immune system geared for defence against Schistosoma parasites, their potential relevance for the immunopathology of IgE-mediated asthma is quite obvious. Indeed, the same group has shown activation of alveolar macrophages by IgE-anti-IgE mechanisms in vitro. Considering the abundance of alveolar macrophages in bronchial secretions and the numerous mediators produced by these cells in inflammatory reactions, there is little doubt that further studies on the role of IgE-activated macrophages in asthma should be considered with priority. The stimulation of IgE-loaded blood monocytes by anti-IgE has recently been confirmed by our group [M. Maly, B. Stadler, A. de Weck, unpublished].

IgE-mediated reactions by eosinophils: As indicated above, the induction of cytotoxicity for Schistosoma through an IgE-mediated mechanism has been demonstrated [59]. The prominent presence of eosinophils in IgE-mediated reactions is well-known. However, eosinophils have usually been considered as secondary cells, called to the reaction site by chemotactic factors produced by triggered basophils and mast cells. Their role at the reaction site is still somewhat disputed: While some see in them primarily scavenging cells mopping up inflammatory products [60], others have demonstrated the cytotoxic effect of eosinophil products, in particular of their major basic protein [61]. The finding that Schistosoma-specific IgE may trigger eosinophils to cytotoxicity opens the possibility that similar mechanisms may operate in triggering inflammatory reactions in allergic diseases. However, definite demonstrations for this are still lacking.

IgE-mediated reactions by platelets: The presence of IgE on platelets in Schistosoma-infected rats, the triggering of platelets by anti-IgE and the cytotoxicity of IgE-loaded platelets in vitro and in vivo for Schistosoma have all been demonstrated recently by Capron's group [62]. Interestingly, similar mechanisms seem to operate in man; anti-IgE triggering stimulates platelets to produce an oxidative burst (detected by chemoluminescence) and to become cytotoxic for Schistosoma. The activation, however, does not proceed until platelet aggregation and mediator release. In atopic patients, the triggering of platelets by an IgE-mediated mechanism also occurs. In pseudoallergic reactions to aspirin, aspirin has also been demonstrated to activate platelets from aspirin-intolerant patients, although investigations performed so far do not plead for an IgE-mediated mechanism [63]. Although the possible role of platelets in immediate-type allergic reactions has been recently emphasized [64], it has been considered there too, that platelets would be secondary cells, triggered at the site of the reaction by mediators released from other inflammatory cells (e.g., platelet activating factor). The recent findings by Capron's group open the possibility that platelets could react primarily with allergen and initiate a reaction. However, the activation of platelets by anti-IgE has not yet revealed the release of some platelet mediators, which seems to be a prerequisite if these cells were to play a major role in the development or modulation of immediate-type allergic reactions.

IgE-mediated reactions by lymphocytes: The presence of IgE antibodies on IgE-bearing B-cells is known by definition; these cells appear to be the precursors of IgE-secreting plasma cells [65]. Since they are present in the circulation in only minute amounts, it is doubtful that the interaction of antigen (or experimentally with anti-IgE) would be able to induce any significant release of B-cell-produced mediators causing or modulating an inflammatory reaction. At sites of local accumulation of such cells, such as lymph nodes or the intestinal mucosa, however, this may be different. Up to now, studies on the production of lymphokines by B-cells triggered by anti-IgE appear to be largely missing.

A small proportion of T-lymphocytes possess low affinity receptors for IgE; their existence is difficult to demonstrate and was first definitely established by Spiegelberg and Frische [66]. Since T-lymphocytes are producers of a wide variety of lymphokines, serving as effector or regulatory molecules, it is conceivable that triggering by antigen and/or by anti-IgE would initiate the production of such inflammatory substances. In the case of antigen, however, it would be, at first glance, very difficult to decide whether triggering has occurred via the IgE receptor or via the T-cell receptor, since actively sensitized individuals may possibly possess T-lymphocytes carrying both of these specific recognition molecules. Experiments using the passive loading of IgE specific for an antigen towards which the lymphocyte donor is not sensitized might resolve that question. Using anti-IgE triggering on T-lymphocytes from atopic patients, we have recently observed limited proliferation, as demonstrated by ^{3}H-thymidine uptake and the development of some clones, which, however, could not be maintained. Evaluation of lymphokine production following triggering by anti-IgE has not yet been attempted; in view of the scarcity of IgE-bearing T-cells, it is unlikely that conclusions could be drawn, unless clones of IgE-bearing T-lymphocytes are used. The interpretation of such experiments is made difficult by the fact that the Fc portion of the anti-IgE antibodies used might itself, upon polymerisation, trigger cells carrying Ig Fc receptors (T-cells and macrophages/monocytes).

13.3 Conclusions

In conclusion, it may be stated that IgE-mediated reactions appear to be much more complex and to involve many more cell types and mechanisms as was dreamed even a few years ago. A considerable amount of immunopharmacological and clinical research needs to be done in man, in order to assess the respective importance of the putative immunopathological pathways, which have been recently established experimentally.

References

1. Prausnitz C, Küstner J (1921) Studien über die Überempfindlichkeit 2. Zentralbl Bakteriol 86: 120
2. Ishizaka K, Ishizaka T, Hornbrook MM (1966) Physicochemical properties of reaginic antibody. V. Correlation of reaginic activity with E globulin antibody. J Immunol 97: 840
3. Johannson SGO, Bennich H (1967) Immunological studies of an atypical (myeloma) immunoglobulin. Immunology 73: 381
4. Farah FS, Kern M, Eisen HN (1960) Specific inhibition of wheal and erythema responses with univalent haptens and univalent antibody fragments. J Exp Med 112: 1211
5. Ovary Z, Karush F (1960) Studies on the immunologic mechanisms of anaphylaxis. I. Antibody-hapten interactions studied by passive cutaneous anaphylaxis in the guinea pig. J Immunol 84: 409
6. de Weck AL, Schneider CH (1969) Molecular and stereochemical properties required of antigens for the elicitation of allergic reactions. In: Westphal O, Bock HE, Grundmann E (eds) Current Problems in Immunology. Springer, Berlin Heidelberg New York, p 32
7. Portier P, Richet CH (1902) De l'action anaphylactique de certains venins. CR Soc Biol 54: 170
8. Ovary Z, Taranta A (1963) Passive cutaneous anaphylaxis with antibody fragments. Science 140: 193
9. Mota I (1964) The mechanism of anaphylaxis. I. Production and biological properties of mast cell sensitizing antibody. Immunology 1: 681
10. Levine BB, Vaz NM (1970) Effect of combinations of inbred strain, antigen and antigen dose on immune responsiveness and reagin production in the mouse: a potential mouse model for immune aspects of human atopic allergy. Int Arch Allergy 39: 156
11. Clausen JT, Spärck JV, Werdelin O, Larsen SO, Lundberg L (1985) Immunogenetic studies of respiratory anaphylaxis in selectively bred guinea pigs. Allergy 40: 15
12. Mota I, Perini A, Trinade VS (1974) The mechanism of the adjuvant effect of Bordetella pertussis: the substance responsible for the selective enhancement of IgE antibody production. Int Arch Allergy 47: 425–432
13. Vaz NM, Phillips-Quagliata JM, Levine BB, Vaz EM (1971) H-2 linked genetic control of immune responsiveness to ovalbumin and ovomucoid. J Exp Med 134: 1335

14. Lundberg L (1979) Guinea pig inbred for studies of respiratory anaphylaxis. Acta Pathol Microbiol Immunol Scand [C] 87:55
15. Rousseaux-Prévost R, Bazin H, Capron A (1977) IgE in experimental schistosomiasis. I. Serum IgE levels after infection by Schistosoma mansoni in various strains of rats. J Immunol 33:501
16. McDevitt HO, Chinitz A (1969) Genetic control of the antibody response: relationship between immune response and histocompatibility (H-2) type. Science 163:1207
17. Katz DH (1984) Regulation of the IgE system: experimental and clinical aspects. Allergy 39:81–106
18. Ishizaka K, Ishizaka T (1983) Immunology of IgE-mediated hypersensitivity. In: Middleton E Jr, Reed CE, Ellis EF (eds) Allergy: Principles and Practice, 2nd edn. Mosby, St. Louis, pp 43–73
19. Frick OL (1982) Viral infections as triggers of allergy. In: Steffen C, Ludwig H (eds) Clinical Immunology and Allergology. Elsevier, Amsterdam, pp 283–292
20. Blaser K, de Weck AL (1982) Regulation of the IgE antibody response by idiotype-anti-idiotype network. Prog Allergy 32:203–264
21. Tada T (1975) Regulation of reaginic antibody formation in animals. Prog Allergy 19:122
22. Kishimoto T, Hirai Y, Suemura M, Nakanishi K (1978) Regulation of antibody response in different immunoglobulin classes. IV. Properties and functions of IgE class specific suppressor factor(s) released from DNP-mycobacterium primed T cells. J Immunol 121:2106
23. Chiorazzi N, Vaz DA, Katz DH (1977) Hapten-specific IgE antibody responses in mice. VII. Conversion of IgE "non responder" strains to IgE "responders" by elimination of suppressor T cell activity. J Immunol 118:48
24. Hirashima M, Yodoi I, Ishizaka K (1981) Regulatory role of IgE-binding factors from rat T lymphocytes. V. Formation of IgE-potentiating factors by T lymphocytes from rats treated with Bordetella pertussis vaccine. J Immunol 126:838
25. Marsh DG (1975) Allergens and the genetics of allergy. In: Sela M (ed) The Antigens, vol. 3. Academic Press, New York, p 227
26. Neftel KA, Wälti M, Spengler H, de Weck AL (1982) Effect of storage of penicillin G solutions on sensitization to penicillin G after intravenous administration. Lancet I: 986–988
27. Gerrard GW (1979) Allergy in breast-fed babies to ingredients in breast milk. Ann Allergy 42:169–172
28. Marsh D, Chase G, Friedhoff L (1979) Association of HLA antigens and total serum immunoglobulin E level with allergic response and failure to respond to ragweed allergen Ra3. Proc Natl Acad Sci USA 76:2903
29. de Weck AL, Blumenthal M, Yunis E, Jeannet M (1977) HLA and Allergy. In: Dausset J, Svjegaard W (eds) HLA and Disease. Williams and Wilkins, Baltimore
30. Fineman SM, Mudawwar FB, Geha RS (1979) Characteristics and mechanisms of action of the concanavalin A-activated suppressor cell in man. Cell Immunol 45:120
31. Geha RS, Reinherz E, Leung D, McKee KT, Schlossman S, Rosen FS (1981) Deficiency of suppressor T cells in the hyperimmunoglobulin E syndrome. J Clin Invest 68:783
32. Katz DH (1978) Control of IgE antibody production by suppressor substances. J Allergy Clin Immunol 62:44–55
33. Saryan JA, Rappaport J, Leung D, Parkman R, Geha RS (1983) Regulation of human immunoglobulin E synthesis in acute graft versus host disease. J Clin Invest 71:556
34. Leung D, Brosek C, Frankel R, Geha RS (1983) IgE specific suppressor factors in normal human serum: in vitro and in vivo effects. Clin Res 31:164A
35. Geha RA, Twarog F, Rappaport J, Parkman R, Rosen S (1980) Increased serum IgE levels following allogeneic bone marrow transplantation. J Allergy Clin Immunol 66:78
36. Saryan JA, Leung D, Geha RS (1983) Induction of human IgE synthesis by a factor derived from T cells of patients with hyper-IgE states. J Immunol 130:242–247
37. Capron A, Dessaint JP, Capron M, Bazin H (1975) Specific IgE antibodies in immune adherence of normal macrophages to S. mansoni schistosomules. Nature 253:474
38. Ovary Z (1963) In vitro and in vivo interactions of anti-hapten antibodies with monovalent and bivalent haptens. In: Conceptual Advances in Immunology and Oncology. Hober and Harper, New York, p 206
39. Parker CW, Kern M, Eisen HN (1962) Polyfunctional dinitrophenyl haptens as reagents for elicitation of immediate-type allergic responses. J Exp Med 115:789
40. Levine BB, Redmond AP (1968) The nature of the antigen-antibody complexes initiating the specific wheal-and-flare reaction in sensitized man. J Clin Invest 47:556
41. Levine BB (1965) The nature of antigen-antibody complexes which initiate anaphylactic reactions. II. The effect of molecular size on the abilities of homologous multivalent penicilloyl haptens to evoke PCA and pas-

sive Arthus reactions in the guinea pig. J Immunol 94:121
42. de Weck AL, Schneider CH (1972) Specific inhibition of allergic reactions to penicillin in man by a monovalent hapten. I. Experimental studies. Int Arch Allergy 42:782
43. de Weck AL, Girard JP (1972) Specific inhibition of allergic reactions to penicillin in man by a monovalent hapten. II. Clinical studies. Int Arch Allergy 42:798
44. de Weck AL, Jeunet F (1975) Clinical trial of Ro 6-0787, a monovalent specific hapten inhibitor of penicillin allergy. Immunobiology 150:138
45. Ishizaka T, Tomioka H, Ishizaka K (1971) Degranulation of human basophil leukocytes by anti-IgE antibody. J Immunol 106:705
46. Ishizaka T, Ishizaka K, Bennich H, Johansson SGO (1970) Biologic activities of aggregated immunoglobulin E. J Immunol 104:854
47. Ishizaka T, Ishizaka K (1978) Triggering of histamine release from rat mast cells by divalent antibodies against IgE receptors. J Immunol 120:800
48. de Weck AL, Schneider CH, Gutersohn J (1968) The role of penicilloylated protein impurities, penicillin polymers and dimers in penicillin allergy. Int Arch Allergy 33:535
49. Sullivan TJ, Parker KL, Kulczycki A Jr, Parker CW (1976) Modulation of cyclic AMP in purified rat mast cells. III. Studies on the effect of concanavalin A and anti-IgE on cyclic AMP concentration during histamine release. J Immunol 117:713
50. Jensen C, Norn S, Stahl Skov P, Espersen F, Koch C, Permin H (1984) Bacterial histamine release by immunological and non immunological lectin-mediated reactions. Allergy 39:371
51. Ishizaka K, Soto S, Ishizaka K (1973) Mechanisms of passive sensitization. III. Number of IgE molecules and their receptor sites on human basophil granulocytes. J Immunol 111:500
52. Conroy MC, Adkinson NF Jr, Lichtenstein LM (1977) Measurement of IgE on human basophils: Relation to serum IgE and anti-IgE induced histamine release. J Immunol 118:1317
53. May CD, Remigio L (1982) Observations on high spontaneous release of histamine from leukocytes in vitro. Clin Allergy 12:229
54. Conroy MC, de Weck AL (1981) The effect of aspirin and indomethacin on histamine release from leukocytes of patients with suspected intolerance to aspirin. Int Arch Allergy Appl Immunol 66 [Suppl I]: 152
55. Ida S, Hooks JJ, Siraganian RP, Notkins AL (1977) Enhancement of IgE-mediated histamine release from human basophils by viruses: role of interferon. J Exp Med 145:892
56. Foreman J, Jordan C (1983) Histamine release and vascular changes induced by neuropeptides. Agents Actions 13:105
57. Capron A, Dessaint JP, Capron M, Bazin H (1975) Specific IgE antibodies in immune adherence of normal macrophages to Schistosoma mansoni schistosomules. Nature 253:474–475
58. Dessaint JP, Capron A, Joseph M, Bazin H (1979) Cytophilic binding of IgE to the macrophage. II. Immunologic release of lysosomal enzyme from macrophages by IgE and anti-IgE in the rat: A new mechanism of macrophage activation. Cell Immunol 46:24–36
59. Capron M, Rousseaux J, Mazingue C, Bazin H, Capron A (1978) Rats' mast cell eosinophil interaction in antibody dependent eosinophil cytotoxicity to Schistosoma mansoni. J Immunol 121:2518
60. Wenge P (1981) The eosinophil granulocyte and its role in the inflammatory process. In: Wenge A, Lindbom A (eds) The Inflammatory Process. An introduction to the study of cellular and humoral mechanisms. Almqvist and Wiksell, Stockholm, pp 305–327
61. Zheutlin LM, Ackerman SJ, Gleich GH, Thomas LL (1984) Stimulation of basophil and rat mast cell histamine release by eosinophil granule-derived cationic proteins. J Immunol 133:2180
62. Joseph M, Auriaults C, Capron A, Vorng H, Viens P (1983) A new function for platelets: IgE-dependent killing of schistosomes. Nature 303:310
63. Ameisen JC, Capron M, Joseph M, Maclouf J, Vorng H, Pancré V, Fournier E, Wallaert B, Tonnel AB (1985) Aspirin-sensitive Asthma: Abnormal platelet response to drugs inducing asthmatic attacks. Int Arch Allergy Appl Immunol 78:438
64. Knauer KA, Lichtenstein LM, Adkinson NF Jr, Fish JE (1981) Platelet activation during antigen-induced airway reactions in asthmatic subjects. N Engl J Med 304:1404
65. Ishizaka K (1976) Cellular events in the IgE antibody response. Adv Immunol 23:1
66. Frische R, Spiegelberg HL (1978) Fc receptors for IgE on normal rat lymphocytes. J Immunol 121:471
67. Gell PGH, Coombs RRA (1963) The classification of allergic reactions underlying diseases. In: Gell PGH, Coombs RRA (eds) Clinical Aspects of Immunology. Blackwell, Oxford, p 317

14. Properties of Short-term Sensitizing IgG Antibodies (IgG S-TS) in Asthma

W. E. Parish

Most anaphylactic hypersensitivity and disorders are mediated by IgE, but in some patients little or no IgE antibody to the relevant antigen is detected and tests on the basophils with antigen do not show the characteristic morphological changes though some histamine is released. In such patients another antibody may mediate anaphylactic changes; it occurs in the IgG fraction of sera proved to be free of all contaminating IgE. It differs from IgE in that the tissue sensitizing property is unchanged after heating at 56 °C or after treatment with a chemical reducing agent. It occurs in low titer only, and on passive transfer sensitizes skin for about four hours. It has therefore been designated IgG short-term sensitizing (IgG S-TS) antibody [15, 17–19].

IgG S-TS activity is found most frequently in persons with gastrointestinal food allergy and in asthma. This antibody, or antibody with similar properties, has also been detected in patients with generalized anaphylaxis following the injection of tetanus toxoid [15, 17], horse γ-globulin [17], protamine sulfate [12] and the neuromuscular blocking agent, succinylcholine [14]. It also occurs in persons showing skin test responses to antigens to which they are not clinically allergic.

In asthma, IgG S-TS may occur with and without IgE to the same antigen [20]. It appears to have a significant role in the pathogenesis of some cases of cryptogenic asthma, and in nonatopic asthmatic persons whose sera contain little or no specific IgE to the relevant inhalant antigen. The following reviews the properties of IgG S-TS relevant to asthma.

14.1 Properties of IgG S-TS Activity

IgG S-TS differs in many properties from IgE. Even without the evidence of short-term sensitizing antibody activity in sera or IgG fractions treated with immunoadsorbents to remove all IgE, the differences in duration of sensitization, and the resistance of the IgG antibody sensitizing ability to heat or to chemical reduction, distinguishes between the two classes of antibody. The properties of IgE and IgG S-TS are compared below.

IgE	IgG S-TS
1. Tissue sensitization mediated by IgE or fractions containing it.	Tissue sensitization by fraction of pure IgG not contaminated by IgE.
2. Very firm binding to tissue *in vitro.*	Weak binding to tissue *in vitro,* eluted by washing, though individual variation in affinity.
3. Passive cutaneous sensitization *in vivo* may persist in man 4 to 5 weeks, and in monkey 1 to 3 weeks. Sensitization is transferred by high titers in some sera. Challenge by prick test effective.	Passive sensitization *in vivo* in man or monkey persists 2 to 4 hours only. Titers are low, rarely above 1/16 dilution. Challenge responses are seen by prick test, but are more evident following intracutaneous injection.
4. Antigen-challenged sites show wheal and flare.	Wheal and flare but less intense than IgE, and about 5 min slower in reaching maximum response.

5. Skin response much reduced by antihistamine drugs.	Much reduced by same antihistamine drugs.
6. Cutaneous anaphylaxis in monkeys not suppressed by depletion of complement or neutrophils.	Not suppressed by complement or neutrophil depletion.
7. IgE blocks binding of IgE antibody by human basophils *in vitro* and in human and monkey skin *in vivo.*	IgG S-TS fraction blocks IgG S-TS antibody in monkey skin, and impedes sensitization by IgE for about 2 to 4 hours in human and monkey skin.
8. Passive sensitizing potential destroyed by heating at 56 °C for 30 min to 1 hour, and by treatment with 0.1 M 2-mercaptoethanol.	Passive sensitization potential not abolished at 56 °C for 4 hours and resistant to 2-mercaptoethanol.

The noninvolvement of IgE in the passive transfer sensitization tests to the skin of man or monkey was shown by treating IgG fractions or whole serum containing S-TS activity, with anti-IgE immunoadsorbents capable of removing IgE reagin from sera or serum fractions containing it. In no instance did the removal of IgE affect the S-TS activity; a result observed in three different laboratories [5, 12, 17, 19, 20].

IgE has strong binding affinity to sensitize mast cells in human tissues on treatment *in vitro.* The antibody is not easily eluted by washing with various salt solutions. Slices of human IgE-sensitized lung and skin on antigen challenge, release histamine; bronchial rings and strips of small intestine contract. In contrast IgG S-TS shows weak sensitizing affinity for slices of lung and skin and none for human bronchial rings or small intestine in the Schultz-Dale technique (Table 14.1). The low sensitizing titers of IgG S-TS together with its weak affinity, being easily eluted by washing, probably account for its failure to sensitize the bronchial and intestinal tissue *in vitro.*

Suspensions of human leukocytes containing many basophils are readily sensitized by IgE *in vitro* to release histamine and other anaphylactic mediators on challenge with anti-IgE or with specific antigen. IgG fractions containing S-TS activity contain an IgG component that binds to basophils, and treatment with anti-IgG antibody releases histamine, but treatment with the relevant antigen, eliciting a passive cutaneous anaphylactic response with the same serum in man, does not. The tests repeated on several occasions are consistent in that some IgG binds to the basophil membrane and is capable of mediating histamine release, but not by antigen specific for the IgG antibody [17, 18]. Some sera from normal, nonallergic persons, also have IgG binding to basophils, but in the absence of clinical evidence, any S-TS activity is unknown.

A strict criterion of an anaphylactic antibody is that it binds to the mast cell or basophil membrane by the Fc portion; bridging across the free Fab portions by two or more antibody molecules by antigen initiates the release or generation of the mediators of tissue anaphylactic change.

Table 14.1. IgE and IgG S-TS. Comparison of the sensitization of tissues for passive anaphylaxis

Test	Ability of	
	IgE	IgG S-TS
P.K. man	+	+
PCA monkey	+	+
Human skin *in vitro*	+	±
Human lung *in vivo*	+	±
Human leukocytes	+	– [a]
Monkey leukocytes	+	–
SD [b] human bronchus	+	–
SD [b] monkey ileum	+	–

[a] IgG binds to basophils but no anaphylactic release of histamine with antigen

[b] SD = Schultz-Dale technique for anaphylactic contraction of passively sensitized strips of human bronchus or monkey ileum

This is a property of IgE. So far, IgG S-TS has not been demonstrated to have this activity on isolated basophils or mast cells.

14.2 IgG S-TS in Asthma

There are several reports of IgG S-TS occurring in the sera of patients with asthma, both with and without IgE to the same antigen. Antigens inducing formation of IgG S-TS in asthma are *Dermatophagoides pteronyssinus* [4, 5], house dust [1], grass pollen [1, 20], milk, egg, and budgerigar serum [20], *Aspergillus fumigatus* [20] and platinum [21].

The clinical signs of asthma in patients with both IgG S-TS and IgE antibody to the same antigen do not differ from those of patients whose asthma is mediated by IgE alone. Similar clinical signs occurred in patients with IgG S-TS antibody to *D. pteronyssinus* and normal total amounts of IgE, as were seen in patients with increased total and antigen-specific IgE [4]. The coexistence of IgG S-TS and IgE antibodies to one or more of milk, grass pollen and hen egg antigens and also to *Aspergillus fumigatus* was found in some patients with extrinsic asthma [20]. In another group of persons suspected to be hypersensitive to foods, the coexistence of IgG S-TS and IgE antibodies was reported [2]. In these patients IgG S-TS may have augmented the activity of IgE, increasing the severity of the allergic response. The patients whose asthma was associated with IgG S-TS alone were reported to differ from those with the IgE-mediated condition in that they did not respond to treatment with disodium cromoglycate [4, 5].

In cryptogenic asthma, or asthma in nonatopic persons hypersensitive to a known antigen, IgG S-TS appears to have a more significant role in mediating the disorder, and usually occurs without, or with only small amounts of IgE to the relevant antigen. Four of nine patients with cryptogenic asthma (late age of onset, negative prick test reactions to 22 routine common allergens and no definite association with a particular antigen) had no IgE antibodies, but IgG S-TS only to milk, pollen or hen egg, and to *Candida albicans* or *Aspergillus fumigatus* [20]. In this group of cryptogenic asthmatic patients it would appear that IgG S-TS was the only anaphylactic antibody, and possibly mediated or contributed to the asthma.

IgG S-TS antibodies also occur in asthmatic nonatopic persons who are hypersensitive to a known antigen and who have a clear history of exposure to the antigen usually for several years. In eleven patients with asthma, hypersensitive to budgerigar antigens and with one exception, a history of long exposure to the birds (Table 14.2), none of them responded to prick tests with a battery of twenty common allergens and showed no response to prick tests with undiluted or diluted budgerigar, pigeon or hen sera [20]. The prick test would detect any normal atopic subjects. Furthermore seven of the patients had 50 IU or less, total IgE, and two had 290 IU IgE or less (Table 14.2).

These 11 nonatopic asthmatic patients showed several features differing from those of atopic extrinsic asthmatics. In tests done *blind* in three separate laboratories without knowledge of the results obtained elsewhere, fairly consistent findings were observed for the group (Table 14.3) [20]. Though they were prick test-negative to common environmental and to the asthma inducing antigens, on intracutaneous injection of the avian antigens, positive responses were observed in all ten patients tested, of which five showed dual immediate and late responses and three showed late responses only. Positive responses to intracutaneous injection and not by prick test are consistent with the experimental passive transfer tests in which much stronger reactions are elicited when the sensitized skin site is challenged by intracutaneous injection than by prick tests.

Susceptibility to asthma by inhalation of budgerigar serum antigen was demonstrated by bronchial challenge, in which all six tested developed asthma two to three hours later, i.e., typical late responses.

Examination for serum antibodies (Table 14.2) showed that nine had precipitins to budgerigar antigen and one had IgE to this antigen, detected by RAST (radioallergosorbent test), but only 1.3 times the background control, which would normally be

Table 14.2. Results of tests on eleven nonatopic patients with asthma induced by sensitivity to budgerigar serum antigens. [From 20]

Patient	Years exposed to budgerigars	Routine prick test	Avian Ag		Bronchial challenge-budgerigar serum	PCA no. +/3 baboons			RAST budgerigar sorbent units	IgE total units	PPTNS budgerigar serum	Blocking antibody
			Prick test	Intra-cutaneous		24 h unheated	Un-heated	Heated				
B.A.	10	–	–	Late	Late	3	0	0	0.54	488	+	Yes
B.U.L.	8	–	Na	Dual	Na	0	0	0	Nil	147	+	
B.U.R.	1	–	–	Dual	Late	0	0	1	0.64	9.5	+	
B.U.S.	13	–	–	Dual	Late	0	1	1	1.30	10.5	+	
C.A.	25	–	Na	Dual	Na	3	2	2	Nil	16.4	+	
C.O.	1	–	–	Late	Late	1	0	0	Nil	34.6	+	Yes
D.	15	–	–	Dual	Late	1	0	0	0.70	290	+	
G.	4	–	–	Late	Late	0	0	0	0.49	50	+	
M.A.	29	–	–	Imm	Na	3	2	2	0.80	650	–	No
M.I.	2	–	–	Na	Na	0	0	0	0.57	1.6	–	
P.	13	–	–	Imm	Na	3	2	1	Nil	33.5	+	Yes

Na = not available; Imm = immediate

designated as doubtful (normal positive value > 2-fold). Two other patients showed positive RAST to one of five other avian antigens. Three of four sera examined had blocking antibody for IgE-binding in RAST. All three had precipitating antibody, the fourth did not. This could account for the positive 24-hour PCA tests in which, in four sera, there was evidence of both IgE and IgG S-TS antibodies. In the skin of the monkey challenged 24 hours after sensitization, any blocking antibody could diffuse away during the sensitization period, leaving the long-persisting IgE antibody sensitizing the mast cells.

The total evidence indicates that heat-stable, short-term sensitizing IgG antibody has a significant role in mediating asthma in nonatopic persons, in some of whom either no or very little IgE to the relevant antigen is detected. These patients appear to develop asthmatic sensitivity after long and frequent exposure to the antigens, and most, but not all, develop IgG precipitins.

Asthma is a common occupational disorder in workers in platinum refining plants, irrespective of any atopic susceptibility. The patients have strong prick test reactions to platinum salts, and asthma following bronchial challenge inhalation with very small amounts of platinum dusts. The asthma has all the clinical features of a typical IgE-mediated hypersensitivity. During the development of an *in vitro* test to detect antiplatinum IgE antibodies, the presence of a sensitizing antibody was confirmed by passive transfer tests in man and monkey. IgE antibody was detected in three persons. Furthermore, three of six sera heated at 56 °C for 2 hours immediately before injection into skin of the human volunteers, and challenged 3 to 4 hours later by prick tests with ammonium tetrachloroplatinite, mediated a flare response in one of the three test subjects, though all three subjects were receptive to sensitization by IgE [21]. The short-term sensitizing activity of these sera is attributed to heat-stable IgG S-TS, though the IgG fraction was not separated from the sera. The test also indicates that the formation of antibody to metals is not confined to IgE, though IgE appears to be formed more readily than IgG.

Table 14.3. Summary of the results of tests made on eleven nonatopic persons with asthma due to sensitivity to budgerigar serum antigen. [From 20]

Test	No. positive/ No. tested
Prick test response to routine and to avian antigens	0/11
Intracutaneous injection of avian antigen responses: immediate – two, late – three, dual – five persons	10/10
Bronchial challenge to budgerigar antigen (all late responses)	6/ 6
Precipitins to budgerigar antigen	9/11
RAST-sorbent units 1 to budgerigar antigen	1/11
RAST-sorbent units 1 to one of five other avian antigens (one antigen positive in each of two persons)	2/11
Blocking antibody for RAST antibody to budgerigar	2/ 3
Monkey PCA tests: 24 h alone – two, S-TS alone – two, 24 h + S-TS, four persons	8/11

14.3 Extrinsic Allergic Alveolitis and Allergic Pulmonary Aspergillosis

Extrinsic allergic alveolitis and allergic pulmonary aspergillosis are chronic lung disorders with impaired pulmonary function. Patients form precipitins to the inducing antigens which are a diagnostic feature. IgG S-TS is usually, but not always, found in sera with precipitins to the relevant antigen and it was considered possible that IgG S-TS contributed to the pathogenesis of these disorders.

In six patients with extrinsic allergic alveolitis and no immediate asthmatic signs on challenge by inhalation, all had precipitins to avian antigens, three to budgerigar, two to chicken and one to pigeon. None of the patients were atopic; they did not respond to any of thirty common allergens by prick test, and did not have above normal amounts of total IgE. The sera of all six examined by Prausnitz-Küstner (P-K) transfer to normal persons contained antibodies sensitizing skin in low titre for 3 but not 24 hours, and resistant to heat and alkylation [25]. These are the properties of IgG S-TS.

On examination of thirty-four patients with allergic pulmonary aspergillosis, all had precipitins to *Aspergillus fumigatus*, thirty-one had IgE antibody detected by monkey PCA, of which ten also had heat-stable short-term sensitizing antibody. Two of these sera containing both IgE and IgG S-TS, were treated with an anti-IgE immunoadsorbent which removed all the IgE and potential to sensitive monkey skin for 24 hours, but left the IgG S-TS antibody titer unchanged in one, and slightly decreased in the other, due to the technical procedure [20].

This association with pulmonary disease, precipitins, and IgG S-TS activity is not consistent. In twenty-two patients with aspergilloma, all had antigen-specific precipitins, and none showed any IgG S-TS activity [20]. Similarly, 214 sera from cases of extrinsic allergic alveolitis (farmer's lung) had precipitins to *Micropolyspora faeni*, without any IgG S-TS activity [19].

Persons with a long exposure to potent antigens tend to form precipitins, and may develop chronic pulmonary disorders. Though IgG S-TS is usually found in sera with precipitins, not all patients with extrinsic allergic alveolitis and precipitins have demonstrable IgG S-TS. It is therefore unlikely that the IgG sensitizing antibody is an essential prerequisite to the alveolitis, but based on its known biological activity, if present it is likely to exacerbate allergic episodes.

14.4 In Vitro Passive Sensitization of Human Lung

Slices of fresh human lung have been sensitized by IgG S-TS *in vitro* and on antigenic challenge released histamine [16–18]. Much less histamine is released by IgG S-TS-sensitized lung, e.g., 8.8 and 6.7% of total histamine, than by IgE-sensitized lung in the same tests, e.g., 22.3 and 23.9%. The procedure gives inconsistent results in tests with IgG S-TS, but this is partly due to technical features, among which are thickness of lung slices, as slices greater than 1 mm fragment thickness are more effective, individual variation in samples which varies as it does for IgE sensitization, the duration of sensitization, 30 min to 1 hour is optimal, and the number of washes, as IgG S-TS appears to be easily removed by washing [18].

Apart from histamine, other pharmacological mediators detected in the supernatant fluid are eosinophil chemotactic factor (ECF-A) and the ECF oligopeptides attracting eosinophils and neutrophils. The leukotriene complex SRS-A was not detected.

Within the technical limitation of tests with an antibody easily eluted from the tissue, it has been possible to sensitize lung with a heat-stable IgG antibody which on antigenic challenge releases histamine and some other pharmacological mediators associated with anaphylaxis, but the activity is very much less than that of IgE.

14.5 IgG Blocking Sensitization of Human Lung by IgE

In monkey passive cutaneous anaphylaxis by human sera containing IgE, some sera partially inhibit sensitization by IgE for about 2 to 4 hours. The reaction is a ring with a pale center that does not completely fill with the blue indicator dye. If challenged at 24 hours the reaction site shows a well-defined homogeneous blue colour. Other sera do not show the spontaneous partial inhibition if challenged at 2 hours. The blocking activity at the 2- to 4-hour period is due to the IgG content [11]. Similarly, IgG S-TS [17] and IgG_4 [22, 23] will block sensitization of IgE for 2 to 4 hours, and IgG S-TS responses frequently show a ring form [17].

IgG was tested for any blocking of IgE sensitization of human lung slices *in vitro,* to examine any property of IgG, to regulate IgE sensitization by blocking, and possibly as indirect evidence of any sensitizing properties of IgG subclasses. Blocking in these tests refers to competition by Fc at the cell surface whereby IgG may prevent the binding of IgE. It is unrelated to antigen specificity.

Table 14.4. Inhibition of IgE sensitization of human lung slices by serum proteins assayed by a decrease in histamine release after challenge by β-lactoglobulin antigen

Diluent conc/ml	Net % histamine release by antigen	% Inhibition
Hank's salt solution	20	0
IgE 0.01 g	11	45
IgE 0.05 g	9.6	52
IgG (N) 1 mg	17.6	12
IgG (S-TS) 1 mg	17.1	14.5
IgGl 1 mg	17.9	10.5
IgG4 1 mg	17.7	11.5
IgG (horse) 1 mg	17.2	14
IgG (seal) 1 mg	17.8	11
Albumin (human) 1 mg	18.5	7.5

IgG (N) = IgG fraction from normal person; IgG (S-TS) = IgG fraction from person with S-TS antitetanus titer 1:8. Net % histamine release: the % of release greater than spontaneous release of lung treated with same diluent, but without antigen challenge

A serum fraction containing 0.04 μg IgE/ml depleted of IgG, IgA and most albumin, and which had anti-β-lactoglobulin RAST titer of 2.6 absorbent units was diluted in Hank's salt solution (the standard histamine release preparation) or diluted in total IgG or IgG subclass fractions (Table 14.4). These antibody solutions were incubated with slices of lung in triplicate for 4 hours. The lung was washed thrice and challenged with 100 μg β-lactoglobulin/ml for 15 min. The amount of histamine released in the supernatant fluid, and the amount remaining in the lung, were assayed to determine the percentage of anaphylactic release.

Table 14.4 is an abbreviated summary of the results, but illustrates that IgG significantly impeded sensitization by IgE, but the IgG preparations had little blocking activity and there was no evidence of a selective inhibition. Human serum albumin, a nonsensitizing protein, appeared to impede sensitization by 7.5% though an alternative interpretation of the result is that albumin stabilized the tissue fragments, whereas the Hank's balanced salt solution with HEPES buffer enhanced histamine release by antigen. The globulin preparations were more effective at reducing IgE sensitization, possibly reflecting a greater adherence of globulin to the cells, though not by selective binding to receptors. This requires further examination. Total IgG preparations impeded sensitization more than the IgG_1 and IgG_4 fractions, but the variation in results from each of the samples examined in triplicate does not provide firm evidence of selective activity. Horse γ-globulin which does not sensitize human tissue anaphylactically also impeded sensitization, as did a total globulin preparation of seal serum to which very few persons would be exposed, which was included as a second control preparation should the lung or IgE donor have had weak sensitivity to horse serum.

Further tests were made with the IgE sensitizing antibody, diluted, and the duration of sensitization reduced, in order to find conditions that would show more definite evidence of inhibition. The results of the most conclusive test show that in optimal conditions to show reduced IgE sensitizing potency, by diluting the IgE and using the short duration of 1 hour sensitization, IgG_4 could impede sensitization more than IgG_1. However, the results after sensitization at 30 min and 2 hours were not so conclusive. There was no IgG S-TS preparation available for comparison.

Evidence thus far available indicates that an IgG preparation containing IgG S-TS appeared to have more ability to impede sensitization of lung by IgE than did IgG of normal serum, but analysis of the spread of the amounts of histamine released does not indicate definite selective activity. However, IgG_4 in optimal conditions of test, impeded sensitization by IgE more than IgG_1, but the impeding activity is not strong, and is very dependent upon test conditions and individual lung preparations.

14.6 IgG_4 in Asthma

Though the total amount of IgG does not usually increase in atopic disorders, there is quite often an increase in the subclass IgG_4, usually associated with an increase in total IgE. Increased total and antigen-specific IgG_4 occur in some asthmatic patients [3, 4, 9, 10, 13]. It has been suggested that in asthmatic patients with little or no increase in total IgE and a significant increase in IgG_4, that IgG_4 mediates the asthma. Furthermore, these patients are reported not to respond to treatment with disodium cromoglycate effective against immediate IgE-mediated asthma [8, 9]. The IgG_4-associated asthma in persons without allergen-specific IgE on bronchial provocation tests was a late response, 2 to 4 hours after challenge [10].

In a study of IgE and IgG_4 antibody assays by RAST, a high proportion of persons allergic to guinea pig dander had no specific IgE antibody, but had IgG_4, which also occurred in a smaller proportion of persons with allergy to cat dander [3]. In another study 6% of 26 patients allergic to several antigens, or to mold only, had positive skin (intracutaneous) tests and no IgE by RAST. The leukocytes of these patients released histamine on treatment with anti-IgG_4, and also with specific allergen [24]. This cannot be interpreted to show that the allergen-binding was due to the IgG_4.

Despite the clinical association between atopic disorders and increased total and allergen-specific IgG_4 there is as yet no certain evidence that IgG_4 is an anaphylactic antibody, or that IgG S-TS activity is mediated by IgG_4. Preparations of purified IgG_4 have not sensitized skin *in vivo* or tissue or basophils *in vitro*, to antigen-induced anaphylaxis. Nevertheless, IgG_4 binds to human basophils, presumably by Fc receptors, so that subsequent treatment with anti-IgG_4, polyclonal [19, 23, 24] or monoclonal [7], releases histamine, but the relevant antigen does not. It therefore fails to show the essential property of an anaphylactic antibody.

Another phenomenon associated with the binding of IgG_4 to mast cells and basophils is the blocking or impeding sensitization by IgE. In this context blocking refers to competition of the two classes of molecule on the cell surface irrespective of antigenic specificity. Myeloma IgG_4 injected into monkey skin will block sensitization at the site for about 4 hours [22, 23]. In tests *in vitro* with human basophils, if treated with enough IgG_4, passive sensitization by IgE is impeded or reduced for a short time thereby decreasing the amount of histamine released on challenge by antigen specific for the IgE [19]. No blocking was seen with equal amounts of IgG_1. Human basophils treated with IgG_4 also failed to form rosettes with antigen-linked particles, indicating the inability to bind antigen [6]. It is believed that the IgG_4 receptors are separate from those for IgE, but the excess of IgG_4 on the cell surface reduces the access of IgE to its receptor. This could occur *in vivo* as the amount of free IgG_4, particularly in persons with increased amounts of IgG_4 is much greater than that of IgE.

Present evidence indicates that IgG_4, or the greater part of IgG_4, is not an anaphylactic antibody, and is not IgG S-TS. IgG_4 can nevertheless bind to basophils and presumably to mast cells. In sufficient amount it impedes sensitization by IgE, though this activity is of short duration on basophils *in vitro*. The significance of increased amounts of IgG_4 in atopic persons, including some asthmatics, has not been ascertained. If it regulates IgE sensitization by swamping the cell membrane impeding IgE-binding, it is not a very effective system, though the much greater amount of IgG_4 than IgE could provide the excess needed.

References

1. Berry JB, Brighton WD (1977) Familial human short-term sensitizing (IgG S-TS) antibody. Clin Allergy 7:401–406
2. Brighton WD (1980) Frequency of occurrence of IgG (S-TS). Clin Allergy 10:97–100
3. Bruynzeel PLB, Berrens L (1979) IgE and IgG4 antibodies in specific human allergies. Int Arch Allergy Appl Immunol 58:344–350
4. Bryant DH, Burns MW, Lazarus L (1973) New type of allergic asthma due to IgG 'reaginic' antibody. Br Med J IV:589–592
5. Bryant DH, Burns MW, Lazarus L (1975) Identification of IgG antibody as a carrier of reaginic activity in asthmatic patients. J Allergy Clin Immunol 56:417–428
6. Devey ME, Panzani R (1975) The IgG subclasses of antibodies to castor bean allergen in patients with allergic asthma. Detection of a high incidence of antibodies of the IgG4 subclass. Clin Allergy 5:353–361
7. Faga DL, Slaughter CA, Capra JD, Sullivan TJ (1982) Monoclonal antibodies to immunoglobulin G4 induce histamine release from human basophils in vitro. J Allergy Clin Immunol 70:399–404
8. Gwynn CM, Morrison Smith J, Leon GL, Stanworth DR (1978) Role of IgG4 subclass in childhood allergy. Lancet I:910–911
9. Gwynn CM, Morrison Smith J, Leon GL, Stanworth DR (1979) IgE and IgG4 subclass in atopic families. Clin Allergy 9:119–123
10. Gwynn CM, Ingram J, Almousauri T, Stanworth DR (1982) Bronchial provocation tests in atopic patients with allergen-specific IgG4 antibodies. Lancet I:254–256
11. Hutchcroft BJ, Moore EG, Orange RP, Underdown BJ (1980) Short and long latency skin sensitizing antibody in passive cutaneous anaphylaxis in the monkey. Clin Allergy 10:631–637
12. Lakin JD, Blocker TJ, Strong M, Yocum W (1978) Anaphylaxis to protamine sulfate mediated by a complement-dependent IgG antibody. J Allergy Clin Immunol 61:102–107
13. Merrett TG, Lee T, Barnetson RSC, Burr ME, Merrett J, Kay AB (1982) Role of IgG4 in asthma: a comparison of polyclonal and monoclonal anti-IgG4 for assay of total and specific IgG4. In: Kemeny DM, Lessof MH (eds) Recent developments in RAST and other solid-phase immunoassay systems. Excerpta Medica, Amsterdam, pp 44–52
14. Moneret-Vautrin DA, Laxenaire MC, Moeller R (1981) Anaphylaxis due to succinylcholine. Immunoallergological study of thirteen cases. Clin Allery 11:175–183
15. Parish WE (1970) Short-term anaphylactic IgG antibodies in human sera. Lancet II:591–592
16. Parish WE (1971) Detection of reaginic and short-term sensitizing anaphylactic or anaphylactoid antibodies to milk in sera of allergic and normal persons. Clin Allergy 1:369–380
17. Parish WE (1973) A human heat-stable anaphylactic or anaphylactoid antibody which may participate in pulmonary disorders. In: Austen KF, Lichtenstein LM (eds) Asthma: Physiology, Immunopharmacology and

Treatment. Academic Press, New York, pp 71–89
18. Parish WE (1978) Evidence for human IgG antibodies anaphylactically sensitizing man. In: Bach MK (ed) Immediate hypersensitivity: modern concepts and developments. Marcel Dekker, New York, pp 277–299
19. Parish WE (1981) The clinical relevance of heat-stable, short-term sensitizing anaphylactic IgG antibodies (IgG S-TS) and of related activities of IgG4 and IgG2. Br J Dermatol 105:223–231
20. Pepys J, Parish WE, Stenius-Aarniala B, Wide L (1979) Clinical correlations between long-term (IgE) and short-term (IgG S-TS) anaphylactic antibodies in atopic and 'non-atopic' subjects with respiratory allergic disease. Clin Allergy 9:645–658
21. Pepys J, Parish WE, Cromwell O, Hughes EG (1979) Passive transfer in man and the monkey of Type 1 allergy due to heat labile and heat stable antibody to complex salts of platinum. Clin Allergy 9:99–108
22. Stanworth DR, Smith AK (1973) Inhibition of reagin-mediated PCA reactions in baboons by the human IgG4 sub-class. Clin Allergy 3:37–41
23. Vijay HM, Perelmutter L (1977) Inhibition of reagin-mediated PCA reactions in monkeys and histamine release from human leukocytes by human IgG4 subclass. Int Arch Allergy Appl Immunol 53:78–87
24. Vijay HM, Perelmutter L, Bernstein IL (1978) Possible role of IgG4 in discordant correlations between intracutaneous skin tests and RAST. Int Arch Allergy Appl Immunol 56:517–522
25. Warren CPW, Cherniack RM, Tse KS (1977) Extrinsic allergic alveolitis from bird exposure. Clin Allergy 7:303–314

15. The Role of Lymphocytes and of their Abnormalities in Atopic Diseases

M. Ricci, E. Maggi, G. F. del Prete, S. Romagnani

This work was supported by funds of Ministero Pubblica Istruzione (grants 12.02.00550 and 12.01.03447) and C.N.R. grant CT 83.02556.04.

The understanding of cellular and molecular interactions involved in the regulation of IgE biosynthesis can allow an actual progress in the control of IgE antibody system that promises to lead to more successful therapy and even prevention of atopic diseases. A considerable body of experimental data pertaining to the regulation of IgE antibody system is derived from studies performed in animal models. *In vivo* and *in vitro* studies in rodents suggest that IgE synthesis, while requiring T helper cells and factors for initiation, is also under active T suppressor cell control. Antigen-specific, as well as idiotype-specific and isotype-specific suppressor T-lymphocytes which regulate IgE antibody responses have been described [1, 2]. A regulatory role of cells possessing receptor for the Fc fragment of IgE ($Fc_\varepsilon R^+$ cells) has also been demonstrated; latest results seem to suggest that $BFc_\varepsilon R^+$ cells exert a major role rather than $TFc_\varepsilon R^+$ cells in the isotype-restricted regulation [3]. However, the investigations in humans have been hampered until now by the obvious impossibility to carry out *in vivo* studies and by the difficulties encountered in *in vitro* studies, essentially due to the extremely small amounts of IgE and regulatory factors produced by lymphocytes.

In this chapter the studies performed in order to clarify the mechanisms responsible for IgE disregulation in atopic patients will be reviewed; in particular, the following aspects related to the role of lymphocytes in atopic diseases will be discussed: possible alterations of the T-cell system in atopic patients; *in vitro* lymphocyte responses to allergens; *in vitro* models of IgE production by human lymphocytes.

15.1 Possible Alterations of the T-cell System in Atopic Patients

An impairment of the T-cell system as responsible for the increased IgE production in atopy has been suggested mainly by animal experiments and by the clinical associations between certain types of T-cell immunodeficiency diseases and hyper-IgE states. In animal models selective reduction in suppressor T-cell function increases the IgE responses [1–3]. IgE levels are often elevated in deficiencies of T-cell system, such as Wiskott-Aldrich, Di George's syndrome and Hodgkin's disease (HD). However, the clinical findings are not fully convincing. First, abnormalities in IgE synthesis are detectable in some but not all patients with T-cell immunodeficiencies. Second, increased IgE levels in patients with HD cannot be simply interpreted as a consequence of suppressor T-cell deficiency. We were unable to show any relationship between raised IgE levels and changes of T-cell number and function in untreated patients with HD. Moreover, the treatment of patients with radiotherapy resulted in a noticeable fall in IgE concentrations and T-cell number and function [4].

Some reports have described depressed lymphocyte proliferation to phytomitogens and subnormal absolute or relative numbers of T-cells in atopics [5]. Infants with a family history of atopy have significantly lower numbers of T-cells than infants lacking this heredity [6]. However, in other studies atopic diseases have not been associated with low T-cell numbers or reduced proliferative responses to mitogens [7, 8]. The absolute and relative number of T-cell subsets detectable in peripheral blood (PB) of atopic patients has also been evaluated. Reduced percentages of T-lymphocytes possessing receptor for the Fc fragment of IgG (T_γ-cells) were found in patients with common atopy [8, 9], but the ratio between T4- and T8-positive cells in patients with common atopy was usually normal [10]. Concanavalin A-activated T-cell suppressor system was functionally equivalent in atopic subjects and nonatopic individuals. Atopic subjects have recently been documented to have reduced histamine-induced suppressor T-cell function and to have decreased phenotypic expression of T-cell H_2 receptors when compared to nonatopic controls. T suppressor cells from atopics produce fewer suppressor signals than cells from nonatopics and their monocytes produce less prostaglandin E_2 even if the suppressor signals are provided [11].

The alterations of the T-cell system are much more evident in patients with atopic dermatitis. These patients have a lot of T-cell abnormalities, which include reduced delayed hypersensitivity response to antigens *in vivo,* depressed response in autologous mixed lymphocyte reaction (AMLR), depressed T-cell proliferation to antigens *in vitro* and a decreased capacity to generate cytotoxic T-cells. These abnormalities have been associated with a decrease in the number of T8-positive cells, and of T29-positive cells and in a decreased capacity to generate help for cytotoxic cells [12]. Patients with moderate to severe atopic dermatitis and highly elevated IgE levels have low percentages of T_ε-cells and lower percentages of T-cells than nonatopic controls and atopic patients in remission [13]. It is of interest that in infants in whom eczema subsequently developed, the number of T8-positive cells was reduced and functional suppressor activity was lower than in nonatopic infants [14]. This finding, if confirmed, would indicate that a defect of T-cell regulation could precede clinically atopic disease and could be of primary pathogenetic importance. Detection of low levels of T8-positive cells in the PB of infants might have predictive value of atopy.

Thus, it is reasonable to conclude that although phenotypic and/or functional alterations of the T-cell system have been demonstrated in patients with atopic dermatitis and elevated serum-IgE, further work is still necessary to get clear-cut evidence of such T-cell deficiency in patients with common atopy (patients suffering from allergic rhinitis and/or bronchial asthma). More sensitive assays are required to identify abnormal T-cell function (possibly genetic) in common atopy and the definite relationship between the T-cell dysfunction and IgE hyperproduction.

15.2 In Vitro Lymphocyte Responses to Allergens

It has been shown that T-cells from atopic patients usually develop a greater proliferative response and lymphokine production than T-cells from nonatopics, when challenged *in vitro* with the appropriate allergen [15–17]. These findings have been confirmed more recently with the use of purified grass Rye I and *Dermatophagoides pteronyssinus* P_1 antigens [18, 19]. Allergen-specific T-cell lines and clones usually characterized by the helper/inducer phenotype have been obtained from PB of atopic subjects. The proliferative response of these lines and clones required antigen presentation by autologous antigen presenting cells (APC) or by APC from unrelated but histocompatible individuals. The restriction was probably at a level of HLA class II (DR) histocompatibility antigens, since the proliferative response to the allergen was significantly lowered by anti-DR monoclonal antibodies, but not by antibodies to Class I or β-2 microglobulin determinants [20].

All these data are in favor of a T-lymphocyte hyperresponsiveness to allergen epitopes in atopics. Class II histocompatibility antigens at a level of APC and their recognition by T-cell receptors are involved in the control of specific immune responses to allergen. The degree of genetic control of the response to allergen epitopes may depend at individual levels on 'immune response' (Ir) genes and related major histocompatibility complex (MHC) class II molecules.

15.3 In Vitro Models of IgE Production and Regulation by Human Lymphocytes

The *in vitro* models recently developed for the study of IgE production and regulation in humans are of interest since they could have the potential to allow an understanding of cellular and molecular mechanisms responsible for the IgE antibody hyperproduction. Models of spontaneous IgE production in vitro and IgE production induced by signals delivered *in vitro* have been reported.

In vitro spontaneous IgE production: Spontaneous IgE production *in vitro* has been demonstrated in cultures of PB-lymphocytes from patients with severe atopic disease [21] and also from a proportion of patients with common atopy and slightly elevated serum-IgE levels [22]. Of interest are the results obtained in our laboratory by studying in the last three years the spontaneous IgE production *in vitro* in a total number of 143 individuals. B-cell-rich, instead of unfractionated mononuclear cell, suspensions were used, since in our experience this allows a better evaluation of the *de novo* synthesized IgE. *De novo* synthesized IgE was never observed in cultures of B-cell populations from normal donors and only occasionally from patients with pollenosis tested out of the pollination season. The frequency of cases showing IgE synthesis *in vitro* was progressively higher from grass-sensitive patients studied during the pollination season, mite-sensitive patients, patients with multiple sensitivities and patients with atopic dermatitis [18]. Thus, it is evident that atopic patients can have circulating IgE-producing cells and the presence of these cells seems to be related to the entity and number of allergen stimulations. It may, indeed, be considered as a parameter of high atopic status. The spontaneously IgE-producing cells present in the circulation of a proportion of atopic patients are faster sedimenting and lighter than the majority of PB-lymphocytes, appear to be resistant to antimitotic agents and bear on their surface DR determinants and IgE, but not IgM [22, 23]. They are no longer capable of responding to activation signals delivered *in vitro* and can be influenced by signals, such as autologous or allogeneic T-cells, antigen, anti-ε monoclonal antibodies and lectins, only in a negative way [24, 25]. Normal T-cells seem to be more consistently inhibitory than atopic T-cells when added to the cultures containing spontaneously IgE-producing B-cells. Moreover a proportion of atopic patients seems to be lacking in T-cells capable of lowering the spontaneous IgE production *in vitro* by autologous B-cells [25]. Of interest are the recent results obtained by studying the effect of anti-idiotype antibody on the IgE production in vitro by human B-lymphocytes. Evidence for the importance of idiotype(Id)/anti-idiotype (anti-Id) interactions in the regulation of IgE responses has been previously given in animal models. In some experimental systems manipulation through the Id/anti-Id network (such as immunization with IgG idiotypes or administration of antigen coupled to syngeneic spleen cells) has been shown to lead to the production of (auto)anti-Id antibodies and to the suppression of IgE antibody responses [26, 27]. The results obtained in experiments carried out in man indicate that in vitro synthesis of antigen-specific IgE is under regulation by Id/anti-Id interactions that can involve both T- and B-lymphocytes [28].

IgE produced by signals delivered in vitro: Models in which IgE production by normal or atopic cells is induced by signals delivered *in vitro* and is not the simple reflex of an activation which has already occurred *in vivo* are undoubtedly more suitable for the study of activity of early and late memory B-cells and possibly of their precursors. To do this, some models have been studied, such as production induced by polyclonal B-cell activators (PBA), soluble T-cell factors and alloreactive T-cell clones.

Conflicting results have been reported by using classic PBA to stimulate IgE production by human lymphocytes *in vitro*. The difficulty to obtain reproducible results with PBA probably reflects the scarcity of B-cells capable of differentiating into IgE-secreting cells in the PB of nonatopic subjects or the failure of such cells to respond to PBA. Better results have been reported with the use of soluble factors derived from cells of patients with severe atopy. T-cell supernatants (TCS) from patients elevated serum-IgE levels were found to be capable of inducing IgE production in vitro by normal B-cells [29] and of potentiating the IgE production by B-cells from atopic patients [30]. IgE potentiating factors seem to be glycoprotein in nature and apparently isotype (IgE)-specific [29]. IgE potentiating activity was also demonstrated in the serum ultrafiltrates of some patients with atopic dermatitis and elevated IgE serum levels [18]. The existence and role of human IgE potentiating factors have been confirmed by establishing T-T-cell hybridomas capable of releasing factors with the same activity [31]. The mechanisms by which the IgE helper factors potentiate IgE synthesis are at present unclear. These factors probably act as differentiation signals for IgE-bearing cells but the possibility that they cause a switch in isotype synthesis cannot be excluded.

Recently, it has been shown that an alloreactive T-cell clone (ATCC) induced a high rate production *in vitro* of all the Ig isotypes, including IgE, when challenged with B-cells from the original donor of stimulating cells or from other donors possessing the appropriate alloantigen [32]. The release of IgE in the supernatants of PB-lymphocyte cultures stimulated with the ATCC started after 4 days and peak IgE concentrations were found between 7 and 12 days. Depletion from B-cell suspensions of DR^+ and IgE^+, but also of IgM^+, cells lowered the IgE production induced by the ATCC, thus suggesting that at least a proportion of cells activated by the clone possessed IgM on their surface [18]. These data indicate that PB-lymphocytes from both atopic and nonatopic subjects can be activated *in vitro* to differentiate in IgE-producing cells, provided that suitable stimulation is achieved.

15.4 Conclusions

Excessive and persistent production of IgE antibody represents the cardinal immunological feature of the allergic phenotype. At least two main independent immunological alterations may be proposed as responsible for the allergic phenotype: the increase of specific immune responses to allergen epitopes and the preferential expression of the IgE isotype in the antibody response. These alterations can be acquired as independent genetic traits. The T-cell hyperresponsiveness to allergens has been demonstrated in atopic patients. Atopic patients have a greater number of T-cells with specific receptors for allergen epitopes, which persist in the circulation even a long time after allergen exposure. The expansion of T-cell clones specific for allergens may be secondary to the preferential exposure at a level of APC, of complexes formed by allergen epitopes and corresponding class II histocompatibility molecules. The expansion of specific $T_{H/I}$ cells and their persistence may be modulated by antigen- and Id-specific T suppressor cells (Fig. 15.1).

Two main mechanisms have been suggested to explain the preferential expression of the IgE isotype in immune responses of atopic people: an impairment of IgE class-specific regulatory T-lymphocytes (Fig. 15.1), and a primary hyperactivity of the T helper (T_H)-B-cell system involved in the IgE production (Fig. 15.2).

The findings that may suggest the alterations of the T-cell system and particularly the impairment of IgE-specific regulatory T-cells in atopic subjects have already been reviewed and discussed. Clear-cut evidence of phenotypic and/or functional alterations of the T-cell suppressor system has been given only in patients with atopic dermatitis. On the other hand, the presence in atopic patients (particularly in those with severe atopic disease) of circulating spontaneously IgE-producing cells, as well as circulating T-lymphocytes able to release IgE potentiating factors, which has been documented by the application of *in vitro* models for the study of IgE production, seem to suggest a selective hyperactivity of the T_H-B-cell system involved in the IgE production at least in a proportion of atopic patients. Obviously, the possibility that this hyperactivity is at least in part the reflex of an impairment of regulatory T-cells cannot be excluded. Both the impairment of regulatory T-lymphocytes and primary hyperactivity of the T_H-B-cell system involved in the IgE antibody pro-

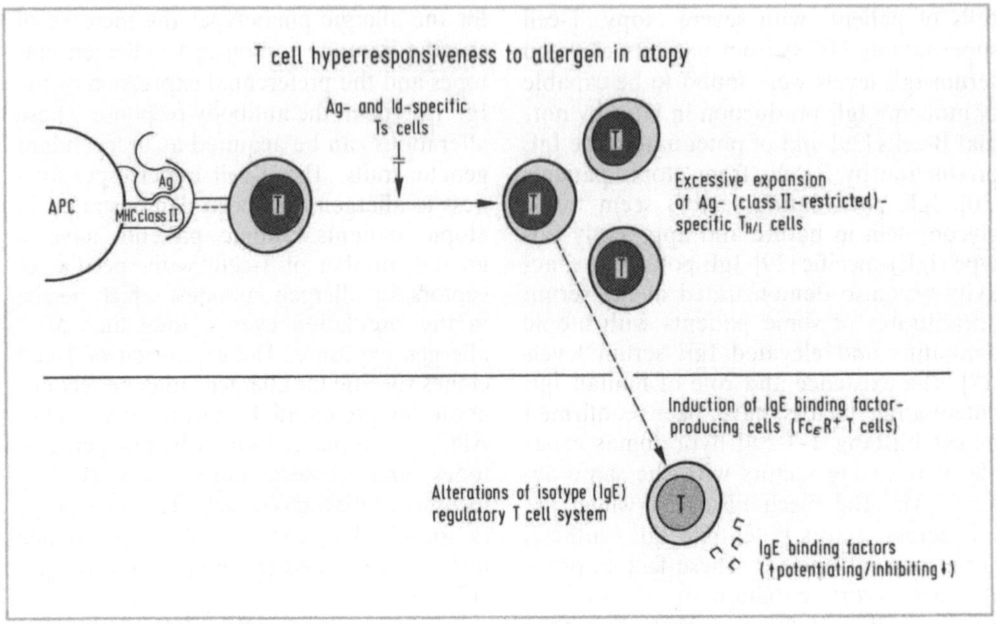

Fig. 15.1. Possible alterations in atopic phenotype leading to T-cell hyperresponsiveness to antigen (Ag). A first selection of Ag can occur at a level of Ag presenting cells (APC) because of the binding of a site of class II molecule to a corresponding site of Ag. Activation and proliferation of Ag-specific T-cell clones are made possible since T-cell receptors can corecognize Ag site (epitope) and a site of class II molecule at a level of APC. This interaction may be facilitated by the persistence on the membrane of APC, of stable complexes formed by Ag and corresponding class II molecules. Thus, the *selection* of Ag by class II molecules appears as an initial important step in the events leading to Ag-specific T-cell hyperresponsiveness. MHC-associated Ir genes can control the specific immune responses by related class II molecules. The expansion of specific $T_{H/I}$ cells and their persistence may be modulated by Ag- and idiotype (Id)-specific T suppressor cells. A defect of this regulatory system may constitute another alteration in atopy. The excessive expansion of Ag (class II-restricted)-specific $T_{H/I}$ cells may also induce the formation of IgE-binding factor-producing cells ($Fc_\varepsilon R^+$ T-cells) involved in the isotype (IgE)-specific regulatory system. Alterations of this system may be present in atopic phenotype

duction could coexist. The studies performed with anti-Id antibody raise the possibility that idiotypic network plays an important role in the modulation of IgE responses. Thus, it could be of interest to determine whether there are differences between atopic and nonatopic individuals in terms of regulation of IgE synthesis by anti-Id antibodies.

Finally, it should be noted that several recent data indicate meaningful physiological participation of lymphoid cells capable of binding IgE through Fc receptors in the regulation of IgE responses [3, 33]. The number of $Fc_\varepsilon R^+$ cells markedly increases in atopic individuals with active disease. The great majority of $Fc_\varepsilon R^+$ cells can be detected when purified B-lymphocyte suspensions are screened [33]. A number of human B-cell lines expressing $Fc_\varepsilon R$ secrete IgE-binding factors capable of enhancing the spontaneous synthesis of IgE [34]. These findings provide some new insights into the possible levels of cellular alterations related to the expression of the allergic phenotype.

References

1. Tada T (1975) Regulation of reagin formation. Prog Allergy 19: 122–186
2. Ishizaka K (1980) Regulation of the IgE response. In: Fougerau M, Dausset J (eds) Im-

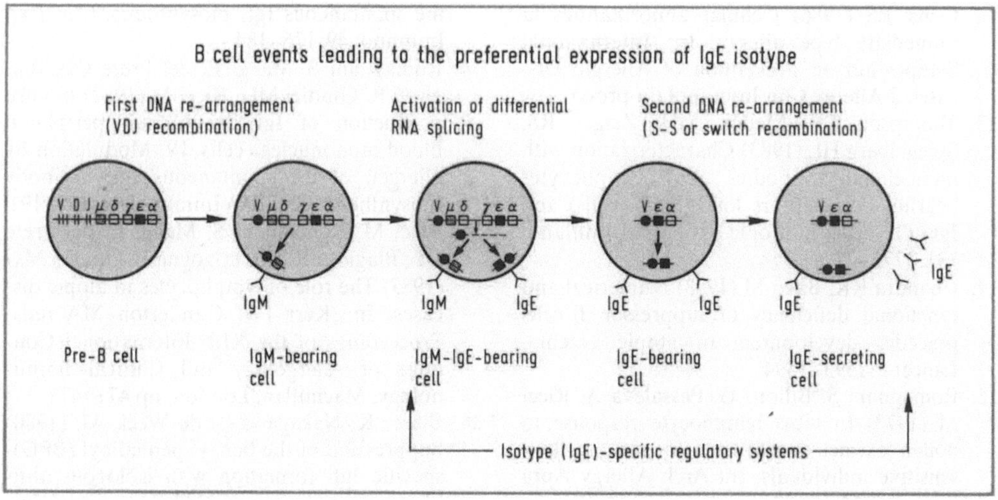

Fig. 15.2. B-cell events leading to the preferential expression of IgE isotype in atopy. IgM-IgE double bearing B-cells derive from B-cells bearing surface-IgM. Antigenic stimulation causes the maturation of precursor cells into memory B-cells that bear exclusively IgE. T-cells appear to participate in the development of IgE memory B-cells and IgE-secreting cells. As shown in mice, the differentiation of IgM-bearing B-cells into IgM-IgE-bearing B-cells can involve the activation of differential RNA processing of a single large transcript containing VH, Cμ, Cδ, Cγ and Cε gene sequences. The large transcript can be spliced into μ or ε mRNA by specific enzymes. IgM-IgE-bearing B-cells differentiate into IgE-bearing cells and IgE-secreting cells by a second DNA rearrangement or switch recombination with simultaneous DNA deletion. Isotype (IgE)-specific regulatory systems, acting on B-cells bearing IgE, play a very important role in the regulation of B-lymphocyte differentiation from IgE memory cells and IgE-secreting cells. These systems comprise of a complex web of cellular and molecular interactions involving $Fc_{\varepsilon}R^+$ T- and B-cells, related IgE-binding factors with potentiating or suppressive activity, and, as shown in mice, factors inducing such biologic activities and IgE-induced regulants. The preferential expression of IgE isotype in atopic patients could depend on possible alterations at different levels of cellular and molecular interactions of IgE regulatory systems leading to the excessive formation of IgE-secreting cells

munology 80. Academic Press, London, p 815–828
3. Katz DH (1984) Regulation of the IgE system: experimental and clinical aspects. Allergy 39:81–106
4. Romagnani S, Biagiotti R, Amadori A, Maggi E, Biti G, Bellesi G, Ricci M (1980) Hyperproduction of IgE and T-cell dysfunction in Hodgkin's disease. Int Arch Allergy Appl Immunol 63:64–72
5. Strannegard O, Strannegard IL (1978) T lymphocyte number and function in human IgE-mediated allergy. Immunol Rev 41:149–170
6. Juto P (1980) Immune responses, type of feeding and atopic allergy in infants. Medical dissertation, Umea University, pp 7–50
7. Neiburger RG, Neiburger JB, Dockhorn RJ (1978) Distribution of peripheral blood T and B lymphocyte markers in atopic children and changes during immunotherapy. J Allergy Clin Immunol 61:88–92
8. Romagnani S, Biagiotti R, Maggi E, Amadori A, Giudizi MG, Ricci M (1978) Lymphocyte responsiveness in atopy. In: Ricci M, Fauci AS, Arcangeli P, Torzuoli P (eds) Developments in Clinical Immunology. Academic Press, London, pp 185–191
9. Canonica GW, Mingari MC, Melioli G, Colombatti M, Moretta L (1979) Imbalances of T cell subpopulations in patients with atopic diseases and effect of specific immunotherapy. J Immunol 123:2669–2672
10. Leung D, Rhodes AR, Geha RS (1981) Enumeration of T cell subsets in atopic dermatitis using monoclonal antibodies. J Allergy Clin Immunol 67:450–455
11. Matloff SM, Kiselis IK, Rocklin RE (1983) Reduced production of histamine-induced suppressor factor (HSF) by atopic mononuclear cells and decreased prostaglandin E2 output by HSF-stimulated atopic monocytes. J Allergy Clin Immunol 72:359–364

12. Geha RS (1986) Cellular abnormalities in immediate type allergy. In: International Symposium on Prevention of Allergic Diseases. J Allergy Clin Immunol (in press)
13. Thompson LF, Mellon MH, Zeiger RS, Spiegelberg HL (1983) Characterization with monoclonal antibodies of T lymphocytes bearing Fc receptors for IgE (T_ε cells) and IgG (T_γ cells) in atopic patients. J Immunol 131:2772–2776
14. Chandra RK, Baka M (1983) Numerical and functional deficiency of suppressor T cells precedes development of atopic eczema. Lancet 2:1393–1394
15. Romagnani S, Biliotti G, Passaleva A, Ricci M (1973) In vitro lymphocyte response to pollen extract constituents in grass pollen-sensitive individuals. Int Arch Allergy Appl Immunol 44:40–50
16. Rocklin RE, Sheffer AL, Greineder DK, Melmon KL (1980) Generation of antigen-specific suppressor cells during allergy desensitization. N Engl J Med 302:1213–1219
17. Ricci M, Romagnani S, Amadori A, Maggi E (1976) Hyposensitization and lymphocyte responsiveness. In: Allergy and Clinical Immunology. Proceedings of the IXth International Congress of Allergology, Buenos Aires. Excerpta Medica, Amsterdam, pp 495–501
18. Ricci M, del Prete GF, Maggi E, Lanzavecchia A, Romagnani S (1986) Advances in understanding of mechanisms of IgE disregulation in atopy by the application of in vitro methods. J Allergy Clin Immunol (in press)
19. Rawle FC, Mitchell EB, Platts-Mills AC (1984) T cell sensitization to D. pteronyssinus antigen P1. J Allergy Clin Immunol 73 [Suppl]: 119–129
20. Lanzavecchia A, Santini P, Maggi E, del Prete GF, Falagiani P, Romagnani S, Ferrarini M (1983) In vitro selective expansion of allergen specific T cells from atopic patients. Clin Exp Immunol 52:21–28
21. Fiser PM, Buckley RH (1979) Human IgE biosynthesis in vitro: studies with atopic and normal blood mononuclear cells and subpopulations. J Immunol 123:1788–1794
22. Romagnani S, Maggi E, del Prete GF, Troncone R, Ricci M (1980) In vitro production of IgE by human peripheral blood mononuclear cells. I. Rate of IgE biosynthesis. Clin Exp Immunol 42:167–174
23. Romagnani S, Damiani G, Giudizi MG, Biagiotti R, Almerigogna F, del Prete GF, Maggi E, Bargellesi A, Ricci M (1982) In vitro production of IgE by human peripheral blood mononuclear cells. III. Demonstration of a circulating IgE-bearing cell involved in the spontaneous IgE biosynthesis. Clin Exp Immunol 49:176–184
24. Romagnani S, Maggi E, del Prete GF, Biagiotti R, Giudizi MG, Ricci M (1982) In vitro production of IgE by human peripheral blood mononuclear cells. IV. Modulation by allergen of the spontaneous IgE antibody biosynthesis. Clin Exp Immunol 49:185–191
25. Ricci M, Romagnani S, Maggi E, del Prete GF, Biagiotti R, Almerigogna F, Giudizi MG (1983) The role of lymphocytes in atopic diseases. In: Kerr IW, Ganderton MA (eds) Proceedings of the XIth International Congress of Allergology and Clinical Immunology. Macmillan, London, pp 471–477
26. Blaser K, Nakagawa T, de Weck AL (1980) Suppression of the benzyl penicilloyl (BPO)-specific IgE formation with isologous anti-idiotypic antibodies in BALB/c mice. J Immunol 125:24–30
27. de Weck AL, Blaser K (1983) Idiotypic regulation of the IgE response. In: Kerr IW, Ganderton MA (eds) Proceedings of the XIth International Congress of Allergology and Clinical Immunology. Macmillan, London, pp 371–376
28. Geha RS, Comunale M (1983) Regulation of immunoglobulin E antibody synthesis in man by antiidiotypic antibodies. J Clin Invest 71:46–54
29. Sarjan JA, Leung D, Geha RS (1983) Induction of human IgE synthesis by a factor derived from T cells of patients with hyper-IgE states. J Immunol 130:242–247
30. Romagnani S, Maggi E, del Prete GF, Ricci M (1983) IgE synthesis in vitro induced by T cell factors from patients with elevated serum IgE levels. Clin Exp Immunol 52: 85–88
31. Young MC, Leung D, Geha RS (1984) Production of human T-T hybridoma secreting IgE specific helper factors. J Allergy Clin Immunol 73 [Suppl]: 172
32. Lanzavecchia A (1984) One out of five peripheral blood B lymphocytes is activated to high-rate Ig production by human alloreactive T cell clones. Eur J Immunol 13:820–824
33. Spiegelberg HL (1984) Structure and function of Fc receptors for IgE on lymphocytes, monocytes and macrophages. Adv Immunol 35:61–88
34. Delespesse G, Sarfati M, Rocha G, Rector E, Sehon AH (1984) In vitro synthesis of human IgE. In: International Symposium on Prevention of Allergic Diseases, Florence, June 24–27. O.I.C. Medical, Florence, p 12

16. Delayed-type Hypersensitivity Responses to Inhalant Allergens: a Form of Cutaneous Basophil Hypersensitivity (CBH)

E. B. Mitchell

16.1 Cutaneous Basophil Hypersensitivity (CBH)

When considering the immune mechanisms involved in immune inflammation it is important to recognize that in disease such inflammation is chronic, and as such cannot be explained by acute self-limited reactions. This is particularly true of the allergic diseases. The atopic individual develops an immune response which in addition to IgE-specific antibody usually includes IgG antibody of various subclasses and sensitized T-lymphocytes [1, 2]. These T-cells presumably have the potential to contribute to allergen-induced cell-mediated immune events.

Since the early work of Jones and Mote [3], it has been evident that a complex relationship between immediate and delayed hypersensitivity responses at the same reaction site can exist. In 1969 [4], Dvorak and his colleagues recognized that, in guinea pigs, "Jones-Mote"-type responses induced by the injection of a protein antigen in saline, involved the recruitment of basophils to the delayed reaction site in the skin. The reactions, termed cutaneous basophil hypersensitivity (CBH), are now known to occur widely in biology, both in man [5] and in experimental animals [6, 7]. The presence of the basophil appears to be regulated by the function of sensitized T-cells in the guinea pig model [8, 9]. Furthermore the recruited basophil has the capacity to anaphylactically degranulate at the delayed reaction site, indicating that more than one type of reaction [10] may potentially develop concurrently.

16.2 Skin Response to Inhalant Allergens

The recognition that the induced response to contact allergens in the skin of sensitive individuals represents cutaneous basophil hypersensitivity [11] in which both T-cells and basophils are present in the skin lesions gave rise to the search for a similar reactivity to inhalant allergens. The application of crude allergen in high concentration to the skin of atopic dermatitis patients, sensitive to this allergen, gives rise to a delayed eczematous reaction. This response is present at 24 hours and lasts 72 hours or longer [12]. Prior sensitization, determined by the presence of immediate hypersensitivity skin test responses, was essential in achieving the eczematous reaction. Using the purified house dust mite allergen, antigen P_1, it is apparent that the quantity of antigen required to elicit the delayed eczematous response was approximately 6 times that required to elicit the immediate reaction. However, it should be remembered that delayed hypersensitivity responses in experimental animals and in man require the introduction of μg quantities of antigen and not ng or pg quantities for their elicitation. Furthermore, it was necessary to gently abrade the skin prior to the application of allergen via the patch test technique. This was necessary as the keratinized layers of the skin would not normally allow the entry of a water-soluble allergen (unlike the situation with the lipid-soluble contact sensitizers).

Biopsy of the positive reactions to inhalant allergen at 48 hours indicated that the reactions were infiltrated by basophils as well as mononuclear cells, eosinophils, and neutrophils. Inhalant allergens, therefore, are capable of inducing cutaneous basophil hypersensitivity responses. In contrast, neither saline applied to atopic dermatitis skin, or allergen to nonatopic skin was able to induce a similar cellular infiltrate. It should be remembered that appropriate fixation and embedding procedures are necessary to allow basophil identification [12]. In this circumstance glutaraldehyde fixation, plastic embedding, followed by Giemsa staining was used [13].

16.3 Cell-mediated Immunity to Allergen

Patients with atopic dermatitis, who have immediate hypersensitivity to the house dust mite antigen (antigen P_1) can be shown to possess circulating T-cells which will proliferate following allergen exposure *in vitro* [14]. Patients with both asthma and rhinitis who show a similar immediate sensitivity also possess these sensitized T-cells. The response induced is dose-dependent, requiring μg quantities of allergen, and can be shown to involve cells having a T helper cell phenotype, as identified by the monoclonal antibody Leu 3a (Bectonand Dickenson) and fluorescence-activated cell sorting (FACS). Furthermore, in these experiments the presence of peripheral blood monocytes, acting as antigen presenting cells was required. To implicate cell-mediated immunity in the inhalant allergen-induced patch test lesions, the possibility that T-cells and antigen presenting cells are recruited to or expanded at this site must be considered. There is now preliminary evidence from experiments using immunoperoxidase labeling techniques and monoclonal antibodies that cells bearing both T helper and suppressor phenotypes infiltrate these lesions [Zachary et al, unpublished observations; 15]. Furthermore, cells bearing both Ia and OKT-6 (ortho) antigens, presumably Langerhans cells are also expanded. These results support the concept that allergen-induced basophil containing lesions are examples of cell-mediated immune events.

16.4 Chronic Allergen Exposure

The naturally occurring lichenified lesions of atopic dermatitis patients have not been shown to be infiltrated by basophils [16]. These lesions are, however, infiltrated by mononuclear cells and have an expanded number of mast cells. To attempt recreating natural exposure to house dust mite allergen, antigen P_1 was repeatedly applied to the same skin site, again using the modified patch test technique, over a period of 10 days. The differential cell counts over this period of time indicated that the early basophil infiltration that developed was replaced by a subsequent mast cell hyperplasia or recruitment, this mast cell expansion developing at a time when other infiltrating cells were disappearing [17]. It is known from other studies that a complex relationship between basophils and mast cells at inflammatory sites can develop, usually involving an early basophil infiltrate being replaced by a later mast cell recruitment [18]. It appears therefore that chronic inhalant allergen exposure results in lesions which are infiltrated by cells similar to those present in naturally developing eczematous skin lesions.

Recently there has been some evidence that mast cell heterogeneity exists in rodents and perhaps in man [19, 20]. Careful analysis of the mast cell expansion in the allergen-induced patch test lesions failed to show any structural or morphological differences [17].

16.5 Basophil Recruitment

The mechanisms involved in basophil recruitment to the skin are unclear. It is known that the mast cell-dependent late phase skin response (LPR) is associated with an infiltration of eosinophils, mononuclear cells and neutrophils, as well as basophils [21, 22]. While it has been shown that following antigen challenge, the mast cell releases mediators which give rise to cell recruitment, passive transfer studies have failed to conclusively show that these mediators can recruit basophils [23].

In vivo: Using the patch test technique, before and after the infusion of large volumes of IgE containing plasma to patients with hypo-γ-globulinemia, it was possible to transfer the ability to elicit a delayed reaction at 48 hours. The plasma used had been harvested from patients with atopic dermatitis who were known to give a positive patch test reaction to antigen P_1 and to have high levels of IgE antibody specific for this antigen. The results of differential cell counting following biopsy of these lesions indicated that it was possible to transfer an ability to recruit eosinophils, neutrophils and mononuclear cells in this manner but not basophils [24]. Similar local transfer studies in normal nonatopic subjects with pre- and postallergen patch testing indicated that serum from sensitive atopic dermatitis subjects did have the ability to recruit basophils as well as the other cell types, but that this ability did not reside in the IgE antibody fraction. From these experiments it appears that the delayed cellular. response to allergen cannot be explained by IgE mast cell-mediated events alone.

In vitro: It has been clearly demonstrated, in the past, that both activated complement components [25] and lymphocyte products [26, 27] are capable of chemoattracting basophils. Using the blind well chamber technique (a modified Boyden chamber) we have demonstrated that the supernatants from lymphocytes cultured with allergen for 3 days *in vitro* are capable of inducing basophils to migrate across a polycarbonate membrane [28]. This was true when the lymphocytes were those of house dust mite sensitive subjects cultured with its major allergen, antigen P_1. The effect was not, however, specific for basophils as it was also active against neutrophils and mononuclear cells. When the arachidonic acid metabolite, leukotriene B_4 was used the results were different. This agent is known to chemoattract eosinophils, neutrophils and mononuclear cells [29, 30]. However, it was shown to have only a weak effect against basophils [28]. Furthermore, when leukotriene B_4 and the lymphocyte-derived supernatant were directly compared, the degree of cell migration was comparable for neutrophils and mononuclear cells but not for basophils.

It would appear that the results of both *in vivo* and *in vitro* experiments indicate that the action of lymphocytes, presumably T-cells (the cells known to respond to allergen) represents a more likely explanation of basophil recruitment to the skin site than does mast cell mediator release.

If we directly compare leukotriene B_4 activity with the lymphocyte-derived supernatant activity, we can see that the two preparations are roughly comparable for cells such as mononuclear cells and neutrophils, but that in the case of the basophil a marked difference is present. In this situation the lymphocyte-derived supernatant is much more potent at chemoattracting the basophil than is leukotriene B_4. Therefore it would appear that the results of both our *in vivo* and our *in vitro* experiments suggest that mast cell mediators cannot explain the recruitment of basophils to the skin site, and that it is much more likely to be due to T-cells which are known to be present in these induced lesions.

Finally, it should be noted that in some very recent experiments in mice, Askenase and his colleagues [31, 32] have been able to show that delayed hypersensitivity involves a T-cell that can produce an antigen-specific factor which directly acts on mast cells to induce mediator release. In other words, both IgE antibody and T-cell products can give rise to mast cell mediator release. In humans the identification of a T-cell-derived basophil histamine releasing activity (HRA) [33] would appear to indicate the potential for identifying similar type factors. In conclusion therefore, it appears that in the skin at least the response to allergen involves sensitized T-cells as well as IgE antibody, and that the reactions occurring have more in common with cell-mediated immunity than they do with immediate hypersensitivity alone. What probably occurs is a complex overlapping between immediate hypersensitivity, a delayed phase skin response dependent upon the release of mast cell mediators, and cutaneous basophil hypersensitivity dependent upon T-cell function. There is no reason to presuppose that such reactions do not occur in the airway, and indeed one of the most important recruited cells in allergic rhinitis is the basophil. Indeed, it has been shown that the mediators released in induced late phase responses in the nose are more likely to be due to basophils than mast cells. It has yet to be shown that these rules apply to the lower airway, namely in asthma. When considering how desensitization might work, it is necessary to look at all the mechanisms that are underway in allergen-induced inflammation. It may well be that we will have to totally rethink our approaches to this treatment modality before we will end up with a successful approach.

References

1. Chapman MD, Rowntree S, Mitchell EB, di Prisco de Fuenmajor MC, Platts-Mills TAE (1983) Quantitative assessments of IgG and IgE antibodies to inhalant allergens in patients with atopic dermatitis. J Allergy Clin Immunol 72:27–33
2. Rocklin RE, Sheffer AL, Greineder DK, Melmon KL (1980) Generation of antigen specific suppressor cells during allergy desensitization. N Engl J Med 302:1213–1216
3. Jones TD, Mote JR (1934) The phases of foreign protein sensitization in human beings. N Engl J Med 210:120–123
4. Dvorak HF, Dvorak AM, Simpson BA, Richerson HB, Leskowitz S, Karnovsky MJ (1970) Cutaneous basophil hypersensitivity. II. A light and electron microscopic description. J Exp Med 132:558–582
5. Dvorak HF (1976) Cutaneous basophil hypersensitivity. J Allergy Clin Immunol 58: 229–240
6. Askenase PW (1977) Role of basophils, mast cells and vasoamines in hypersensitivity reactions with a delayed time course. Prog Allergy 23:199
7. Mitchell EB, Askenase PW (1983) Basophils in human disease. Clin Rev Allergy 1:427–448
8. Askenase PW (1976) Cutaneous basophil hypersensitivity uncovered in the cell transfer of classical tuberculin hypersensitivity. J Immunol 117:741–747
9. Mitchell EB, Askenase PW (1982) Suppression of T cell mediated cutaneous basophil hypersensitivity by serum from guinea pigs immunized with mycobacterial adjuvant. J Exp Med 156:159–172
10. Coombs RRA, Gell PGH (1975) Classification of allergic reactions responsible for clinical hypersensitivity and disease. In: Gell PGH, Coombs RRA, Lachman PJ (eds) Clinical Aspects of Immunology, 3rd edn. Blackwell, Oxford Edinburgh Carlton Boston Palo Alto
11. Dvorak HF, Mihm MC (1972) Basophilic leukocytes in allergic contact dermatitis. J Exp Med 135:235–254
12. Mitchell EB, Crow J, Chapman MD, Jouhal SS, Pope FM, Platts-Mills TAE (1982) Basophils in allergen induced patch test sites in atopic dermatitis. Lancet I:127–130
13. Godfrey HP, Pastore MS, Askenase PW (1981) A modified Giemsa stain for demonstrating basophils in glycol methacrylate. J Histotech 125:587–592
14. Rawle FC, Mitchell EB, Platts-Mills TAE (1984) T cell responses to the major allergen from the house dust mite, *D. pteronyssinus*, antigen P_1: comparison of patients with asthma, atopic dermatitis and perennial rhinitis. J Immunol 133:195–201
15. Zachary CB, MacDonald DM, Mitchel EB (unpublished observation)
16. Mihm MC, Soter NA, Dvorak HF, Austen KF (1976) The structure of normal skin and the morphology of atopic eczema. J Invest Dermatol 67:305
17. Mitchell EB, Crow J, Williams G, Platts-Mills TAE (1986) Increase in skin mast cells following chronic house dust mite exposure. Br J Dermatol 114:65
18. Dvorak HF, Mihm MC, Dvorak AM, Johnson RA, Manseau EJ, Morgan E, Colvin RB (1974) Morphology of delayed type hypersensitivity reactions in man. I. Quantitative description of the inflammatory response. Lab Invest 31:111–130
19. Befus AD, Pearce FL, Gauldie J, Horsewood P, Bienenstock J (1982) Mucosal mast cells. I. Isolation and functional characteristics of rat intestinal mast cells. J Immunol 128:2475–2480
20. Strobel S, Miller HRP, Ferguson A (1981) Human intestinal mucosal mast cells: evaluation of fixation and staining techniques. J Clin Pathol 34:851–858
21. Dolovich J, Hargreave FE, Chalmers R, Shier KJ, Gauldie J, Bienenstock J (1973) Late cutaneous allergic responses in isolated IgE-dependent reactions. J Allergy Clin Immunol 52:38–46
22. Richerson HB, Rajtora DW, Penick GD, Dick FR, Yoo TJ, Kammermeyer JK, Anuras JS (1979) Cutaneous and nasal allergic responses in ragweed hay fever; lack of clinical and histopathological correlations with late phase reactions. J Allergy Clin Immunol 64:67–77
23. Solley GO, Gleich GJ, Jordan RE, Schroeter AL (1976) The late phase of the immediate wheal and flare skin reaction. J Clin Invest 58:408–420
24. Mitchell EB, Crow J, Rowntree S, Webster ADB, Platts-Mills TAE (1984) Cutaneous basophil hypersensitivity to inhalant allergens: local transfer of basophil accumulation with immune serum but not IgE antibody. J Invest Dermatol 83:290–295
25. Ward PA, Dvorak HK, Cohen S, Yoshida T, Data R, Selvaggio SS (1975) Chemotaxis of basophils by lymphocyte-dependent and lymphocyte-independent mechanisms. J Immunol 114:1523–1531

26. Lett-Brown MA, Boetcher DA, Leonard EJ (1976) Chemotactic responses of normal human basophils to C5a and to lymphocyte-derived chemotactic factor. J Immunol 117:246–252
27. Lett-Brown MA, Aelvoet M, Hooks JJ, Georgiades JA, Theuson DO, Grant JA (1981) Enhancement of basophil chemotaxis *in vitro* by virus induced interferon. J Clin Invest 67:547–552
28. Mitchell EB, Jouhal SS, Rawle FC (1984) Basophil recruitment in allergic subjects: basophil chemotactic activity produced by allergen stimulated peripheral blood mononuclear cells. J Allergy Clin Immunol 73:149
29. Lewis RA, Austen KF (1981) Mediation of local homeostasis and inflammation by leukotrienes and other mast cell-dependent compounds. Nature 293:103–106
30. Atkins PC, Wasserman SI (1983) Chemotactic mediators. Clin Rev Allergy 1:385–395
31. Ptak W, Askenase PW, Rosenstein RW, Gershon RK (1982) Transfer of an antigen specific immediate hypersensitivity-like reaction with an antigen binding factor produced by T cells. Proc Natl Acad Sci USA 79:1969–1971
32. Askenase PW, Rosenstein R, Ptak W, Gershon RW (1983) T cells produce an antigen binding factor with *in vivo* activity analogous to IgE antibody. J Exp Med 157:862–866
33. Theuson DO, Speck LS, Lett-Brown MA, Grant JA (1979) Histamine-releasing activity (HRA). I. Production by mitogen or antigen stimulated human mononuclear cells. J Immunol 123:626–632

E. Mediator Release and Bronchial Obstruction

17. Physiological and Pharmacological Control of Inflammatory Mediator Release in Bronchial Asthma

S. T. Holgate

Bronchial asthma is a disease of complex etiology. Over the last 5 years the recognition that widespread reversible airways' obstruction characteristic of bronchial asthma, is associated with enhanced reactivity of the airways to specific and nonspecific stimuli has stimulated new approaches to its diagnosis and an increased understanding of the pathogenetic nature of the disease. It is now generally accepted that enhanced bronchial reactivity is the central physiological abnormality of the airways in asthma [1], but the mechanism underlying this abnormal responsiveness remains to be defined. From a pathological standpoint the airways in asthma are infiltrated with inflammatory cells, particularly eosinophils, neutrophils and monocytes, there is hypersecretion of mucus and desquamation of the surface respiratory epithelium with plugging of the airways, thickening of the basement membrane, hypertrophy of airways smooth muscle and mucosal and submucosal edema [2]. These features, which are tantamount to an obliterative bronchiolitis, are reversible both spontaneously and with treatment. Indeed, the reversibility of the airway obstruction has formed the major part of the clinical definition of asthma [3] and separates it from those forms of bronchial obstruction which characterize chronic bronchitis and emphysema.

From a clinical standpoint asthma is conveniently subdivided into allergic (extrinsic) or nonallergic (intrinsic) forms, and although there may be differences in the way these disease variants may present clinically and respond to treatment, the basic underlying abnormality of bronchial inflammation and hyperreactivity remains [1]. A number of studies have shown that following treatment with sodium cromoglycate or corticosteroids a component of bronchial reactivity in asthma is reversible [4]. It is therefore tempting to speculate that hyperreactivity in asthma relates directly to airway inflammation irrespective of the precipitating factor(s) [1]. The majority of asthma in children and young adults is associated with an atopic status, with seasonal and perennial exposure to environmental allergens being closely correlated with increased airway reactivity and exacerbation of asthma [5], whereas removal from offending antigens results in clinical improvement [6].

It is now recognized that in patients with allergic asthma inhalation of antigen extracts to which the subjects are specifically sensitive, causes an immediate bronchoconstriction, reaching a maximum 5–15 min after challenge [7]. This early reaction is not infrequently followed by a late bronchoconstrictor response occurring 6 or more hours later, which on occasions may occur repeatedly over several days [8]. Thus, in allergic asthma, antigen bronchial provocation provides a useful clinical model to investigate the pathogenesis of allergic asthma and to study the effects of therapeutic agents on the ensuing response.

17.1 Control of Mast Cell Mediator Secretion

It is now widely recognized that following antigen provocation of patients with allergic asthma airway narrowing results from the release of inflammatory mediators. Mast cells within the bronchial wall play a sentinel role in initiating this response and have provided a logical focus for recent investigations.

Human lung tissue is a particularly rich source of mast cells, most of which are found in the airways superficial to the basement membrane [9]. On occasion, mast cells are located within the ciliated respiratory epithelium where they are able to interact with inhaled antigens. Using mechanical [10] and enzymatic [11] techniques it is possible to disperse viable mast cells from human lung tissue for further investigation. Human dispersed lung mast cells are heterogeneous with respect to their size and content of granules [12]. The membrane-bound granules of mast cells are specialized in this cell to be secreted upon cell stimulation [13].

Human mast cells contain in excess of 130,000 cell surface receptors which bind specifically to the C4 domain of the Fc fragment of the reaginic antibody, IgE [14]. In the immediate hypersensitivity reaction it is the cross-linkage of cell-bound IgE, through interaction with specific antigen, that results in the secretion of preformed and newly generated inflammatory mediators [15].

Activated mast cells undergo rapid degranulation which reaches completion within 5 min of immunological stimulation [10]. The cell membrane events which underlie the coupling of mast cell activation to secretion of mediators has been intensively investigated. Following the cross-linkage of cell-associated IgE a membrane serine esterase activity is revealed with consequent activation of two methyltransferase enzymes which are stereochemically orientated within the mast cell membrane [16]. It is proposed that a methyltransferase situated on the cytoplasmic face of the cell membrane, donates a single methyl group to phosphatidylethanolamine (PE), forming monomethylphosphatidylethanolamine (MPE). This phospholipid, in being less polar than PE, is thought to move within the membrane, bringing it into contact with a second methyltransferase which adds two further methyl groups to MPE, converting it to phosphatidylcholine (PC) (Fig. 17.1). It is further suggested that alteration of the annular lipids in the region of IgE receptors is fundamental to the exposure of channels which facilitate the influx of extracellular calcium ions. While most of the experimental work which has incriminated phospholipid methylation in activation-secretion coupling of mast cells has been carried out on rat basophil leukemic cells [17] and rat serosal mast cells [18], a recent study has reported similar changes following immunological activation of isolated and human lung mast cells [19].

Despite repeated attempts, a number of independent groups have had difficulty demonstrating stimulus-related phospholipid methylation [20, 21]. However, that methylation reactions are involved in mast cell secretion also accrues from evidence that methyltransferase inhibitors such as 3-deazaadenosine and its S-isobuteryl analogue, either alone or in the presence of homocysteine thiolactone, are potent inhibitors of immunological mediator release [16–19, 22]. These pharmacological agents are also able to inhibit histamine release from human lung mast cells activated with the calcium ionophore A23187, a secretagogue which activates mast cells by directly inserting calcium into the cell membrane, thereby bypassing the IgE-Fc receptor mechanism [22]. However, in experiments on human mast cells isolated from the same lungs, 3-deazaadenosine in the presence of homocysteine thiolactone has been shown to be 17 times more potent at inhibiting mediator release when the cells were activated immunologically compared to A23187 [22]. From these results it seems reasonable to conclude that methylation reactions may be involved at several stages of mast cell activation-secretion coupling.

Two other early cellular events have also been described in association with IgE receptor bridging which are considered relevant to mast cell activation. The first of these is the stimulation of the phosphatidylinosotol phosphatidic acid cycle mediated through the calcium-independent stimulation of phospholipase C (Fig. 17.1). With a wide variety of secretagogues such as calcium ionophore A23187, compound 48/80 and antihuman IgE, pulse labeling of membrane phospholipids of rat mast cells with P^{32} has demonstrated a rapid degradation of phosphatidylinosotol to diacylglycerol and inosotol monophosphate which precedes mediator secretion [23]. Diacylglycerol may undergo further cleavage under the enzymatic control of diglyceride lipase (a calcium-dependent enzyme) which generates arachidonic acid for subsequent oxidative metabolism and the

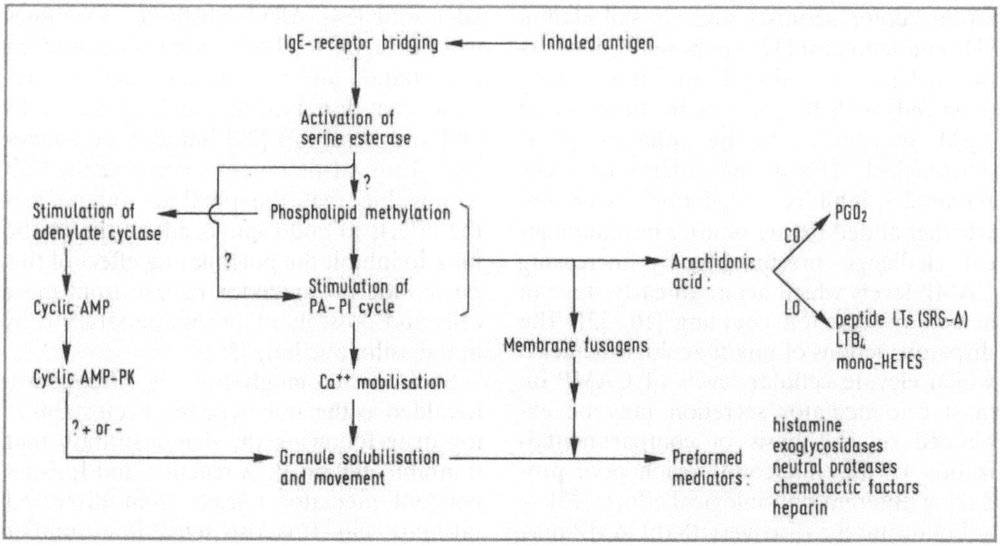

Fig. 17.1. Proposed sequence of biochemical events involved in mast cell activation-secretion coupling

membrane fusagen monoacylglycerol. Diacylglycerol may also undergo a condensation reaction with ATP to phosphatidic acid which when followed by sequential adduction with CDP and inosotol reforms phosphatidylinosotol. Stimulation of the phosphatidylinosotol phosphatidic acid cycle has been incriminated in the opening of calcium channels which is common to a number of secretory cell types [24].

A second cellular event which occurs 5–15 s after stimulation of rodent mast cells for mediator secretion is an early rise in the cellular levels of CAMP due to receptor-stimulated activation of membrane adenylate cyclase (Fig. 17.1) [25]. In activated rodent mast cells this transient increase in CAMP activates both isoenzymes of intracellular CAMP-dependent protein kinase which may be involved in the progression of the secretory response [26]. However, on the basis that pharmacological increases in CAMP or the dibutyryl analogue of CAMP have been shown to inhibit mediator secretion from mast cells [27], an IgE-dependent increase in the levels of this cyclic nucleotide may represent some form of intrinsic cell regulation (Fig. 17.1) [16]. Recent studies on isolated human lung mast cells have also shown that cell activation is accompanied by a transient increase in cellular levels of CAMP that precedes the onset of mediator secretion [19].

In human basophils, adenosine also stimulates adenylate cyclase to increase cellular levels of CAMP through activation of cell surface A_2 purinoceptors [28, 29]. In human basophils and mast cells this nucleoside and related analogues have been shown to inhibit mediator release if added before immunological challenge, but enhance release when added while mediator secretion is ongoing [29, 30]. This data may be interpreted as CAMP being obligatory for the coupling of cell activation to secretion. Thus, preincubation of mast cells with adenosine, which increases cellular levels of CAMP, could prematurely activate CAMP-dependent protein kinase, thereby depriving the mast cell of this enzyme obligatory for immunological stimulation. In contrast, adenosine-induced stimulation of adenylate cyclase in parallel with immunological stimulation could increase the pool of CAMP required for activation-secretion coupling and therefore lead to enhanced mediator secretion.

Not all agents which increase mast cell levels of CAMP, however, have this diverse effect on human lung mast cells. β_2-

adrenoceptor agonists such as salbutamol [31] and fenoterol [32] are potent inhibitors of mediator secretion from human lung mast cells with IC_{50} values in the range of 1 μM. In contrast to the opposing pharmacological effects of adenosine, salbutamol inhibits mediator secretion whether added before or after immunological challenge presumably by increasing CAMP levels which act at an early stage of activation-secretion coupling [16, 23]. The disparate actions of pharmacological agents which elevate cellular levels of CAMP on mast cell mediator secretion may be explained on the basis of compartmentalization of this nucleotide, each pool producing different physiological effects [25].

Following the discovery that CAMP may act as a second messenger to exert a modulatory function on mast cell mediator secretion, a number of drugs have been developed which inhibit the breakdown of CAMP to adenosine monophosphate (AMP) by phosphodiesterase. Methylxanthines such as theophylline and its diethylamine salt aminophylline, have been most intensively investigated in this regard and are widely heralded as producing their pharmacological effects by phosphodiesterase inhibition. It should be noted, however, that these drugs produce their inhibitory effect on CAMP phosphodiesterase at concentrations which are beyond those that are achieved therapeutically in the treatment of asthma (10–20 μg/ml). Recently we have demonstrated that plasma concentrations of theophylline within the therapeutic range have the capacity to increase cellular levels of CAMP in dispersed human lung cells and isolated human leukocytes, although we were unable to demonstrate significant synergism with the β-adrenoceptor agonist isoprenaline [unpublished observation]. This, together with other observations [summarized in 33], casts doubt on whether methylxanthines exert their major pharmacological activity in asthma through inhibition of phosphodiesterase and alternative pharmacological mechanisms must be considered. Within the therapeutic range, theophylline and related methylxanthines are potent competitive antagonists of the receptor-mediated effects of adenosine [34]. Alkyl-substituted xanthines will antagonize both adenosine-induced potentiation and inhibition of mediator release from dispersed human lung mast cells [30] and basophils [29] induced by adenosine. Thus, at therapeutic concentrations it is possible that theophylline antagonizes the effects of endogenous adenosine in the lung to inhibit the potentiating effect of this nucleoside on mediator release from mast cells and possibly other inflammatory cells in the asthmatic lung [35].

Sodium cromoglycate is frequently heralded as the archetype mast cell stabilizing drug following the demonstration that it inhibits the rat PCA reaction and IgE-dependent mediator release from dispersed rat mast cells. It is also active in a number of *in vivo* animal bronchoconstrictor models [36]. Sodium cromoglycate is an effective inhibitor of antigen- and exercise-induced bronchoconstriction in asthma, and has a therapeutic application particularly in the prophylaxis of asthma in children and young adults. On the basis of its proposed mast cell stabilizing effect, it is surprising to find that sodium cromoglycate has inconsistent inhibitory effects on mediator release from human dispersed lung mast cells *in vitro* (IC_{30}, 10^{-3} M) [32]. However, sodium cromoglycate is more effective at inhibiting immunological mediator release from human lung fragments [37] and mast cells of bronchoalveolar lavage (IC_{30}, 10^{-5} M), suggesting that pharmacological heterogeneity of mast cells may exist within the human lung.

The concept of mast cell heterogeneity within the human lung is of particular interest since it has been suggested that most of the mast cells identified superficial to the basement membrane of the airway have characteristic staining properties with Alcian Blue and fail to stain with saffranin or berberine sulfate, identifying them with the so-called mucosal-type mast cell as described in the gastrointestinal tract [38]. In animal models enteric mast cells have morphological, biochemical and pharmacological differences when compared to the classical connective tissue mast cells, although at present there is insufficient information to fully extend this concept to the human respiratory tract.

In rat mast cells, sodium cromoglycate produces its inhibitory effect through stimulation of cell surface receptors which activate guanalate cyclase to increase cellular levels of cyclic GMP, activate cyclic GMP-dependent protein kinase and phosphorylate an inhibitory cytoplasmic protein of molecular weight 68,000 daltons [39]. Phosphorylation of this protein exhibits both concentration response and kinetic relationships with the inhibitory effect of sodium cromoglycate on IgE-dependent mediator secretion and may represent an intrinsic down-regulation mechanism of the mast cell secretory response.

In addition to releasing preformed mediators, the coupling of mast cell IgE-Fc receptors stimulates phospholipases A_2 and C in concert with other membrane-active enzymes to liberate substantial quantities of the polyunsaturated fatty acid, arachidonic acid (Fig. 17.1). Arachidonic acid released from the *sn*-2 position of membrane phospholipids is rapidly oxidized to a number of highly potent, newly generated chemical mediators pertinent to the immediate hypersensitivity reaction. Two pathways have been described, the cyclooxygenase pathway leading to prostanoid release and the 5-lipoxygenase pathway with release of hydroxy acids and the sulfidopeptide leukotrienes of a slow reacting substance of anaphylaxis (SRS-A). Following immunological stimulation human lung mast cells cyclooxygenize arachidonic acid almost entirely to prostaglandin (PG) D_2 [40, 41]. The potent bronchoconstrictor activity of this prostanoid on asthmatic airways [42] suggests that it plays an important role in bronchoconstriction following antigen bronchial provocation. Substantial amounts of thromboxane A_2 are also released from activated dispersed human lung cells, although this is now known to originate from activated monocytes and macrophages rather than mast cells [41]. Immunological stimulation of human lung fragments releases a further array of prostanoids including $PGF_{2\alpha}$, PGE_2 and PGI_2 [43], however, only small amounts of these prostanoids are generated from activated human dispersed lung cells, suggesting they originate from cells which are not dispersed upon proteolytic digestion of lung tissue, such as smooth muscle, fibroblasts and endothelial cells.

In addition to generating prostanoids, activation of human lung cells releases substantial quantities of 5-hydroxyeicosatetraenoic acid (5-HETE), leukotriene (LT) B_4, and the 6-sulfidopeptide leukotrienes of SRS-A, LTC_4 and LTD_4, derived from the 5-lipoxygenase pathway [44, 45]. Since all of these arachidonic acid metabolites are pro-inflammatory it is of interest to observe the effect of pharmacological agents that might modulate their formation and release. One such compound, U-60,257 (piriprost), inhibits the *in vitro* generation of sulfidopeptide leukotrienes from antigen-challenged human lung fragments of birch pollen-sensitive asthmatic patients [46] and is also inhibitory, over the micromolar range, on the generation of LTB_4 and 5-HETE from ionophore-stimulated rat mononuclear cells and human neutrophils [47]. Incubation of dispersed human lung mast cells with 0.1–200 μM piriprost prior to activation with calcium ionophore A23187 inhibits leukotriene generation but this is accompanied by an enhanced release of the cyclooxygenase product, PGD_2 [48, 49]. A simplistic explanation for this phenomenon is the diversion of arachidonic acid generated by mast cells from the lipoxygenase to the cyclooxygenase pathway.

The inhibition of generation and release of lipid mediators may also explain the potent anti-inflammatory action of corticosteroids in asthma. In a number of animal models it has been shown that prolonged incubation of cells with corticosteroids stimulates the release of a peptide of molecular weight 16,000–40,000 daltons (lipomodulin or macrocortin) that inhibits membrane phospholipase A_2 activity [50]. Thus, the release of this peptide, which reaches a maximum 3–6 hours after corticosteroid exposure, inhibits the generation of arachidonic acid and therefore the synthesis and release of its oxidative metabolites. This effect of steroids has been demonstrated *in vitro* on neutrophils, basophils and monocytes, which contribute toward the airway inflammatory response in asthma [50], but not on isolated human lung mast cells [51].

In addition to IgE-dependent stimulation, mast cell activation may also occur by specific interaction with the complement anaphylatoxic peptides, C3a, C4a and C5a [52], and with complex bacterial cell wall lectins [unpublished observation]. Both these mechanisms may be pertinent to the pathogenesis of nonallergic asthma, while the ability of hypertonicity to induce mast cell secretion may be relevant to the pathogenesis of exercise-induced asthma.

17.2 Secondary Effector Cells in the Pathogenesis of Bronchoconstriction

The mast cell secretory granules contain a number of peptides and proteins which are chemotactic for eosinophils and neutrophils. In addition, activated mast cells release substantial amounts of LTB_4 and mono-HETEs which exhibit potent chemotactic activities. It is suggested that these chemotactic factors interact causing the selective migration of neutrophils, eosinophils and monocytes into the area of mast cell degranulation, whereupon these cells become activated to release their own inflammatory products [53]. A number of pharmacological agents have been shown to interfere with these responses. Among its many other effects, sodium cromoglycate interferes with the stimulus-related expression of monocyte complement receptors at concentrations in the region of 10^{-9} M [54]. In addition corticosteroids are highly effective at inhibiting antigen-induced late phase reactions in human skin and asthma.

While secondary effector cells such as monocytes, neutrophils and eosinophils contribute towards the airway inflammatory response of asthma, there is increasing evidence that some of these cells, once in the airways, may be stimulated directly by IgE-dependent mechanisms. In particular, macrophages and eosinophils possess low affinity receptors for IgE and release both preformed and newly generated mediators upon cell activation [55–57]. Thus, primary activation of these cells provides a mechanism by which airway obstruction may occur without invoking the participation of mast cells.

17.3 Relationship Between Bronchial Reactivity and Mast Cell Mediator Release

The cause(s) of bronchial hyperreactivity in asthma have so far eluded a definition. A fundamental abnormality in the contractile behaviour of airway smooth muscle is unlikely, since the contractile responsiveness of isolated human airway smooth muscle *in vitro* bears no correlation with measurements of bronchial responsiveness *in vivo* [58]. It has, however, been suggested that smooth muscle of asthmatic airways behaves as a single rather than a multiple unit [59]. The release of mast cell-derived and other inflammatory mediators onto the surface of the airway increases permeability of the epithelium, enabling antigens and large molecular weight mediators to propagate the bronchoconstrictor response by gaining access to subepithelial inflammatory cells [60]. It is plausible that, in asthma, bronchial mast cells and possibly other inflammatory cells are continually stimulated to secrete inflammatory mediators and that this leads to altered smooth muscle behavior characterized by bronchial hyperreactivity. Recent studies have shown that in asthma mast cells are recovered from bronchoalveolar lavage in increased numbers [61]. There is also some evidence that circulating basophils and bronchoalveolar lavage mast cells from patients with asthma demonstrate increased spontaneous mediator release [61, 62] which correlates with nonspecific airway reactivity [63]. If these observations are confirmed then enhanced mediator secretion could provide the missing link in proposing an inflammatory mediator model for the pathogenesis of bronchial hyperreactivity.

In allergic asthma, the bronchoconstrictor response to inhaled antigens in allergic asthma depends upon two factors: nonspecific bronchial reactivity and mast cell sensitivity [64, 65]. Thus, in patients with marked airway hyperreactivity only a small amount of mediator release would be necessary to induce significant bronchoconstriction, whereas in patients with normal airway reactivity greater mediator release would be necessary to produce an equivalent physiological response (Fig. 17.2). We have recently confirmed this hypothesis by

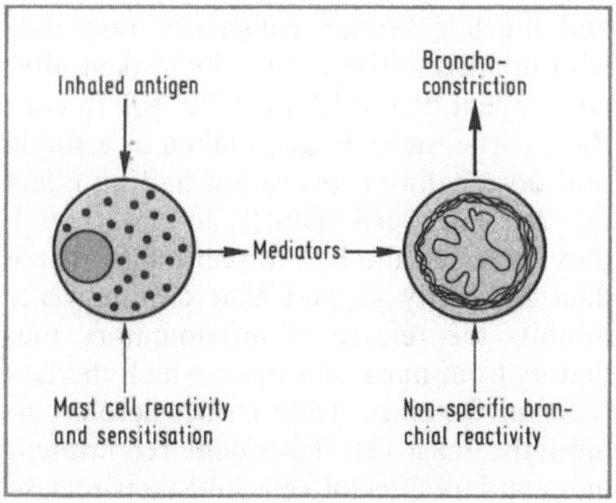

Fig. 17.2. Relationship between mast cell mediator release and nonspecific bronchial reactivity as determinants of the airway response to inhaled antigen in asthma

showing that in perennial asthmatics with hyperreactive airways (PC_{20} methacholine 0.09 mg/ml) antigen provocation, producing a 30% fall in FEV_1, caused a less than twofold increase in circulating neutrophil chemotactic factor (NCF) and no detectable increase in plasma histamine [66]. However, in a group of seasonal asthmatic patients whose airway reactivity was almost normal (PC_{20} methacholine 4.0 mg/ml) antigen provocation required to produce the same degree of bronchoconstriction resulted in a 10–15-fold increase in NCF [unpublished observation] and a 3–4-fold increase in plasma histamine [65], which in peaking 5 min following challenge preceded maximum bronchoconstriction at 15–20 min [67]. These observations provide strong evidence incriminating bronchial mast cells in the initial airway response to inhaled antigen. The reported finding that NCF and histamine are released into the circulation during late asthmatic responses suggests that mast cells and basophils might also be involved in the pathogenesis of this reaction [68].

17.4 Pharmacological Modulation of Bronchial Mast Cell Mediator Release In Vivo

The ability to detect increments in circulating mediators following antigen provocation in asthma has provided a useful model to investigate the comparative effects of antiasthma drugs on airway caliber and mediator release. Thus, in a group of seasonal asthmatic patients, in whom antigen provocation produced an immediate 3–4-fold rise in plasma histamine levels, we have shown that inhaled salbutamol 200 µg (sufficient to produce bronchodilatation) totally inhibited the antigen-induced release of mast cell-derived histamine and NCF [69]. Sodium cromoglycate in a dose of 20 mg by inhalation only partially inhibited the immediate airway response and the release of histamine with antigen challenge, but completely inhibited the release of NCF. Ipratropium bromide, 1 mg inhaled, which produced the same degree of bronchodilatation as achieved with salbutamol, failed to influence either antigen-induced bronchoconstriction or the release of mast cell mediators measured in the circulation. This finding is in contrast to some *in vitro* studies demonstrating that cholinergic agonists stimulate IgE-dependent mediator release from human lung fragments [70].

The role of histamine in the pathogenesis of asthma is controversial. Human lung is an organ containing particularly high levels of histamine, almost entirely located in mast cell secretory granules [70, 71]. Previous studies investigating the effect of H_1-antihistamines on bronchial provocation have been hampered by their very low antihistaminic activity and lack of pharmacological specificity [72]. In an attempt to overcome these problems a number of investigators, using high concentrations of inhaled, oral or intravenous H_1-antagonists, have demonstrated a variable protective effect against bronchoconstriction with inhaled antigen, though the precise concentrations of the drug achieved in the airways is difficult to define [73]. We have recently shown that the potent nonsedative and specific H_1-antihistamine, astemizole, when given in a dose of 10 mg daily for a period of 2 weeks, inhibited the skin wheal response to histamine (10 µg/ml), by greater than 95%, produced a 17-fold reduction in the airway response to inhaled histamine and protected the airways from antigen-induced bronchoconstriction by reducing the maximum fall in FEV_1 from 30% to 8% without having any effect on the release of histamine [unpublished data]. Thus, a potent antihistamine such as astemizole might be of benefit to patients with allergic asthma. In a placebo-controlled study astemizole 10 mg daily has indeed been shown to provide a useful protective effect against seasonal symptoms of hay fever and of asthma [74]. It is, however, unlikely that antihistamines will be of benefit to patients with perennial asthma symptoms and marked airway hyperreactivity.

The influence of corticosteroids on immediate antigen-induced bronchoconstriction and release of inflammatory mediators has produced conflicting results. The general consensus of a number of studies is that corticosteroids cause a reduction in nonspecific airway reactivity which protects the airways against all forms of bronchial provocation including antigen without affecting the release of mast cell mediators [4, 75].

On a theoretical basis, calcium antagonists should also provide a protective effect in patients with bronchial asthma, and certainly a number of studies employing exercise, isocapnic hyperventilation and histamine bronchial provocation suggest that dihydropyridine derivatives such as verapamil and nifedipine are pharmacologically active in asthma [reviewed in 76]. However, calcium antagonists appear to be relatively ineffective in blocking the immediate airway response to inhaled antigen. We have recently demonstrated that nifedipine and nicardipine have inhibitory effects on IgE-dependent mast cell mediator release, but at concentrations in excess of 10 μM, which are far in excess of plasma levels achieved therapeutically (0.05–0.1 μM) [77]. Although calcium-blocking drugs attenuate bronchoconstriction induced by various provocations they are of relatively little use in the long-term treatment of asthma [76], though one study has reported some protection against nocturnal bronchoconstriction [78].

There have been few studies reporting the effect of drugs on the late asthmatic reaction. Early studies demonstrated that sodium cromoglycate when taken before antigen provocation, blocked both the early and the late bronchoconstrictor responses with inhaled antigen, but when taken after challenge it had little effect [79, 80]. In contrast, corticosteroids when taken as a single oral dose before provocation had no effect on the early asthmatic reaction, though they inhibited the late response [80]. These data indirectly suggest that cromoglycate inhibits the release of inflammatory mediators from mast cells upon which the late reaction depends, while corticosteroids inhibit the mast cell-dependent recruitment of secondary effector cells and their release of mediators.

Anecdotal observations indicate that β-adrenoceptor agonists, when administered before antigen provocation have little effect on the late asthmatic reaction. If this is confirmed, then it is of particular interest because these drugs are highly active in inhibiting the immediate airway response to inhaled antigen. These contradictory observations on the early and late reactions may be reconciled on the basis that β_2-adrenoceptor agonists inhibit mediator secretion from mast cells intimately involved in the pathogenesis of the early asthmatic reaction but fail to inhibit a secondary activated cell type (e.g., macrophages) which may be fundamental to the late asthmatic response.

We have recently demonstrated that a small dose of inhaled salbutamol 10 μg, is approximately equipotent with oral salbutamol, 8 mg, in blocking the airway response to inhaled methacholine. However, inhaled salbutamol was twice as effective in blocking bronchoconstriction induced by antigen than was oral salbutamol. These data may be interpreted as a preferential effect of inhaled salbutamol on bronchial mucosal mast cells [81]. Since β_2-adrenoceptor agonists also have the capacity to inhibit the opening of epithelium tight junctions by a CAMP-dependent mechanism [82], it is also possible that drugs of this type, when taken by inhalation, may protect the bronchi from penetration of inhaled antigen and high molecular weight inflammatory mediators to subepithelial effector cells.

The last 5 years have seen enormous advances in the understanding of the pathogenesis of asthma, though as yet the precise factor(s) which contribute to the central abnormality of bronchial hyperreactivity have not been clearly defined. Nevertheless, the knowledge that inflammatory mediators play an important role in the pathogenesis of asthma should lead to a further increase in our understanding of the disease and hopefully reveal other mechanisms at which to direct therapeutic pharmacological agents.

References

1. McFadden ER (1984) Pathogenesis of Asthma. J Allergy Clin Immunol 73:413–424
2. Hogg JC, Pare PD, Boucher R, Michoud MC, Guerzon G, Moroz L (1977) Pathologic abnormalities in asthma. In: Lichtenstein LM, Austen KF (eds) Asthma: Physiology, Immunopharmacology and Treatment, vol. 2. Academic Press, New York London, pp 1–14
3. Porter R, Birch J (eds) (1971) The Identification of Asthma. Ciba Foundation Study Group No. 38. Churchill Livingstone, Edinburgh London
4. Löwhagen O, Rak S (1985) Modification of bronchial reactivity after treatment with sodium cromoglycate during pollen season. J Allergy Clin Immunol 75:460–467
5. Boulet LP, Cartier A, Thompson NC, Roberts RS, Dolovitch J, Hargreave FE (1983) Asthma and increases in non-allergic bronchial responsiveness from seasonal pollen exposure. J Allergy Clin Immunol 74:399–406
6. Platts-Mills TAE, Mitchell EB, Nock P, Tovey ER, Moszaro H, Wilkins SR (1982) Reduction in bronchial hyperreactivity during prolonged allergen avoidance. Lancet II:675–678
7. Pepys J (1967) Hypersensitivity to inhaled organic antigen. J R Coll Physicians Lond 2:42–48
8. Warner JO (1976) Significance of late reactions after bronchial challenge with house dust mite. Arch Dis Child 51:905–911
9. Cutz E, Levison H, Cooper DM (1978) Ultrastructure of airways in children with asthma. Histopathology 2:407–421
10. Church MK, Pao GJ-K, Holgate ST (1982) Characterization of histamine secretion from mechanically dispersed human lung mast cells: effects of anti-IgE, calcium ionophore A23187, compound 48/80, and basic polypeptides. J Immunol 129:2116–2121
11. Paterson NAM, Wasserman SI, Said JW, Austen KF (1976) Release of chemical mediators from partially purified human lung mast cells. J Immunol 117:1356–1362
12. Schulman ES, Kagey-Sabotka A, MacGlashan DW, Adkinson NF, Peters SP, Schleimer RP, Lichtenstein LM (1983) Heterogeneity of human mast cells. J Immunol 131: 1936–1941
13. Schwartz LB, Austen KF (1980) Enzymes of the mast cell granule. J Invest Dermatol 74:349–353
14. Coleman JW, Godfrey RC (1981) The number and affinity of IgE receptors on dispersed human lung mast cells. Immunology 44:859–863
15. Ishizaka R, Chang TH, Taggart M, Ishizaka K (1977) Histamine release from rat mast cells by antibodies against rat basophil leukaemia cell membrane. J Immunol 119:1589–1596
16. Ishizaka T (1981) Analysis of triggering events in mast cells for immunoglobulin E-mediated histamine release. J Allergy Clin Immunol 67:90–96
17. Morita Y, Chiang PK, Siraganian RP (1981) Effect of inhibitors of transmethylation on histamine release from human basophils. Biochem Pharmacol 30:785–791
18. Ishizaka T, Hirata F, Ishizaka K, Axelrod J (1980) Stimulation of phospholipid methylation, Ca^{2+} influx and histamine release by bridging of IgE receptors on rat mast cells. Proc Natl Acad Sci USA 77:1903–1906
19. Ishizaka T, Conrad DH, Schulman ES, Sterk AR, Ishizaka K (1983) Biochemical analysis of initial triggering events of IgE-mediated histamine release from human lung mast cells. J Immunol 130:2397–2362
20. Moore JP, Johannsson A, Hesketh TR, Smith GA, Metcalf JC (1984) Calcium signals and phospholipid methylation in eukaryotic cells. Biochem J 221:675–684
21. Benyon RC, Church MK, Holgate ST (1986) IgE dependent activation of mast cells is not associated with enhanced phospholipid methylation. Biochem Pharmacol 35:2535–2544
22. Benyon RC, Church MK, Holgate ST (1984) The effect of methyltransferase inhibitors on histamine release from human dispersed lung mast cells activated with anti-human IgE and calcium ionophore A23187. Biochem Pharmacol 33:2881–2886
23. Sullivan TJ (1982) Diacyl-glycerol metabolism and the release of mediators from mast cells. In: Becker EL, Simon AS, Austen KF (eds) Biochemistry of the Acute Allergic Reactions. Alan R. Liss, New York, pp 229–238

24. Cockcroft S, Gomperts BD (1979) Evidence for a role of phosphatidyl-inositol turnover in stimulus-secretion coupling. Studies with rat peritoneal mast cells. Biochem J 178:681–685
25. Holgate ST, Lewis RA, Austen KF (1980) Role of cyclic nucleotides in mast cell activation and secretion. Prog Immunol 4:846–859
26. Winslow CM, Lewis RA, Austen KF (1981) Mast cell mediator release as a function of cyclic AMP-dependent protein kinase activation. J Exp Med 154:1125–1133
27. Sullivan TJ, Parker KL, Eiser SA, Parker CW (1975) Modulation of cyclic AMP in purified rat mast cells. II. Studies on the relationship between intracellular cyclic AMP concentrations and histamine release. J Immunol 114:1480–1485
28. Hughes PJ, Holgate ST, Roath S, Church MK (1983) The relationship between cyclic AMP changes and histamine release from basophil rich human leucocytes. Biochem Pharmacol 32:2557–2563
29. Church MK, Holgate ST, Hughes PJ (1983) Adenosine inhibits and potentiates IgE-dependent histamine release from human basophils by an A_2-receptor mediated mechanism. Br J Pharmacol 80:719–726
30. Hughes PJ, Holgate ST, Church MK (1984) Adenosine inhibits and potentiates IgE-dependent histamine release from human lung mast cells by an A_2-purinoceptor mediated mechanism. Biochem Pharmacol 33:3847–3852
31. Peters SP, Schulman ES, Schleimer RP, MacGlashan DW, Newball HH, Lichtenstein LM (1982) Dispersed human lung mast cells: pharmacologic aspects and comparison with human lung fragments. Am Rev Respir Dis 126:1034–1038
32. Holgate ST, Church MK, Cushley MJ, Robinson C, Mann JS, Howarth PH (1984) Pharmacological modulation of airway calibre and mediator release in human models of bronchial asthma. In: Kay AB, Austen KF, Lichtenstein LM (eds) Asthma: Physiology, Immunopharmacology and Treatment. Academic Press, London, pp 319–345
33. Cushley MJ, Holgate ST (1984) Development of Theophylline Preparations. In: Buckle DR, Smith H (eds) Butterworth, Edinburgh, pp 205–223
34. Fredholm BB (1980) Are methylxanthines' effects due to antagonism of endogenous adenosine. Trends Pharmacol Sci 1:129–132
35. Holgate ST, Mann JS, Cushley MJ (1984) Adenosine as a bronchoconstrictor mediator in asthma and its antagonism by methylxanthines. J Allergy Clin Immunol 74:302–306
36. Stokes TC, Morley J (1981) Prospects for an oral Intal. Br J Dis Chest 75:1–14
37. Church MK, Young KD (1983) The characteristics of inhibition of mediator release from human lung fragments by sodium cromoglycate, salbutamol and chlorpromazine. Br J Pharmacol 78:671–679
38. Strobel S, Miller HRP, Ferguson A (1981) Human intestinal mast cells: evaluation of fixation and staining techniques. J Clin Pathol 34:851–858
39. Wells E, Mann J (1983) Phosphorylation of a mast cell protein in response to treatment with anti-allergic compounds. Implications for the mode of action of sodium cromoglycate. Biochem Pharmacol 32:837–842
40. Lewis RA, Soter NA, Diamond PT, Austen KF, Oates JA, Roberts JL II (1982) Prostaglandin D_2 generation after activation of rat and human mast cells with anti-IgE. J Immunol 129:1627–1631
41. Holgate ST, Burns GB, Robinson C, Church MK (1984) Anaphylactic- and calcium-dependent generation of prostaglandin D_2 (PGD_2), thromboxane B_2, and other cyclooxygenase products of arachidonic acid by dispersed human lung cells and relationship to histamine release. J Immunol 133:2138–2144
42. Hardy CC, Robinson C, Tattersfield AE, Holgate ST (1984) The bronchoconstrictor effect of inhaled prostaglandin D_2 in normal and asthmatic men. N Engl J Med 311:209–213
43. Schulman ES, Newball HH, Demers LM, Fitzpatrick FA, Adkinson NF (1981) Anaphylactic release of thromboxane A_2, prostaglandin D_2 and prostacyclin from human lung parenchyma. Am Rev Respir Dis 124:402–406
44. Lewis RA, Austen KF (1981) Mediators of local homeostasis and inflammation by leukotrienes and other mast cell dependent compounds. Nature 293:103–108
45. MacGlashan DW, Schleimer RP, Peters SP, Schulman ES, Adams GK III, Newball HH, Lichtenstein LM (1982) Generation of leukotrienes by purified human lung mast cells. J Clin Invest 70:747–751
46. Dahlen SE, Hansson G, Hedqvist P, Björck T, Granstrom E, Dahlen B (1984) Allergen challenge of lung tissue from asthmatics elicits bronchial contraction that correlates with release of leukotrienes C_4, D_4 and E_4. Proc Natl Acad Sci USA 80:1712–1716
47. Bach M (1984) Prospects for the inhibition of leukotriene synthesis. Biochem Pharmacol 33:515–521

48. Robinson C, Holgate ST (1986) Ionophore-dependent generation of eicosanoids in human dispersed lung cells: modulation by 6,9-deepoxy-6,9-(phenylimino)-delta-6,8-prostaglandin I, (U-60,257). Biochem Pharmacol 35:1903–1908
49. Holgate ST, Robinson C (1984) 6,9-de-epoxy-6,9-(Phenylimino)-$\Delta^{6,8}$-prostaglandin I, (U-60,257) stimulates prostaglandin D_2 and inhibits thromboxane B_2 release from ionophore changed human dispersed lung cells. Br J Pharmacol 83:603–605
50. Hirata F, Schiffman E, Venkatasubramanian K, Solomon D, Axelrod J (1980) A phospholipase A_2 inhibitory protein in rabbit neutrophils induced by glucocorticoids. Proc Natl Acad Sci USA 77:2533–2536
51. Schleimer RP, MacGlashan DW, Schulman ES, Peters SP, Adkinson NF, Newball HH, Adams GK, Lichtenstein LM (1982) The effect of glucocorticoids on mediator release from human basophils and mast cells. Fed Proc 41:487
52. Hugli TE (1981) The structural basis for anaphyl toxin in chemotactic functions of $C3_a$ and $C5_a$. In: Critical Views in Immunology. CRC Press, Boca Raton, pp 321–366
53. Holgate ST, Kay AB (1985) Mast cells, mediators and asthma. Clin Allergy 15:221–233
54. Kay AB, Nagakura T, Walsh G, Carroll M (1984) Disodium cromoglycate as an anti-inflammatory agent. Thorax 39:233
55. Dessaint J-P, Capron A, Joseph M, Bazin H (1979) Cytophilic binding of IgE to the macrophage. II. Immunologic release of lysosomal enzyme from macrophage by IgE and anti-IgE in the rat: a new mechanism of macrophage activation. Cell Immunol 46:24–34
56. Capron M, Capron A, Dessaint J-P, Torpier G, Johansson SGO, Prin A (1981) Fc receptors for IgE on human and rat eosinophils. J Immunol 126:2087–2092
57. Shaw RJ, Cromwell O, Kay AB (1984) Preferential generation of leukotriene C_4 by human eosinophils. Clin Exp Immunol 56: 716–722
58. Armour CL, Lazar NM, Schellenburg RR, Taylor SM, Chan N, Hogy JC, Paré PD (1984) A comparison of *in vivo* and *in vitro* airway reactivity to histamine. Am Rev Respir Dis 129:907–910
59. Daniel EE, Davis C, Jones T, Kannan MS (1980) Control of airway smooth muscle. In: Hargreave FE (ed) Airway Reactivity. Astra Pharmaceuticals, Missisauga, Ontario, pp 80–109
60. Hogg JC (1981) Bronchial mucosal permeability and its relationship to airways hyperreactivity. J Allergy Clin Immunol 67: 421–425
61. Tomioka M, Ida S, Yuriko S, Ishihara T, Takishima T (1984) Mast cells in bronchoalveolar lumen of patients with bronchial asthma. Am Rev Respir Dis 129:1000–1005
62. Howarth PH, Pao GJ-K, Church MK, Holgate ST (1984) Exercise and isocapnic hyperventilation-induced bronchoconstriction in asthma: relevance of circulating basophils to measurements of plasma histamine. J Allergy Clin Immunol 73:391–394
63. Neijens HJ, Raatgeep HC, Degenhart HJ, Karrebijn KF (1982) Release of histamine from leucocytes and its determinants *in vitro* in relation to bronchial responsiveness to inhaled histamine and exercise *in vivo.* Clin Allergy 12:577–586
64. Cockcroft DW, Ruffin RE, Frith PA, Cartier A, Juniper EF, Dolovich J, Hargreave FE (1982) Determinants of allergen-induced asthma: Dose of allergen circulating IgE antibody concentrations and bronchial responsiveness to inhaled histamine. Am Rev Respir Dis 120:1053–1058
65. Mann JS, Holgate ST, Howarth PH (1984) Influence of non-specific airway reactivity on the immediate airway response to inhaled allergen in asthma. Thorax 39:706
66. Howarth PH, Pao GJ-K, Holgate ST (in press) The relationship between mast cell mediator release and bronchial reactivity in allergic asthma. J Allergy Clin Immunol
67. Holgate ST, Church MK, Cushley MJ, Robinson C, Mann JS, Howarth PH (1984) Pharmacologic modulation of airway calibre and mediator release in human models of bronchial asthma. In: Kay AB, Austen KF, Lichtenstein CM (eds) Asthma: Physiology, Immunopharmacology and Treatment. IIIrd International Symposium. Academic Press, London, pp 391–415
68. Durham SR, Lee TH, Merrett TG, Merrett J, Brown MJ, Causon R, Kay AB (1983) Immunological studies of antigen-induced late asthmatic reactions. Thorax 38:224
69. Howarth PH, Durham SR, Kay AB, Church MK, Holgate ST (1985) Influence of albuterol, cromolyn sodium and ipratropium bromide on the airway and circulating mediator responses to antigen bronchial provocation in asthma. Am Rev Respir Dis 132: 986–992
70. Kaliner M, Orange RP, Austen KF (1982) Immunological release of histamine and slow reacting substance of anaphylaxis from human lung. IV. Enhancement by cholinergic and alpha adrenergic stimulation. J Exp Med 136:556–567

71. Morr H (1979) Immunological release of histamine from human lung. 2. Studies on acetylcholine and the anticholinergic agent ipratropium bromide. Respiration 38:273–279
72. White J, Eiser NM (1983) The role of histamine and its receptors in the pathogenesis of asthma. Br J Dis Chest 77:215–226
73. Eiser NM, Mills J, Snashall PD, Guz A (1981) The role of histamine receptors in asthma. Clin Sci 60:363–370
74. Howarth PH, Holgate ST (1984) Comparative trial of two non-sedative H_1-antihistamines, terfenadine and astemizole, for hay fever. Thorax 39:668–672
75. Kraar J, Koëter GH, Mark VDM, Sluiter HJ, deVries K (1985) Changes in bronchial hyperreactivity induced by 4 weeks of treatment with antiasthmatic drugs in patients with allergic asthma: A comparison between budesonide and terbutaline. J Allergy Clin Immunol 76:628–636
76. Barnes PJ (1983) Calcium channel blockers and asthma. Thorax 38:481–485
77. Church MK, Holgate ST, Kim Y-Y (1984) Inhibition of histamine release from human mast cells by nifedipine and nicardipine. Br J Pharmacol 82 [Suppl]: 2648
78. Patakas D, Vlachoianni E, Tsara V, Louridas G, Agiropoulou P (1983) Nifedipine in bronchial asthma. J Allergy Clin Immunol 72:932–933
79. Pepys J, Hargreave FE, McCarthy DJ (1968) Inhibitory effects of disodium cromoglycate on allergen inhalation tests. Lancet II:134–137
80. Booij-Noord H, Orie NG, deVries K (1971) Immediate and late bronchial obstructive reactions to inhalation of house dust and protective effects of disodium cromoglycate and prednisolone. J Allergy Clin Immunol 48:344–354
81. Holgate ST, Benyon RC, Howarth PH, Agins R, Hardy C, Robinson C, Durham SR, Kay AB, Church MK (1985) Relationship between mediator release from human lung mast cells *in vitro* and *in vivo*. Int Arch Allergy Appl Immunol 77:47–56
82. Duffy ME, Hainan B, Ho S, Bentzel CJ (1981) Regulation of epithelial tight junctions permeability by cyclic AMP. Nature 294:451–453

18. Mast Cells and Basophils

S. P. Peters, J. A. Grant, A. M. Dvorak, L. M. Lichtenstein

Supported by grants AI 07290, AI 12621, CA 28834 and CIRID AI 20135 from the National Institute of Allergy and Infectious Diseases, and National Cancer Institute, National Institutes of Health, Department of Health and Human Services, Bethesda, Maryland.
Publication No. 000 from the O'Neill Research Laboratories at The Good Samaritan Hospital, Baltimore, Maryland.

That mast cells and allergic mechanisms play at least some role in bronchial asthma has been suggested for at least 75 years [92]. The *incidence* of these mechanisms in a cross section of all asthmatics [31, 77], and the *importance* of allergic mechanisms as compared with neural mechanisms is controversial, however, and has been discussed and debated for at least as long [16, 113].

This chapter will review data suggesting that mast cells and their circulating counterpart, the basophilic leukocyte, play an important role in bronchial asthma. Anatomical considerations, mechanisms and agents producing cellular activation, mediators produced by these cells, physiological and pharmacological control mechanisms, interactions of mast cells and basophils with other cells, and information gained using experimental models *in vivo* will be discussed. Information obtained using human cells and models will be stressed. However, data from other experimental models will also be included when general principles, potentially applicable to the human system, can be illustrated.

18.1 Anatomical Considerations

Mast cells are prominent in skin, the gastrointestinal tract, and the respiratory system where their concentration has been estimated to be 7,000–12,000/mm^3 [96], 20,000/mm^3 [102], and 20,000/mm^3 [160], respectively. They appear most frequently around blood vessels and nerves.

The most comprehensive survey of mast cells in mammalian lung has been performed by Guerzon et al [47] using monkey lung. By both quantitative histologic examination and measurement of total lung histamine (assuming 3–8 pg of histamine per mast cell), the total number of mast cells per lung was estimated at between 10^7 and 10^8. Approximately 83% of the cells were located in conducting airways with the remaining 17% in parenchyma. The number of mast cells in different airway generations varied from 60,000 in the trachea to 8,000,000 in terminal bronchioles. The number of superficial mast cells (superficial to the basement membrane) varied from 0–0.4% of total mast cells in the trachea to 0–27% of total mast cells in the terminal bronchioles, with an overall average of 12%.

Human lung mast cells have been shown to be heterogeneous in terms of size (9.9 –18.4 microns in diameter), histamine content (2.5–10.1 pg per mast cell), and function in terms of their ability to release histamine and prostaglandin D_2 (large cells release more histamine and PGD_2 than small cells) [133]. In addition, a more extreme mast cell heterogeneity has been well characterized in rodents with the suggestion that similar diversity also exists in humans. The two forms of rodent mast cells have been termed *typical* or *connective tissue*, and *atypical* or *mucosal* [5, 7, 112]. The connective tissue mast cell is prominent in connective tissue, lung, skin, and serosal surfaces (including the peritoneal cavity of rodents), stains with usual mast cell stains, and appears T-lymphocyte-independent. The rodent mucosal mast cell is most prominent in mucosal surfaces such as the gastrointestinal tract, requires special staining techniques, and is T-lymphocyte-dependent. These two cell types differ not only in location and staining characteristics, but also in ultrastructure, response to mast cell triggering agents, and the effect of antiallergic compounds [5, 7, 112]. However, work performed to date with human lung and human intestinal mast cells does not suggest a similar heterogeneity in humans. Studies performed with human intestinal mast cells show these cells to be similar to human lung mast cells in a number of properties [33]. These include histamine content, staining characteristics, ultrastructure by electron microscopy, response to anti-IgE and other mast cell triggering agents, and quantitative aspects of the release of the inflammatory mediators histamine, prostaglandin D_2, and sulfidopeptide leukotrienes [33]. Whether distinct subpopulations of human mast cells exist, remains to be established.

The circulating counterpart of the mast cell, the basophilic leukocyte, represents the least common type of granulocyte in human blood. The mean concentration of basophils in human blood, $40/mm^3$ ($20–45/mm^3$) suggests that the total circulating pool of basophils represents approximately 180,000,000 cells [109].

Histological and morphological information implicating mast cells in the pathogenesis of bronchial asthma comes from studies employing bronchial and bronchoalveolar lavage [111, 153] and from autopsy studies [12]. Histamine containing mast cells or basophils has been identified free in the lumen of human bronchi [111], and mast cells of two morphological types (small and round versus large and pleomorphic or oval) have been identified in bronchoalveolar lavage fluid [153]. The number of mast cells recovered from asthmatic subjects (0.25%) has been reported to be greater than in control subjects (0.08%), but similar to that recovered from patients with other pulmonary diseases (0.23%). The histamine content of asthmatic mast cells (8.2 ± 6.0 pg/cell) was lower than control mast cells (15.3 ± 10.8 pg/cell) [153]. In addition, the number of mast cells in the bronchial walls of patients who died of asthma has been reported to be decreased when compared with bronchial tissue from patients who died from other causes [12]. Taken together, these two observations suggest that mast cells in asthmatics have been activated to release chemical mediators and to degranulate.

The importance of basophils in the pathogenesis of bronchial asthma is less clear. Kimura et al [65], studying sputum from asthmatic subjects, reported that the number of basophils increased just before the onset of an asthmatic attack, and that the number of basophils seen was related to the severity of the relapse. Functional differences have also been observed in basophils from asthmatic subjects when compared to control subjects [29, 156] (to be discussed below). In addition, considerable evidence is available linking basophils to the pathogenesis of other inflammatory disorders [105]. For example, basophils are prominent in delayed hypersensitivity reactions such as allergic contact dermatitis reactions and delayed "Jones-Mote" reactions in man [2, 22, 34], and have been observed in nasal secretions of allergic patients where a close relationship between the presence of basophils, nasal provocation, and clinical symptoms was seen [49, 88]. An increase in basophil chemotactic activity in the blood of patients with allergic rhinitis has also been described [52]. In vitro, the migration of basophils is controlled by many factors including complement-derived peptides, lymphokines, and interferon [71, 72]. It is reasonable to suggest that basophils, like other granulocytes such as the polymorphonuclear leukocyte, migrate into areas of active inflammation in response to chemotactic factors released from mast cells and other cells. In that way, they may participate in prolonging the inflammatory response in conditions such as bronchial asthma and other allergic disorders.

18.2 Cellular Activation

The number of agents that can trigger mast cells and basophils to release inflammatory mediators is long, diverse, and summarized in Table 18.1. The classic mechanism by which mast cells and basophils are activated involves the cross-linking of IgE receptors on the surface of these cells by antigen or antigen equivalent (anti-IgE or anti-IgE receptor) [57, 60, 140]. IgG (probably of the subclass IgG_4) is also present on the surface of basophils and the cross-linking of these surface molecules also results in mediator release [26, 44]. Numerous other

Table 18.1. Agents that can activate mast cells and basophils

This table contains most of the agents known to activate human mast cells and basophils. The absence of a specific agent under the mast cell or basophil column implies *either* that the substance does not activate that cell type *or* that the substance has not been rigorously examined in that system. The section of the table containing nonhuman cells lists only *additional* agents not already present under the human cell section.

Mast cells	Basophils
Human cells	
Antigen	Antigen
Anti-IgE	Anti-IgE
Anti-IgG	Anti-IgG
Ionophores (e.g., A23187)	Ionophores
Hyperosmolarity	Hyperosmolarity
Gastrin (cutaneous mast cells)	C3a, C5a
Macrophage-derived factors	Macrophage-derived factors
	Lymphocyte-derived factors (e.g., HRA)
	Formyl methionine peptide
	Eosinophil major basic protein
	Pepstatin A
	Deuterium oxide
	Phorbol esters
	Phospholipase A
	Platelet factor 4 and other platelet products
	5-Hydroperoxyeicosatetraenoic acid [a]
	Prostaglandin D_2 [a]
	Leukotriene B_4 [a]
Nonhuman cells	
Phospholipase A	
Compound 48/80	
15-Hydroxyeicosatetraenoic acid	
Substance P	
Somatostatin	
Eosinophil major basic protein	

[a] Require the presence of cytochalasin B

substances can also activate these cells. They include macrophage and lymphocyte products, such as histamine releasing activity (HRA) [73, 139, 150, 151], ionophores [76, 99], hyperosmolar stimuli [24, 28], deuterium oxide [29, 156], phorbol esters [128], and platelet factor 4 and other uncharacterized platelet-derived products [9, 66]. The cationic protein, major basic protein derived from eosinophils, stimulates the noncytotoxic release of histamine from human basophils and rat mast cells as well [103], suggesting that eosinophils may be able to enhance inflammatory reactions generated by basophils and perhaps mast cells in certain situations. Also noteworthy are peptide triggers including anaphylatoxins C3a and C5a [39, 42], formyl methionine containing peptide analogues of bacterial products [143], pepstatin A [86], peptide hormones and candidates for neurotransmitters such as gastrin [148], substance P [91], and somatostatin [149], and enzymes such as phospholipase A_2 [127, 161]. Finally, lipid products, particularly those derived from arachidonic acid such as 5-hydroperoxyeicosatetraenoic acid, prostaglandin D_2, leukotriene B_4, and 15-hydroxyeicosatetraenoic acid can also activate mast cells and basophils under certain conditions [117, 118].

As shown on Table 18.1, mast cells and basophils differ in the compounds which produce activation in some cases. In addition, human and nonhuman cells may also show such differences.

Because a wide variety of substances can activate these cells, mast cells and basophils can be tentatively implicated in bronchial asthma initiated by numerous mechanisms besides classic *allergic* or IgE-mediated reactions.

Early events in the release process initiated by the bridging of IgE receptors include a transient rise in intracellular CAMP concentration, activation of a CAMP-dependent protein kinase, phospholipid methylation, phospholipid turnover, and calcium influx [57, 58, 74, 116, 145]. In addition, a diisopropyl fluorophosphate inhibitable serine protease(s) appears to be involved in both the release mechanism and the process of desensitization, at least in the basophil [63, 64, 123]. Considerable effort has been directed toward defining these and other early events, and those efforts are continuing. Less is known about late events in the release process although evidence has been obtained to suggest that microtubules may be involved [37, 38, 78, 119].

Morphologically, human mast cells and basophils degranulate by different mechanisms [19, 23, 28, 35]. Mast cell granules appear to swell, lose electron density, and then fuse with other granules before the contents are extruded. Stimulation of basophils results in the fusion of individual granules with the plasma membrane and extrusion of their unaltered contents, without prior fusion of granules with each other as seen in mast cells. The appearance of basophils activated by antigens, C5a, and the lymphokine HRA appears similar [21] (Figs. 18.1, 18.2). The ultrastructure of basophil and mast cell degranulation recently has been reviewed in detail by Galli et al [35].

Morphological events associated with newly generated mediators have not been as well studied as the release of preformed mediators. Recent electron microscopic autoradiographic studies have shown that lipid bodies, osmiophilic structures found in variable numbers in the cytoplasm of human lung mast cells, are heavily labeled with ^3H-arachidonic acid during overnight culture [18, 20] (Fig. 18.2c). No labeling (above background) of other cell compartments or organelles such as the plasma membrane was observed in these studies [18, 20]. While these observations appear to run counter to the prevailing view that arachidonic acid used to generate inflammatory metabolites described below, is derived largely from sources within the plasma membrane, the precise role (if any) lipid bodies play in the generation of inflammatory mediators remains to be determined. Label (presumably AA metabolite(s)) has been seen in degranulation channels of activated cells (Fig. 18.2d), but these channels, in aggregation, were not significantly labelled with ^3H [20] (Fig. 18.2d).

18.3 Mediators

The classic mediator associated with mast cells and basophils is *histamine* [6, 59] (Table 18.2). This substance is bound to intracellular proteoglycan, heparin in the case of mast cells, and *chondroitin sulfate* in basophils in concentrations of approximately 2–10 pg/mast cell and 1 pg/basophil [95, 133, 159]. Histamine constricts smooth muscle, increases vascular permeability, and can modulate lymphocyte function [121].

Other potent inflammatory mediators produced by these cells are metabolites of *arachidonic acid.* Mast cells have been demonstrated to synthesize and release *prostaglandin D_2, thromboxane B_2, leukotriene C_4*, and *5-hydroxyeicosatetraenoic acid* after IgE-mediated activation [68, 75, 116, 131]. Whether human lung mast cells also release *leukotriene B_4* has not been conclusively established, although mast cells derived from rodents do synthesize this potent chemotactic substance [94]. To date, human basophils have been shown to release only leukotriene C_4 in response to antigens or

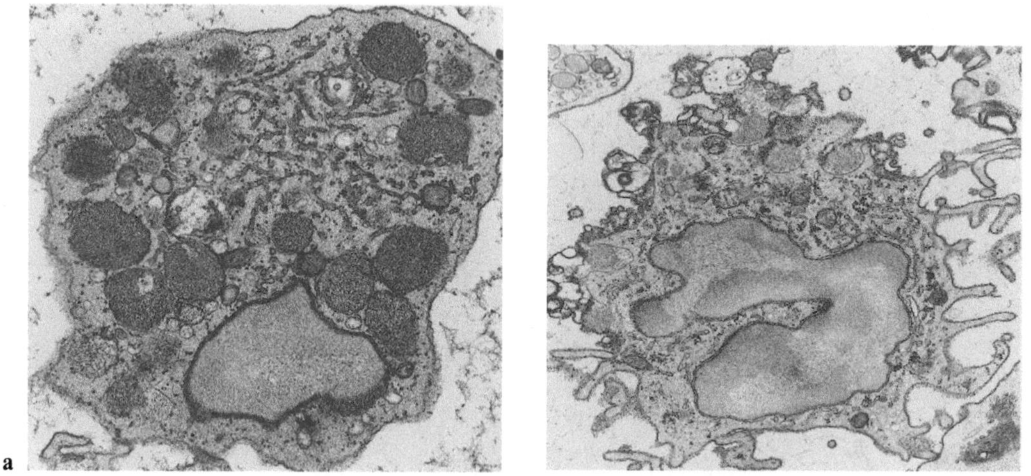

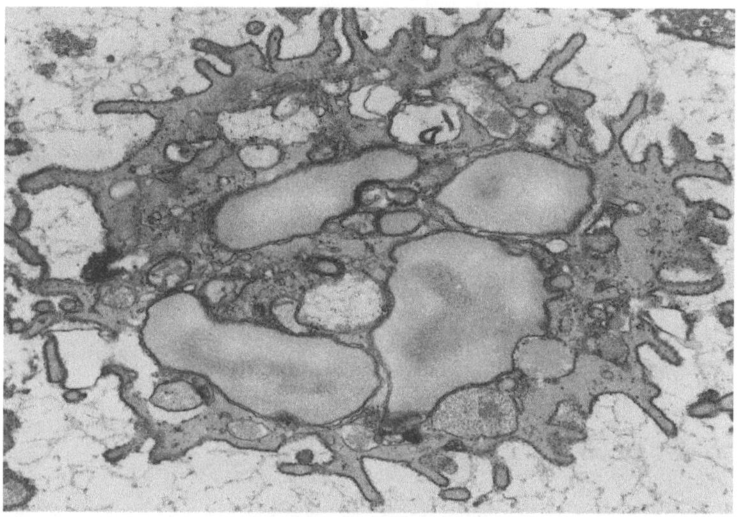

Fig. 18.1 a–c. Human basophils. **a** Control (× 19,190). **b** Degranulated with antigen (× 12,780). **c** Degranulated by hyperosmotic stimuli (× 22,000)

anti-IgE, but not when activated with C5a [30, 82].

Prostaglandin D_2 has been shown to constrict smooth muscle, increase pulmonary artery pressure, and produce bronchoconstriction in humans [48, 54, 158]. In these bronchoconstrictor effects, PGD_2 was 3.5 times more potent than $PGF_{2\alpha}$ and more potent in asthmatic than in normal subjects [48]. Increased production of PGD_2 has been observed in patients with systemic mastocytosis [125].

Leukotriene C_4 is the parent component of slow reacting substance of anaphylaxis (SRS-A, or leukotrienes C_4, D_4, and E_4). These sulfidopeptide leukotrienes also produce potent smooth muscle constriction *in vitro* and *in vivo,* affect vascular permeability, and enhance mucus secretion [17, 46, 62, 85]. As noted above, leukotriene B_4, and to a lesser extent, *5-hydroxyeicosatetraenoic acid (5-HETE),* are potent chemoattractants for human polymorphonuclear leukocytes [32, 40].

The platelet activating factor, *acetyl-glyceryl-ether-phosphorylcholine (AGEPC),* is also a product of the human lung mast cell [120], and evidence has been obtained for

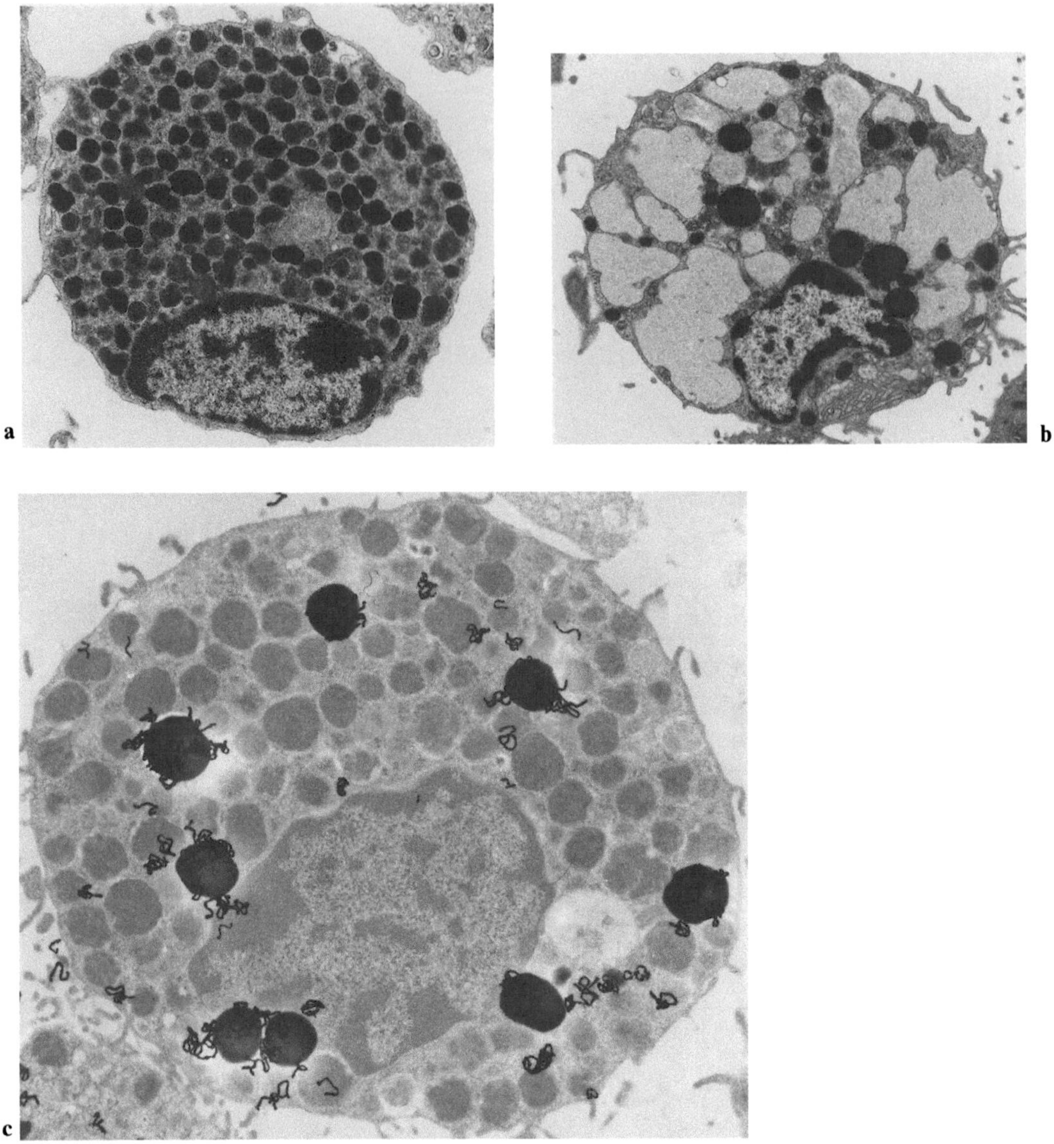

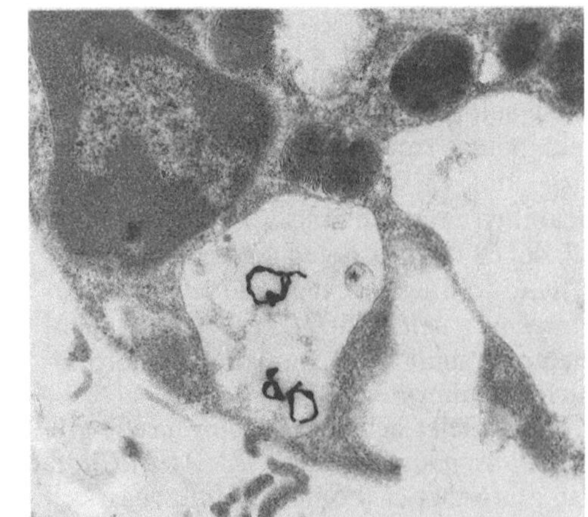

Fig. 18.2a–d. Human lung mast cells. **a** Control (×9,240). **b** Challenged with anti-IgE (×7,800). **c** Autoradiograph after prelabeling with ^{3}H-arachidonic acid showing labeling of osmiophilic bodies (×13,500). **d** With similar ^{3}H-AA labeling after activation by anti-IgE showing grains of ^{3}H in degranulation channels (×21,600)

Table 18.2. Mediators produced by mast cells and basophils

The same qualifications stated in Table 18.1 apply to the mediators listed here.

Mast cells	Basophils
Human cells	
Histamine	Histamine
Prostaglandin D_2	Leukotriene C_4
Thromboxane A_2	Lysosomal hydrolases
Leukotriene C_4	? Kallikrein-like enzyme
5-Hydroxyeicosatetraenoic acid	Proteoglycan (chondroitin 4 and 6 sulfates)
Platelet activating factor (AGEPC, perhaps others)	
Chemotactic factors	
Eosinophil chemotactic factors	
Leukotriene B_4	
Lysosomal hydrolases (e.g., hexosaminidase, β-glucuronidase, arylsulfatase)	
Tryptase	
Proteoglycan (heparin)	
Kininogenase	
Nonhuman cells	
Leukotriene B_4	
12-Hydroxyeicosatetraenoic acid	
Myeloperoxidase	
Superoxide dismutase	

Table 18.3. Preparations of mast cells and basophils in common use

Human cells	Rodent cells
Human blood basophils	Rat serosal mast cells
Human cord blood basophils	Lines of rat leukemic basophils
Human lung mast cells	Rat intestinal mast cells
Human intestinal mast cells	Mouse bone marrow-derived mast cells
Human skin mast cells	

platelet activation following antigen bronchial challenge in humans *in vivo* [67]. Other platelet activating factors besides AGEPC may also be released by mast cells [93]. In addition, AGEPC has been shown to cause the release of leukotrienes C_4 and D_4 from isolated perfused rat lungs [157].

Other mast cell and basophil mediators are proteins and include chemotactic molecules [3, 110], lysosomal enzymes (hexosaminidase, β-glucuronidase, arylsulfatase) [138], proteoglycans (as noted above) [95, 159], and enzymes with protease activity (tryptase which may be identical to a recently described kininogenase) [122, 137, 138]. Myeloperoxidase and superoxide dismutase have also been identified in rodent mast cells [50, 51].

18.4 Physiological and Pharmacological Control Mechanisms

Mast cells and basophils from a number of different tissues and species are under active investigation (Table 18.3). Cells from rodent sources such as rat serosal mast cells and lines of leukemic basophils [4, 126] have had the traditional advantages of ready availability, and the ability to obtain relatively large quantities of cells in a highly purified form. These have recently been supplemented by lines of mouse bone marrow-derived mast cells [35, 36, 97, 163]. In addition, since issues of mast cell heterogeneity have been raised, preparations of rat intestinal mast cells, as compared with serosal mast cells, have been the source of active investigation [5, 7, 112].

Human cells have the advantage of relevance, but until recently were unable to be obtained in large quantities in a relatively pure form. Many earlier studies have been performed with preparations of mixed leukocytes or crude dispersed human lung mast cells [59, 110, 119]. Recently, human skin and intestinal mast cells have been studied [33, 147], and methods have been obtained for purifying human basophils and human lung mast cells [81, 135]. A preparation of cells enriched in basophils derived from umbilical cord blood has also been described [104]. Although a number of different preparations of mast cells and basophils are now available for study including preparations of human cells which approach homogeneity, not all preparations respond to drugs and modulating factors in the same way; therefore, generalization from cell type to cell type, particularly between species, is hazardous.

A number of agents have been shown to be almost uniformly effective in inhibiting mediator release from mast cells and basophils initiated by bridging IgE receptors (Table 18.4). They include phospholipase *inhibitors,* many lipoxygenase inhibitors, inhibitors of serine proteases, and agents such as colchicine [38, 64, 84, 89, 123]. Agents which increase cellular CAMP concentrations, either through adenylate cyclase activation or by other means, also inhibit mediator release [8, 107, 119, 135, 146, 159]. Differences in the response of mast cells and basophils as far as their response to adenylate cyclase agonists appear to reside in the presence (or absence) of a specific receptor. For example, human basophils have an apparent histamine type 2 receptor as shown by their response to the H_2-agonist dimaprit and to exogenous histamine, while dispersed human lung mast cells show no such response [80, 119, 155]. Inhibitors of phospholipid methylation are also effective in inhibiting mediator release [57, 58].

Table 18.4. Physiological and pharmacological control mechanisms

Agents that inhibit mediator release from human mast cells and basophils

Putative phospholipase A_2 inhibitors (mepacrine, phenidone, *p*-bromophenacyl bromide)
Lipoxygenase inhibitors (eicosatetraynoic acid (ETYA), eicosatriynoic acid (ETI), nordihydroguaiaretic acid (NDGA))
Protease inhibitors (diisopropyl fluorophosphate (DFP))
Colchicine

Agents that increase cellular CAMP concentrations

Adenylate cyclase agonists (β-agonists, certain prostaglandins (e.g., PGE, adenosine))

Agents that increase CAMP levels by other mechanisms (phosphodiesterase inhibitors, dibutyryl CAMP)
Inhibitors of phospholipid methylation (3-deaza-adenosine (3-deaza-ADO))

Agents that enhance mediator release from human mast cells and basophils

Deuterium oxide
Cytochalasins
Hyperosmolar stimuli
Interferon
Lymphokines

Deuterium oxide, cytochalasins, and hyperosmolar stimuli all are effective in enhancing mediator release from mast cells and basophils [24, 28, 29, 37, 38, 106, 119, 156]. Of particular interest is the ability of leukocyte products such as interferon and lymphokines to enhance mediator release from basophils [55, 56], as well as the ability of macrophage-derived and lymphocyte-derived products to cause mediator release as described above [134, 139, 150, 151].

Other control mechanisms of pharmacological, and in some instances of perhaps physiological importance, are listed in Table 18.5. These observations have been listed so that *differences* between human lung mast cells and human basophils, and between human lung mast cells and rat serosal mast cells, are highlighted.

Human lung mast cells and human basophils differ in their response to H_2-agonists, indomethacin, 5-HPETE, 5-HETE, PGD_2,

Table 18.5. Variations in mediator release from different preparations of mast cells and basophils

Differences between human lung mast cells and human basophils

1. H_2-agonists inhibit histamine release from human basophils but not human lung mast cells.
2. Indomethacin, 5-hydroperoxyeicosatetraenoic acid (5-HPETE), 5-hydroxyeicosatetraenoic acid (5-HETE), and prostaglandin D_2 (PGD_2) enhance antigen-induced histamine release from basophils but not mast cells.
3. 5-HPETE, PGD_2, and LTB_4 induce histamine release from human basophils but not mast cells (in the presence of cytochalasin B).
4. Anti-inflammatory steroids inhibit mediator release from basophils but not mast cells.
5. Low concentrations of adenosine (1–10 μM) inhibit histamine release from basophils but enhance histamine release from mast cells.

Differences between human lung mast cells and rat serosal mast cells

1. Phosphatidylserine enhances histamine release from rat serosal mast cells but not human lung mast cells.
2. Disodium cromoglycate is a more potent and consistent inhibitor of histamine release from rat than human mast cells.
3. Leukotriene C is a major arachidonic acid metabolite in human lung mast cells but has no or little importance in rat serosal mast cells.
4. Cytochalasins enhance mediator release from human mast cells but inhibit release from rat serosal mast cells.
5. Anti-inflammatory steroids inhibit mediator release from rat serosal mast cells but not human lung mast cells.

LTB_4, anti-inflammatory steroids, and adenosine. As noted above, stimulation of H_2-receptors inhibits histamine release from human basophils but not from human lung mast cells [80, 119, 155]. Indomethacin (and other nonsteroidal anti-inflammatory agents), 5-HPETE, 5-HETE, and PGD_2 all enhance antigen-induced histamine release from basophils but not from mast cells [84, 88, 114, 115]. Such enhancement of histamine release appears to be stimulus-specific as release initiated by C5a is inhibited by indomethacin [27]. 5-HPETE, PGD_2, and LTB_4 induce histamine release in the presence of cytochalasin B from human basophils but not from mast cells [117, 118]. Anti-inflammatory steroids inhibit mediator release from basophils but not from mast cells [129, 131]. And finally, low concentrations of adenosine inhibit histamine release from basophils but enhance release from mast cells [87, 119]. Based on these differences we may presume that mechanisms involved in the release of inflammatory mediators may be different in these two cell types, and that pharmacological agents may be developed with a similar selectivity of action.

The regulation of mediator release from human basophils stimulated by allergens or by C5a is similar in terms of response to extracellular calcium, need for active glycolysis, microtubule polymerization, and response to drugs that can affect cellular levels of CAMP [43, 45]. Pharmacological concentrations of indomethacin inhibit C5a-dependent release of histamine, in contrast to the stimulatory effect of this drug on allergen-induced mediator release [27, 88].

A number of differences also exist between human lung mast cells and rat serosal (peritoneal) mast cells, until recently the most common source of mast cells or basophils in general use for drug development (Table 18.5). Phosphatidyl serine enhances histamine release from rat serosal mast cells but not from human lung mast cells [119, 144]. Disodium cromoglycate is a more potent and consistent inhibitor of histamine release from rat than human cells [10, 79]. Leukotriene C_4 appears to be generated in much larger quantities by human lung mast cells than rat peritoneal mast cells [83, 116, 124, 162]. Cytochalasins enhance mediator release from human mast cells but inhibit release from rat mast cells [79, 106, 108]. And anti-inflammatory steroids inhibit mediator release from rat and mouse mast cells but not from human lung fragments or purified human lung mast cells [15, 90, 131].

18.5 Cell-cell Interactions

The anaphylactic or IgE-mediated release of mediators, particularly primary cyclooxygenase products of arachidonic acid, has been studied in detail in preparations of chopped human lung and purified human lung mast cells [1, 83, 131, 136]. From these studies it is clear that the mast cell is the major source of histamine, prostaglandin D_2 and perhaps thromboxane B_2 released from human lung tissue [130]. Other primary cyclooxygenase products including the prostacyclin metabolite, 6-keto-prostaglandin $F_{1\alpha}$, and prostaglandin E_2 and $F_{2\alpha}$ apparently arise from other cells besides mast cells, perhaps through activation of these cells by mast cell mediators. Differences between human lung parenchyma and airway tissue have been noted in their ability to generate cyclooxygenase products [132]. In parenchyma the rank order of generation was 6-keto-$PGF_{1\alpha} \sim PGD_2 > PGF_{2\alpha} > TxB_2 \sim PGE$; in airway 6-keto-$PGF_{1\alpha} > PGE \sim PGF_{2\alpha} > PGD_2 > TxB_2$.

In addition, it has been shown that other human cells besides mast cells, such as alveolar macrophages, can be activated by antigen through IgE-dependent mechanisms to release inflammatory mediators [61, 154]. Although the mast cell is a major (and perhaps the primary) contributor of sulfidopeptide leukotrienes (leukotrienes C_4, D_4, and E_4 or components of SRS-A) after IgE-mediated stimulation [83, 116, 130, 131], human alveolar macrophages have been shown to generate leukotriene D_4 *in vitro* [11]. Recent studies have also suggested that arachidonic acid or arachidonic acid metabolites produced by one cell type can be used as substrate for further metabolism by other cells. The lymphocytes of pollen-sensitive individuals can be activated *in vitro* [25], and could release lymphokines that might affect mast cells, basophils, and other cells. Clearly the sociology of inflammatory mediator production by different cell types in complex tissues, such as the lung, is just beginning to be investigated.

Based on the actions of the metabolites known to be released by activated mast cells and basophils, scenarios of the inflammatory reaction initiated by these cells can be developed. For example, mast cell activation by antigen results in the release of histamine, a kininogenase, lysosomal enzymes and other granule constituents, prostaglandin D_2, thromboxane B_2, leukotriene

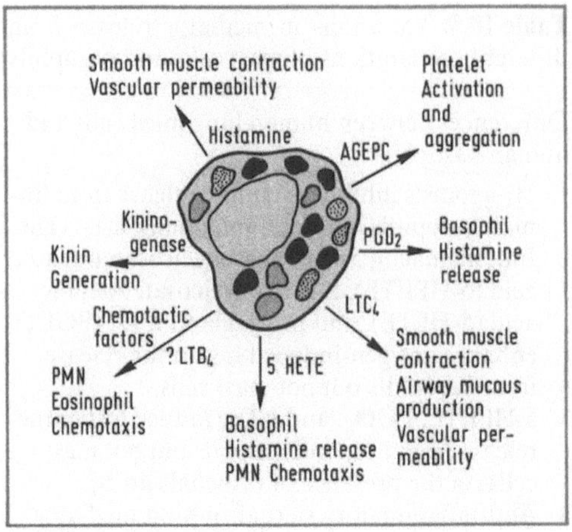

Fig. 18.3. Mediators produced by purified human lung mast cells and their physiologic effects

C_4, 5-HETE, platelet activating factor, factors chemotactic for neutrophils and eosinophils including, perhaps, leukotriene B_4 (Fig. 18.3). These compounds begin a localized inflammatory reaction with an increase in vascular permeability (edema), smooth muscle constriction, and a stimulation of mucus production. In the lung such an inflammatory reaction can be amplified by resident lung cells such as macrophages, if they too have been activated. Platelets, neutrophils, eosinophils, lymphocytes, and perhaps basophils migrate into the area because of the increase in permeability under the direction of chemotactic factors and are activated: platelets by AGEPC or platelet activating factor, neutrophils by phagocytic stimuli and leukotriene B_4, lymphocytes perhaps by antigen and mononuclear cells such as monocytes and macrophages, and basophils by prostaglandin D_2 and 5-HETE; physiological stimuli for eosinophil activation have not been completely defined.

Because the initial mast cell activation and mediator release is followed by recruitment of other inflammatory cells into the area, the potential for amplification of the initial response and for *late* reactions, reactions that occur hours after initial mast cell activation, is great. Neutrophils have the ability to amplify the inflammatory response as they respond to a wide variety of stimuli, generate or release a wide variety of inflammatory mediators after activation including lysosomal enzymes, active oxygen species, and oxygenated products of arachidonic acid, particularly leukotriene B_4 [41, 141]. In addition, they can be important in the termination of such reactions as they have the ability to metabolize sulfidopeptide (leukotrienes C_4, D_4, and E_4) and dihydroxy leukotrienes (leukotriene B_4) by myeloperoxidase-dependent and ω-oxidative mechanisms, respectively [67, 142]. Factors which control the balance between the amplicative and terminative phases of this inflammatory response are largely unknown.

18.6 Experimental Models

Several *in vivo* models of human diseases of the airways and nose are in common use. These models include bronchospastic disease with early and/or late changes in lung function initiated by antigen, exercise (or cold dry air), and oral challenge, and diseases of the nose initiated by similar challenge procedures. Diseases of the nose including allergic and vasomotor rhinitis are important sources of morbidity in man. In addition, the nose is a readily accessible portion of the upper airway whose secretions after specific challenge can be collected easily; it may provide a useful model for the study of diseases of the lower airways (the bronchi), as well. Efforts to link mast cells with diseases of the airways and nose demand a combination of *in vitro* and *in vivo* observations. The spectrum of mediators produced by human cells *in vitro* must be determined, together with a profile of their biologic activities. In addition,

Table 18.6. Release of mediators in *in vivo* models of asthma and rhinitis

Bronchoprovocation		
Antigen challenge		
	Immediate reactions	– Neutrophil chemotactic factor
		Histamine
		Platelet factor 4
	Late reactions	– Neutrophil chemotactic factor
Exercise challenge		
	Immediate reactions	– Neutrophil chemotactic factor
		Histamine
	Late reactions	– Neutrophil chemotactic factor
Aspirin challenge (aspirin-sensitive asthmatics)		
	Immediate reactions	– Neutrophil chemotactic factor
Nasal provocation		
Antigen challenge		
	Immediate reactions	– Histamine
		TAME esterase activity
		Kinins
		Prostaglandin D_2
		Sulfidopeptide leukotrienes (C_4, D_4, E_4)
	Late reactions	– Histamine
		TAME esterase activity
		Kinins
		(Prostaglandin D_2 *not* found)
Cold dry air challenge		
	Immediate reactions	– Histamine
		TAME esterase activity
		Kinins
		Prostaglandin D_2
		Sulfidopeptide leukotrienes

such mediators must be found in models of the human disease, and ultimately, in the disease itself. Such an association does not provide a causal link between particular cellular functions and mediators and the disease process, but is consistent with that hypothesis. Such a causal link can be strongly inferred only when pathophysiologic events can be interrupted by *specific* pharmacologic agents.

Table 18.6 lists human *in vivo* models in which mast cell or putative mast cell mediators have been observed; in blood when the lung has been challenged, and in nasal secretions when the nose has been the target organ. Neutrophil chemotactic factor (presumably mast cell-derived) has been observed immediately after antigen, exercise, and oral aspirin challenge, and in late reactions after antigen or exercise challenge [3, 53, 69, 70, 101]. Histamine has been observed acutely after antigen and exercise challenge, and platelet factor 4 after antigen challenge [67, 69, 70]. Antigen challenge of the nose resulted in the acute release of histamine, TAME esterase activity, kinins, prostaglandin D_2, and sulfidopeptide leukotrienes in nasal secretions [14, 98]. Late reactions initiated by antigen resulted in a similar profile of mediators, except that prostaglandin D_2 was not found [100]; whether leukotrienes occur in this situation is under investigation. Challenge of the nose with cold dry air in individuals who report symptoms after similar natural exposure, results in a similar profile of mediators in nasal secretions, but quantitatively less than that seen after antigen challenge [152].

These data strongly suggest that mast cells in the airways and nose are activated by a variety of different stimuli *in vivo* in man. In addition, we have shown that interventions such as drug treatment or immunotherapy which produce symptomatic relief, are associated with a decrease in mediators released after specific challenge [13, 99]. From these data we conclude that mast cells and basophils play an important role in asthma in humans.

18.7 Conclusions

The observations reviewed here strongly suggest that mast cells and perhaps basophils play an important role in the pathogenesis of diseases of both the upper and lower airways, the nose and the bronchi, respectively. They are located at the interface of the individual and his environment (mucosal surfaces) and in key areas to sense invasion (around nerves and blood vessels). Evidence has been obtained to suggest that mast cells and basophils have been activated in asthmatic subjects, and we now know a long list of both immunologic and nonimmunologic triggers that can activate these cells. These cells release a large variety of preformed mediators and synthesize and release at least as many newly formed mediators after activation. These mediators have the ability to initiate an immediate response including smooth muscle spasm, edema formation, and mucus secretion, and can call in additional inflammatory cells such as neutrophils, eosinophils, and perhaps basophils to continue this inflammatory reaction. Because it has clearly been shown that nonimmunologic, physical stimuli, as well as IgE-mediated stimuli can activate mast cells and basophils, they are likely to play an important role in *nonallergic* as well as in *allergic* asthma. Efforts to gain further insight into pathophysiological events produced by these cells and to control their function pharmacologically, will likely produce important benefits for individuals suffering from these disorders. In addition, since mast cells have been observed to proliferate in sites of inflammation in a number of different disorders such as inflammatory disorders of the joints, intestines, and in interstitial diseases of the lung, such insights may eventually prove helpful in these disorders as well.

Acknowledgements: We would like to thank Stephen J. Galli, M. D., for his many helpful suggestions and his critical reading of the manuscript. We thank Stephanie Peters for secretarial assistance.

References

1. Adkinson NF Jr, Newball H, Findlay SR, Adams GK, Lichtenstein LM (1980) Anaphylactic release of prostaglandins from human lung in vitro. Am Rev Respir Dis 121:911–920
2. Askenase PW, Atwood JE (1976) Basophils in tuberculin and "Jones-Mote" delayed reactions in humans. J Clin Invest 58:1145–1154
3. Atkins PC, Norman M, Weiner H, Zweiman B (1977) Release of neutrophil chemotactic activity during immediate hypersensitivity reactions in humans. Ann Intern Med 86:415–418
4. Barsumian EL, Isersky C, Petrino MG, Siraganian RP (1981) IgE-induced histamine release from rat basophilic leukemia cell lines: isolation of releasing and non-releasing clones. Eur J Immunol 11:317–323
5. Befus AD, Pearce FL, Gauldie J, Horsewood P, Bienenstock J (1982) Mucosal mast cells. I. Isolation and functional characteristics of rat intestinal mast cells. J Immunol 128:2475–2480
6. Bhat KN, Arroyave CM, Marney SR Jr, Stevenson DD, Tan EM (1976) Plasma histamine changes during provoked bronchospasm in asthmatic patients. J Allergy Clin Immunol 58:647–656
7. Bienstock J, Befus AD, Pearce F, Denburg J, Goodacre R (1982) Mast cell heterogeneity: derivatization and function, with emphasis on the intestine. J Allergy Clin Immunol 70:407–412
8. Bourne HR, Lichtenstein LM, Melmon KL, Henney CS, Weinstein Y, Shearer GM (1974) Modulation of inflammation and immunity by cyclic AMP. Receptors for vasoactive hormones and mediators of inflammation regulate many leukocyte functions. Science 184:19–28
9. Brindley LL, Sweet JM, Goetzl EJ (1983) Stimulation of histamine release from human basophils by human platelet factor 4. J Clin Invest 72:1218–1223
10. Butchers PR, Fullarton JR, Skidmore IF, Thompson LE, Vardey CJ, Wheeldon A (1979) A comparison of the anti-anaphylactic activities of salbutamol and disodium cromoglycate in the rat, the rat mast cell and in human lung. Br J Pharmacol 67:23–32
11. Chavis DM, Godard P, Michel FB, de Paulet AC (1983) Purification and mass spectrometry identification of leukotriene D_4 synthesized by human alveolar macrophages. Biochem Biophys Res Commun 111:518–524
12. Connell JT (1971) Asthmatic deaths, role of the mast cell. JAMA 215:769–776
13. Creticos PS, Marsh DG, Adkinson NF, Proud D, Naclerio RM, Kagey-Sobotka A, Lichtenstein LM, Norman PS (1984) Evaluation by nasal pollen challenge of immunotherapy with rapidly released ragweed allergens. J Allergy Clin Immunol 73:141 (abstract)
14. Creticos PS, Peters SP, Adkinson NF Jr, Naclerio RM, Hayes EC, Norman PS, Lichtenstein LM (1984) Peptide leukotriene release after antigen challenge in patients sensitive to ragweed. N Engl J Med 310:1626–1630
15. Daeron M, Sterk AR, Hirata F, Ishizaka T (1982) Biochemical analysis of glucocorticoid-induced inhibition of IgE-mediated histamine release from mouse mast cells. J Immunol 129:1212–1218
16. Dixon WE, Brodie TG (1902) Contributions to the physiology of the lungs. 1. The bronchial muscles, their innervation, and the action of drug upon them. Physiol: 97–173
17. Drazen JM, Austen KF, Lewis RA, Clark DA, Goto G, Marfat A, Corey EJ (1980) Comparative airway and vascular activities of leukotrienes C-1 and D *in vivo* and *in vitro*. Proc Natl Acad Sci USA 77:4354–4358
18. Dvorak AM, Dvorak HF, Peters SP, Schulman ES, MacGlashan DW Jr, Pyne K, Galli SJ, Lichtenstein LM (1983) Lipid bodies: Cytoplasmic organelles important to arachidonate metabolism in macrophages and mast cells. J Immunol 131:2965–2976
19. Dvorak AM, Galli SJ, Schulman ES, Lichtenstein LM, Dvorak HF (1983) Basophil and mast cell degranulation: Ultrastructural analysis of mechanisms of mediator release. Fed Proc 42:2510–2515
20. Dvorak AM, Hammel I, Schulman ES, Peters SP, MacGlashan DW Jr, Schleimer RP, Newball HH, Pyne K, Dvorak HF, Lichtenstein LM, Galli SJ (1984) Differences in the behavior of cytoplasmic granules and lipid bodies during human lung mast cell degranulation. J Cell Biol 99:1678–1687
21. Dvorak AM, Lett-Brown MA, Thueson DO, Pyne K, Raghuprasad PK, Galli SJ, Grant JA (1984) Histamine-releasing activity (HRA). III. HRA induces human basophil histamine release by provoking noncytotoxic granule exocytosis. Clin Immunol Immunopathol 32:142–150
22. Dvorak AM, Mihm MC Jr, Dvorak HF (1976) Degranulation of basophilic leukocytes in allergic contact dermatitis reactions in man. J Immunol 116:687–695

23. Dvorak AM, Newball HH, Dvorak HF, Lichtenstein LM (1980) Antigen-induced IgE-mediated degranulation of human basophils. Lab Invest 43:126–139
24. Eggleston PA, Kagey-Sobotka A, Schleimer RP, Lichtenstein LM (1984) Interaction between hyperosmolar and IgE-mediated histamine release from basophils and mast cells. Am Rev Respir Dis 130:86–91
25. Evans R, Pence H, Kaplan H, Rocklin RE (1976) The effect of immunotherapy on humeral and cellular responses in ragweed hayfever. J Clin Invest 57:1378–1385
26. Fagan DL, Slaughter CA, Capra JD, Sullivan TJ (1982) Monoclonal antibodies to immunoglobulin G_4 induce histamine release from human basophils in vitro. J Allergy Clin Immunol 70:399–404
27. Farnam J, Grant JA, Lett-Brown MA, Hunt C, Thueson DO, Giclas PC (1985) Complement-mediated release of histamine from basophils in vitro. V. Differential effects of drugs modulating arachidonic acid metabolism. J Immunol 134:541–547
28. Findlay SR, Dvorak AM, Kagey-Sobotka A, Lichtenstein LM (1981) Hyperosmolar triggering of histamine release from human basophils. J Clin Invest 67:1604–1613
29. Findlay SR, Lichtenstein LM (1980) Basophil "releasibility" in patients with asthma. Am Rev Respir Dis 122:53–59
30. Findlay SR, Lichtenstein LM, Grant JA (1980) Generation of slow reacting substance by human leukocytes. II. Comparison of stimulation by antigen, anti-IgE, calcium ionophore, and C5-peptide. J Immunol 124:238–242
31. Ford RM (1969) Aetiology of asthma: a review of 11,551 cases (1958 to 1968). Med J Aust 1:629–631
32. Ford-Hutchinson AW, Bray MA, Doig MV, Shipley ME, Smith MJH (1980) Leukotriene B, a potent chemokinetic and aggregating substance released from polymorphonuclear leukocytes. Nature 286:264–265
33. Fox CC, Dvorak AM, Peters SP, Lichtenstein LM (1985) Isolation and characterization of human intestinal mucosal mast cells. J Immunol 135:483–491
34. Galli SJ, Dvorak AM (1984) Editorial. What do mast cells have to do with delayed hypersensitivity? Lab Invest 50:365–368
35. Galli SJ, Dvorak AM, Dvorak HF (1984) Basophils and mast cells: Morphologic insights into their biology, secretory patterns, and function. In: Ishizaka K (ed) Mast Cell Activation and Mediator Release. Prog Allergy, vol. 34. Karger, Basel, pp 1–141
36. Galli SJ, Dvorak AM, Marcum JA, Ishizaka T, Nabel G, Der Simonian H, Pyne K, Goldin JM, Rosenberg RD, Cantor H, Dvorak HF (1982) Mast cell clones: A model for the analysis of cellular maturation. J Cell Biol 95:435–444
37. Gillespie E, Lichtenstein LM (1972) Heavy water enhances IgE-mediated histamine release from human leukocytes: Evidence for microtubule involvement. Proc Soc Exp Biol Med 140:1228–1230
38. Gillespie E, Lichtenstein LM (1972) Histamine release from human leukocytes: Studies with deuterium oxide, colchicine, and cytochalasin B. J Clin Invest 51:2941–2947
39. Glovsky MM, Higli TE, Ishizaka T, Lichtenstein LM, Erickson BW (1979) Anaphylatoxin-induced histamine release with human leukocytes. Studies of C3a leukocyte binding and histamine release. J Clin Invest 64:804–811
40. Goetzl EJ, Pickett WC (1980) The human PMN leukocyte chemotactic activity of complex hydroxy-eicosatetraenoic acids (HETEs). J Immunol 125:1789–1791
41. Goldyne ME, Burrish GF, Poubelle P, Borgeat P (1984) Arachidonic acid metabolism among human mononuclear leukocytes. Lipoxygenase-related pathways. J Biol Chem 259:8815–8819
42. Grant JA, Dupree E, Goldman AS (1975) Complement-mediated release of histamine from human leukocytes. J Immunol 114:1101–1105
43. Grant JA, Dupree E, Thueson DO (1977) Complement-mediated release of histamine from human basophils. III. Possible regulatory role of microtubules and microfilaments. J Allergy Clin Immunol 60:306–311
44. Grant JA, Lichtenstein LM (1972) Reversed in vitro anaphylaxis induced by anti-IgG: Specificity of the reaction and comparison with antigen-induced histamine release. J Immunol 109:20–25
45. Grant JA, Settle L, Whorton EB, Dupree E (1976) Complement-mediated release of histamine from human basophils. II. Biochemical characterization of the reaction. J Immunol 117:450–456
46. Griffin M, Weiss JW, Leitch AG, McFadden ER Jr, Corey EJ, Austen KF, Drazen JM (1983) Effects of leukotriene D on the airways in asthma. N Engl J Med 308:436–439
47. Guerzon GM, Paré PD, Michoud M-C, Hogg JC (1979) The number and distribution of mast cells in monkey lung. Am Rev Respir Dis 119:59–66
48. Hardy CC, Robinson C, Tattersfield E, Hol-

gate ST (1984) The bronchoconstrictor effect of prostaglandin D_2 in normal and asthmatic men. N Engl J Med 311:209–213
49. Hastie R, Heroy JH III, Levy DA (1979) Basophil leukocytes and mast cells in human nasal secretions and scrapings studied by light microscopy. Lab Invest 40:554–561
50. Henderson WR, Kaliner M (1978) Immunologic and non-immunologic generation of superoxide from mast cells and basophils. J Clin Invest 61:187–196
51. Henderson WR, Kaliner M (1979) Mast cell granule peroxidase: location, secretion, and SRS-A inactivation. J Immunol 122:1322–1328
52. Hirsch SR, Kalbfleisch JH (1980) Existence of basophil chemotaxis in subjects with hay fever. J Allergy Clin Immunol 65:274–277
53. Hollingsworth HM, Downing ET, Braham SS, Glassroth J, Binder R, Center DM (1984) Identification and characterization of neutrophil chemotactic activity in aspirin-induced asthma. Am Rev Respir Dis 130:373–379
54. Horton EW, Jones RL (1974) Biological activity of prostaglandin D_2 on smooth muscle. Br J Pharmacol [Proc BPS] 52: 110P–111P
55. Ida S, Hooks JJ, Siraganian RP, Notkins AL (1977) Enhancement of IgE-mediated histamine release from human basophils by viruses: role of interferon. J Exp Med 145:892–906
56. Ida S, Hooks JJ, Siraganian RP, Notkins AL (1980) Enhancement of IgE-mediated histamine release from human basophils by immune-specific lymphokines. Clin Exp Immunol 41:380–387
57. Ishizaka T, Conrad DH, Schulman ES, Sterk AR, Ishizaka K (1983) Biochemical analysis of initial triggering events of IgE-mediated histamine release from human lung mast cells. J Immunol 130:2357–2362
58. Ishizaka T, Conrad DH, Schulman ES, Sterk AR, Ko CGL, Ishizaka K (1984) IgE-mediated triggering signals for mediator release from human mast cells and basophils. Fed Proc 43:2840–2845
59. Ishizaka T, de Bernardo R, Tomioka H, Lichtenstein LM, Ishizaka K (1972) Identification of basophil granulocytes as a site of allergic histamine release. J Immunol 108:1000–1008
60. Ishizaka K, Ishizaka T, Orange RP, Austen KF (1970) The capacity of human immunoglobulin E to mediate the release of histamine and slow reacting substance of anaphylaxis (SRS-A) from monkey lung. J Immunol 104:335–343
61. Joseph M, Tonnel AB, Topier G, Capron A, Arnoux B, Benveniste J (1983) Involvement of immunoglobulin E in the secretory process of alveolar macrophages from asthmatic patients. J Clin Invest 71:221–230
62. Juhlin L, Hammarstrom S (1982) Effects of intradermally injected leukotriene C_4 and histamine in patients with urticaria, psoriasis and atopic dermatitis. Br J Dermatol 107 [Suppl] 23:106–110
63. Kaliner M, Austen KF (1973) A sequence of biochemical events in the antigen-induced release of chemical mediators from sensitized human lung tissue. J Exp Med 138:1077–1094
64. Kazimierczak W, Meier HL, MacGlashan DW Jr, Lichtenstein LM (1984) An antigen-activated DFP-inhibitable enzyme controls basophil desensitization. J Immunol 132: 399–405
65. Kimura I, Tanizaki Y, Saito K, Takahashi K, Ueda N, Sato S (1975) Appearance of basophils in the sputum of patients with bronchial asthma. Clin Allergy 5:95–98
66. Knauer KA, Kagey-Sobotka A, Adkinson NF Jr, Lichtenstein LM (1984) Platelet augmentation of IgE-dependent histamine release from human basophils and mast cells. Int Arch Allergy Appl Immunol 74:29–35
67. Knauer KA, Lichtenstein LM, Adkinson NF Jr, Fish JE (1981) Platelet activation during antigen-induced airway reactions in asthmatic subjects. N Engl J Med 304:1404–1407
68. Lee CW, Lewis RA, Tauber AI, Mehrotra M, Corey EJ, Austen KF (1983) The myeloperoxidase-dependent metabolism of leukotrienes C_4, D_4, and E_4 to 6-*trans*-leukotriene B_4 diastereoisomers and the subclass-specific S-diastereoisomeric sulfoxides. J Biol Chem 258:15004–15010
69. Lee TH, Brown MJ, Nagy L, Causon R, Walport MJ, Kay AB (1982) Exercise-induced release of histamine and neutrophil chemotactic factor in atopic asthmatics. J Allergy Clin Immunol 70:73–81
70. Lee TH, Nagakura T, Papageorgiou N, Iikura Y, Kay AB (1983) Exercise-induced late asthmatic reactions with neutrophil chemotactic activity. N Engl J Med 308: 1502–1505
71. Lett-Brown MA, Aelvoet M, Hooks JJ, Georgiades JA, Thueson DO, Grant JA (1981) Enhancement of basophil chemotaxis in vitro by virus-induced interferon. J Clin Invest 67:547–552
72. Lett-Brown MA, Boetcher DA, Leonard EJ (1976) Chemotactic responses of normal human basophils to C5a and to lympho-

cyte-derived chemotactic factor. J Immunol 117:246–252
73. Lett-Brown MA, Thueson DO, Plank DE, Duffy L, Grant JA (1984) Histamine-releasing activity. V. Characterization and purification using high-performance liquid chromatography. Cell Immunol 87:445–451
74. Lewis RA, Holgate ST, Roberts LJ II, Maguire JF, Oates JA, Austen KF (1979) Effects of indomethacin on cyclic nucleotide levels and histamine release from rat serosal mast cells. J Immunol 123:1663–1668
75. Lewis RA, Soter NA, Diamond PT, Austen KF, Oates JA, Roberts LJ II (1982) Prostaglandin D_2 generation after activation of rat and human mast cells with anti-IgE. J Immunol 129:1627–1631
76. Lichtenstein LM (1975) The mechanism of basophil histamine release induced by antigen and by the calcium ionophore A23187. J Immunol 114:1692–1699
77. Lichtenstein LM (1978) An evaluation of the role of immunotherapy in asthma. Am Rev Respir Dis 117:191–197
78. Lichtenstein LM, de Bernardo R (1971) IgE mediated histamine release: In vitro separation into two phases. Int Arch Allergy Appl Immunol 41:56–71
79. Lichtenstein LM, Foreman JC, Conroy MC, Marone G, Newball HH (1979) Difference between histamine release from rat mast cells and human basophils and mast cells. In: Pepys J, Edwards AM (eds) The Mast Cell: Its Role in Health and Disease. Pitman, Kent, pp 83–96
80. Lichtenstein LM, Gillespie E (1973) Inhibition of histamine release by histamine controlled by H2 receptor. Nature 244:287–288
81. MacGlashan DW Jr, Lichtenstein LM (1980) The purification of human basophils. J Immunol 124:2519–2521
82. MacGlashan DW Jr, Lichtenstein LM (1984) Dimeric IgE may not represent the unit signal for the release of all mediators in human basophils. Fed Proc 43:1663 (abstract)
83. MacGlashan DW Jr, Schleimer RP, Peters SP, Schulman ES, Adams GK III, Newball HH, Lichtenstein LM (1982) Generation of leukotrienes by purified human lung mast cells. J Clin Invest 70:747–751
84. MacGlashan DW Jr, Schleimer RP, Peters SP, Schulman ES, Adams GK, Sobotka AK, Newball HH, Lichtenstein LM (1983) Comparative studies of human basophils and mast cells. Fed Proc 42:2504–2509
85. Marom Z, Shelhamer JH, Bach MK, Morton DR, Kaliner M (1982) Slow-reacting substances, leukotriene C_4 and D_4, increase the release of mucus from human airways *in vitro*. Am Rev Respir Dis 126:449–451
86. Marone G, Columbo M, Soppelsa L, Condorelli M (1984) The mechanism of basophil histamine release induced by pepstatin A. J Immunol 133:1542–1546
87. Marone G, Findlay SR, Lichtenstein LM (1979) Adenosine receptor on human basophils: Modulation of histamine release. J Immunol 123:1473–1477
88. Marone G, Kagey-Sobotka A, Lichtenstein LM (1979) Effects of arachidonic acid and its metabolites on antigen-induced histamine release from human basophils *in vitro*. J Immunol 123:1669–1677
89. Marone G, Kagey-Sobotka A, Lichtenstein LM (1981) Possible role of phospholipase A_2 in triggering histamine secretion from human basophils *in vitro*. Clin Immunol Immunopathol 20:231–239
90. Marquardt DL, Wasserman SI (1983) Modulation of rat serosal mast cell biochemistry by *in vivo* dexamethasone administration. J Immunol 131:934–939
91. Mazurek N, Pecht I, Teichberg VI, Blumberg S (1981) The role of N-terminal tetrapeptide in the histamine-releasing action of substance P. Neuropharmacology 20:1025–1027
92. Meltzer SJ (1910) Bronchial asthma as a phenomenon of anaphylaxis. JAMA 55:1021–1024
93. Mencia-Huerta J-M, Lewis RA, Razin E, Austen KF (1983) Antigen-initiated release of platelet-activating factor (PAF-acether) from mouse bone marrow-derived mast cells sensitized with monoclonal IgE. J Immunol 131:2958–2964
94. Mencia-Huerta J-M, Razin E, Ringel EW, Corey EJ, Hoover D, Austen KF, Lewis RA (1983) Immunologic and ionophore-induced generation of leukotriene B_4 from mouse bone marrow-derived mast cells. J Immunol 130:1885–1890
95. Metcalf DD, Lewis RA, Silbert JE, Rosenberg RD, Wasserman SI, Austen KF (1979) Isolation and characterization of heparin from human lung. J Clin Invest 64:1537–1543
96. Mikhail GR, Miller-Milinska M (1964) Mast cell population in human skin. J Invest Dermatol 43:249–256
97. Nabel G, Galli SJ, Dvorak AM, Dvorak HF, Cantor H (1981) Inducer T lymphocytes synthesize a factor that stimulates proliferation of cloned mast cells. Nature 291:332–334
98. Naclerio RM, Meier HL, Kagey-Sobotka A, Adkinson NF Jr, Meyers DA, Norman PS, Lichtenstein LM (1983) Mediator release

after nasal airway challenge with allergen. Am Rev Respir Dis 128:597–602
99. Naclerio RM, Meier HL, Kagey-Sobotka A, Norman PS, Lichtenstein LM (1984) *In vivo* model for the evaluation of topical anti-allergic medications. Arch Otolaryngol 110:25–27
100. Naclerio R, Togias A, Proud D, Kagey-Sobotka A, Adkinson NF Jr, Norman PS, Lichtenstein LM (1985) Inflammatory mediators in late antigen-induced rhinitis. N Engl J Med 313:65–70
101. Nagy L, Lee TH, Kay AB (1982) Neutrophil chemotactic activity in antigen-induced late asthmatic reactions. N Engl J Med 306:497–501
102. Norris HT, Zamchek N, Gottlieb L (1963) The presence and distribution of mast cells in the human gastrointestinal tract at autopsy. Gastroenterology 44:448–455
103. O'Donnell MC, Ackerman SJ, Gleich GJ, Thomas LL (1983) Activation of basophil and mast cell histamine release by eosinophil granule major basic protein. J Exp Med 157:1981–1991
104. Ogawa M, Nakahata T, Leary AG, Sterk AR, Ishizaka K, Ishizaka T (1983) Suspension culture of human mast cells/basophils from umbilical cord blood mononuclear cells. Proc Natl Acad Sci USA 80:4494–4498
105. Okuda M, Ohtsuka H, Kawabori S (1979) The role of the blood basophil in allergic nasal manifestations. In: Pepys J, Edwards AM (eds) The mast cell, its role in health and disease. Pitman, Kent, pp 767–771
106. Orange RP (1975) Dissociation of the immunological release of histamine and slow reacting substance of anaphylaxis from human lung using cytochalasins A and B. J Immunol 114:182–186
107. Orange RP, Austen WG, Austen KF (1971) Immunological release of histamine and slow-reacting substance of anaphylaxis from human lung. J Exp Med 134:136s–148s
108. Orr TSC, Hall DE, Allison A (1972) Role of contractile microfilaments in release of histamine from mast cells. Nature 236:350–351
109. Parwaresch MR (1976) The human blood basophil. Springer, Berlin Heidelberg New York, pp 3–4
110. Paterson NAM, Wasserman SI, Said JW, Austen KF (1976) Release of chemical mediators from partially purified human lung mast cells. J Immunol 117:1356–1362
111. Patterson R, McKenna JM, Suszko IM, Solliday NH, Pruzansky JJ, Roberts M, Kehoe TJ (1977) Living histamine-containing cells from the bronchial lumens of humans. J Clin Invest 59:217–225
112. Pearce FL, Befus AD, Gauldie J, Bienenstock J (1982) Mucosal mast cells. II. Effects of anti-allergic compounds on histamine secretion by isolated intestinal mast cells. J Immunol 128:2481–2486
113. Permutt S (1980) Irritability and allergy: The neuron and the mast cell. Am Rev Respir Dis 122:187–189
114. Peters SP, Kagey-Sobotka A, MacGlashan DW Jr, Lichtenstein LM (1984) Effect of prostaglandin D_2 in modulating histamine release from human basophils. J Pharmacol Exp Ther 228:400–406
115. Peters SP, Kagey-Sobotka A, MacGlashan DW Jr, Siegel MI, Lichtenstein LM (1982) The modulation of human basophil histamine release by products of the 5-lipoxygenase pathway. J Immunol 129:797–803
116. Peters SP, MacGlashan DW Jr, Schulman ES, Schleimer RP, Hayes EC, Rokach J, Adkinson NF Jr, Lichtenstein LM (1984) Arachidonic acid metabolism in purified human lung mast cells. J Immunol 132:1972–1979
117. Peters SP, Schleimer RP, Kagey-Sobotka A, Naclerio RM, MacGlashan DW Jr, Schulman ES, Adkinson NF Jr, Lichtenstein LM (1982) The role of prostaglandin D_2 in IgE-mediated reactions in man. Trans Assoc Am Physicians XCV:221–228
118. Peters SP, Schleimer RP, MacGlashan DW Jr, Schulman ES, Kagey-Sobotka A, Adams GK III, Lichtenstein LM (1983) Lipoxygenase products of arachidonic acid: Their role in inflammatory events mediated by human basophils and mast cells. In: Hadden JW, Chedid L, Dukor P, Spreafico F, Willoughby D (eds) Advances in immunopharmacology 2. Pergamon Press, Oxford, pp 617–622
119. Peters SP, Schulman ES, Schleimer RP, MacGlashan DW Jr, Newball HH, Lichtenstein LM (1982) Dispersed human lung mast cells: Pharmacologic aspects and comparison with human lung tissue fragments. Am Rev Respir Dis 126:1034–1039
120. Schleimer RP, MacGlashan DW Jr, Peters SP, Pinckard RN, Adkinson NF Jr, Lichtenstein LM (1986) Characterization of inflammatory mediator release from purified human lung mast cells. Am Rev Respir Dis 133:614–617
121. Plaut M, Lichtenstein LM (1982) Histamine and immune responses. In: Ganellin CR, Parsons ME (eds) Pharmacology of Histamine Receptors. John Wright, London, pp 392–435

122. Proud D, Lichtenstein LM (1984) Human lung mast cell kininogenase: apparent identity to kininogenase. Fed Proc 43:1807 (abstract)
123. Pruzansky JJ, Paterson R (1975) The diisopropylfluorophosphate inhibitable step in antigen-induced histamine release from human leukocytes. J Immunol 114:939–943
124. Razin E, Mencia-Huerta M, Lewis RA, Corey EJ, Austen KF (1982) Generation of leukotriene C_4 from a subclass of mast cells differentiated *in vitro* from mouse bone marrow. Proc Natl Acad Sci USA 79:4665–4667
125. Roberts LJ II, Sweetman BJ, Lewis RA, Austen KF, Oares JA (1980) Increased production of prostaglandin D_2 in patients with systemic mastocytosis. N Engl J Med 303:1400–1404
126. Rohlich P, Anderson P, Uvnas B (1971) Electron microscopic observations on compound 48/80-induced degranulation in rat mast cells. J Cell Biol 51:465–483
127. Schleimer RP et al (unpublished observation)
128. Schleimer RP, Gillespie E, Lichtenstein LM (1981) Release of histamine from human leukocytes with the tumor-promoting phorbol diesters. I. Characterization of the response. J Immunol 126:570–574
129. Schleimer RP, Lichtenstein LM, Gillespie E (1981) Inhibition of basophils histamine release by anti-inflammatory steroids. Nature 292:454–455
130. Schleimer RP, MacGlashan DW Jr, Peters SP, Naclerio RM, Proud D, Adkinson NF Jr, Lichtenstein LM (1984) Inflammatory mediators and mechanisms of release from purified human basophils and mast cells. J Allergy Clin Immunol 74:473–481
131. Schleimer RP, Schulman ES, MacGlashan DW Jr, Peters SP, Hayes EC, Adams GK III, Lichtenstein LM, Adkinson NF Jr (1983) Effects of dexamethasone on mediator release from human lung fragments and purified human lung mast cells. J Clin Invest 71:1830–1835
132. Schulman ES, Adkinson NF Jr, Newball HH (1982) Cyclooxygenase metabolites in human lung anaphylaxis: airway vs. parenchyma. J Appl Physiol 53:589–595
133. Schulman ES, Kagey-Sobotka A, MacGlashan DW Jr, Adkinson NF Jr, Peters SP, Schleimer RP, Lichtenstein LM (1983) Heterogeneity of human mast cells. J Immunol 131:1936–1941
134. Schulman ES, Liu MC, Proud D, MacGlashan DW Jr, Lichtenstein LM, Plaut M (1985) Human lung macrophages induce histamine release from basophils and mast cells. Am Rev Respir Dis 131:230–235
135. Schulman ES, MacGlashan DW Jr, Peters SP, Schleimer RP, Newball HH, Lichtenstein LM (1982) Human lung mast cells: Purification and characterization. J Immunol 129:2662–2667
136. Schulman ES, Newball HH, Demers LM, Fitzpatrick FA, Adkinson NF Jr (1981) Anaphylactic release of thromboxane A_2, prostaglandin D_2, and prostacyclin from human lung parenchyma. Am Rev Respir Dis 124:402–406
137. Schwartz LB, Lewis RA, Austen KF (1981) Tryptase from human pulmonary mast cells. Purification and characterization. J Biol Chem 256:11939–11943
138. Schwartz LB, Lewis RA, Seldin D, Austen KF (1981) Acid hydrolases and tryptase from secretory granules of dispersed human lung mast cells. J Immunol 126:1290–1294
139. Sedgwick JD, Holt PG, Turner KJ (1981) Production of a histamine-releasing lymphokine by antigen- or mitogen-stimulated human peripheral T cells. Clin Exp Immunol 45:409–418
140. Segal DM, Taurog JD, Metzger H (1977) Dimeric immunoglobulin E serves as a unit signal for mast cell degranulation. Proc Natl Acad Sci USA 74:2993–2997
141. Serhan CN, Radin A, Smolen JE, Korchak H, Samuelsson B, Weissmann G (1982) Leukotriene B_4 is a complete secretagogue in human neutrophils: A kinetic analysis. Biochem Biophys Res Commun 107:1006–1012
142. Shak S, Goldstein IM (1984) ω-oxidation is the major pathway for the catabolism of leukotriene B_4 in human polymorphonuclear leukocytes. J Biol Chem 259:10181–10187
143. Siraganian RP, Hook WA (1977) Mechanism of histamine release by formyl methionine-containing peptides. J Immunol 119:2078–2083
144. Stechschulte DJ, Austen KF (1974) Phosphatidyl serine enhancement of antigen-induced mediator release from rat mast cells. J Immunol 112:970–978
145. Sullivan TJ, Parker KL, Kulczycki A Jr, Parker CW (1976) Modulation of cyclic AMP in purified rat mast cells. III. Studies of the effect of concanavalin A and anti-IgE on cyclic AMP concentration during histamine release. J Immunol 117:713–716
146. Tauber AI, Kaliner M, Stechschulte DJ, Austen KF (1973) Immunological release of histamine and slow reacting substance of anaphylaxis from human lung. V. Effects of

prostaglandins on release of histamine. J Immunol 111:27–32
147. Tharp MD, Suvunrungsi RT, Sullivan TJ (1983) IgE-mediated release of histamine from human cutaneous mast cells. J Immunol 130:1896–1901
148. Tharp MD, Thirlby R, Sullivan TJ (1984) Gastrin induces histamine release from human cutaneous mast cells. J Allergy Clin Immunol 74:159–165
149. Theoharides TC, Douglas WW (1981) Mast cell histamine secretion in response to somatostatin analogues: structural considerations. Eur J Pharmacol 73:131–136
150. Thueson DO, Speck LS, Lett-Brown MA, Grant JA (1979) Histamine releasing activity (HRA). I. Production by mitogen- or antigen-stimulated human mononuclear cells. J Immunol 123:626–632
151. Thueson DO, Speck LS, Lett-Brown MA, Grant JA (1979) Histamine releasing activity (HRA). II. Interaction with basophils and physiochemical characterization. J Immunol 123:633–639
152. Togias A, Naclerio R, Proud D, Fish J, Adkinson NF Jr, Kagey-Sobotka A, Norman PS, Lichtenstein LM (1984) Mast cell mediators are released *in vivo* following nasal challenge with cold dry air. Clin Res 32:540 A (abstract)
153. Tomioka M, Ida S, Shindoh Y, Ishihara T, Takishima T (1984) Mast cells in bronchoalveolar lumen of patients with bronchial asthma. Am Rev Respir Dis 129:1000–1005
154. Tonnel AB, Gosset P, Joseph M, Fournier E, Capron A (1983) Stimulation of alveolar macrophages in asthmatic patients after local provocation test. Lancet 1:1406–1408
155. Tung R, Kagey-Sobotka A, Plaut M, Lichtenstein LM (1982) H_2 antihistamines augment antigen-induced histamine release from human basophils *in vitro*. J Immunol 129:2113–2115
156. Tung R, Lichtenstein LM (1982) *In vitro* histamine release from basophils of asthmatic and atopic individuals in D_2O. J Immunol 128:2067–2072
157. Voelkel NF, Worthen S, Reeves JT, Henson PM, Murphy RC (1982) Nonimmunological production of leukotrienes induced by platelet-activating factor. Science 218:286–288
158. Wasserman MA, duCharme DW, Grifin RL, deGraaf GL, Robinson FG (1977) Bronchopulmonary and cardiovascular effects of prostaglandin D_2 in the dog. Prostaglandins 13:255–269
159. Wasserman SI (1983) Mediators of immediate hypersensitivity. J Allergy Clin Immunol 72:101–115
160. Wasserman SI (1984) The mast cell and synovial inflammation. Arthritis Rheum 27:841–844
161. Whelan CJ (1978) Histamine release from rat peritoneal mast cells by phospholipase A. The "activation" of phospholipase A by phospholipids. Biochem Pharmacol 27:2115–2118
162. Yecies LD, Wedner HJ, Johnson SM, Jakschik BA, Parker CW (1979) Slow reacting substance (SRS) from ionophore A23187-stimulated peritoneal cells of the normal rat. I. Conditions of generation and initial characterization. J Immunol 122:2083–2089
163. Yung Y-P, Eger R, Tertian G, Moore MAS (1981) Long-term *in vitro* culture of murine mast cells. II. Purification of a mast cell growth factor and its dissociation from TCGF. J Immunol 127:794–799

19. Alveolar Macrophages

Ph. Godard, M. Damon, Ph. Vago

This work was in part supported by the Fonds Spécial du Comité National de Lutte contre les Maladies Respiratoires.

Alveolar macrophages (AM) are the principal resident phagocytes in the human lung and play a major role in the local defense against environmental agents. The first event that occurs when foreign material enters the body is its uptake by phagocytes, generally by nonimmunological mechanisms (Ilya Metchnikoff, 1882). But we know now that this cell is involved in the development and expression of humoral and cell-mediated immune responses [22]; AM has been considered for a long time as an accessory cell; in fact it plays a central role by handling and presenting the antigen and by regulating the immune response; moreover AM is an important secretory cell involved in the production of a number of bioactive materials that regulate other cellular functions [29].

Some lines of evidence suggest that AM could play an important role in the pathophysiology of lung hypersensitivity diseases, such as bronchial asthma [8]. For example, AM can be specifically activated by an IgE-dependent mechanism [9, 28] in vitro as well as in vivo, to release a number of inflammatory mediators. Besides, the functional activity of AM appears to be impaired in cases of bronchial asthma, such as their suppressor activity in allergic asthmatics [1] or their ability to release some prostanoids in asthma with aspirin idiosyncrasy [8].

The bronchoalveolar lavage (BAL) method, which is well tolerated by asthmatic patients, allows us to obtain AM in great number and to study them in vitro. In this chapter we will summarize some knowledge concerning the AM from asthmatic patients; most of the studies have been made with allergic asthmatic patients.

19.1 Studies of AM In Vitro

BAL in asthmatic patients: Details about performing BAL have been given in many papers, and owing to the popularity of this method of obtaining the so-called bronchoalveolar cells, extensive literature is developing. Our own experience demonstrates that fiberoptic bronchoscopy with BAL can be safely performed (for research purposes) in patients with (mild) asthma. Differential cell counts of Wright's stained preparations after cytocentrifugation indicate that 80 to 95% of the cells from each lavage are macrophages. The cellular composition of BAL fluids in asthmatics has been reported in Chapter 26.

AM culture: Cells were sedimented from the BAL fluid by centrifugation at 250 g for 10 min at 25 °C and the cell pellet was resuspended in a medium (199 for example; Gibco Chemical Co, Glasgow, Scotland) with 100 U/ml penicillin and 50 µg/ml streptomycin. Cells (0.5 to 1.0×10^6) were plated in 35 mm diameter plastic petri dishes and allowed to adhere for 2 hours at 37 °C in a 5% CO_2 incubator. After elimination of nonadherent cells by extensive washing, AM were purified up to 95% (as assessed by morphology and specific staining) and could be studied from a morphological or functional point of view.

Morphology: Heterogeneity of AM is an important feature of these cells and appears on light and electron microscopic studies. After a 24-hours culture, two types of mononuclear cells could be distinguished morphologically by light microscope study. In normal subjects, the small cells (10 to 20 µm) accounted for 69% and the large cells (30 to 45 µm) for 31% of the mononuclear cells. In allergic asthmatic patients, there were 63 and 37%, and in aspirin-sensitive asthmatic patients, there were 43 and 57% respectively of small and large mononuclear cells [8].

Electron microscopy studies: For electron microscopy, 15 ml of recovered BAL fluid (at least 10 ml) were immediately fixed in cacodylate-buffered cold glutaraldehyde. 12–48 hours after, the sample was washed with cacodylate buffer, post-fixed in 1% osmium tetroxide for 60 min, dehydrated in a graded series of ethyl alcohol, and embedded in an Epon resin. Ultrathin sections (0.05–0.1 µm), prepared with a IKB Ultrotome II (Uppsala, Sweden) and stained with uranyl acetate and lead citrate, were examined with a Hitachi HU 11C electron microscope (Tokyo, Japan).

From a morphological point of view, AM heterogeneity had been confirmed; some of them appeared normal, the others were activated, with numerous pseudopodes. In asthmatic patients, all these cells could be observed in BAL fluids. The percentage of each type had to be checked carefully, in relation to asthma since some evidence of AM activation after specific challenge had been observed (Fig. 19.1).

AM viability: The AM viability must be assessed at all steps of the culture; this can be performed by morphological means (i.e., using the trypan blue exclusion test), or by biochemical means (i.e., analyzing the level of the cytoplasmic marker lactate dehydrogenase in the supernatants).

After a 24-hours culture the AM viability was significantly lower in cultures from asthmatic patients than in those from normal subjects; there was an inverse relationship between the AM viability and the number of eosinophils in the BAL fluid [8]; we suggest that this impaired viability could be due to an interaction between eosinophil and AM in the bronchoalveolar lumen. The cytotoxicity of this cell is indeed well-known. In a collaborative study with Dr G. J. Gleich, we have shown [unpublished data] that AM contain small quantities of immunoreactive major basic protein (MBP): from 200 to 1,000 ng/10^6 cells, in quantities correlated to the number of eosinophils in the BAL fluid. On the other hand, we know that 100 µg/ml MBP is able to induce a desquamation of the tracheal epithelium in a 19-hours culture in vitro, and that 10^{-6} M MBP is able to induce an enhancement of histamine release from mast cells.

It is important to know the cell-to-cell interrelations in the bronchoalveolar lumen in order to understand better the inflammatory cascade which occurs during asthma.

19.2 Alveolar Macrophages Membrane Receptors

The expression on AM of determinants encoded by the I region (Ia antigens) of the major histocompatibility complex is required for the presentation of antigen to T-cells in antigen-specific lymphoproliferation [11, 19]. Ia expression is sensitive to environmental regulation [18]. Ia expression in normal nonsmokers and normal cigarette smokers was characterized, using three concentrations of anti-Ia antibodies and immunofluorescence: Ia expression by smoker AM was less than that of nonsmoker AM at all antibody concentrations; Ia was variably reexpressed by smoker AM after 4 days of in vitro culture indicating that the mechanism for Ia expression was intact [E. C. Lawrence, oral communication].

We investigated the proportion of AM bearing HLA-DR antigens in allergic asthmatic patients; half of AM (52 to 61%) expressed HLA-DR antigens as detected by a monoclonal antibody BL-2 to monomorphic HLA-DR in both the asthmatic and the control groups [1].

Interleukin 1 (IL-1), first identified as a lymphocyte activating factor, can replace Ia+ cells and restore the proliferative response in cultures blocked by anti-Ia, but it must act in concert with the specific antigen [4, 10].

The AM from asthmatic patients have surface-bound IgE molecules in vivo and can be specifically triggered by contact with the sensitizing allergens. The presence of IgE-specific receptors on the macrophage surfaces has been demonstrated by Spiegelberg et al [24] and Joseph and colleagues [9] both at the ultrastructural level with im-

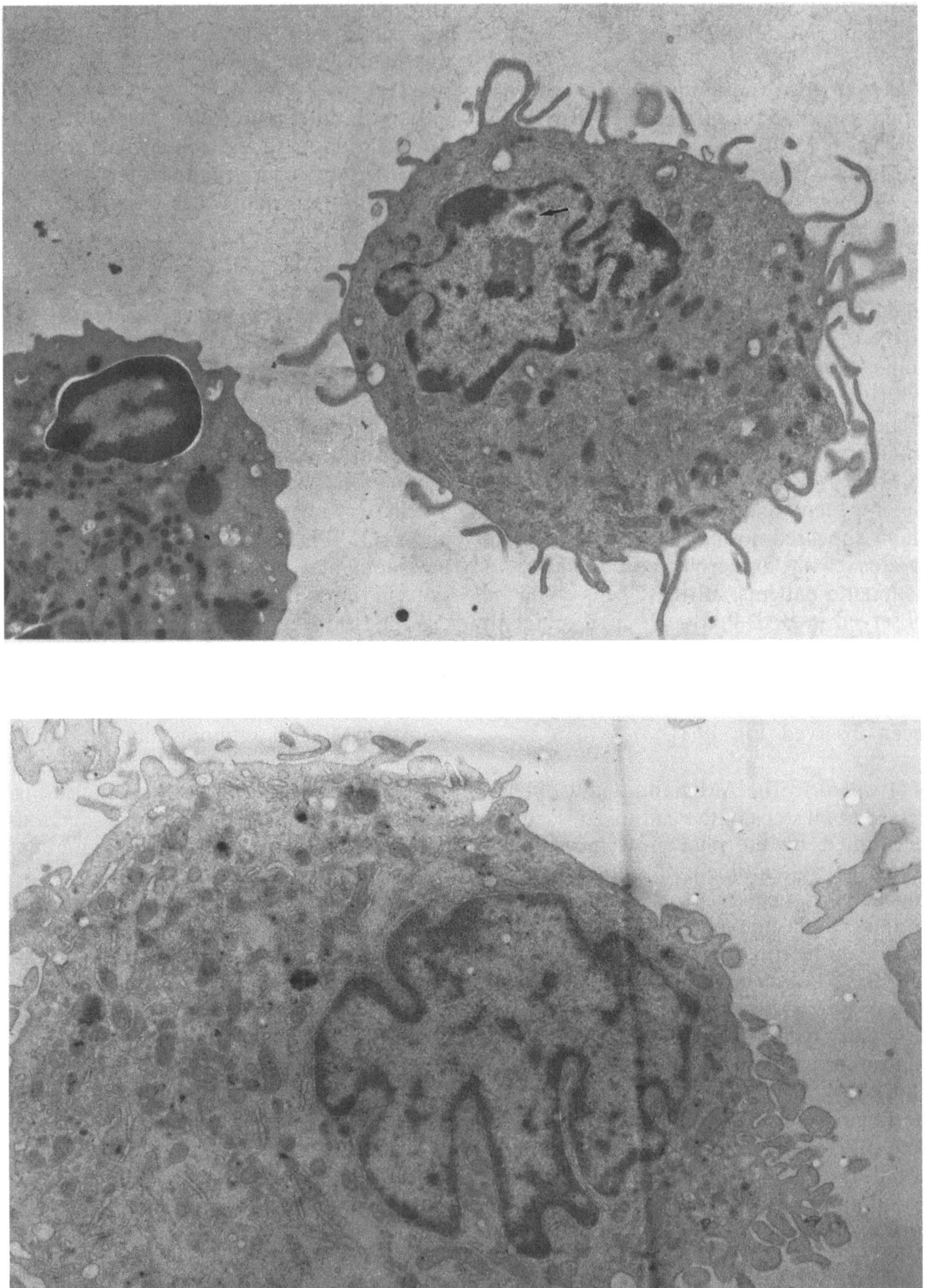

a

b

Fig. 19.1 a, b. Alveolar macrophage of an allergic asthmatic patient (man, 25 years old, without symptoms at the time of the first BAL, IgE = 250 UI/ml, specific IgE +). **a** Electron microscopic study – before specific challenge, AM appear normal. **b** Electron microscopic study – after specific challenge, the BAL has been performed 2 hours after the onset of the airway obstruction which was spontaneously reversible within 1 hour. AM appears with some evidence of activation

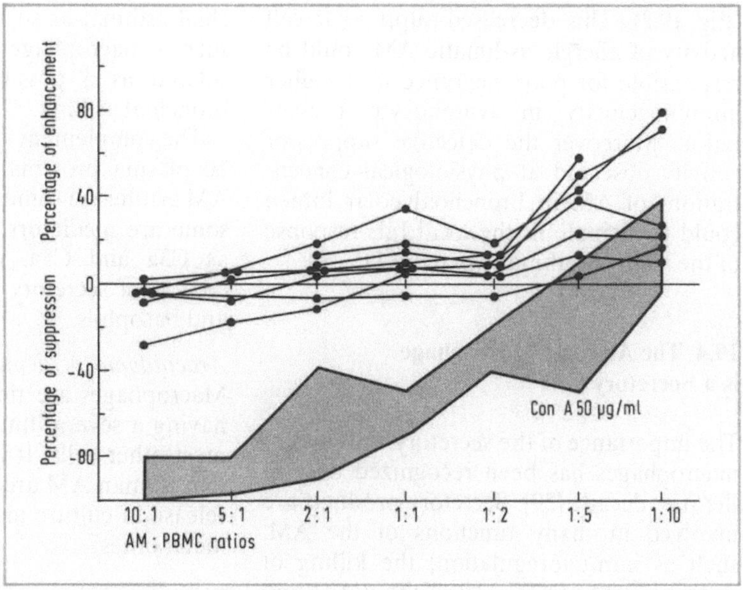

Fig. 19.2. Effect of asthmatic alveolar macrophages (AM) on autologous peripheral blood mononuclear cells (PBMC). PBMC from eight allergic asthmatic patients and twelve healthy subjects were cultured in the presence of con A (50 μg/ml) and various quantities of AM. The control group range is shown by the hatched area (mean ± SD): At high ratio, AM from normal subjects were able to suppress the lymphoproliferative responses of autologous PBMC to con A. For asthmatic patients (indicated by continuous lines), no significant variation was observed whatever the AM : PBMC ratios

munoperoxidase labeling, and at low magnification by the formation of 15–18% rosettes with human IgE-coated erythrocytes. The formation of such rosettes was inhibited after incubation of AM with aggregated myeloma IgE. In comparison with normal subjects, there was an increased number of IgE-Fc receptors and a higher density of bound IgE on AM from allergic asthmatics. Fc receptors for IgE ($Fc_{\varepsilon}R$) on mast cells and basophils have been extensively studied; the major reason why $Fc_{\varepsilon}R$ on AM were not recognized earlier is the much lower affinity with which monomeric IgE bind to these cells as compared to mast cells and basophilic granulocytes.

19.3 Involvement of AM in the Immune Response

Immunologically specific mechanisms of host defense are operative in the lung; while such specificity is ultimately provided by lymphocytes, interactions of lymphocytes with AM appear necessary for initiation, modulation and expression of pulmonary immune reactivity. Many functional properties of AM are well documented in the regulation of the immune response, such as antigen presentation [25], release of soluble factors [27] and modulation of lymphocyte activation [26].

Lymphocyte activation triggered by a variety of antigens and mitogens on the one hand results in local elaboration of lymphokines which activates AM, but also on the other hand requires the presence of mononuclear phagocytes. In man these cells play a role in supporting optimal B- and T-cell activation. In peripheral blood and in the lung, monocytes and AM respectively appear to be the major population subserving this function [5].

A well-known AM accessory cell function is the augmentation of mitogen-induced proliferation [15, 23]. In fact, this modulation is dependent on the ratio between AM and lymphocytes. When this ratio is high the AM have an inhibitory effect activity, whereas when the ratio is low an enhanced response of the lymphocyte proliferation induced by the mitogens is observed [14].

In the allergic asthmatic patients we studied, this suppressive activity at high ratio did not exist, whereas at low ratio a higher enhancing effect had been observed

(Fig. 19.2). This decreased suppressor cell activity of allergic asthmatic AM could be responsible for poor clearance to a higher immunogenicity in lymphocyte presentation. Moreover the defective suppressor activity observed at physiological concentrations of AM in bronchoalveolar lumen could participate in the local IgE response of the allergic asthmatic patients [1].

19.4 The Alveolar Macrophage is a Secretory Cell

The importance of the secretory activities of macrophages has been recognized only in the past decade [29]. Secretory products are involved in many functions of the AM, such as immunoregulation, the killing of microbes and tumors. All of these AM mediators are not secreted by a single AM simultaneously because cells display distinct secretion phenotypes under developmental and environmental regulators. AM heterogeneity could probably explain the wide range of results which are obtained with human AM.

AM enzymes: AM secrete a number of enzymes which participate in a wide range of functions. Some enzymes are constitutively secreted, some are secreted by inflammatory AM, others by activated AM.

In allergic asthmatic patients, the β-glucuronidase is released by AM as a consequence of a specific activation by the (specific) allergen; this has been demonstrated in vitro as well as in vivo by Tonnel and colleagues [28].

It is most likely that enzymes and enzyme inhibitors are involved in the pathophysiology of bronchial asthma but their significance is not known.

Proteins: AM secrete certain plasma proteins which participate in inflammation, tissue repair [2], immune regulation, and molecular transport.

An AM-derived mucus secretagogue has recently been described by Marom and colleagues, which caused cultured human airways to release increased amounts of radiolabeled mucus glycoproteins [16]. Hypersecretion of mucus accompanies bronchial asthma; as suggested by Kaliner [16], such a macrophage factor should be considered as a possible agent involved in bronchial asthma.

The complement system consists of about 20 plasma proteins. It is most likely that AM synthesize some of them. Among them, some are mediators of inflammation, such as C3a and C5a, which can induce secretion of secretory granules of mast cells and basophils.

Arachidonic acid metabolites [3, 6–8, 12]: Macrophages are rich in arachidonic acid, having a several times higher content than most other cells. It is now well established that human AM are able to synthesize and release in culture most of the arachidonate metabolites:

- by the cyclooxygenase pathway: PGE_2 – $PGF_{2\alpha}$ – and TxB_2 (Fig. 19.3) [8], and also PGI_2,
- by the lipoxygenase pathway: HETEs (mainly at the 5-position), LTB_4 and sulfidopeptide leukotrienes (LTC_4 + LTD_4, that is to say the SRS-A) (Fig. 19.4).

Arachidonate metabolites have potent bioactive activities [13]: characteristically slow contraction of the smooth muscle cells, inflammation with erythema, edema and pain (probably in concert with histamine and bradykinin), hypersecretion, chemotaxis of neutrophils and eosinophils [17].

Arachidonate metabolites are not truly secretory products, in the sense that they are not secreted by the fusion of secretory vesicles to plasma membranes, but they are released extracellularly after the triggering by phagocytosis, other chemical stimuli and also by an IgE-dependent mechanism according to experiments conducted by Rankin with LTC_4 [21].

Platelet activating factor: PAF is a unique class of lipid which derives from the membrane phospholipids. It aggregates platelets and induces the release of their vasoactive amines, induces an important bronchoconstriction and has some pro-inflammatory properties due to eosinophils which it is able to attract into the airways.

Reactive metabolites of oxygen: Inflammatory and activated AM are capable of a re-

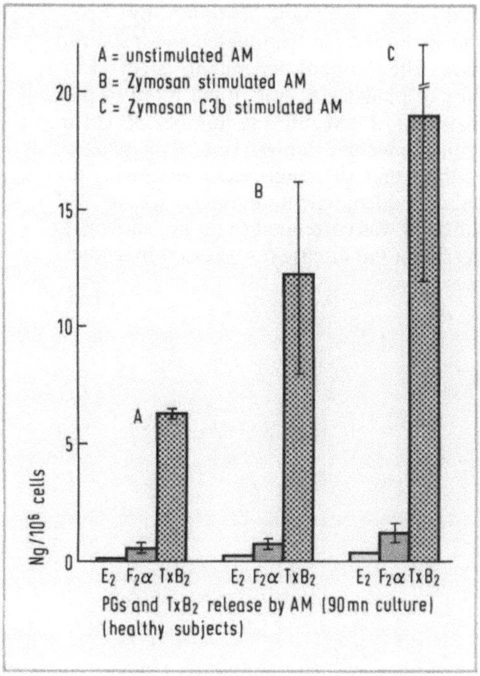

Fig. 19.3. PGE_2–$F_{2\alpha}$ and TxB_2 generation by AM

spiratory burst leading to the production of reactive metabolites of oxygen. These include superoxide anion ($O_2^{\cdot -}$), hydrogen peroxide (H_2O_2), hydroxyl radical ($OH^{\cdot}$) and singlet oxygen ($^1O_2$).

The metabolites of oxygen induce a denaturation of the proteins, a lipid peroxidation. Their metabolism is probably linked to that of arachidonic acid. They play an important role in some pathological conditions such as the pulmonary toxicity of oxygen, ozone and cigarette smoke.

In bronchial asthma (Fig. 19.5) some preliminary data suggest that they are involved in the pathophysiology of bronchial hyperreactivity and bronchial inflammation.

19.5 Conclusions

The alveolar macrophage is probably one of the most important cells in the pathophysiology of the human airways and lung. Studies in vitro, and some in vivo suggest

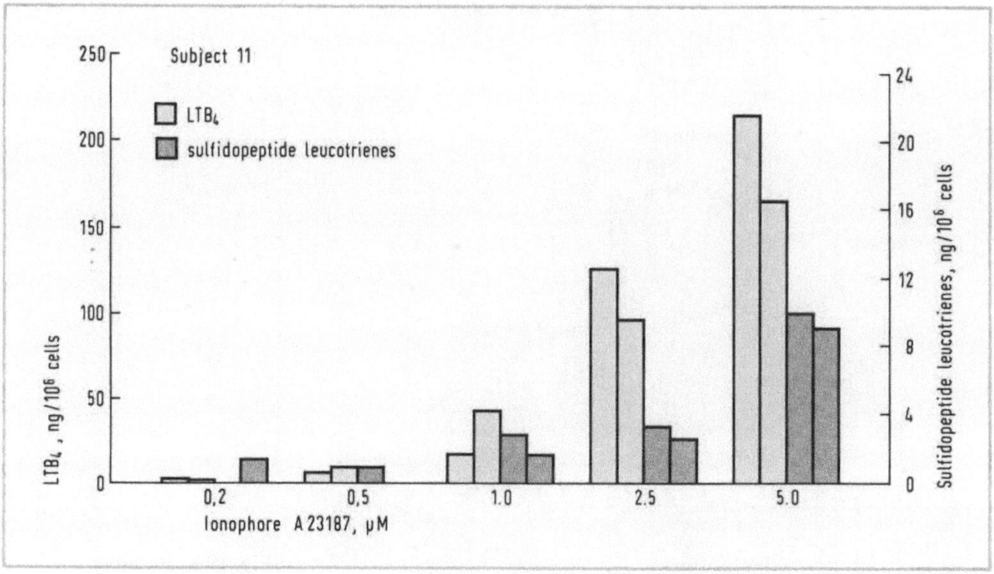

Fig. 19.4. LTB_4 and sulfidopeptide LTs generation by AM in an asthmatic patient. AM have been cultured for a 30 min period of time in the presence of calcium ionophore. LTs have been assessed in culture medium, using specific RIA (Prof. R. A. Lewis, Boston, USA)

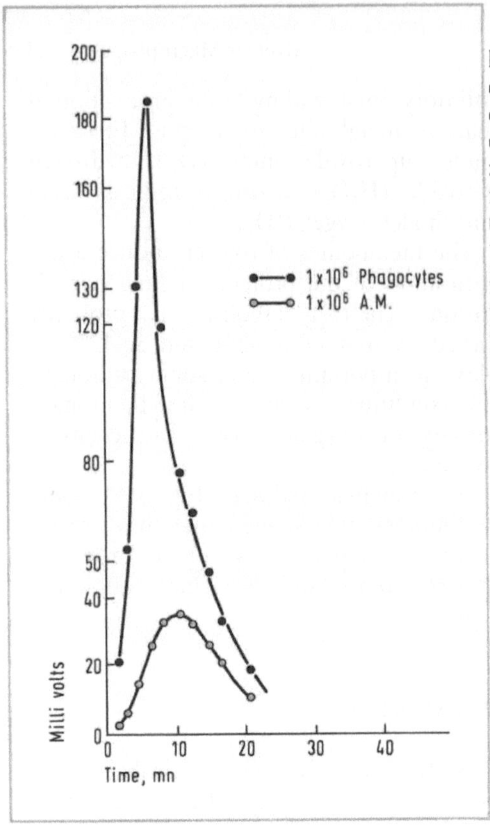

Fig. 19.5. Luminol-dependent chemoluminescence of AM and phagocytes. The cells were obtained from asthmatic patients by bronchoalveolar lavage and stimulated by opsonized zymosan. The luminol-dependent chemoluminescence of phagocytes was much more important than that of AM. But the number of AM in the bronchoalveolar lumen was always much higher than that of phagocytes. Moreover, the luminol-dependent chemoluminescence of AM in asthmatics was correlated (data not shown) to the severity of the disease (as assessed by clinical score)

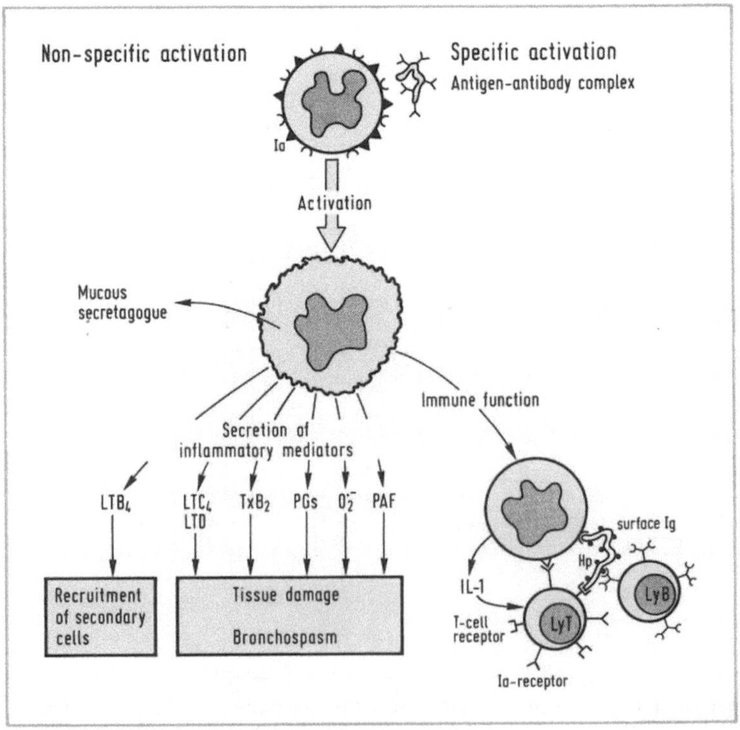

Fig. 19.6. Putative role of alveolar macrophages in the asthmatic reactions

that this cell is involved in all steps of the pathogenesis of bronchial asthma (Fig. 19.6):

- release of bronchospastic mediators,
- release of inflammatory mediators,
- activation by a lot of mechanisms, specific or not, and
- decreased suppressor activity suggesting a role in the immune response.

But if all these abnormalities suggest that AM could play a role in bronchial asthma, no demonstration has yet been made to show that it is the reality. In the near future we will have some liposomes to treat our patients; at that time and in this way we will be able to demonstrate that the AM really is an important cell.

Acknowledgements: We are indebted to: Prof. J. Clot (Montpellier, France), Prof. R. A. Lewis (Harvard Medical School, Boston) and Prof. G. J. Gleich (Mayo Clinic Foundation) for their helpful collaboration.

References

1. Aubas P, Cosso B, Godard P et al (1984) Decreased suppressor cell activity of alveolar macrophages in bronchial asthma. Am Rev Respir Dis 130:875–878
2. Bitterman PB, Rennard SI, Hunninghake GW, Crystal RG (1982) Human alveolar macrophage growth factor for fibroblasts. J Clin Invest 70:806–822
3. Damon M, Chavis C, Godard P et al (1983) Purification and mass spectrometry identification of leukotriene D4 synthetised by human alveolar macrophages. Biochem Biophys Res Commun 111:518–524
4. Durum SK, Gershon RK (1982) Interleukin 1 can replace the requirement for I-A positive cells in the proliferation of antigen-primed T cells. Proc Natl Acad Sci USA 79:4747–4750
5. Eibl MM, Mannhalter JW, Zlabinger G et al (1982) Defective macrophage function in a patient with common variable immunodeficiency. N Engl J Med 307:803–806
6. Fels OS, Pawlowski NA, Cramer EB et al (1982) Human alveolar macrophages produce leukotriene B4. Proc Natl Acad Sci USA 79:7866–7870
7. Godard P, Damon M, Michel FB et al (1983) Leukotriene B4 production from human alveolar macrophages. Clin Res 31:548 A
8. Godard P, Chaintreuil J, Damon M et al (1982) Functional assessment of alveolar macrophages: comparison of cells from asthmatics and normal subjects. J Allergy Clin Immunol 70:88–93
9. Joseph M, Tonnel AB, Torpier G, Capron A et al (1983) Involvement of immunoglobulin E in the secretory processes of alveolar macrophages from asthmatic patients. J Clin Invest 71:221–230
10. Koretsky GA, Elias JA, Kay SL et al (1983) Spontaneous production of interleukin-1 by human alveolar macrophages. Clin Immunol Immunopathol 29:443–450
11. Lattime C, Gillis S, Pecoraro G, Stutman O (1982) Ia-dependent interleukin 2 production in syngeneic cellular interactions. J Immunol 128:480–485
12. Laviolette M, Picard S, Braquet P, Borgeat P (1984) In vitro defective alveolar macrophages release of leukotriene B4 and 5-hydroxyeicosatetraenoic acid in smokers. Am Rev Respir Dis 129:A316
13. Lewis RA, Austen KF (1984) The biologically active leukotrienes. J Clin Invest 73: 889–897
14. Lilker RA (1982) Alveolar macrophages. Enhancers or suppressors of pulmonary immune reactivity? Chest 82:261
15. Liu MC, Proud D, Schleimer RP, Plaut M (1984) Human pulmonary macrophage enhance and inhibit lymphocyte proliferation. J Immunol 132:2895–2903
16. Marom Z, Shelhamer JH, Kaliner M (1984) Human pulmonary macrophage-derived mucus secretagogue. J Exp Med 159:844–860
17. Martin TR, Altman LC, Albert RK, Henderson WR (1984) Leukotriene B4 production by the human alveolar macrophage: a potential mechanism for amplifying inflammation in the lung. Am Rev Respir Dis 129:106–111
18. Mason R, Austin H, Brodsky F, Gordon S (1982) Monoclonal antimacrophage antibodies: human pulmonary macrophages express HLA-DR (Ia-like) antigens in culture. Am Rev Respir Dis 125:586–593
19. Moore L, Myrvik O (1977) The role of normal alveolar macrophages in cell-mediated immunity. J Reticuloendothel Soc 21:131–139
20. Pawlowski NA, Kaplan G, Hamill AL, Cohn ZA, Scott WA (1983) Arachidonic acid metabolism by human monocytes. J Exp Med 158:393–412
21. Rankin JA, Hitchcock M, Merril WW et al (1982) IgE-dependent release of leukotriene C4 from alveolar macrophage. Nature 297:329–331

22. Rosenberg SA, Lipski PE (1980) The role of monocyte factors in the differentiation of immunoglobulin secreting cells from human peripheral blood B cells. J Immunol 125:232–237
23. Schuyler MR, Todd LS (1981) Accessory cell function of rabbit alveolar macrophages. Am Rev Respir Dis 123:53–57
24. Spiegelberg HL, Boltz-Nitulescu G, Plummer JA, Melewicz FM (1983) Characterization of the IgE Fc receptors on monocytes and macrophages. Fed Proc 42:124–128
25. Stadecker MJ, Wyler DJ, Wright JA (1982) Ia antigen expression and antigen-presenting function by macrophages isolated from hypersensitivity granulomas. J Immunol 128:2739–2744
26. Thiele DL, Lipski PE (1982) The accessory function of phagocytic cells in human T cell and B cell responses. J Immunol 129:1033–1040
27. Takemura R, Werb Z (1984) Secretory products of macrophages and their physiological functions. Am J Physiol 246:C1–C9
28. Tonnel AB, Gosset P, Joseph M, Fournier E, Capron A (1983) Stimulation of alveolar macrophages in asthmatic patients after local provocation test. Lancet I:1406–1408
29. Unanue ER (1976) Secretory function of mononuclear phagocytes: a review. Am J Pathol 83:396–417

20. Neutrophils and the Asthmatic Response

A. B. Kay

20.1 Neutrophils in Allergic Tissue Reactions

The infiltration of neutrophils is an early event following tissue mast cell degranulation. The kinetics of inflammatory cell infiltration following allergic tissue reactions are similar in IgE-mediated reactions in human skin [1], as well as models of anaphylaxis in the skin and lung of guinea pigs [2]. The initial infiltration of neutrophils is rapid, i.e., within a few hours. This is followed by an accumulation of eosinophils which, in the case of passive cutaneous anaphylaxis in guinea pig skin, was maximal at 8 hours [2]. After this time macrophages become the predominant cell and persist at the site of the IgE-allergen interaction for several days.

Neutrophils have a number of characteristic properties. For instance, they bind the Ig (Fc) portion of IgG_1, IgG_2, IgG_3, IgG_4, IgA_1 and IgA_2 and possess complement (CR1 and CR3) receptors. Recent work indicates that there is also a recognition unit for serum transferrin (which is distinct from the conventional transferrin receptor) since plasma protein selectively promotes the firm adhesion of neutrophils to a wide range of pollen grains [3]. Although it is uncertain at the present time as to the precise nature of this specific transferrin recognition unit, it has been established that the reaction is time-, temperature- and concentration-dependent and involves magnesium, but not calcium ions. This phenomenon may have relevance to the way in which certain organic particles are cleared from the lung and nasal passages.

There are two major types of granule, the azurophil (or primary) granule, and the specific (or secondary) granule. Both granule types contain a wide range of pro-inflammatory enzymes. These include myeloperoxidase, acid hydrolases, neutral proteases, lysozyme and cationic proteins from the primary granules and lactoferrin, lysozyme and the vitamin B_{12}-binding protein from the secondary granules.

20.2 Mast Cell-associated Neutrophil Chemotactic Factors

Mast cells elaborate a number of chemical mediators and these are conventionally divided into those that are preformed in granules and those that are newly generated from the plasma membrane as the result of either immunologic or nonimmunologic stimuli (Fig. 20.1). Many of these agents are chemotactic for the neutrophil. The most potent appear to be PAF-acether, leukotriene B_4 and a high molecular weight neutrophil chemotactic factor (or activity) termed NCF or NCA. NCA is of particular interest because it can be readily identified both in the serum of asthmatic individuals and in patients with physical urticarias who have undergone an appropriate challenge procedure [4]. The factor is heat-stable and has a high molecular weight (600,000 to 700,000 daltons). It appears to be related to mast cell activation since NCA was released together with histamine and was inhibited by prior administration of disodium cromoglycate (DSCG) [5]. NCA is also released after exercise-induced asthma (EIA) [6] and this has led to speculation that mast cells are also involved in EIA and that the stimulus for mediator release is either respiratory heat exchange or hyperosmolarity resulting from loss of water [7]. It has also been shown that NCA is released in antigen-induced and exercise-induced early and late phase asthmatic responses [8, 9]. The identification of NCA in late reactions indicates that mast cells might undergo a second degranulation possibly as a result of histamine releasing agents derived from in-

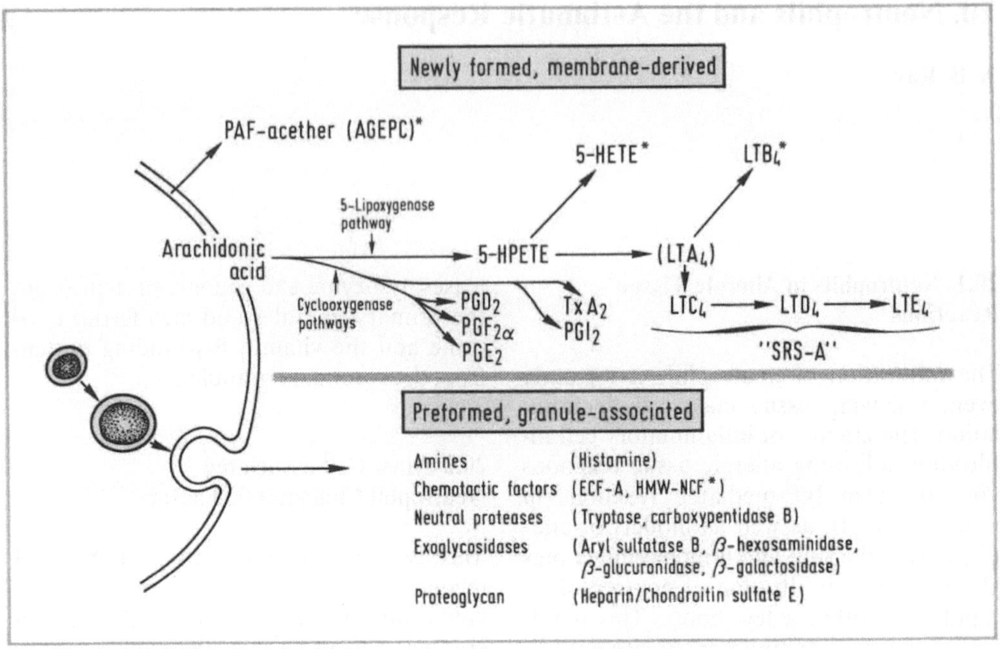

Fig. 20.1. Mast cell-associated mediators of hypersensitivity. The principal neutrophil chemotactic factors, i.e. PAF-acether, LTB_4, HMW-NCF and 5-HETE are indicated

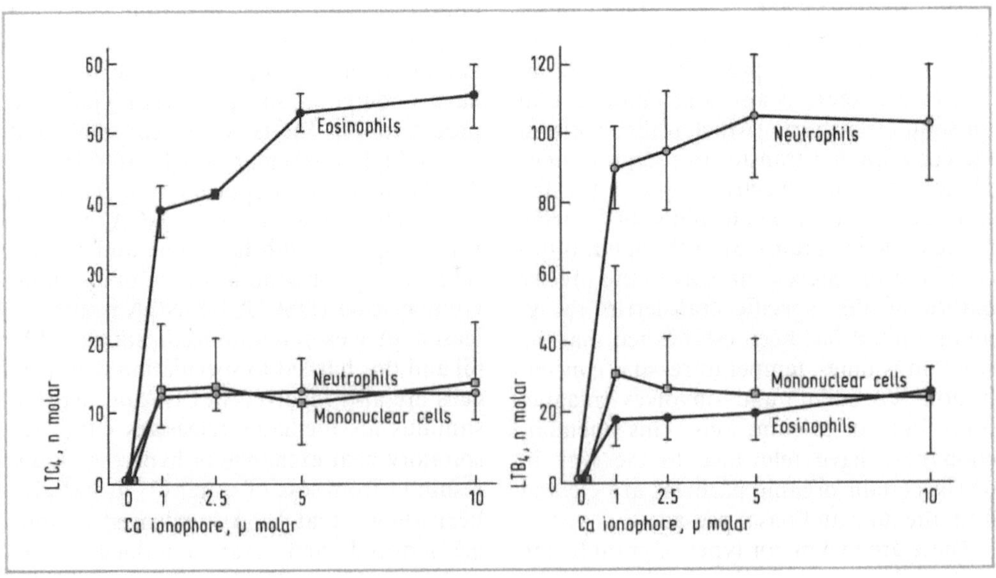

Fig. 20.2. Preferential generation of LTB_4 by neutrophils and LTC_4 by eosinophils from human leukocytes separated on metrizamide gradients and stimulated by the calcium ionophore. (Reproduced by permission of Clinical and Experimental Immunology)

flammatory cells. Both atopic and nonatopic asthmatics with EIA release NCA into the circulation indicating that in these situations mast cell degranulation can proceed independently of IgE [10]. Heat-stable neutrophil chemotactic activity was also identified after challenge of isolated human lung fragments with anti-IgE [11]. The major NCA released following this procedure had similar physicochemical properties to the NCA detected in the circulation of asthmatic subjects after bronchial challenge with specific antigen, i.e., a molecular size of approximately 600,000 daltons (as estimated by Sephacryl S300 gel filtration chromatography), elution from DEAE-Sephacel (pH 7.8) between 0.1 and 0.2 molar NaCl, and an isoelectric point of between 6.5 and 6.8 as determined by chromatofocusing on polybuffer exchanger 94.

20.3 Neutrophils and Leukotrienes

Leukotriene (LT) B_4 is chemotactic for neutrophils and eosinophils. Interestingly, neutrophils themselves also preferentially generate LTB_4 as their principal 5-lipoxygenase product after stimulation with the calcium ionophore. Eosinophils, on the other hand, produce predominantly LTC_4 [12]. For instance, the leukocyte generating capacities of ionophore-stimulated human eosinophils and neutrophils were compared using specific radioimmunoassays for LTC_4 and LTB_4. Mixed granulocyte preparations (neutrophils and eosinophils) produced both LTB_4 and LTC_4 in a time-dependent fashion which was maximal at 10 and 15 min respectively. After the separation of eosinophils and neutrophils by metrizamide gradients, LTC_4 production was predominantly from eosinophils whereas neutrophils were the principal source of LTB_4 (Fig. 20.2). These findings were confirmed by reverse phase high performance liquid chromatography (HPLC) and gas chromatography-mass spectrometry (GC-MS).

20.4 Neutrophils and Asthma

There is now evidence that neutrophils are recruited and activated in clinical models of bronchial asthma indicating that mast cell mediators might have both a direct action on bronchial tissue as well as indirect effects as a result of recruitment and activation of inflammatory cells. We have been able to support these ideas by studying changes in the expression of neutrophil complement receptors (as a marker of activation) in asthma after allergen challenge [13]. Asthmatics who had a fall in the forced expiratory volume in one second (FEV_1) after the inhalation of histamine served as controls. Allergen-induced bronchoconstriction was followed by a rise in NCA which in turn was associated with neutrophil activation as shown by an increase in the percentage of neutrophil complement rosettes. These changes were not observed with histamine-induced bronchospasm. This suggests that allergen-induced asthmatic reactions are accompanied by activation of leukocytes and that these alterations appear to be associated with the release of mast cell-associated mediators rather than the effect of bronchoconstriction, per se. Similar findings have been observed in EIA, supporting the view that mast cell activation occurs in this situation either as a result of thermal changes or alterations in osmolarity [7, 14]. In these experiments we were able to inhibit neutrophil activation and the elevations in NCA by prior administration of DSCG [14] (Figs. 20.3, 20.4). Neutrophil (and monocyte) activation has also been observed during allergen-induced late phase asthmatic reactions [15].

A scheme is proposed of how these mediators and cells might interact in asthma (Fig. 20.5). It is known that mast cells generate LTB_4 and NCA and these in turn activate neutrophils. Neutrophils have been shown to preferentially generate LTB_4 which in turn activates eosinophils in directional locomotion. LTC_4 is produced predominantly by eosinophils (although the physiologic stimulus is yet to be defined). Two of the cardinal features of asthma, that is bronchial smooth muscle constriction and increased mucus production, can be explained on the basis of the recognized actions of LTC_4. Furthermore, LTC_4 is also produced directly from mast cells as well as LTB_4 and eosinophil chemotactic factor of

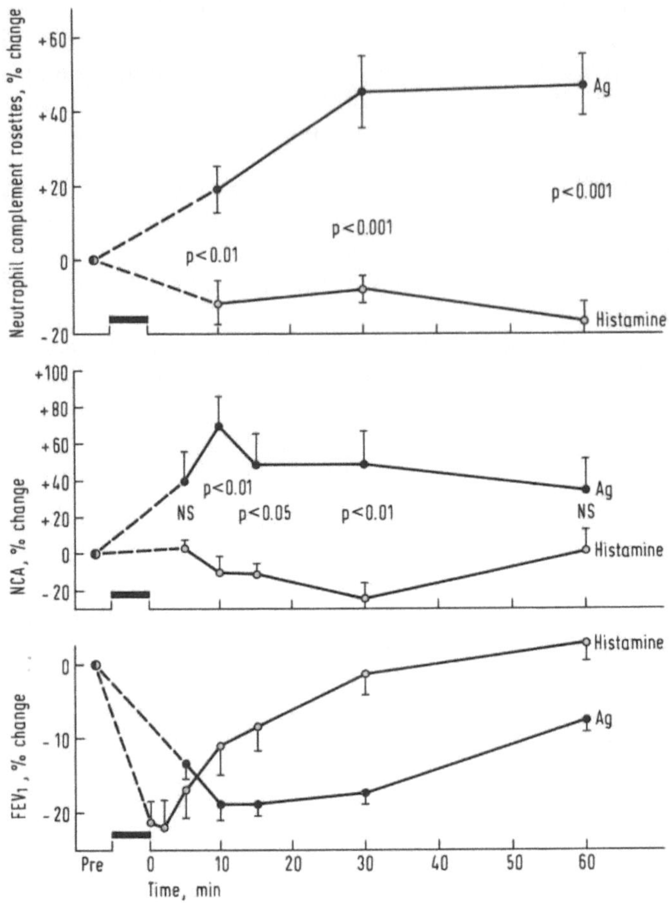

Fig. 20.3. Changes in neutrophil C3b rosettes (CR) and neutrophil chemotactic activity (NCA) compared with changes in FEV_1 after allergen (Ag) and histamine challenge. The solid bars represent the period of inhalational challenge. The data were analyzed by the Student's unpaired t test

anaphylaxis (ECF-A) which in turn stimulate eosinophils directly. Thus, neutrophils can be regarded as early pro-inflammatory cells in the asthmatic response but they in turn interact with other leukocytes to produce a cascade of mediators and other chemical agents which contribute in a critical fashion to the pathogenesis of the disease.

20.5 Conclusions

Infiltration of neutrophils is an early event following tissue mast cell degranulation and the more potent mast cell-associated chemotactic factors include NCA, LTB_4 and PAF-acether. Neutrophils are activated *in vitro* by several chemotactic factors including NCA. *In vivo* neutrophil activation is demonstrable after allergen-induced asthma and this was preceded by elevations in serum NCA. After ionophore stimulation, neutrophils preferentially generate LTB_4 whereas eosinophils produce LTC_4. These studies indicate that neutrophils probably contribute to allergic tissue reactions both by the secretion of their potent inflammatory enzymes and also by the recruitment of additional inflammatory cells.

Fig. 20.4. Changes in monocyte C3b rosettes (CR) and neutrophil chemotactic activity (NCA) compared with changes in FEV_1 after allergen (Ag) and histamine challenge. The solid bars represent the period of inhalational challenge. The data were analyzed by the Student's unpaired t test

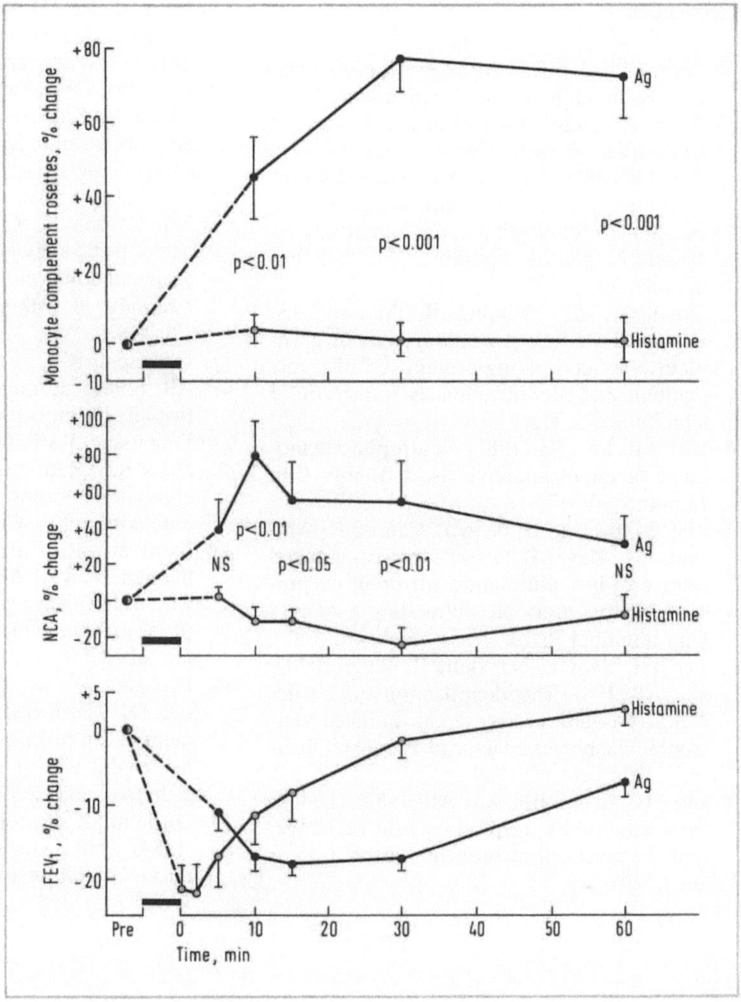

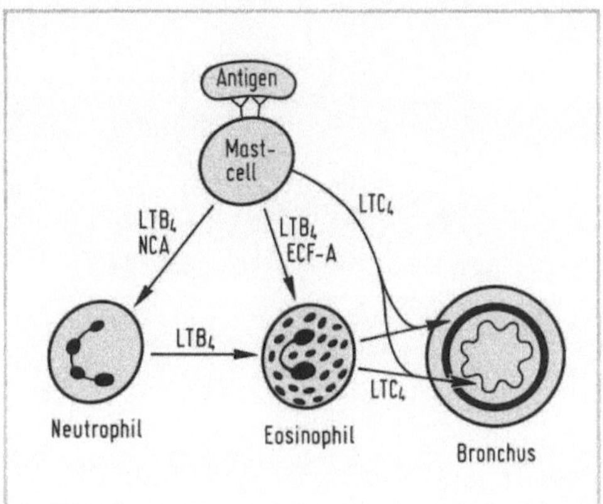

Fig. 20.5. A diagrammatic representation of some interactions between mast cells, neutrophils and eosinophils in bronchial asthma

References

1. Turnbull LW, Evans DP, Kay AB (1977) Human eosinophils, acidic tetrapeptides (ECF-A) and histamine. Interactions *in vitro* and *in vivo*. Immunology 32:57
2. Kay AB (1970) Studies on eosinophil leucocyte migration. I. Eosinophil and neutrophil accumulation following antigen-antibody reactions in guinea pig skin. Clin Exp Immunol 6:75
3. Sass-Kuhn SP, Moqbel R, Mackay JA, Cromwell O, Kay AB (1984) Human granulocyte pollen binding protein (GPBP); recognition and identification as transferrin. J Clin Invest 73:202
4. Kay AB, Lee TH (1982) Neutrophil chemotactic factor of anaphylaxis. J Allergy Clin Immunol 70:317
5. Lee TH, Brown MJ, Nagy L, Causon R, Walport JM, Kay AB (1982) Exercise-induced release of histamine and neutrophil chemotactic factors in atopic asthmatics. J Allergy Clin Immunol 70:73
6. Lee TH, Nagy L, Nagakura T, Walport MJ, Kay AB (1982) The identification and partial characterisation of an exercise-induced neutrophil chemotactic factor in bronchial asthma. J Clin Invest 69:889
7. Lee TH, Assoufi BK, Kay AB (1983) The link between exercise, respiratory heat exchange, and the mast cell in bronchial asthma. Lancet 1:520
8. Nagy L, Lee TH, Kay AB (1982) Neutrophil chemotactic activity in antigen-induced late asthmatic reactions. N Engl J Med 306:497
9. Lee TH, Nagakura T, Papageorgiou N, Iikura Y, Kay AB (1983) Exercise-induced late asthmatic reactions with neutrophil chemotactic activity. N Engl J Med 308:1502
10. Lee TH, Nagakura T, Cromwell O, Brown MJ, Causon R, Kay AB (1984) Neutrophil chemotactic activity (NCA) and histamine in atopic and non-atopic individuals after exercise-induced asthma. Am Rev Respir Dis 129:409
11. O'Driscoll BRC, Lee TH, Cromwell O, Kay AB (1983) Immunologic release of neutrophil chemotactic activity from human lung tissue. J Allergy Clin Immunol 72:695
12. Shaw RJ, Cromwell O, Kay AB (1984) Preferential generation of leukotriene C_4 by human eosinophils. Clin Exp Immunol 56:716
13. Durham SR, Carroll M, Walsh G, Boghossian S, Kay AB (1984) Leucocyte activation during antigen-induced early and late phase asthmatic reactions. J Allergy Clin Immunol 73:146–152 (abstract)
14. Papageorgiou N, Carroll M, Durham SR, Lee TH, Walsh GM, Kay AB (1983) Complement receptor enhancement as evidence of neutrophil activation after exercise-induced asthma. Lancet 2:1220
15. Durham SR, Carroll M, Walsh GM, Kay AB (1984) Leucocyte activation in allergen-induced late-phase asthmatic reactions. N Engl J Med 311:1398

21. Eosinophils in Bronchial Asthma

E. Frigas, G. J. Gleich

Supported by grants from the National Institute of Health, AI 09728, AI 15231, AI 11483 and from the Mayo Foundation.

During the past decade, the role of the eosinophil in the pathogenesis of bronchial asthma has been intensely investigated and a considerable number of new findings have provided fresh insights into the function of the eosinophil in asthma. To bring this field into perspective, we will

- summarize our current views of the pathology of asthma,
- review the new findings linking the eosinophil with the pathogenesis of asthma, and
- discuss the implications that the eosinophil is an effector cell for organ dysfunction in asthma.

21.1 The Pathology of Bronchial Asthma

A major contribution to our knowledge of the pathology of asthma has been derived from autopsy studies of patients who died in status asthmaticus [7, 15, 16, 29, 34, 35]. Additional information has been obtained from studies of sputum, endobronchial aspirates, and biopsy specimens from asthmatic patients [6, 10, 28]. These studies have delineated the pathology of asthma and have highlighted the shedding of epithelial cells from the bronchi of asthmatic patients, either singly or in clumps [6, 7, 10, 15, 16, 28, 29, 34, 35, 47], leading to denudation of the respiratory epithelium. In addition, abnormal cilia and cytoplasmic blebs [10], microscopic plugs and casts (like the Curschmann's spirals) [9], eosinophils and eosinophil by-products (like the Charcot-Leyden crystal protein) [43] have been described. Below the basement membrane which is per se intact, there is a 5–10 μm thick hyaline-like layer composed of collagen and immunoglobulin deposits [5, 7, 10, 24, 34, 45]. The lamina propria is edematous with marked increase of the collagen fibrils which appear separated and in disarray [10, 45]. Within the bronchial wall, the glands and peribronchial muscle appear hypertrophic, the goblet cells are hyperplastic, and the capillaries are dilated [7, 16, 34, 35]. Finally, there is a striking inflammatory infiltrate which penetrates the entire thickness of the bronchial wall and the nearby pulmonary parenchyma. In this inflammatory infiltrate, which overflows into the bronchial lumen, eosinophils predominate [6, 7, 10, 15, 16, 28, 29, 34, 35]. Neutrophils have been noted only when there is a coexisting bacterial infection [7, 16, 34, 35]; and lymphocytes, plasma cells, and mast cells are found incidentally and rarely [10].

21.2 The Effect of Eosinophil Granule Major Basic Protein (MBP) on the Bronchial Epithelium

Studies of eosinophil granules have revealed the presence of several cationic proteins [27]. One of these, the MBP, is an arginine-rich, strongly basic protein, with a molecular weight of about 11,000 in the guinea pig and 9,300 in humans. It has two reactive sulfhydryl groups per molecule, and these readily oxidize to yield disulfide-linked polymers. MBP accounts for greater than 50% of the granule protein in the guinea pig, and the crystalline core of the secondary eosinophil granule is composed entirely of MBP [42] (Fig. 21.1).

The ability of the eosinophil to damage tumor cells in vitro [52] and of the MBP to directly injure parasites in vitro [4] raised the possibility that MBP may also damage other cells. To study the potential role of eosinophil in asthma, we tested the effect of MBP on a number of cells in vitro [25]. When bronchial epithelial, intestinal, splenic, endothelial, and cutaneous cells

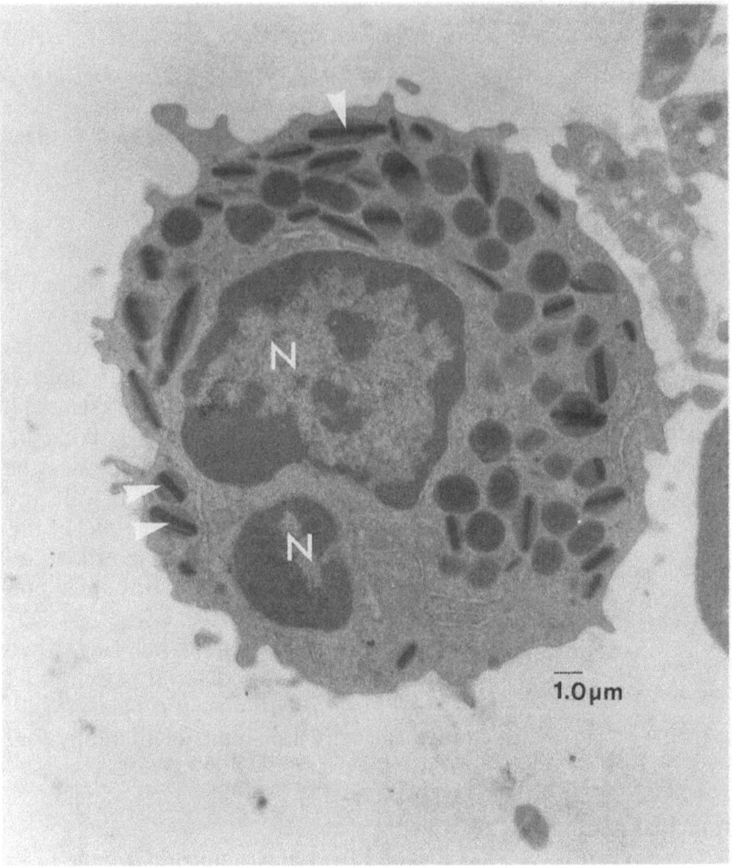

Fig. 21.1. Transmission electron photomicrograph of a mature eosinophil leukocyte, with its characteristic secondary or specific granules (arrowheads) made of dense quadrangular crystalloid cores embedded in a less dense matrix. The crystalloid cores are made entirely by MBP. N = nucleus. (Original magnification ×2,500)

were exposed to guinea pig-derived MBP in vitro, all cell types were damaged in a dose-related manner [25]. Subsequently, we studied the changes produced by the MBP on guinea pig respiratory epithelium in vitro [22]. MBP concentrations as low as 10 μg/ml produced ciliostasis at 48 hours, while 100 μg/ml caused the slowing of ciliary beating within 3 hours and cessation of ciliary motion within 23 hours. Examination by microscopy of this tissue showed varying degrees of epithelial damage, which were directly related to the dose and the length of exposure to MBP. With the lowest concentration of MBP tested (10 μg/ml), the epithelium was disrupted, and damaged cells were free in the lumen. With MBP levels of 50 μg/ml and 100 μg/ml the epithelium was extensively damaged, showing detachment of ciliated and brush cells and destruction of individual cells leaving behind only basal cells; with higher MBP levels, the entire mucosal layer was sloughed off down to the level of the lamina propria. The exfoliated cells were severely damaged with lysis of the cellular membrane, the cilia were stripped from cells, and characteristic cytoplasmic blebs on the shaft of the cilia were seen [22]. A test of the effect of human MBP on human bronchial tissue cultures showed that human MBP produced damage in a dose-related manner, and the damage consisted of desquamation and frank destruction of the bronchial epithelium [23] (Fig. 21.2). Both guinea pig and human MBP were able to damage respiratory epithelium of both species. These experiments established that MBP is destructive to the bronchial epithelium and that the changes produced in vitro by the MBP mimicked those seen in bronchial asthma.

21.2.1 Levels of MBP in Sputum of Patients With Bronchial Asthma

We next tested whether MBP was detectable in human sputum [23], using the radioimmunoassay (RIA) for human eosinophil MBP established by Wassom et al [61]. Fig. 21.3 shows the sputum MBP levels in 204 patients with various respiratory diseases [14, 21]. These sputa were consecutive samples sent to the laboratory for microbiological analyses. Among the patients without measurable MBP (Group A) and those with concentrations of sputum MBP below 0.1 μg/ml (Group B), only two were diagnosed by their physicians as having asthma. Among the patients with concentrations of sputum MBP greater than 0.1 μg/ml (Group C), 28 of 40 patients were diagnosed as having asthma. Of the remaining 12 patients, 7 carried the diagnosis of bronchopneumonia, 2 cardiac insufficiency, 2 cancer, and 1 epileptic coma. 8 of these 12 patients had previous diagnoses of chronic obstructive lung disease (COPD) in their histories. The geometric mean of the MBP concentrations for the asthmatic patients differed significantly from the patients without a diagnosis of asthma ($p < 0.001$) by the Mann-Whitney rank sum test. These results indicated that an elevated concentration of sputum MBP is a good marker for asthma [14, 23].

The finding that an elevated sputum MBP level was associated with asthma led us to determine the sputum MBP levels in patients hospitalized with asthma. We studied 25 consecutive patients with asthma admitted for treatment of acute exacerbation of their asthma [14, 23]. Fig. 21.4 shows their highest concentrations of sputum MBP on the right; for comparison, the sputum MBP levels of the patients with asthma shown in Fig. 21.3 are shown again to the left in Fig. 21.4. The hospitalized asthmatic patient group had significantly ($p < 0.001$) elevated concentrations of sputum MBP when compared with the outpatient asthmatic patient group (to the left of Fig. 21.4), suggesting that during an acute attack of asthma the sputum MBP concentration increases [14, 23]. Also, in 7 of the 25 hospitalized asthmatics, their MBP levels in sputum were greater than 10 μg/ml (1.1×10^6 M), the lowest level found toxic in vitro to respiratory epithelium [22]. Following treatment of asthma in each of the hospitalized asthmatic patients, the sputum concentration of MBP decreased significantly ($p < 0.005$, t test) from admission to dismissal [14, 23].

21.2.2 Localization of MBP in Lung Tissues of Patients with Bronchial Asthma

We next tested whether MBP was present at the site of damage to the epithelium in patients dying of asthma. To do this, we developed an immunofluorescence technique for analysis of formalin-fixed, paraffin-embedded tissue [19], and we studied lung tissues from patients with asthma and from control patients deceased from other causes [20]. Lung tissue specimens from 22 autopsy cases at the Mayo Clinic between 1967 and 1979 were studied. Examination of sections stained with hematoxylin and eosin (H & E) showed that all patients with asthma had a thickened basement membrane zone, goblet cell hyperplasia, and peribronchial inflammatory infiltrates with eosinophils in the lamina propria. Examination of the same sections by immunofluorescence showed MBP staining which was cell-associated as well as extracellular. Some eosinophils were intact, others partially intact, others partially degranulated surrounded by their extruded granules, and others totally disrupted and unrecognizable by the usual H & E stain. Patients with death not due to asthma showed neither epithelial damage nor extracellular MBP immunofluorescence, while intracellular MBP was noted on occasion. Figs. 21.5 and 21.6 show examples of certain patterns of MBP immunofluorescence seen in asthmatic patients. Fig. 21.5 shows diffuse staining of a mucus plug with streaks and whirls of brilliant glowing. In addition, the epithelial surface of this bronchiole is stained in a patchy, scalloped manner. Fig. 21.6b shows diffuse extracellular MBP immunofluorescence in the lamina propria. This area of intense glowing corresponds to the presence of necrotic, amorphous, eosinophilic material on the H & E-stained section (Fig. 21.6a).

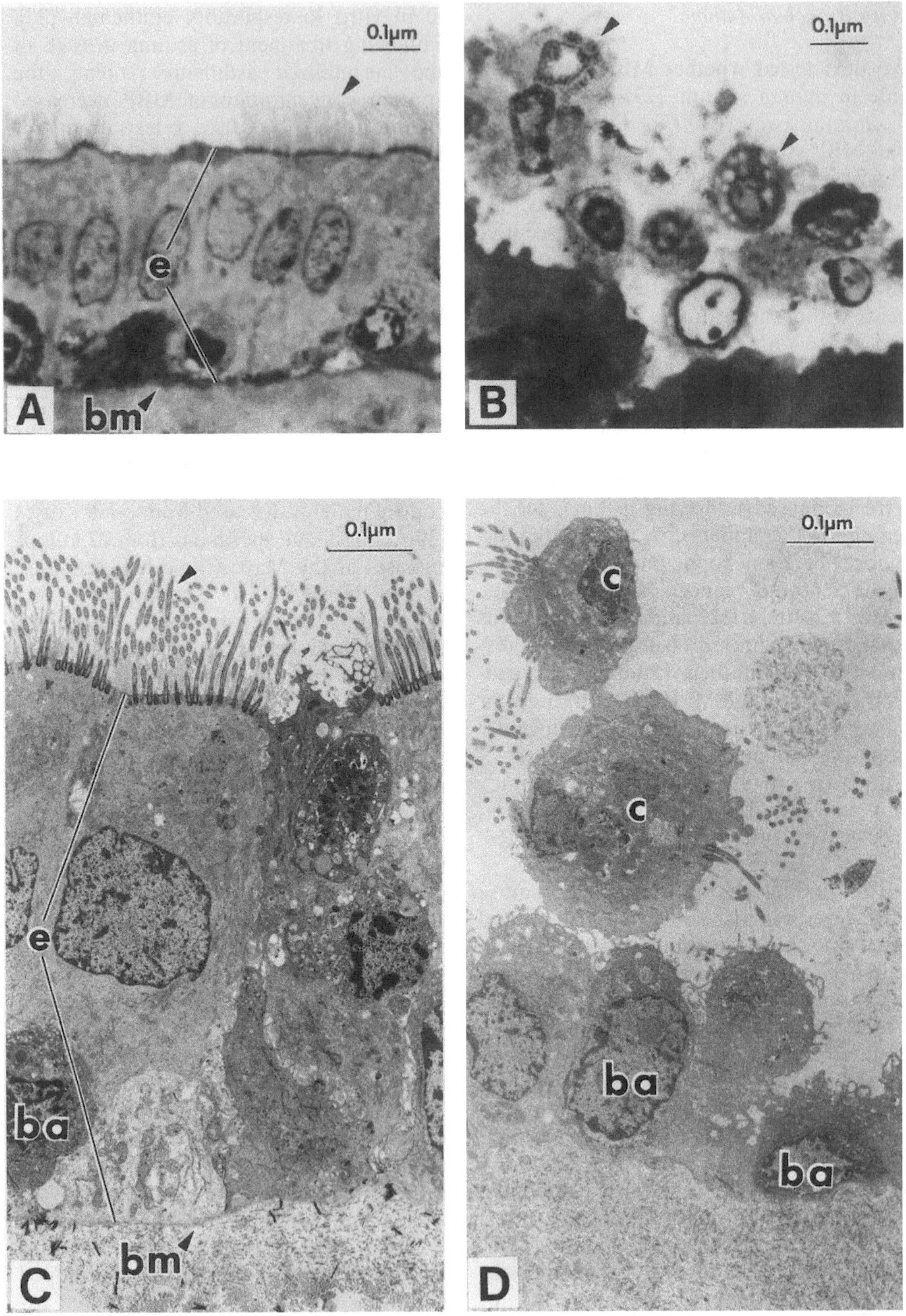
0.1μm
e
A
bm
0.1μm
B
0.1μm
e
ba
bm
C
0.1μm
c
c
ba
ba
D

◀ **Fig. 21.2A–D.** Effect of human MBP on human bronchial epithelium. **A** and **B** Observations of fixed tissue, stained with hematoxylin and eosin, by light microscopy. **A** Control human bronchial ring after 68 hours in culture; note cilia (arrowhead) of surface epithelium (e) and its basement membrane (bm) (× 1,000). **B** Treatment with 100 μg/ml of human MBP for 19 hours. Surface epithelium has been detached from lamina propria. Damaged epithelial cells are seen free in lumen (arrowheads) (× 1,000). **C** and **D** Transmission electron photomicrographs. **C** Control specimen. Note surface epithelium (e) and its basement membrane (bm). Note cilia on the luminal surface (arrowhead); ba = basal cell (× 1,500). **D** Treatment with 100 μg/ml of human MBP for 19 hours. Note disruption of epithelial layer and damage to ciliated cells (c) and basal cells (ba) (× 1,500). [From 22]

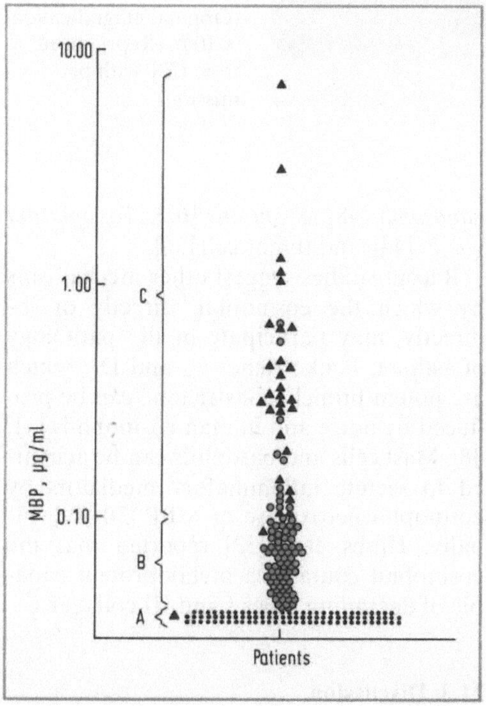

Fig. 21.3. Sputum MBP levels in 204 patients with various respiratory diseases including asthma. Each symbol represents one patient. The ordinate shows the concentration of MBP in sputum in μg/ml. The triangles identify the 30 patients diagnosed as having asthma. The green circles identify the patients with measurable MBP but without asthma. The black circles identify the patients without measurable MBP and without asthma. These latter sputa were assigned the lowest detectable MBP level. The symbols bracketed by A at the bottom of the figure had levels of MBP below the limit of sensitivity of the RIA. The symbols bracketed by B had sputum MBP concentrations below 0.1 μg/ml. The symbols bracketed by C had sputum MBP concentrations between 0.1 μg/ml and 10.0 μg/ml [21].

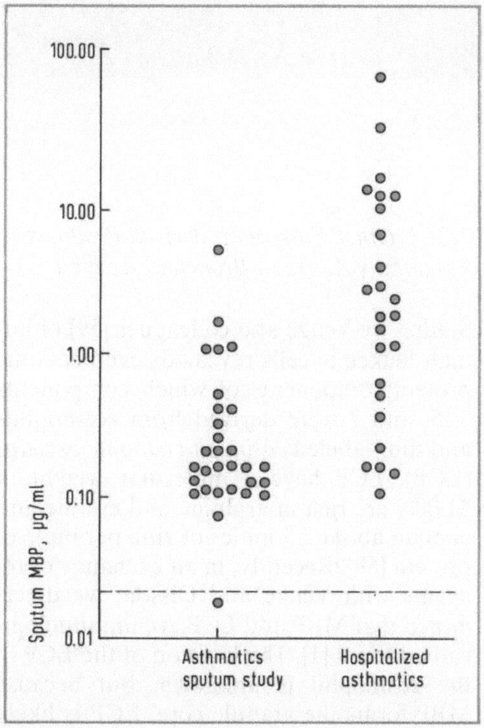

Fig. 21.4. Sputum MBP levels from the 30 patients with asthma (see Fig. 21.3) on the left and from 25 hospitalized patients with an acute flare of asthma on the right. The ordinate shows the sputum concentration of MBP in μg/ml. The dashed line at the bottom of the figure designates the limit of sensitivity of the RIA for sputum MBP

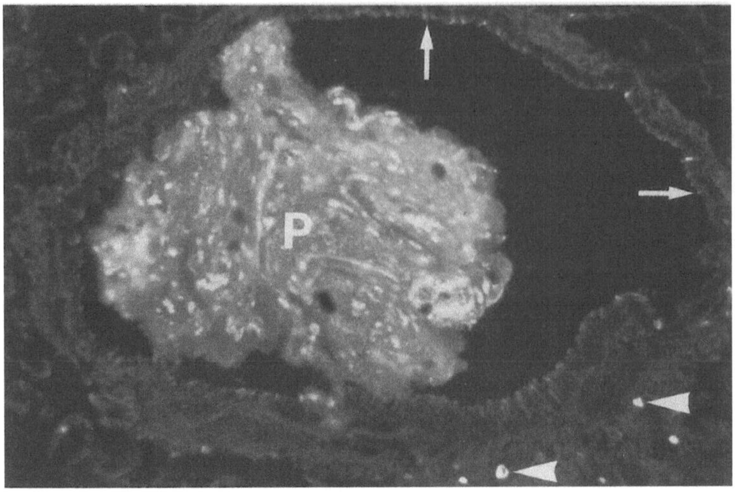

Fig. 21.5. Section of a bronchiole with mucus plug (P) from a patient with asthma, stained with anti-MBP. Note the diffuse staining of the plug (P) with brilliant swirls as well as the patchy, scalloped, less intense glowing of the luminal surface of the respiratory epithelium (arrows). There are also discrete eosinophils in the peribronchiolar area (arrowheads). (Original magnification ×100). (Reproduced from [20], with permission)

21.2.3 Other Eosinophil-derived Products Potentially Active in Bronchial Asthma

Studies by Venge and colleagues [59] of human leukemic cells revealed seven cationic protein components of which components 5, 6, and 7 were derived from eosinophils and thus labeled *eosinophil cationic proteins* (ECP). ECP have a molecular weight of 21,000, are rich in arginine and cystine and contain about 2.5 moles of zinc per mole of protein [59]. Recently, in an exchange of reagents with Venge and Olsson, we determined that MBP and ECP are immunologically distinct [1]. The location of the ECP in the eosinophil is unknown, but because MBP forms the granule core, ECP is likely in the matrix. ECP kills *schistosomules* [46], and in comparative experiments it is tenfold more potent than MBP. ECP and MBP neutralize heparin [59]. ECP also accelerates the normal plasma recalcification time by interaction of factor XII [58]. Allergen-provoked asthma increases serum-ECP [12], and treatment with β-agonists and theophylline lowers the serum-ECP levels [11].

Eosinophil peroxidase (EPO) [13] is localized in the granule matrix [17] and consists of a single polypeptide chain [14]. EPO in the presence of H_2O_2 and halide can induce mast cell degranulation [30] and enhances killing of *schistosomula* [37], *trypanosoma* [48], *S. aureus* [62], *Toxoplasma gondii* [44], and tumor cell [36].

Recent studies suggest other mechanisms by which the eosinophil, directly or indirectly, may participate in the pathology of asthma. Leukotrienes C_4 and D_4, which are potent bronchoconstrictors, can be produced by horse and human eosinophils [31, 38]. Mast cells and basophils can be activated to secrete inflammatory mediators by eosinophil peroxidase or MBP [30, 49]. Finally, Hibbs et al [32] reported that the eosinophil contains a metaloprotein capable of degrading types I and III collagens.

21.3 Discussion

Bronchial asthma has a specific pathology, and the hallmarks are a massive infiltration of the lung parenchyma by eosinophils and destruction of the mucociliary apparatus [6, 7, 10, 15, 16, 28, 29, 34, 35, 47]. It is estimated that during an asthmatic attack more than half a billion eosinophil cells could accumulate in the lung tissues [35, 56].

The idea that the eosinophil should function to the benefit of the host was first proposed by Schlecht at the turn of this century with his studies on anaphylaxis. On the basis of this work, eosinophilia could be considered as a protective reaction of the organism against certain decomposition

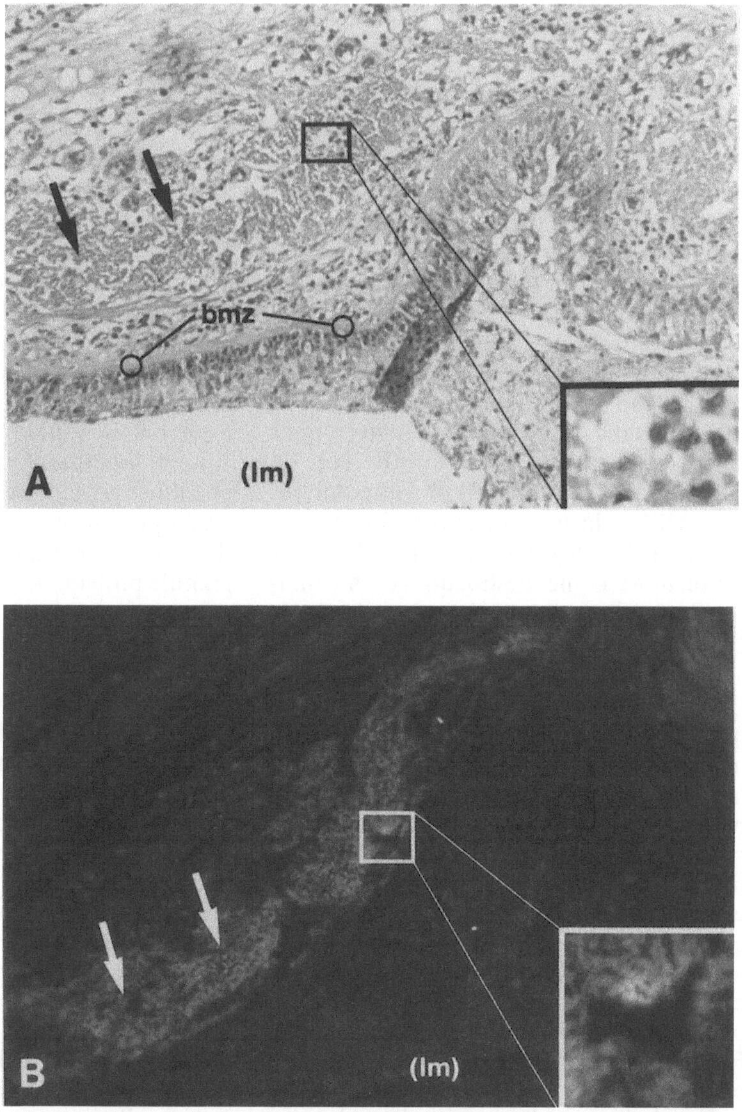

Fig. 21.6. Section of a bronchus from a patient with asthma. **A** H & E staining reveals an inflammatory cell infiltrate in the lamina propria with large patches of amorphous necrotic eosinophilic material (arrows) and a thick hyaline layer below the basement membrane (bmz). **B** When stained for MBP, these areas below the basement membrane in the lamina propria glow intensely for extracellular MBP; lm = bronchial lumen. Although some discrete eosinophils can be seen when stained by H & E (insert A), the entire area glows diffusely when stained with anti-MBP (insert B). (Original magnification × 100 and inserts A and B × 400). (Modified and reproduced from [20])

products of heterogeneous and even homologous proteins [54]. Subsequently, with the discovery of the various enzymatic constituents of the eosinophil granules, the theory was developed that the eosinophil neutralizes and switches off the reaction that elicited the eosinophilia. According to this theory, the eosinophil is attracted at the level of the bronchus to enzymatically neutralize the harmful mediators released by the mast cell [40, 63]. Because it possesses histaminase, arylsulfatase B, phospholipase D, and lysophospholipase [65], the eosinophil should inactivate, respectively, histamine [67], the leukotrienes C_4 and D_4 [60], the platelet activating factors [39] secreted by the mast cell, and the lysophosphatides [64]. Austin, whose laboratory has done much of this work, has been quoted: "The eosinophil can undo whatever the mast cell does" [53]. It remains to be shown that such events occur in vivo. One experiment, testing the effect of eosinophils on the levels of histamine released in vivo, did not find any increase in the quantity of histamine released in the absence of the eosinophil as it would have been expected by this theory. In fact, in the absence of eosinophils, a reduction in the quantity of histamine released was observed [26].

What then is the role of the eosinophil in asthma? We suggest that the eosinophils are attracted to the bronchial wall and lumen, either through a preceding allergen-IgE reaction and various chemotactic factors [26], as in allergic (extrinsic) asthma, or through unknown stimuli and chemotactic factors as in patients with non-IgE-mediated (intrinsic) asthma. By whichever chemotactic mechanism ultimately responsible for the accumulation of eosinophils in the asthmatic bronchus and lumen, once there, the eosinophils release MBP [14, 20, 23] either by secretion [3] or via autolysis. The MBP which is cytotoxic for human bronchial epithelium in vitro [23] may cause in vivo the destruction of the mucociliary apparatus seen in asthma [6, 7, 10, 15, 16, 28, 29, 34, 35, 47] leading to the inability to clear the bronchial secretions. Certainly, large quantities of MBP are detectable in the damaged areas of asthmatics' lungs [20] and high concentrations of MBP can be measured in the sputa of patients with asthma [14, 23]. Destruction of the epithelial barrier of the bronchus by the MBP, activation of basophils and mast cells by the MBP [49], eosinophil-induced capillary vasodilatation [66], may constitute amplification mechanisms by which even more eosinophils are attracted in the asthmatic bronchi, establishing a vicious cycle. Furthermore, eosinophil-derived LTC_4 [38] may contribute to the obstruction of the asthmatic bronchi by causing bronchoconstriction. The role of ECP in asthma remains uncertain, while the recently described eosinophil-derived zinc containing metaloprotein [32] may contribute to the edema and the disarray of the collagen fibers of the lamina propria described in asthmatics [10, 28, 45]. It remains, however, to be demonstrated that this metaloprotein is detectable in the lamina propria of asthmatic bronchi. This hypothesis for a harmful role of the eosinophil in asthma is consistent with the well-established direct correlation between the degree of blood and tissue eosinophilia in asthma and the severity of this disease, i.e., the more severe the asthma, the more pronounced the eosinophilia [33, 55]. In our clinical practice, in adjusting the dose of glucocorticoids used for treatment of asthma, we take into consideration the total blood eosinophil count [33], and the sputum concentration of MBP [14]. In addition, this model provides an explanation for the benefit from therapy with adrenergic agonists [41, 50] and especially glucocorticoids [2, 18, 50] which reduce the numbers of eosinophils in the blood and tissues. Also, the glucocorticoids inhibit degranulation of eosinophils [51], and prevent the expression of Fc receptors in the cell surface of the eosinophils [8, 57]. Research is needed to develop more specific anti-eosinophil drugs which would possibly prevent the migration of the eosinophils in the bronchi of asthmatics or that would neutralize eosinophil-derived granule proteins.

21.4 Conclusions

Peripheral blood and tissue eosinophilia are hallmarks of both allergic and nonallergic asthma. Analyses of the in vitro activities of the eosinophil granule major basic protein (MBP) revealed that MBP is toxic both to helminthic parasites and to mammalian cells, including human respiratory epithelium in vitro. The in vitro damage to respiratory epithelium consisted of desquamation and frank destruction of cells. Analysis of 204 random sputum samples for MBP showed that elevated concentrations of MBP are a good marker for asthma. Patients treated for acute asthma have even higher levels of MBP in their sputa, and these levels decreased after treatment. Finally, MBP is present outside the eosinophil in the lesions of the asthmatic lungs of patients who had died of asthma. Overall, these results are in keeping with the hypothesis that in asthma the eosinophil damages respiratory tissues.

Acknowledgements: The authors gratefully acknowledge the secretarial assistance of the Mayo Typing Service and Cheryl R. Adolphson for her comments and suggestions in the review of this manuscript.

References

1. Ackerman SJ, Loegering DA, Venge P, Olsson I, Harley JB, Fauci AS, Gleich GJ (1983) Distinctive cationic proteins of the human eosinophil granule: major basic protein, eosinophil cationic protein, and eosinophil-derived neurotoxin. J Immunol 131: 2977–2982
2. Andersen V, Bro-Rasmussen F, Hougard K (1968) Autoradiographic studies of eosinophil kinetics: effect of cortisol. In: Proceedings of the XIIth Congress of the International Society of Hematology. International Society of Hematology, New York
3. Butterfield JH, Ackerman SJ, Scott RE, Pierre RV, Gleich GJ (1984) Evidence for secretion of human eosinophil granule major basic protein and Charcot-Leyden crystal protein during eosinophil maturation. Exp Hematol 12:163–170
4. Butterworth AE, Wassom DL, Gleich GJ, Loegering DA, David JR (1979) Damage to schistosomula of *Schistosoma mansoni* induced directly by eosinophil major basic protein. J Immunol 122:221–229
5. Callerame ML, Condemi JJ, Bohrod MG, Vaughan JH (1971) Immunologic reactions of bronchial tissues in asthma. N Engl J Med 284:459–464
6. Carabelli AA (1958) Cytologic patterns in bronchopulmonary disease. Am Rev Tuberc 77:22–31
7. Cardell BS, Pearson RSB (1959) Death in asthmatics. Thorax 14:341–352
8. Crabtree GR, Munck A, Smith KA (1979) Glucocorticoids inhibit expression of Fc receptors on the human granulocytic cell line HL-60. Nature 279:338–339
9. Curschmann H (1882) Über Bronchiolitis exsudativa und ihr Verhältniss zum Asthma nervosum. Dtsch Arch Klin Med 32:1–34
10. Cutz E, Levison H, Cooper DM (1978) Ultrastructure of airways in children with asthma. Histopathology 2:407–421
11. Dahl R, Venge P (1978) Blood eosinophil leucocyte and eosinophil cationic protein: *in vivo* study of the influence of beta-2-adrenergic drugs and steroid medication. Scand J Respir Dis 59:319–322
12. Dahl R, Venge P, Olsson I (1978) Variations of blood eosinophils and eosinophil cationic protein in serum in patients with bronchial asthma: studies during inhalation challenge test. Allergy 33:211–215
13. Desser RK, Himmelhoch SR, Evans WH, Januska M, Mage M, Shelton E (1972) Guinea pig heterophil and eosinophil peroxidase. Arch Biochem Biophys 148: 452–465
14. Dor PJ, Frigas E (1983) Dosage radioimmunologique de la protéine majeure basique du granule éosinophile dans l'expectoration: un appoint diagnostique dans l'asthme. Rev Fr Mal Respir 11:209–217
15. Dunnill MS (1960) The pathology of asthma, with special reference to changes in the bronchial mucosa. J Clin Pathol 13:27–33
16. Ellis AG (1908) The pathological anatomy of bronchial asthma. Am J Med Sci 136:407–429
17. Enomoto T, Kitani T (1966) Electron microscopic studies on peroxidase and acid phosphatase reaction in human leukocytes (in normal and leukemic cells and on phagocytosis). Acta Haematol Jpn 29:554–570
18. Essellier AF, Jeanneret RL, Morandi L (1954) The mechanism of glucocorticoid eosinopenia: contribution to physiology of eosinophil granulocytes. Blood 9:531–549
19. Filley WV, Ackerman SJ, Gleich GJ (1981) An immunofluorescent method for specific staining of eosinophil granule major basic protein. J Immunol Methods 47:227–238
20. Filley WV, Holley KE, Kephart GM, Gleich GJ (1982) Identification by immunofluorescence of eosinophil granule major basic protein in lung tissues of patients with bronchial asthma. Lancet 2:11–16
21. Frigas E, Dor PJ, Gleich GJ (1983) The usefulness of sputum radioimmunoassay for the eosinophil major basic protein in the diagnosis of asthma. Folia Allergologica et Immunologica Clinica 30 [Suppl 4]:92
22. Frigas E, Loegering DA, Gleich GJ (1980) Cytotoxic effects of the guinea pig eosinophil major basic protein on tracheal epithelium. Lab Invest 42:35–43
23. Frigas E, Loegering DA, Solley GO, Farrow GM, Gleich GJ (1981) Elevated levels of the eosinophil granule major basic protein in the sputum of patients with bronchial asthma. Mayo Clin Proc 56:345–353
24. Gerber MA, Paronetto F, Kochwa S (1971) Immunohistochemical localization of IgE in asthmatic lungs. Am J Pathol 62:339–351
25. Gleich GJ, Frigas E, Loegering DA, Wassom DL, Steinmuller D (1979) Cytotoxic properties of the eosinophil major basic protein. J Immunol 123:2925–2927
26. Gleich GJ, Olson GM, Loegering DA (1979) The effect of ablation of eosinophils on immediate-type hypersensitivity reactions. Immunology 38:343–353
27. Gleich GJ, Loegering DA (1984) Immunobiology of eosinophils. Ann Rev Immunol 2:429–459
28. Glynn AA, Michaels L (1960) Bronchial biopsy in chronic bronchitis and asthma. Thorax 15:142–153

29. Gough J (1961) Post mortem differences in "asthma" and in chronic bronchitis. Acta Allergologica 16:391–399
30. Henderson WR, Chi EY, Klebanoff SJ (1980) Eosinophil peroxidase-induced mast cell secretion. J Exp Med 152:265–279
31. Henderson WR, Harley JB, Fauci AS, Klebanoff SJ (1983) Leukotriene B_4, C_4 and D_4 generation by human eosinophils. J Allergy Clin Immunol 71:138 (abstract)
32. Hibbs MS, Mainardi CL, Kang AH (1982) Type-specific collagen degradation by eosinophils. Biochem J 207:621–624
33. Horn BR, Robin ED, Theodore J, van Kessel A (1975) Total eosinophil counts in the management of bronchial asthma. N Engl J Med 292:1152–1155
34. Houston JC, de Navasquez S, Trounce JR (1953) A clinical and pathological study of fatal cases of status asthmaticus. Thorax 8:207–213
35. Huber HL, Koessler KK (1922) The pathology of bronchial asthma. Arch Intern Med 30:689–760
36. Jong EC, Klebanoff SJ (1980) Eosinophil-mediated mammalian tumor cell cytotoxicity: role of the peroxidase system. J Immunol 124:1949–1953
37. Jong EC, Mahmoud AAF, Klebanoff SJ (1981) Peroxidase-mediated toxicity to schistosomula of *Schistosoma mansoni.* J Immunol 126:468–471
38. Jörg A, Henderson WR, Murphy RC, Klebanoff SJ (1982) Leukotriene generation by eosinophils. J Exp Med 155:390–402
39. Kater LA, Goetzl EJ, Austen KF (1976) Isolation of human eosinophil phospholipase D. J Clin Invest 57:1173–1180
40. Kay AB, Austen KF (1971) The IgE-mediated release of an eosinophil leukocyte chemotactic factor from human lung. J Immunol 107:899–902
41. Koch-Weser J (1968) Beta adrenergic blockade and circulating eosinophils. Arch Intern Med 121:255–258
42. Lewis DM, Lewis JC, Loegering DA, Gleich GJ (1978) Localization of the guinea pig eosinophil major basic protein to the core of the granule. J Cell Biol 77:702–713
43. Leyden zu Königsberg E (1872) Zur Kenntniss des Bronchial-Asthma. Arch Pathol Anat Physiol 54:324–352
44. Locksley RM, Wilson CB, Klebanoff SJ (1982) Role for endogenous and acquired peroxidase in the toxoplasmacidal activity of murine and human mononuclear phagocytes. J Clin Invest 69:1099–1111
45. McCarter JH, Vazquez JJ (1966) The bronchial basement membrane in asthma: immunohistochemical and ultrastructural observations. Arch Pathol 82:328–335
46. McLaren DJ, McKean JR, Olsson I, Venge P, Kay AB (1981) Morphological studies on the killing of schistosomula of *Schistosoma mansoni* by human eosinophil and neutrophil cationic proteins in vitro. Parasite Immunol 3:359–373
47. Naylor B (1962) The shedding of the mucosa of the bronchial tree in asthma. Thorax 17:69–72
48. Nogueira NM, Klebanoff SJ, Cohn ZA (1982) *T. cruzi:* sensitization to macrophage killing by eosinophil peroxidase. J Immunol 128:1705–1708
49. O'Donnell MC, Ackerman SJ, Gleich GJ, Thomas LL (1983) Activation of basophil and mast cell histamine release by eosinophil granule major basic protein. J Exp Med 157:1981–1991
50. Ohman JL Jr, Lawrence M, Lowell FC (1972) Effect of propranolol on the isoproterenol, responses of cortisol, isoproterenol, and aminophylline. J Allergy Clin Immunol 50:151–156
51. Oliver RC, Glauert AM, Thorne KJI (1982) Mechanism of Fc-mediated interaction of eosinophils with immobilized immune complexes. I. Effects of inhibitors and activators of eosinophil function. J Cell Sci 56:337–356
52. Parrillo JE, Fauci AS (1978) Human eosinophils. Purification and cytotoxic capability of eosinophils from patients with the hypereosinophilic syndrome. Blood 51:457–473
53. Samter M (1980) Eosinophils – nominated but not elected. N Engl J Med 303:1175–1176
54. Schlecht H (1912) Über experimentelle Eosinophilie nach parenteraler Zufuhr artfremden Eiweißes und über die Beziehungen der Eosinophilie zur Anaphylaxie. Arch Exp Pathol Pharmakol 67:137–171
55. Schwartz HJ, Lowell FC, Melby JC (1968) Steroid resistance in bronchial asthma. Ann Intern Med 69:493–499
56. Taylor JG (1900) Studies in leukemia. Contribution from the William Pepper Laboratory of Clinical Medicine, Philadelphia
57. Tolone G, Bonasera L, Sajeva R (1979) Effects of hydrocortisone on binding of IgG or C3b-coated erythrocytes to human monocytes and polymorphonuclear leukocytes. J Pharm Pharmacol 31:563–564
58. Venge P, Dahl R, Hällgren R (1979) Enhancement of factor XII dependent reactions by eosinophil cationic protein. Thromb Res 14:641–649
59. Venge P, Dahl R, Hällgren R, Olsson I (1980) Cationic proteins of human eosino-

phils and their role in the inflammatory reaction. In: Mahmoud AAF, Austen KF (eds) The eosinophil in health and disease. Grune and Stratton, New York, pp 131–142
60. Wasserman SI, Goetzl EJ, Austen KF (1975) Inactivation of slow reacting substance of anaphylaxis by human eosinophil arylsulfatase. J Immunol 114:645–649
61. Wassom DL, Loegering DA, Solley GO, Moore SB, Schooley RT, Fauci AS, Gleich GJ (1981) Elevated serum levels of the eosinophil granule major basic protein in patients with eosinophilia. J Clin Invest 67: 651–661
62. Watanabe K, Hasegawa M, Saito Y, Takayama S (1977) Eosinophilic leucocytes in nasal allergy – movement of enzymes. Clin Allergy 7:263–271
63. Weller PF, Goetzl EJ (1979) The regulatory and effector roles of eosinophils. Adv Immunol 27:339–371
64. Weller PF, Goetzl EJ, Austen KF (1980) Identification of human eosinophil lysophospholipase as the constituent of Charcot-Leyden crystals. Proc Natl Acad Sci USA 77:7440–7443
65. Weller PF, Wasserman SI, Austen KF (1980) Selected enzymes preferentially present in the eosinophil. In: Mahmoud AAF, Austen KF (eds) The eosinophil in health and disease. Grune and Stratton, New York, pp 115–128
66. Yoshida H, Anan S, Hori M, Akiyama T, Ushijima N, Tanaka M (1982) Ultrastructural studies of eosinophils in passive cutaneous anaphylaxis. Arch Dermatol Res 272:197–200
67. Zeiger RS, Colten HR (1977) Histaminase release from human eosinophils. J Immunol 118:540–543

22. Mediators of Asthma Derived from Arachidonic Acid

R. A. Lewis, J.-L. Robin

The cell types which are normally resident in the human lung and the variety of inflammatory leukocytes that can infiltrate pulmonary tissue in the course of inflammatory lung diseases each have phospholipids as major plasma membrane components. When a cell is perturbated by a stimulus that alters the relative quantities and spacial distributions of phospholipids, phospholipase A_2 [1] and/or phospholipase C in concert with diglyceride lipase [2, 3] are also activated, resulting in the release of arachidonic acid for oxidative metabolism to prostaglandins (PGs), thromboxane (Tx), monohydroxy derivatives of arachidonic acid (HETEs), and/or leukotrienes (LTs). The spectrum of oxidative products is dictated by the specificities of the enzymes present in the cellular microenvironment; arachidonic acid may be metabolized to products in the cell from which it is released or by other cells in the immediate vicinity. Additionally, the effects of specific oxidative metabolites of arachidonic acid on target cells may include modification of the capacities of those cells to generate and release additional mediators of inflammation.

The oxidative metabolism of arachidonic acid, as it occurs during immediate hypersensitivity reactions in human pulmonary tissue, produces a number of potent pharmacologic mediators, including prostaglandin D_2 (PGD_2), PGE_2, $PGF_{2\alpha}$, PGI_2, thromboxane A_2 (TxA_2), HETEs, LTC_4, and LTD_4 [4–8]; less direct evidence suggests that LTE_4 and LTB_4 would also be generated [9–11]. Although cyclooxygenase, the initial enzyme in the cascade that produces PGs and TxA_2 from arachidonic acid, is ubiquitous among nucleated mammalian cells, at least one additional enzyme is required for the biosynthesis of each specific metabolite [12]. It therefore follows that each cyclooxygenase product is generated preferentially by a limited number of cell types. From human cells, PGI_2 is, for example, the major cyclooxygenase product derived from vascular endothelial cells [13]; TxA_2 is synthesized as the major product of this pathway in platelets [14] and pulmonary alveolar macrophages [15], and PGD_2 is selectively generated from heparin containing mast cells [6, 16]. Although PGE_2 and $PGF_{2\alpha}$ are products of biosynthesis from a diverse number of cell types [17], a significant portion of their generation in pulmonary tissue may arise from smooth muscle of central and peripheral airways respectively [18]. Of the lipoxygenase cascades, the one which generates the arachidonic acid metabolites with greatest pro-inflammatory activity from cells and tissue of activated human lung, i.e., the leukotrienes B_4, C_4, D_4, and E_4, is the 5-lipoxygenase pathway [7, 19, 20]. A limited number of human cell types have been shown to generate 5-lipoxygenase products, and these include pulmonary alveolar macrophages [10, 11], mast cells [21], neutrophils [22], eosinophils [23], and peripheral blood monocytes [24] (Table 22.1). LTB_4 and LTC_4 are products from the same precursor (LTA_4) [19] by the action of separate enzymes and the generated ratios of LTB_4:LTC_4 are determined by their cell of origin. Whereas LTB_4 is the overwhelmingly preferential product of neutrophils and alveolar macrophages, activated by either a divalent cation ionophore A23187 [10, 22] or a physiologically relevant particulate stimulus [11, 20, 25], LTC_4 is the selective product from pulmonary mast cells activated by antigen bridging of their bound IgE molecules [21] and from eosinophils stimulated with A23187 [23]. When the appearance of LTD_4 and LTE_4 is demonstrated, they have been derived from LTC_4 by cleavage of its peptide side chain; these metabolites from human cells are

Table 22.1. Mean leukotriene generation by human cells

Cell type	Activating stimulus	LTB_4 (ng/ 10^6 cells)	LTC_4 (ng/ 10^6 cells)	References
Macrophage (alveolar)	Ca^{++} ionophore	200	10	[10, 11]
	Zymosan	50	2	[11, 69]
	Zymosan (opsonized)	80	5	[11, 69]
Monocyte	Ca^{++} ionophore	34	15	[24]
	Zymosan	5	1	[24]
Neutrophil	Ca^{++} ionophore	25–50	7.5	[22, 23, 70]
	Zymosan	6	1	[70]
Mast cell	IgE/antigen	4	25	[21]
Eosinophil	Ca^{++} ionophore	6	38	[23]
Eosinophil (nonatopic hypereosinophilia)	Ca^{++} ionophore	2	69	[23]

LTC_4 from *neutrophils* may derive mainly from eosinophil contaminants; LTB_4 from *eosinophils* may derive mainly from neutrophil contaminants

probably generated from LTC_4 almost exclusively after LTC_4 is released from its cell of origin. 5-HETE, the monohydroxylated product of the 5-lipoxygenase pathway, is also produced in cells generating the leukotrienes and may have significant regulatory properties for its cell of origin. A structurally, but probably not functionally, analogous monohydroxylated product of the platelet 12-lipoxygenase pathway, 12-HETE [26], and both 15-HETE and dihydroxylated arachidonic acid metabolites from the 15-lipoxygenase pathway of the eosinophil have also been identified [27]. Dihydroxy and trihydroxy metabolites, such as the recently described lipoxins, can be generated *in vitro* from arachidonic acid, and are theoretically produced by the sequential actions of two different lipoxygenase enzymes [28]; these are not yet identified as qualitatively significant naturally occurring products and little is known about their potential as mediators for biological responses.

22.1 Biological Activities of Arachidonic Acid Metabolites for Pulmonary Inflammation

PGD_2 has been shown to be a potent bronchoconstrictor for normal and asthmatic humans after its inhalation from an aerosolized solution [29] (Fig. 22.1). It is additionally a vasodilator in the skin when administered intradermally [30]. Whereas PGD_2 may thus be presumed to dilate pulmonary and bronchial arterioles, one study of mastocytosis patients, who generate large quantities of PGD_2, has suggested that either PGD_2 or a further metabolite thereof might act contrastingly as a central vasoconstrictor [31]. PGD_2 increases random migration (chemokinesis) of granulocytes, but not their directed migration (chemotaxis) [32]; it could be, nonetheless, a significant effector of neutrophil and eosinophil influx during the evolution of inflammatory lung diseases, since its chemokinetic action would presumably enhance the responses to chemotactic factors.

Inhaled aerosols of LTC_4 and LTD_4 are remarkably potent for producing small airway obstruction in normal human lungs. Each compound has 4,000–6,000 times the molar efficacy of inhaled histamine [33, 34] for altering the maximal midexpiratory flow rate following inhalation to 60% of vital capacity ($\dot{v}_{30}$). Whereas LTC_4 and LTD_4 are almost comparable to one another with respect to their inhaled concentrations required to elicit a maximal effect, the responses evolve over significantly different time courses. The effects of inhaled LTC_4

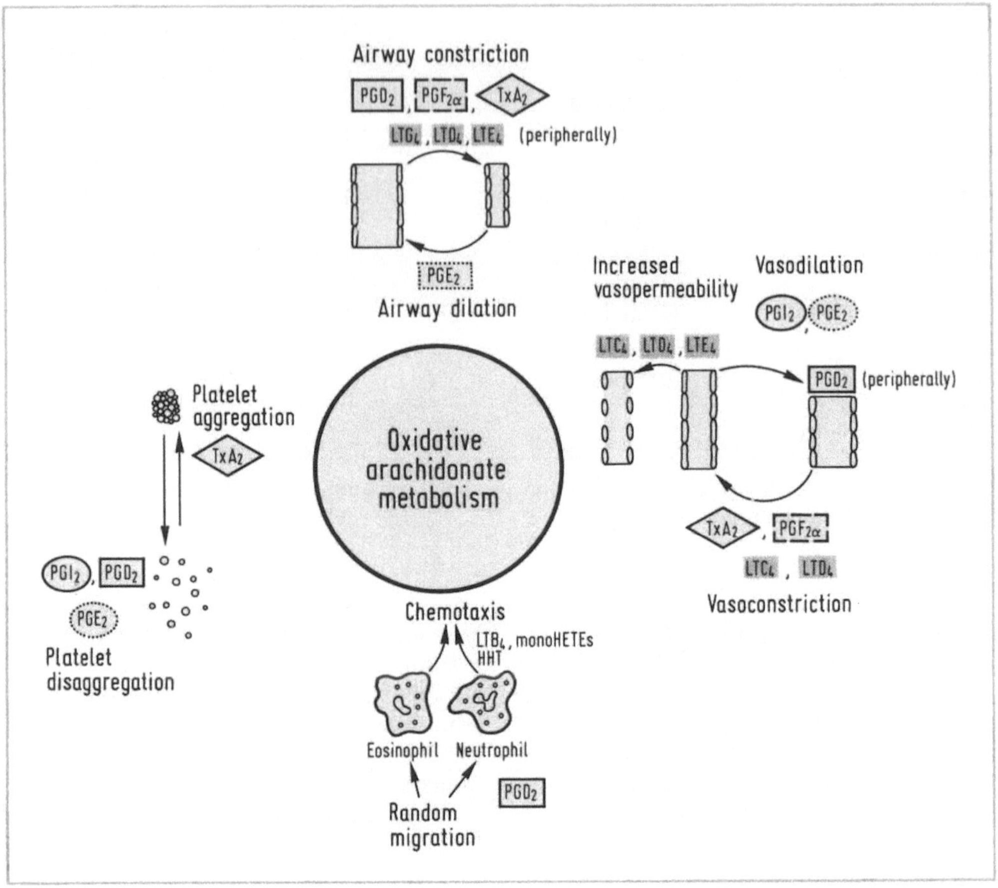

Fig. 22.1. Inflammatory effects of oxidative metabolites of arachidonic acid. HHT = heptadecatrienoic acid

have a much slower onset and are longer-lived than those of LTD_4; for example, the peak response to LTC_4 requires 12 to 17 min at concentrations which produce a 30% fall in $\dot{V}_{30}$, and the response is sustained for an additional 15 min, whereas the peak response to LTD_4 occurs within 2 to 7 min and then begins to diminish by 13 min [33, 34]. The predominating determinant for this difference in time-dependent responses is likely to be the differing characteristics of transduction through separate receptors for LTC_4 and LTD_4; this is suggested by analogy with the differences in time courses for contractions elicited by the same ligands on guinea pig ileum, where the existence of separate receptors is directly supported by assays of specific radioligand binding [35–38]. Additional contributions due to bioconversion of LTC_4 to LTD_4, differing rates of transport of the two leukotrienes across airway mucosa to the responding smooth muscle, and the relative rates of catabolism of LTC_4 and LTD_4 to less active spasmogens (notably LTE_4) are also possible. Furthermore, the continued generation of these leukotrienes during pulmonary inflammation might be expected to increase obstruction of the airways by also increasing mucus secretions [39, 40] and by eliciting postcapillary venopermeability, as demonstrated in buccal mucosa and skin [41–43], with resultant airway mucosal edema. Human bronchial mucosal explants in tissue culture respond to as little as 10^{-9} M LTC_4 or LTD_4 by enhanced mucus glycoprotein secretion [39, 40]. Augmented postcapillary venular permeability by sulfidopeptide leukotrienes, which was initially demonstrated in the dermal microvasculature of guinea pigs following local injections with 10^{-7} M LTC_4, LTD_4, and LTE_4 [41], was confirmed in the hamster cheek pouch by the leakage of fluorescent dye from the circulation following topical application of each leukotriene [42]. In normal humans, the intradermal injection of LTC_4, LTD_4, and LTE_4 produced a wheal and flare response; the wheal, which indicates increased venopermeability, was sustained for 2–4 hours [43].

LTC_4 and, to a lesser extent, LTD_4, have additional vascular effects as arteriolar spasmogens. As for postcapillary venopermeability, the vasoconstrictor response was initially demonstrated at the site of intradermal administration of the leukotrienes in guinea pig skin, and also required a concentration less than 10^{-7} M of each leukotriene [44]; this effect was also confirmed for both the hamster cheek pouch model [42] and in human skin [43]. Vasospasm of coronary arterial vessels is also evoked by these molecules after their intracoronary infusion in sheep [45] or intravenous infusion in rats [46]. In the latter, infusion of LTC_4 also elicited renal vasoconstriction and subsequent limitation of renal blood flow and glomerular filtration [47]. LTC_4-mediated pulmonary vasoconstriction in humans has been suggested by measurement of sulfidopeptide leukotrienes from tracheal aspirates of infants with persistent fetal circulation and pulmonary hypertension [48].

In contrast to PGD_2, LTB_4 and, to a lesser extent, the HETEs, are potent chemotactic factors for neutrophilic and eosinophilic granulocytes. Local administration of LTB_4 causes neutrophilic dermal infiltration in human skin by 4–6 hours [43]. Topical application of LTB_4 to hamster cheek pouch mucosa elicits leukocyte adhesion to the vascular endothelium [42]. A direct effect of LTB_4 on the endothelial cell, which increases neutrophil margination [49] is probably a prerequisite for diapedesis. LTB_4 may additionally be immunoregulatory for lymphocytes by increasing the number of suppressor T-lymphocytes from precursors which lack suppressor surface antigen and function [50]. LTB_4 inhibits mitogen-induced T-cell proliferation [51, 52] as well as immunoglobulin synthesis [50]. LTB_4 has not been tested for its specific immunoregulatory activity on bronchial-associated lymphoid tissue.

22.2 Regulating the Pro-inflammatory Effects of Arachidonic Acid Metabolites

Biosynthesis of prostaglandins and thromboxane from arachidonic acid is interrupted at the level of the cyclooxygenase enzyme by nonsteroidal anti-inflammatory drugs [53]. In contrast, therapeutically achievable concentrations of these drugs are significantly less inhibitory to the lipoxygenases, including the 5-lipoxygenase. In many cases of obstructive lung diseases, and especially asthma, it seems that the generation of cyclooxygenase pathway products would be best preserved since nonsteroidal anti-inflammatory drugs adversely affect a significant percentage of asthmatics. This may reflect the need to conserve the generation of PGE_2 as a bronchodilator and/or as an inhibitor of leukotriene biosynthesis [54]. It seems likely that limitation of 5-lipoxygenase pathway product synthesis or function would generally have an anti-inflammatory effect on obstructive inflammatory lung diseases.

Interruption of the catalytic actions of enzymes in the 5-lipoxygenase cascade would presumably be therapeutic. The 5-lipoxygenase, the initial enzyme of that pathway, can be specifically and irreversibly inhibited in murine bone marrow-derived mast cells by a synthetic arachidonic acid analog, 5,6-dehydroarachidonic acid [55] (Fig. 22.2). Also, conversion of 5-hydroperoxyeicosatetraenoic acid to LTA_4, the immediate precursor of both LTB_4 and LTC_4, can apparently be blocked by diethylcarbamazine, a clinically utilized antihelminthic [55], and the specific glutathione-S-transferase which generates LTC_4 from LTA_4 is inhibited by U-60,257 (Piriprost), an experimental compound (Upjohn, Kalamazoo, MI) [55, 56].

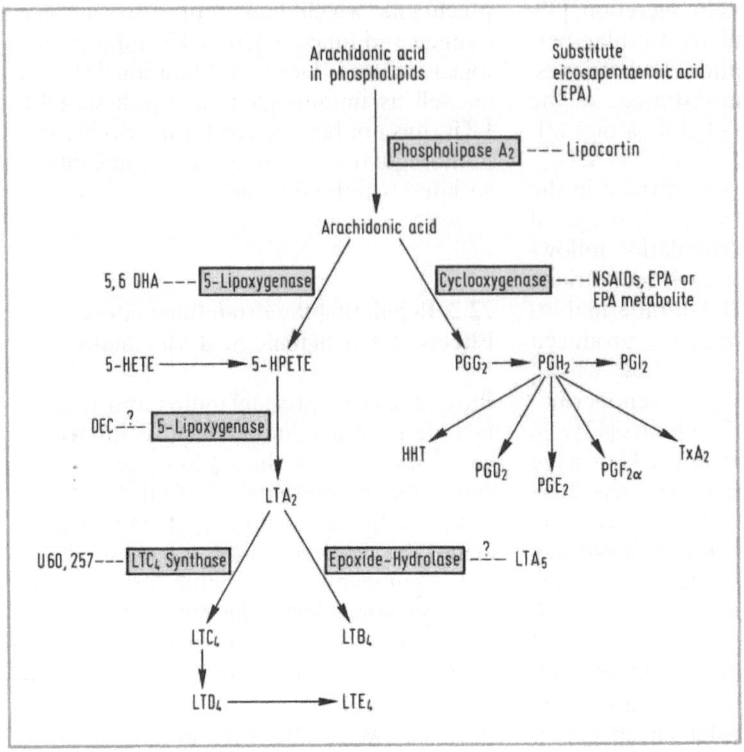

Fig. 22.2. Pharmacological interruption of arachidonic acid metabolism. EPA = eicosapentaenoic acid; NSAIDs = nonsteroidal anti-inflammatory drugs; 5,6-DHA = 5,6-dehydroarachidonic acid; DEC = diethylcarbamazine

Leukotriene effects might alternatively be antagonized at the level of the responding end organ, based upon the existence of specific receptors for LTB_4 on neutrophils [57] as well as for LTC_4 on vascular tissue [58] and nonvascular smooth muscle [36, 37]. However, not all the leukotriene-mediated events are necessarily receptor-mediated; bronchial mucus secretion by arachidonic acid metabolites has few requirements for specific structural domains of the agonist [40].

A more novel therapeutic alternative would be substitution for arachidonic acid with an alternative fatty acid substrate for the 5-lipoxygenase pathway, resulting in a decrease of total leukotriene biosynthesis and/or a reduction in the total pro-inflammatory activities of the products. The consumption of large quantities of fish oils which are rich in triglycerides containing eicosapentaenoic acid and docosahexaenoic acid results in the incorporation of these fatty acids in cellular lipids. Murine mastocytoma cells which were grown in the peritoneal cavities of mice on a fish oil-enriched diet and then stimulated *ex vivo* with calcium ionophore and peritoneal cells of fish oil-fed rats, responding *in vivo* to local immune complex-induced anaphylaxis, each generated LTB_5 and LTC_5 from eicosapentaenoic acid as well as LTB_4 and LTC_4 from arachidonic acid [59, 60]. Although LTC_4 and LTC_5 have comparable spasmogenic activities for airway smooth muscle, as exemplified on guinea pig pulmonary parenchymal strips, LTB_5 is only a weak and partial agonist for neutrophil chemotaxis and aggregation, relative to LTB_4 [61]. Additionally, when neutrophils are activated by calcium ionophore *in vitro* in the presence of eicosapentaenoic acid, the combined biosynthesis of LTB_4 and LTB_5 is less than the generation of LTB_4 in the absence of the marine fatty acid [62].

Finally, it has been suggested that the anti-inflammatory actions of glucocorticosteroids, particularly including decreased arachidonic acid metabolism, occur due to synthesis of an endogenous phospholipase inhibitor, termed *lipocortin* [63–65]. This moiety has been isolated in a number of forms including aggregates and cleavage products, each of which are glycosylated peptides. In its nonphosphorylated forms, lipocortin is alleged to inhibit phospholipases A_2, C, and D. Phosphorylation of the active inhibitor is thought to render secreted lipocortin more resistant to proteolysis; the molecule could then be reactivated by a phosphatase of another cell, wherein arachidonic acid release would thus be inhibited. This hypothesis would suggest that the anti-inflammatory effects of glucocorticosteroids might be reproduced, possibly without steroid side effects, by synthetic lipocortin.

It is overwhelmingly likely, however, that not all of the anti-inflammatory steroid effects that regulate arachidonic acid metabolism would be reproduced by lipocortin as a therapeutic modality. Other data would imply that steroids also act to increase a plasma inhibitor of prostaglandin synthesis [66] and additionally enhance prostaglandin catabolism [67]. Glucocorticosteroids may have additional regulatory effects on specific cell types. In murine bone marrow-derived mast cells, a glucocorticosteroid inhibits the IgE- and antigen-dependent biosynthesis of LTC_4 and LTB_4 by decreasing the total number of cell surface IgE receptors [68]. An additional lipocortin-type mechanism of action is excluded by the lack of steroid effect on calcium ionophore-induced generation of the same products. Furthermore, glucocorticosteroid treatment stimulates increased generation of PGD_2 by both IgE/antigen and ionophore, apparently by inducing increased cyclooxygenase activity; a lipocortin-type action would have predicted decreased PGD_2 biosynthesis.

22.3 Conclusions

Cyclooxygenase products may be pro-inflammatory in some model systems and anti-inflammatory in others, suggesting the possibility that this pathway and its arachidonic acid metabolites could act in either direction according to the particular phase of a specific inflammatory disease. The unfortunate capacity of cyclooxygenase inhibitors to increase certain clinical inflammatory events is consistent with this view. Where 5-lipoxygenase products are likely to be involved, they would appear to be purely pro-inflammatory. It has thus been suggested that the need to control biosynthesis and functional expression of the leukotrienes exists for a variety of inflammatory diseases, particularly including asthma. The test of this proposal with appropriate pharmacotherapies is near at hand.

References

1. Victoria E, van Golde LMG, Hostetler KY, Scherphof GL, van Deenan LLM (1971) Some studies on the metabolism of phospholipids in plasma membranes from rat liver. Biochim Biophys Acta 239:443–457
2. Bell RL, Kennerly DA, Stanford N, Majerus PW (1979) Diglyceride lipase: a pathway for arachidonate release from human platelets. Proc Natl Acad Sci USA 76:3238–3241
3. Kennerly DA, Sullivan TJ, Sylwester P, Parker CW (1979) Diacylglycerol metabolism in mast cells: a potential role in membrane fusion and arachidonic acid release. J Exp Med 150:1039–1044
4. Piper PJ, Walker JL (1973) The release of spasmogenic substances from human chopped lung tissue and its inhibition. Br J Pharmacol 47:291–304
5. Adkinson NF Jr, Schulman ES, Newball HH (1983) Anaphylactic release of arachidonic acid metabolites from the lung. In: Newball HH (ed) Immunopharmacology of the Lung. Marcel Dekker, New York, pp 55–72
6. Lewis RA, Soter NA, Diamond PT, Austen KF, Oates JA, Roberts LJ II (1982) Prostaglandin D_2 generation after activation of rat and human mast cells with anti-IgE. J Immunol 129:1627–1631
7. Marom Z, Shelhammer JH, Sun F, Kaliner M (1983) Human airway monohydroxyeicosatetraenoic acid generation and mucus release. J Clin Invest 72:122–127
8. Lewis RA, Austen KF, Drazen JM, Clark DA, Marfat A, Corey EJ (1980) Slow reacting substance of anaphylaxis: identification of leukotrienes C-1 and D from human and rat sources. Proc Natl Acad Sci USA 77:3710–3714
9. Parker CW, Koch D, Huber MM, Falkenhein SF (1980) Formation of the cysteinyl form of slow reacting substance

(leukotriene E_4) in human plasma. Biochem Biophys Res Commun 97:1038–1046

10. Fels AOS, Pawlowski NA, Cramer EB, King TKC, Cohn ZA, Scott WA (1982) Human alveolar macrophages produce leukotriene B_4. Proc Natl Acad Sci USA 79:7866–7870
11. Godard P, Damon M, Michel FB, Corey EJ, Austen KF, Lewis RA (1983) Leukotriene B_4 production from human alveolar macrophages. Clin Res 31:548 A
12. Samuelsson B, Goldyne M, Granstrom E, Hamberg M, Hammarström S, Malmsten C (1978) Prostaglandins and thromboxanes. Annu Rev Biochem 47:997–1029
13. Moncada S, Higgs EA, Vane JR (1977) Human arterial and venous tissue generates prostacyclin (prostaglandin x), a potent inhibitor of platelet aggregation. Lancet 1: 18–20
14. Hamberg M, Svensson J, Samuelsson B (1975) Thromboxanes: a new group of biologically active compounds derived from prostaglandin endoperoxides. Proc Natl Acad Sci USA 72:2994–2998
15. Godard P, Chantreuil J, Damon M, Coupe M, Flandre O, Crastes de Paulet A, Michel FB (1982) Functional assessment of alveolar macrophages: comparison of cells from asthmatics and normal subjects. J Allergy Clin Immunol 70:88–93
16. Lewis RA, Holgate ST, Roberts LJ II, Oates JA, Austen KF (1981) Preferential generation of prostaglandin D_2 by rat and human mast cells. In: Becker EL, Simon AS, Austen KF (eds) Biochemistry of the Acute Allergic Reactions, 4th International Symposium. Alan R. Liss, New York, pp 239–254
17. Christ EJ, van Dorp DA (1972) Comparative aspects of prostaglandin biosynthesis in animal tissues. Biochim Biophys Acta 270:537–545
18. Gryglewski RJ, Dembinska-Kiec A, Grodzinska L, Panczcyko B (1976) Differential generation of substances with prostaglandin-like and thromboxane-like activities by guinea pig trachea and lung strips. In: Bouhuys A (ed) Lung Cells in Disease. Elsevier, Amsterdam, pp 289–299
19. Samuelsson B (1983) Leukotrienes: mediators of immediate hypersensitivity reactions and inflammation. Science 220:568–575
20. Lewis RA, Austen KF (1984) The biologically active leukotrienes: biosynthesis, metabolism, receptors, functions, and pharmacology. J Clin Invest 73:889–897
21. MacGlashan DW Jr, Schleimer RP, Peters SP, Schulman ES, Adams GK III, Newball HH, Lichtenstein LM (1982) Generation of leukotrienes by purified human lung mast cells. J Clin Invest 70:747–751
22. Borgeat P, Samuelsson B (1979) Arachidonic acid metabolism in polymorphonuclear leukocytes: effects of ionophore A23187. Proc Natl Acad Sci USA 76:2148–2152
23. Weller PF, Lee CW, Foster DW, Corey EJ, Austen KF, Lewis RA (1983) Generation and metabolism of 5-lipoxygenase pathway leukotrienes by human eosinophils: predominant production of leukotriene C_4. Proc Natl Acad Sci USA 80:7626–7630
24. Williams JD, Czop JK, Austen KF (1984) Release of leukotrienes by human monocytes on stimulation of their phagocytic receptor for particulate activators. J Immunol 132:3034–3040
25. Williams JD, Lee TH, Lewis RA, Austen KF (1985) Intracellular retention of the 5-lipoxygenase pathway product, leukotriene B_4, by human neutrophils activated with unopsonized zymosan. J Immunol 134:2624–2630
26. Hamberg M, Samuelsson B (1974) Novel transformation of arachidonic acid in human platelets. Proc Natl Acad Sci USA 71:3400–3404
27. Oates JA (1983) Metabolism of arachidonic acid by the cyclooxygenase pathway in mast cells and by the 15-lipoxygenase pathway in human eosinophils. In: August JT (ed) Biological Response Mediators and Modulators. Academic Press, New York, pp 41–47
28. Serhan CN, Hamberg M, Samuelsson B (1984) Lipoxins: Novel series of biologically active compounds formed from arachidonic acid in human leukocytes. Proc Natl Acad Sci USA 81:5335–5339
29. Hardy C, Robinson C, Tattersfield A, Holgate ST (1984) The bronchoconstrictor effect of inhaled prostaglandin D_2 in normal and asthmatic men. N Engl J Med 311:209–213
30. Flower R, Harvey E, Kingston W (1976) Inflammatory effects of prostaglandin D_2 in rat and human skin. Br J Pharmacol 56:229–233
31. Roberts LJ II, Sweetman B, Lewis RA, Austen KF, Oates J (1980) Increased production of prostaglandin D_2 in patients with systemic mastocytosis. N Engl J Med 303:1400–1404
32. Goetzl EJ, Weller PF, Valone FH (1979) Biochemical and functional basis of the regulatory and protective roles of the human eosinophil. In: Weissmann G, Samuelsson B, Paoletti R (eds) Advances in Inflammation Research, vol. 1. Raven Press, New York, pp 157–167
33. Weiss JW, Drazen JM, Coles N, McFadden ER Jr, Weller P, Corey EJ, Lewis RA, Austen KF (1982) Bronchoconstrictor effects of

leukotriene C in human subjects. Science 216:196–198
34. Weiss JW, Drazen JM, McFadden ER Jr, Weller P, Corey EJ, Lewis RA, Austen KF (1982) Comparative bronchoconstrictor effects of histamine, leukotriene C and leukotriene D in normal human volunteers. Trans Assoc Am Physicians 95:30–35
35. Krilis S, Lewis RA, Corey EJ, Austen KF (1983) Bioconversion of C-6 sulfidopeptide leukotrienes by the responding guinea pig ileum determines the time course of its contraction. J Clin Invest 71:909–915
36. Krilis S, Lewis RA, Corey EJ, Austen KF (1984) Specific binding of leukotriene C_4 to plasma membrane and subcellular receptors of ileal smooth muscle cells. Proc Natl Acad Sci USA 81:4529–4533
37. Krilis S, Lewis RA, Drazen JM, Austen KF (1985) Subclasses of receptors for the sulfidopeptide leukotrienes. In: Braquet P, Garay RP, Frolich JC, Nicosia S (eds) Prostaglandins and Membrane Ion Transport. Raven Press, New York, pp 91–97
38. Hogaboom GK, Mong S, Wu H-L, Crooke S (1983) Peptidoleukotrienes: distinct receptors for leukotrienes C_4 and D_4 in the guinea pig lung. Biochem Biophys Res Commun 116:1136–1143
39. Schelhamer JH, Marom Z, Sun F, Bach MK, Kaliner M (1982) The effects of arachinoids and leukotrienes on the release of mucus from human airways. Chest 81:36S–37S
40. Coles SJ, Neill KH, Reid LM, Austen KF, Nii Y, Corey EJ, Lewis RA (1983) Effects of leukotrienes C_4 and D_4 on glycoprotein and lysozyme secretion by human bronchial mucosa. Prostaglandins 25:155–170
41. Lewis RA, Drazen JM, Austen KF, Clark DA, Corey EJ (1980) Identification of the C(6)-S-conjugate of leukotriene A with cysteine as a naturally occurring slow reacting substance of anaphylaxis (SRS-A). Importance of the 11-*cis* geometry for biological activity. Biochem Biophys Res Commun 96:271–277
42. Dahlen S-E, Bjork J, Hedqvist P, Arfors K-E, Hammarstrom S, Lindgren J-Å, Samuelsson B (1981) Leukotrienes promote plasma leakage and leukocyte adhesion in postcapillary venules: *in vivo* effects with relevance to the acute inflammatory response. Proc Natl Acad Sci USA 78:3887–3891
43. Soter NA, Lewis RA, Corey EJ, Austen KF (1983) Local effects of synthetic leukotrienes (LTC_4, LTD_4, LTE_4, and LTB_4) in human skin. J Invest Dermatol 80:115–119
44. Drazen JM, Austen KF, Lewis RA, Clark DA, Goto G, Marfat A, Corey EJ (1980) Comparative airway and vascular activities of leukotrienes C-1 and D *in vivo* and *in vitro*. Proc Natl Acad Sci USA 77:4354–4358
45. Michelassi F, Landa L, Hill RD, Lowenstein E, Watkins WD, Petkau AJ, Zapol WM (1982) Leukotriene D_4: a potent coronary artery vasoconstrictor associated with impaired ventricular contraction. Science 217:841–843
46. Pfeffer MA, Pfeffer JM, Lewis RA, Braunwald E, Corey EJ, Austen KF (1983) Systemic hemodynamic effects of leukotrienes C_4 and D_4 in the rat. Am J Physiol 244: H628–H633
47. Badr KF, Baylis C, Pfeffer JM, Pfeffer MA, Soberman RJ, Lewis RA, Austen KF, Corey EJ, Brenner BM (1984) Renal and systemic hemodynamic responses to intravenous infusion of leukotriene C_4 in the rat. Circ Res 54:492–499
48. Stenmark KR, James SL, Voelkel NF, Toews WH, Reeves JT, Murphy RC (1983) Leukotriene C_4 and D_4 in neonates with hypoxemia and pulmonary hypertension. N Engl J Med 309:77–80
49. Hoover R, Karnovsky MJ, Austen KF, Corey EJ, Lewis RA (1984) Leukotriene B_4 action on endothelium mediates augmented neutrophil/endothelial adhesion. Proc Natl Acad Sci USA 81:2191–2193
50. Atluru D, Goodwin JS (1984) Control of polyclonal immunoglobulin production from human lymphocytes by leukotrienes; LTB_4 induces an OKT8(+), radiosensitive suppressor cell from resting human OKT8(–) T cells. J Clin Invest 74:1442–1450
51. Payan DG, Goetzl EJ (1983) Specific suppression of human T lymphocyte function by leukotriene B_4. J Immunol 131:551–553
52. Rola-Plezczynski MP, Borgeat P, Sirois P (1982) Leukotriene B_4 induces human suppressor lymphocytes. Biochem Biophys Res Commun 198:1531–1534
53. Vane JR (1978) Inhibitors of prostaglandin, prostacyclin, and thromboxane synthesis. Adv Prostaglandin Thromboxane Leukotriene Res 4:27–44
54. Ham EA, Soderman DD, Zanetti ME, Dougherty HW, McCauley E, Kuehl FA Jr (1983) Inhibition by prostaglandins of leukotriene B_4 release from activated neutrophils. Proc Natl Acad Sci USA 80: 4349–4353
55. Razin E, Romeo LC, Krilis S, Liu F-T, Lewis RA, Corey EJ, Austen KF (1984) An analysis of the relationship between 5-lipoxygenase product generation and the secretion of preformed mediators from mouse bone marrow-derived mast cells. J Immunol 133: 938–945

56. Bach MK, Brashler JR, Smith HW, Fitzpatrick FA, Sun FF, Maguire JC (1982) 6,9-deepoxy-6,9-(phenylimino)-$\Delta^{6,8}$-prostaglandin I_1 (U-60,257), a new inhibitor of leukotriene C and D synthesis: *in vitro* studies. Prostaglandins 23:759–771
57. Goldman DW, Goetzl EJ (1982) Specific binding of leukotriene B_4 to receptors on human polymorphonuclear leukocytes. J Immunol 129:1600–1604
58. Ballermann BJ, Lewis RA, Corey EJ, Austen KF, Brenner BM (1985) Identification and characterization of leukotriene C_4 receptors in isolated rat renal glomeruli. Circ Res 56:324–330
59. Murphy RC, Pickett WC, Culp BR, Lands WEM (1981) Tetraene and pentaene leukotrienes: selective production from murine mastocytoma cells after dietary manipulation. Prostaglandins 22:613–619
60. Leitch AG, Lee TH, Ringel EW, Prickett JD, Robinson DR, Pyne SG, Austen KF, Lewis RA (1984) Immunologically induced generation of tetraene and pentaene leukotrienes in the peritoneal cavities of menhaden-fed rats. J Immunol 132:2559–2565
61. Lee TH, Mencia-Huerta J-M, Shih C, Corey EJ, Lewis RA, Austen KF (1984) Characterization and biological properties of 5,12-dihydroxy derivatives of eicosapentaenoic acid, including leukotriene B_5 and the double lipoxygenase product. J Biol Chem 259:2383–2389
62. Lee TH, Mencia-Huerta J-M, Shih C, Corey EJ, Lewis RA, Austen KF (1984) Effects of exogenous arachidonic, eicosapentaenoic, and docosahexaenoic acids on the generation of 5-lipoxygenase pathway products by ionophore-activated human neutrophils. J Clin Invest 74:1922–1933
63. Hirata F, Notsu Y, Iwata M, Parente L, diRosa M, Flower RJ (1982) Identification of several species of phospholipase inhibiting protein(s) by radioimmunoassay for lipomodulin. Biochem Biophys Res Commun 109:223–230
64. Hirata F, Iwati M (1983) Role of lipomodulin, a phospholipase inhibitory protein in immunoregulation by thymocytes. J Immunol 130:1930–1936
65. Rothhut B, Russo-Marie F, Wood J, diRosa M, Flower RJ (1983) Further characterization of the glucocorticoid-induced antiphospholipase protein 'renocortin.' Biochem Biophys Res Commun 117:878–884
66. Saed SA, McDonald-Gibson WJ, Cuthbert J, Copas JL, Schneider C, Gardiner PJ, Butt NM, Collier HOJ (1977) Endogenous inhibitor of prostaglandin synthetase. Nature 270:32–36
67. Moore PK, Hoult JRS (1980) Anti-inflammatory steroids reduce tissue PG synthetase activity and enhance PG breakdown. Nature 288:269–270
68. Lewis RA, Robin J-L, Austen KF (1985) Pharmacologic regulation of mediator generation and release from the murine bone marrow-derived mast cell. Int Arch Allergy Appl Immunol 77:137–143
69. Godard P, Damon M, Michel FB, Craste de Paulet A, Corey EJ, Ciliberti M, Lewis RA (submitted for publication) Generation of leukotriene B_4, sulfidopeptide leukotrienes, and selected cyclooxygenase products from alveolar macrophages of normal and asthmatic individuals
70. Williams JD, Lee TH, Lewis RA, Austen KF (1985) Intracellular retention of the 5-lipoxygenase pathway product, leukotriene B_4 by human neutrophils activated with opsonized zymosan. J Immunol 134:2624–2630

23. PAF-acether (Platelet Activating Factor)

B. Arnoux, C. Brink, J. Benveniste

When basophils, which were derived from sensitized rabbits, were challenged with a specific allergen a substance was extracted which was capable of aggregating rabbit platelets [3]. Since its initial detection it has been referred to as platelet activating factor (PAF), and more recently acetyl-glyceryl-ether-phosphorylcholine (AGEPC) or PAF-acether. The detection of this ubiquitous compound when various cells or organs are appropriately challenged has led to its acceptance as a pivotal molecule in a variety of pathophysiological conditions.

23.1 Biochemical Structure

Numerous methods can be used for the synthesis of platelet activating factor. In early reports dealing with its preparation, ethanolamine or choline containing plasmalogens from beef hearts were used [10, 23]. The hydrogenation of these choline plasmalogens led to the formation of an alkyl-acyl-glycero-phosphocholine. These compounds were subjected to deacylation by either mild alkaline hydrolysis or methanolysis, a process which yielded a lyso compound (alkyl-glycero-phosphocholine). This latter molecule could then be acetylated to yield 1-O-alkyl-2-acetyl-*sn*-glycero-3-phosphocholine. Recently, total synthesis of platelet activating factor

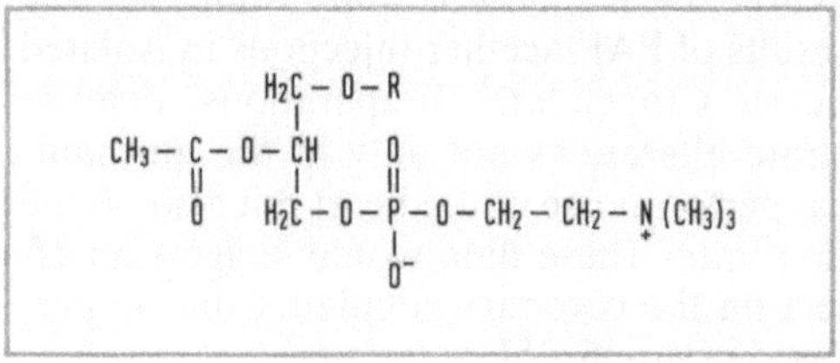

Fig. 23.1. Structure of PAF-acether. R = 16, 18 ...

through the preparation of a lyso compound (lyso PAF) has also been used [27]. In either case the end product (Fig. 23.1) has both the physicochemical and biological properties of the naturally occurring factor. Thus the name PAF-acether was coined as a trivial denomination emphasizing the main structural features of the molecule.

23.2 Detection and Criteria

The acceptance of a biological activity, as being due to PAF-acether, requires some important characterizations [43]. The compound in question should aggregate washed rabbit platelets which have been pretreated with a cyclooxygenase inhibitor (aspirin), in the presence of an ADP enzyme scavenger system (creatine phosphate/creatine phosphokinase). Subsequently, the compound should induce an aggregation that is directly proportional to the amount added to the platelet suspension. The quantity of the putative molecule can be expressed either in weight or in molar concentrations. In addition, the compound must migrate with synthetic PAF-acether in thin layer chromatography as well as elute with it when high performance liquid chromatography (HPLC) methods are employed. The substance must be inactivated by phospholipase A_2 (PLA_2), C and D and exhibit a resistance to *R. arrhizus* lipase challenge [9]. Finally, the compound in question should induce tachyphylaxis when cross-examined against synthetic PAF-acether in washed rabbit platelets. The most preferred way for the detection of PAF-acether is, of course, a structural analysis, but the amount of formed material is usually too low to permit the use of such procedure.

23.3 Source of PAF-acether

The presence of this compound has now been reported for a wide variety of cell types including rodent peritoneal macrophages [32], alveolar macrophages [5] and polymorphonuclear cells [30]. While PAF-acether was first isolated from rabbit basophils [8] its detection in human basophils is still somewhat controversial and results appear to be contradictory [12, 18]. Recently, rabbit platelets have also been shown to produce PAF-acether [2]. When experiments dealing with the formation and detection of PAF-acether in the various cell types are performed, the addition of a stimulatory agent such as the Ca^{2+} ionophore A23187, phagocytable particles, collagen or thrombin, is necessary.

23.4 PAF-acether Metabolism

A series of enzymatic steps appears to be involved in the formation of PAF-acether upon stimulation of the cells. Through the activity of several substrates and enzymes including acyl CoA and acyltransferase, the substrate for PLA_2 is eventually formed, namely 1-alkyl-2-acyl-*sn*-glycero-3-phosphocholine, an analog of phosphatidylcholine that comprises the bulk of membrane phospholipids. The PLA_2 is then capable of hydrolyzing this product to form 1-alkyl-2-lyso-glycero-phosphocholine (2-lyso PAF-acether) which in turn serves as a substrate for the acetyltransferase and for the formation of PAF-acether. The inactivation of PAF-acether depends on acetylhydrolase and acyltransferase activities. Together these two enzymatic systems in activated cells are responsible not only for the formation of the inactive form of PAF-acether, but also the overall rate of biosynthesis of both intracellular and extracellular PAF-acether. The basis for this system has been derived from the experimental evidence gathered in membrane preparations from various cells, namely peritoneal and alveolar macrophages, neutrophils and platelets [1, 2, 7, 29, 35, 48].

23.5 Biological Effects of PAF-acether

Effects on cells: Since the original observation that PAF-acether is a potent aggregatory agent on washed rabbit platelets its activity has also been assessed on platelets [21] from a wide variety of species, including guinea pig, dog and human. It has been known for some time that rat platelets are insensitive to this aggregating agent [34]. Recently, the effect on PAF-acether as an activator of neutrophil aggregation [19], chemotactic activation [22] and lysosomal enzyme and oxygen radical release [36, 41] have been described.

Effect on organs. Vascular effect in vivo: A hypotensive effect of an intravenous injection of PAF-acether in rabbits, guinea pigs, baboons and rats has been reported. In fact, PAF-acether seems to be the same molecule as the antihypertensive polar renomedullary lipid described 25 years ago [14, 33]. In dogs, PAF-acether induces an acute circulatory collapse [11]. In all species the hypotensive effect is independent of platelet aggregation, this is particularly clear in the rat. It has been suggested that this effect may be mediated by adrenolytic activity [17].

Vascular effects in vitro: It is quite surprising that the only direct vascular response to PAF-acether stimulation that has been observed is in the rat portal vein preparation [44]. The absence of effect in isolated vascular muscle preparations has been reported [20]. We were unable to show any direct effect in isolated dog coronary arteries [R. Santamaria, unpublished observations]. It appears that while isolated vessels do not respond to this phosphoether lipid, they do when present in an intact organ such as the heart. The response is quite dramatic. The results of PAF-acether injections in isolated heart Langendorff preparations demonstrate alterations not only in the mechanical performance of the heart but also on the flow rate. These data would suggest an effect on the coronary circulation in the perfused organ [6, 25].

Pro-edematous effects: When PAF-acether was intradermally administered to the rat

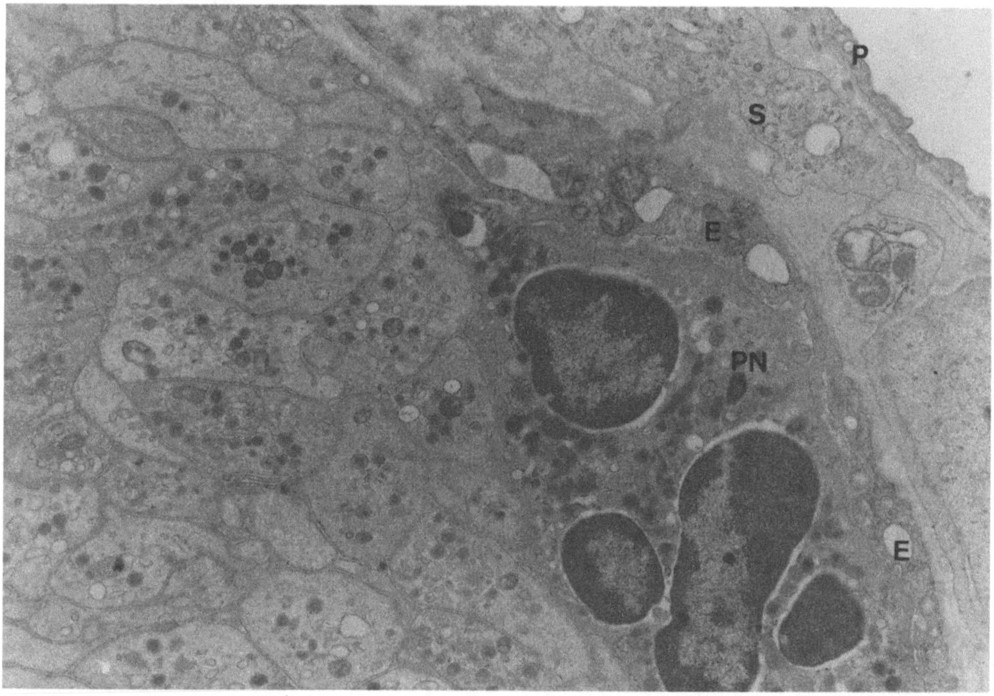

Fig. 23.2. Guinea pig, 90 s after intrajugular injection of 100 ng/kg PAF-acether. Histologic examination of the lung: capillary thrombosis with aggregated platelets, several of which are degranulated. PN = marginated polymorphonuclear neutrophils; E = endothelial cells; S = septal cell; P = pneumocytes (×16,000). (Prof. A. Pfister, Laboratoire d'Histologie et d'Embryologie, Faculté de Médecine Necker-Enfants Malades, 75015 Paris, France)

or in a human it induced edema and in the latter case hyperalgesia [3, 13, 15, 39, 40]. This effect was partially inhibited by a cyclooxygenase inhibitor [15] although this result was not confirmed by other authors [13, 39, 40]. This effect appears to be independent of platelets and neutrophil activation [13, 40]. Recently, a dual response – early and late – was reported in human skin [3].

Lung and PAF-acether

In vivo effect: The capacity of PAF-acether to induce a bronchoconstriction in guinea pigs was first described by Vargaftig et al [46]. Intravenous administration induced an immediate increase of inspiratory pressure, reflecting a bronchoconstriction. This phenomenon is associated with thrombocytopenia and a pretreatment of animals with an anti-platelet serum abolished the effects of PAF-acether [46]. Those mechanisms involved in the bronchoconstriction due to PAF-acether have not been clearly elucidated. However, there appears to be a relationship between the route of administration of this factor and the primary sites of action, that is, either cyclooxygenase-dependent [47] or through a lipoxygenase activity [16]. It is difficult to reconcile these results obtained in the same animal species but it may be partially due to the procedures used in the experimental protocols, namely anesthesia, antagonist medication or the quantity of PAF-acether injected.

Using a radiolabeling technique for platelet analysis the trapping of platelets by the lung was observed in the guinea pig 30 s after the bronchoconstriction [37] (Fig. 23.2). This observation suggested a relationship between the bronchoconstriction and the platelets. Anaphylactic effects of

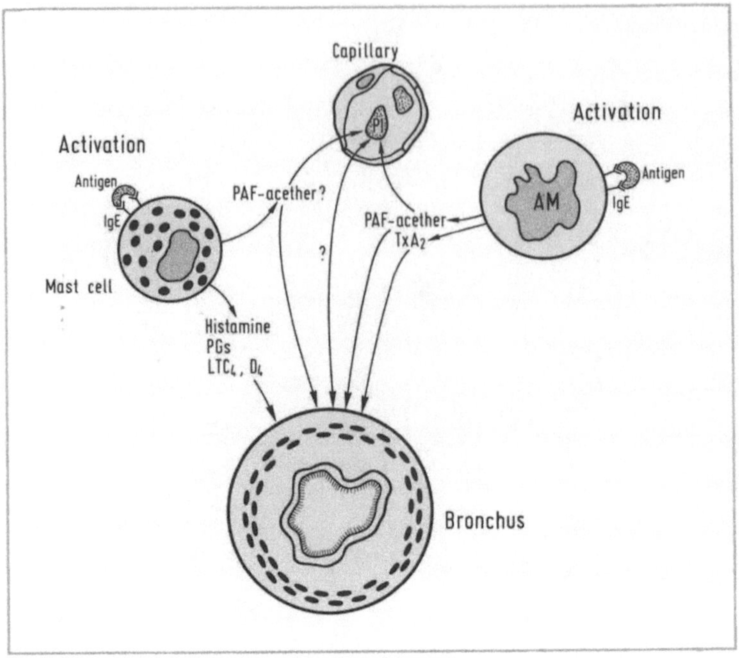

Fig. 23.3. The two possible mechanisms of bronchial obstruction. Pl = platelet

Table 23.1. Release of PAF-acether and lyso PAF-acether from alveolar macrophages by pneumallergens

Macrophages	PAF-acether	Lyso PAF-acether
Nonasthmatic	0 ±0	74±16
Asthmatic	1.2±0.3	110±15
Asthmatic corticoid-treated	0 ±0	15± 1

Results in pmol (mean ± SEM). Alveolar macrophages: 2.5×10^5. Number of experiments: 3–12

PAF-acether have also been described in the rabbit [31].

Recently, the acute effect of PAF-acether was demonstrated on primates, namely the baboon [24] and *Macaca mulatta* [38]. The increase in peak inspiratory pressure after intratracheal deposition of 60 μg/kg of PAF-acether was associated with blood, blood gas and cell modifications. None of these parameter changes were altered if the animal had been pretreated with aspirin, that is, PAF-acether was still effective [24].

A preliminary report of the biological effects of PAF-acether in comatous (cerebral death) patients has recently been published [26]. In these experiments PAF-acether induced an increase in peak inspiratory pressure as well as changes in blood and blood gas values. We also observed significant cardiac modifications, such as a severe drop in the left ventricle stroke work index.

In vitro effect: A direct contractile effect of PAF-acether was reported on guinea pig ileum and lung tissue [45]. However, we were unable to consistently reproduce these results in human and guinea pig lung and ileum tissues [20]. Results using the guinea pig lung parenchymal strip have been especially disappointing since the contractile response, when observed, is extremely small [20]. A small relaxation has been reported for guinea pig tracheal preparations [42]. These data suggest that respiratory muscles are probably not the primary target organ in the pulmonary response to PAF-acether.

Importance of alveolar macrophages: We have recently described the presence of a specific IgE response in alveolar macrophages from atopic patients [28]. These cells are able to release a lysosomal enzyme in the specific allergen challenge as well as PAF-acether. When similar protocols were performed on alveolar macrophages obtained from treated patients (theophylline or corticosteroid) this release was not observed [4] (Table 23.1).

23.6 Conclusions

It is now well accepted that PAF-acether (1-O-alkyl-2-acetyl-*sn*-glycero-phospholipid) can be detected in a variety of cell types which have been stimulated with specific agents. This increase in phosphoether lipid production and/or release can be associated with various inflammatory states. However, the mechanism of its action appears to be quite complex. In fact, the major discrepancies between *in vivo* and *in vitro* observations suggest a multifactorial component for its activity. Within the past few years, cellular components of the human lung, namely alveolar macrophages and mastocytes have been investigated. While their ability to release considerable amounts of smooth muscle contractile and vasoactive substances is well-known, our recent observation that alveolar macrophages release PAF-acether upon specific antigenic stimulation suggests another possible role for these cells and their mediators in pulmonary inflammation and asthma (Fig. 23.3).

References

1. Albert DH, Snyder F (1983) Biosynthesis of 1-alkyl-2-acetyl-*sn*-glycero-phosphocholine by rat alveolar macrophages. J Biol Chem 258:97–102
2. Alonso F, Garcia Gil M, Sanchez-Crespo M, Mato JM (1982) Activation of 1-alkyl-2-lyso-glycero-3-phosphocholine: acetyl-CoA transferase during phagocytosis in human polymorphonuclear leukocytes. J Biol Chem 257:3376–3378
3. Archer CB, Page CP, Paul W, Morley J, McDonald DM (1984) Inflammatory characteristics of platelet-activating factor (PAF-acether) in human skin. Br J Dermatol 110:45–50
4. Arnoux B, Simoes-Caeiro MH, Landes A, Mathieu M, Duroux P, Benveniste J (1982) Alveolar macrophages from asthmatic patients release platelet-activating factor (PAF-acether) and lyso PAF-acether when stimulated with the specific allergen. Am Rev Respir Dis 125:70 (abstract)
5. Arnoux B, Duval D, Benveniste J (1980) Release of platelet-activating (PAF) from alveolar macrophages by calcium ionophore A 23187 and phagocytosis. Eur J Clin Invest 10:437–441
6. Benveniste J, Boullet C, Brink C, Labat C (1983) The actions of PAF-acether (platelet-activating factor) on guinea pig-isolated heart preparations. Br J Pharmacol 80:81–83
7. Benveniste J, Chignard M, Le Couedic JP, Vargaftig BB (1982) Biosynthesis of platelet-activating factor (PAF-acether). II. Involvement of phospholipase A_2 in the formation of PAF-acether and lyso-PAF-acether from rabbit platelets. Thromb Res 25:375–386
8. Benveniste J, Henson PM, Cochrane CG (1972) Leukocyte-dependent histamine release from rabbit platelets: the role of IgE, basophils and a platelet-activating factor. J Exp Med 136:1356–1377
9. Benveniste J, Le Couedic JP, Polonsky J, Tencé M (1977) Structural analysis of purified platelet-activating factor by lipases. Nature 269:170–171
10. Benveniste J, Tencé M, Varenne P, Bidault J, Boullet C, Polonsky J (1979) Semi-synthèse et structure proposée du facteur activant les plaquettes (PAF): PAF-acéther, un alkyl éther analogue de la lysophosphatidylcholine. CR Acad Sc Paris 289D:1037–1040
11. Bessin P, Bonnet J, Apffel D, Soulard C, Desgroux L, Pelas I, Benveniste J (1983) Acute circulatory collapse caused by platelet-activating factor (PAF-acether) in dogs. Eur J Pharmacol 86:403–413
12. Betz SJ, Lotner GZ, Henson PM (1980) Generation and release of platelet-activating factor (PAF) from enriched preparations of rabbit basophils; failure of human basophils to release PAF. J Immunol 125:2749–2755
13. Björk J, Smedegard G (1983) Acute microvascular effects of PAF-acether, as studied by intravital microscopy. Eur J Pharmacol 96:87–94
14. Blank ML, Snyder F, Byers LW, Brooks B, Muirhead EE (1979) Antihypertensive activity of an alkyl ether analog of phosphatidylcholine. Biochem Biophys Res Commun 90:1194–1200
15. Bonnet J, Loiseau AM, Orvaen M, Bessin P (1981) Platelet-activating factor (PAF-acether) involvement in acute inflammatory and pain process. In: Russo-Marie F, Vargaftig BB, Benveniste J (eds) Pharmacology

of Inflammation and Allergy: Lipids and Cells, vol. 100. INSERM, Paris, pp 111–118
16. Bonnet J, Thibaudeau D, Bessin P (1983) Dependency of the PAF-acether-induced bronchospasm on the lipoxygenase pathway in the guinea-pig. Prostaglandins 26:457–466
17. Caillard CC, Mondot S, Julou L (1981) Action hypotensive du PAF-acéther chez le rat. J Pharmacol 12:301 (abstract)
18. Camussi G, Aglietta M, Coda R, Bussolino F, Piacibello W, Tetta C (1981) Release of platelet-activating factor (PAF) and histamine. II. The cellular origin of PAF: monocytes, polymorphonuclear neutrophils and basophils. Immunology 42:191–199
19. Camussi G, Tetta C, Bussolino F, Caligaris Cappio F, Coda R, Masera C, Segoloni G (1981) Mediators of immune complex-induced aggregation of polymorphonuclear neutrophils. II. Platelet-activating factor as the effector substance of immune-induced aggregation. Int Arch Allergy Appl Immunol 64:25–41
20. Cerrina J, Raffestin B, Labat C, Boullet C, Bayol A, Gateau O, Brink C (1983) Effects of PAF-acether on isolated muscle preparations from the rat, guinea pig and human lung. In: Benveniste J, Arnoux B (eds) Platelet-Activating Factor and Structurally-Related Ether Lipids. Elsevier, Amsterdam, pp 205–212 (INSERM Symposium no. 23)
21. Chignard M, Le Couedic JP, Tencé M, Vargaftig BB, Benveniste J (1979) The role of platelet-activating factor in platelet aggregation. Nature 279:799–800
22. Czarnetzki MB, Benveniste J (1981) Effect of 1-O-octadecyl-2-O-acetyl-*sn*-glycero-3-phosphorylcholine (PAF-acether) on leukocytes. I. Analysis of the in vitro migration of human neutrophils. Chem Phys Lipids 29:317–326
23. Demopoulos CA, Pinckard RN, Hanahan DJ (1979) Platelet-activating factor. Evidence for 1-O-alkyl-2-acetyl-*sn*-glyceryl-3-phosphorylcholine as the active component (a new class of lipid chemical mediators). J Biol Chem 254:9355–9358
24. Denjean A, Arnoux B, Masse R, Lockhart A, Benveniste J (1983) Acute effect of intratracheal administration of PAF-acether in baboons. J Appl Physiol 55:799–804
25. Feuerstein G, Boyd LM, Ezra D, Goldstein RE (1984) Effect of platelet-activating factor on coronary circulation of the domestic pig. Am J Physiol 246:H466–H471
26. Gateau O, Arnoux B, Deriaz H, Benveniste J (1984) Acute effects of intratracheal administration of PAF-acether (platelet-activating factor) in humans. Am Rev Respir Dis 129:A3 (abstract)
27. Godfroid JJ, Heymans F, Michel E, Redeuilh C, Steiner E, Benveniste J (1980) Platelet-activating factor (PAF-acether): total synthesis of 1-O-octadecyl-2-O-acetyl-sn-glycero-3-phosphorylcholine. FEBS Lett 116:161–164
28. Joseph M, Tonnel AB, Torpier G, Capron A, Arnoux B, Benveniste J (1983) The involvement of IgG in the secretory processes of alveolar macrophages from asthmatic patients. J Clin Invest 71:221–230
29. Lee T-C, Malone B, Wasserman SI, Fitzgerald V, Snyder F (1982) Activities of enzymes that metabolize platelet-activating factor (1-alkyl-2-acetyl-*sn*-glycero-3-phosphocholine) in neutrophils and eosinophils from humans and the effect of a calcium ionophore. Biochem Biophys Res Commun 105:1303–1308
30. Lotner GZ, Lynch JM, Betz SJ, Henson PM (1980) Human neutrophil-derived platelet-activating factor. J Immunol 124:676–684
31. McManus LM, Hanahan DJ, Demopoulos CA, Pinckard RN (1980) Pathobiology of the intravenous infusion of acetyl-glyceryl-ether-phosphorylcholine (AGEPC), a synthetic platelet-activating factor (PAF) in the rabbit. J Immunol 124:2919–2924
32. Mencia-Huerta JM, Benveniste J (1979) Platelet-activating factor (PAF) and macrophages. I. Evidence for the release from rat and mouse peritoneal macrophages and not from mastocytes. Eur J Immunol 9:409–415
33. Muirhead EE, Stirman JA (1958) Dietary protein and hypertension in the dog: protection by ureterocaval anastomosis with a study of the kidneys so treated. Am J Pathol 34:561 (abstract)
34. Namm DH, Tadepalli AS, High JA (1982) Species specificity of the platelet responses to 1-O-alkyl-2-acetyl-*sn*-glycero-3-phosphocholine. Thromb Res 25:341–350
35. Ninio E, Mencia-Huerta JM, Heymans F, Benveniste J (1982) Biosynthesis of platelet-activating factor (PAF-acether). I. Evidence for an acetyltransferase activity in murine macrophages. Biochim Biophys Acta 710:23–31
36. O'Flaherty JT, Wykle RL, Miller CH, Lewis JC, Waite M, Bass DA, McCall MD, deChatelet LR (1981) 1-O-alkyl-*sn*-glyceryl-3-phosphorylcholines. A novel class of neutrophil stimulants. Am J Pathol 103:70–78
37. Page CP, Paul W, Douglas GJ, Casals-Stenzel J, Morley J (1983) PAF-acether, platelets and bronchospasm. In: Benveniste J, Arnoux B (eds) Platelet-Activating Factor and Struc-

turally-Related Ether-Lipids. Elsevier, Amsterdam, pp 327–334 (INSERM Symposium no. 23)

38. Patterson R, Harris KE (1983) The activity of aerosolized and intracutaneous synthetic platelet-activating factor (AGEPC) in rhesus monkeys with IgE-mediated airway responses and normal monkeys. J Lab Clin Med 102:933–938
39. Pinckard RN, Kniker WT, Lee L, Hanahan DJ, McManus LM (1980) Vasoactive properties of 1-O-alkyl-2-acetyl-*sn*-glyceryl-3-phosphocholine (AcGEPC) in human skin. J Allergy Clin Immunol 63:196 (abstract)
40. Pirotzky E, Page CP, Roubin R, Pfister A, Paul W, Bonnet J, Benveniste J (1984) PAF-acether-induced plasma exudation in rat skin is independent of platelets and neutrophils. Microcirc Endothel Lymph 1:107–122
41. Poitevin B, Roubin R, Benveniste J (1984) PAF-acether generates chemiluminescence in human neutrophils in the absence of cytochalasin B. Immunopharmacology 7:135–144
42. Prancan A, Lefort J, Barton M, Vargaftig BB (1982) Relaxation of the guinea pig trachea induced by platelet-activating factor and by serotonin. Eur J Pharmacol 80:29–35
43. Roubin R, Tencé M, Mencia-Huerta JM, Arnoux B, Ninio E, Benveniste J (1983) A chemically defined monokine-macrophage-defined platelet-activating factor. In: Pick E (ed) Lymphokines, vol. 8. Academic Press, New York, pp 249–276
44. Santamaria R, Pourrias B, Benveniste J (1983) Effet du PAF-acéther sur la veine porte de rat. J Pharmacol 14 [Suppl]:83 (abstract)
45. Stimler NP, Bloor CM, Hugli TE, Wykle RL, McCall CE, O'Flaherty JT (1981) Anaphylactic actions of platelet-activating factor. Am J Pathol 105:64–69
46. Vargaftig BB, Lefort J, Chignard M, Benveniste J (1980) Platelet-activating factor induces a platelet-dependent bronchoconstriction unrelated to the formation of prostaglandin derivatives. Eur J Pharmacol 65:185–192
47. Vargaftig B, Lefort J, Rotilio D (1983) Route-dependent interactions between PAF-acether and guinea-pig bronchopulmonary smooth muscle: relevance of cyclooxygenase mechanism. In: Benveniste J, Arnoux B (eds) Platelet-Activating Factor and Structurally-Related Ether-Lipids. Elsevier, Amsterdam, pp 307–316 (INSERM Symposium no. 23)
48. Wykle RL, Malone B, Snyder F (1980) Enzymatic synthesis of 1-alkyl-2-acetyl-*sn*-glycero-3-phosphocholine, a hypotensive and platelet-aggregating lipid. J Biol Chem 255:10256–10260

24. Immediate-type Reactions

B. Zweiman, P. C. Atkins

It is useful, conceptually, to divide pathological features in asthma into three separate categories:

- smooth muscle spasm;
- airways inflammation with edema; and
- mucous hypersecretion [27].

We will concentrate in this chapter on the mechanisms leading to inflammation of the airway in immediate hypersensitivity reactions.

In the majority of adults presenting with asthma, the disease is chronic and a significant history of allergic reactions accounting for a major portion of the disease is found in no more than 20% of such cases. However, clear-cut asthmatic reactions do occur after antigenic exposure. Recent studies indicate that such reactions can persist for hours. Furthermore, utilizing inhalation challenge of antigen in susceptible subjects, the asthmatic reaction can be initiated in the laboratory and studied in regard to the release of mediators. The latter can then be correlated with pathophysiological events. Utilizing such studies, it has become clear that the asthmatic reaction is a result of the production of inflammatory mediators and cellular inflammatory responses as well as the production of smooth muscle spasm. We will review the current understanding of the importance of the pathways of inflammation in the pathophysiology of asthma, utilizing data accumulated after antigenic challenge of the lung, nose and skin of human allergic subjects.

Since the mast cell plays an important role in the initiation of inflammatory as well as other responses in immediate hypersensitivity reactions, it is important to consider the location of such cells and their relationship to the airway lumen through which inhaled allergens, irritants and microorganisms pass. There are relatively few mast cells in the superficial mucosa [27]. Therefore, it has been questioned how the relatively large airborne molecules which seem to precipitate inflammatory responses in asthma can reach the mast cells and other relevant tissue components. It has been suggested [27] that these antigenic or irritant molecules react with the relatively small number of mast cells on the bronchial epithelial surface. The resultant activation of mast cells and their subsequent release of chemical mediators lead to openings of the tight epithelial junctions, allowing penetration of the exogenous agents to a larger concentration of mast cells in the deeper area.

24.1 Bronchial Hyperreactivity in Asthma

Following exposure of mast cells in the skin or airways of sensitive subjects to antigen, activation starts within minutes. A resultant reaction peaks at 20–30 min and may persist for hours. In most highly sensitive subjects exposed to large concentrations of antigen, this reaction recurs or progresses over a period of 12–24 hours. Although the reaction can be thought of as a continuum, certain differences in response to pharmacologic agents have made it useful to divide the first (immediate) 1–4 hours from the second (late onset) 4–12 hours of this response. We shall focus primarily upon the immediate response; the late onset response will be discussed in the next chapter.

Twenty years ago, inhalation challenge studies documented that allergic subjects with asthma were 3–35 times more sensitive to the inhalation of bronchoconstrictive substances such as histamine or methacholine than allergic subjects without asthma and 75 times more sensitive than nonallergic subjects [57]. In this study, it was also suggested that inhalation challenge with the appropriate antigen would differentiate those atopic subjects with asthma from atopic subjects without asthma. However, follow-up studies indicated that sensitivity to antigen during inhalation challenge could not differentiate rhinitis from asthmatic subjects, but rather that bronchial inhalation sensitivity correlated well with skin and basophil sensitivity to antigen. It appeared that antigen-induced bronchospasm was dependent upon a combination of a) the bronchial lability (measured by sensitivity to inhaled histamine) and, b) the degree of antigen sensitivity (as measured by skin test reactivity) [15, 16, 20, 60]. More recently, there are reports of changes in bronchial lability secondary to naturally occurring antigenic exposure [13, 19, 60]. How do such changes occur? Recent data suggest that infiltration of neutrophilic leukocytes into airways can promote changes in bronchial irritability. Thus, a concept emerges in which a vicious cycle is initiated in patients with increased bronchial irritability and sensitivity to antigen. Following an encounter with antigen, there is a resultant asthmatic episode with associated inflammatory cell infiltration. This results in an increase in bronchial irritability making them more succeptible to further asthmatic episodes. What are the inflammatory events that lead to this vicious cycle during an immediate bronchospastic episode?

24.2 Inflammation in the Airways

To understand these events, we must try to define what we mean by inflammation. In its broadest sense, inflammation results from a combination of vasodilation, increased vascular permeability, and emigration of fluids and cells out of the vessels and into tissues. The typical pathologic findings that may be due to inflammatory reactions in chronic asthma include: markedly edematous mucosa, frequently with detached epithelial cells and cilia; thickened basement membrane and bronchial smooth muscle; and dilated submucosal vessels with prominent accumulation of inflammatory cells both within and around vessels. Eosinophils are most prominent with lesser numbers of neutrophils, lymphocytes and plasma cells; a marked exudative reaction often leading to viscid and tenacious mucous plugs. The latter are composed of mucous, some serum proteins including immunoglobulins, inflammatory cells and their components such as the crystalloids of eosinophils (Charcot-Leyden crystals). Fibrin deposition has not been described as a major feature in the bronchial wall or exudate.

In allergic reactions, inflammation appears to be initiated by the release of mediators as a consequence of mast cell activation leading to these vascular changes and cellular accumulation. Products and/ or components of other cells present in or entering the site may also play a role in perpetuating this reaction. There is now a substantial amount of data to prove that indeed such *mediators of inflammation* are released during ongoing allergic inflammatory reactions in humans.

Using an inhalation challenge model (Table 24.1), it was shown after antigen-induced, but not methacholine-induced, bronchospasm in atopic individuals was accompanied by release into the circulation of a heat-stable, high molecular weight neutrophil chemotactic activity (HMW-NCA) [4]. This activity appeared in the circulation 1 min after inhalation of antigen, peaked at 10 min and persisted for up to 24 hours after the induction of bronchospasm in some subjects [5]. The amount of chemotactic activity appearing in the circulation correlated with the degree of bronchospasm induced, the amount of antigen administered, and the increase in circulating neutrophils that occurred after the antigen-induced bronchospasm [5, 6]. That the source of HMW-NCA is mast cell-related is suggested by a) the inhibition of the appearance of NCA by pretreatment with disodium cromoglycate (a mast cell stabilizer) [5, 39]; b) appearance in the supernatants after antigen challenge of human and guinea pig lung fragments [41, 45]; and c) its correlation with the systemic release of histamine after antigen-induced bronchospasm in humans [2]. HMW-NCA has also been released into the circulation after milk- [43] and house dust-induced [40]

Table 24.1. Mediators of inflammation released *in vivo* after antigen challenge of the airways

Mediator	Organ	Antigen	Action
Histamine	Lung, nose	Challenge dust, milk exercise [a]	Vasodilation, vascular permeability
HMW-NCA	Lung	Pollen, dust milk, exercise [a]	Neutrophil accumulation, neutrophil activation
Heat-labile NCA	Lung	Pollen, dust	Neutrophil accumulation
Leukotriene C_4	Nose	Pollen	Vasodilation, vascular permeability, bronchospasm
PGD_2	Nose	Pollen	Vasodilation, vascular permeability, broncho-spasm
Kallikrein	Nose	Pollen	Activation of coagulation, kinin pathways
Platelet activating factor [b] (PAF, AGEPC)	Lung	Pollen	Platelet activation, activation of coagulation, neutrophil accumulation
Eosinophil cationic protein	Lung	Pollen, dust	? toxicity to bronchomotor reactivity, ? vascular endothelial toxicity

[a] Exercise challenge is included because it is thought that mast cells are activated leading to mediator release (see text)

[b] PAF has not actually been demonstrated, rather a release of platelet factor 4 into the circulation has been found after antigen-, but not methacholine-, induced bronchospasm; HMW-NCA = high molecular weight – neutrophil chemotactic activity; NCA = neutrophil chemotactic activity

bronchospasm and in at least one nonantigenic form of bronchospasm that may be mast cell-mediated in some atopic and nonatopic subjects, exercise-induced bronchospasm [29–31, 38]. In summary then, in bronchospasm of diverse types, after mast cell activation, there appears a potent neutrophil chemotactic activity in the circulation. This HMW-NCA has been demonstrated to have in vivo biologic activity in attracting neutrophils into the circulation and (by inference) locally into the respiratory tract tissue.

Early studies, utilizing radioenzymatic assays sensitive to ng quantities, described increases in plasma histamine during bronchospasm [7, 12, 35] and in naturally occurring asthma [46]. However, these findings were difficult to interpret because of the presence of nonhistamine plasma components which mimicked histamine in these assays [8]. More recently, utilizing a combination of thin layer chromatography and more sensitive (detecting picogram/ml levels) assay procedures, several laboratories have confirmed the earlier observations that increases in circulating levels of histamine do occur during naturally occurring asthma [10], as well as after bronchospasm induced by exercise [29] or after inhalation of antigen [2, 14].

There has been more limited investigation of circulating levels of some other potential pathogenetic mediators during naturally occurring or antigen-induced asthma. Increases in the serum levels of a heat-labile neutrophil chemotactic activity different than the HMW-NCA has been reported [59]. These investigators have also described increased serum levels of an eosinophilic cationic protein during antigen-induced bronchospasm. The latter may be of interest because of the frequent prominent accumulation of eosinophils in the bronchial walls of asthmatics (vide infra) and the reported deleterious in vitro effects of eosinophilic components on such tissues. Although the leukotrienes C_4/D_4 are potent bronchoconstrictors [24], technical factors have limited definition whether the serum levels of these agents increase during asthma. Increased serum levels of platelet factor 4 during asthmatic reactions suggest the possible participation by the potent pro-inflammatory agents, platelet activating factor, AGEPC. It is not yet clear whether intravascular coagulation-kinin pathways are activated in vivo in asthma. Utilizing nasal challenges with pollen grains, immediate reactions occurring in sensitive subjects have been shown to correlate with the presence in nasal washes of histamine, peptide leukotrienes and a kinin activator [21, 36, 44].

Thus, in vivo challenge of the upper and/or lower airways has been shown to result in the immediate appearance of inflammatory mediators that can attract neutrophils, as well as mediators that promote increases in vasodilation and vascular permeability and activation of kinin and coagulation pathways. Although the findings in the plasma/serum of asthmatics may be quite important, it should be recognized that they may not fully reflect events at the asthmatic reaction site itself. Logistic and ethical constraints limit sequential comparisons of local bronchial mediator release and inflammatory responses following inhalation of allergens or irritants by asthmatics. Therefore, studies of allergic inflammatory reactions in the skin have been utilized to shed more light on the local production of mediators and their correlation with histopathologic events.

24.3 Inflammation in Allergic Skin Reactions (Table 24.2)

Table 24.2. Possible mediators in immediate allergic skin reactions[a]

Histamine
Chemotactic factors
Leukotrienes
Other arachidonic acid metabolites
Coagulation – kinin activation components[b]

[a] Based upon *in vivo* studies to date – much of the information is new and requires confirmation/further elucidation

[b] Evidence for role in late cutaneous reaction – role in immediate reactions not defined

Sequential histologic studies of such reaction sites over a 4-hour period [3] have shown: at 20 min there is prominent intercellular edema in the dermis with few inflammatory cells; starting at about one hour, there is an increasing accumulation of inflammatory cells, initially in the perivascular areas and later in the interstitium. These cells are initially mainly neutrophils with eosinophil accumulation becoming prominent between 2–4 hours. Mononuclear cell accumulation becomes more prominent at 6–8 hours [49]. The degree of tissue eosinophil infiltration appears to depend in part on a) the circulating eosinophil count, and b) the degree of antigen sensitivity of the subject [61]. The role of the skin mast cell in initiation of such reactions is underlined by our observations that: a) intradermal injection of compound 48/80 or codeine, nonimmunologic mast cell activators, will induce patterns of gross and histologic cellular inflammatory responses similar to that seen following antigen injection in the same subject [3, 53]; b) ultramicroscopic evidence of mast cell alterations starting at 15 s after antigen injection [53]; c) local application of agents which inhibit mast cell alterations and local release of histamine will also lead to a decreased inflammatory cell accumulation [56].

Studies of exudative cellular inflammatory responses in IgE-mediated reaction sites have also been carried out using various types of skin windows applied to abraded skin. Earlier studies [25, 26] focused mainly on the reactions starting several hours after antigen application to such abraded skin sites. Prominent accumulation of granulocytes, particularly eosinophils, were noted. However, concerns were raised about a) difficulties in quantifying the inflammatory cells which were frequently distorted and clumped on the appended cover glasses and b) the prominent cell exudation even at control sites. More recently, skin blister techniques [28, 53] have at least partially overcome such technical obstacles. For example, we have found [11, 50] that the application of antigen to the base of an unroofed skin blister in sensitive subjects is followed by a progressive increase in first neutrophils and then eosinophils over a 4-hour period. This response is significantly greater than seen at control sites, and does not occur in individuals not sensitive to the particular antigen.

How are such inflammatory responses initiated? As mentioned earlier, prominent alterations of the dermal mast cells occur starting within 15 s after intradermal antigen injection [53]. Thus, it is appropriate to look first at the possible role of mast cell components in such responses.

The injection of purified rat mast cell granules into rat skin reproduces some of the inflammatory responses induced by IgE-dependent mast cell degranulation including a transient local increase in vascular permeability over 30 min, followed by polymorphonuclear infiltrates at 2–8 hours and then mononuclear cell accumulation at 24–48 hours [52]. Injection of solubilized granule components suggests: a) matrix-associated components, particularly a 1,400 MW polypeptide, induce a similar pattern of inflammatory cell responses as does the whole granule; b) no increase in vascular permeability is induced [42]. Analogous studies using granules of human mast cells have not been reported.

The nature of the mediators responsible for the human skin inflammatory findings described above has been a subject of increasing interest and investigation. Histamine has traditionally been considered the major mediator released in IgE-mediated skin reactions. Histamine release has been documented in vitro and in blisters overlying allergic skin reaction sites [23, 28, 33]. Using a skin chamber model that allows sequential monitoring of local in vivo histamine release, such release has been demonstrated, starting within minutes after antigen application and persisting for at least 4 hours in some individuals [11, 50, 53].

Is such released histamine responsible for the inflammatory events observed? Intradermal injection of appropriate histamine concentrations will induce an immediate wheal and flare response but without the more delayed responses also seen at antigen injection sites. Although low histamine concentrations may be modestly chemotactic for eosinophils in vitro [18] most observers have not found prominent eosinophil responses at sites where histamine, by itself, has been injected or applied [3, 17, 55, 58].

Several low molecular mast cell weight components are potential attractants for inflammatory cells in allergic skin reactions [reviewed in 9]. At least 2 tetrapeptides, about 500 MW, termed ECF-A, exist preformed in basophils and mast cells, and preferentially attract eosinophils in vitro. Certain synthetic tetrapeptides (Val-Gly-Ser-Glu and Ala-Gly-Ser-Glu) will attract eosinophils in vitro and induced eosinophil accumulation at sites of intradermal injection [17, 57]. It is of note that increased vascular permeability is not prominent after such reactions. A higher (1,500–3,000) MW component with in vitro eosinophilotactic activity has been found in the blood draining appropriate challenge reactions in individuals with physical urticarias [9]. We [55] have found the in vivo release of a low molecular eosinophil chemotactic factor with skin chambers at the site of allergic skin reactions.

Several of the leukotrienes exhibit both in vitro and in vivo effects on inflammatory responses. LTC_4 and LTD_4 have been released from human lung mast cell suspensions after in vitro anti-IgE challenge [34]. In our skin chamber studies, these leukotrienes accumulate at allergic reaction sites, generally over several hours [51]. Intradermal injection of synthetic LTC_4 or LTD_4 preparations induces vasodilation and a delayed onset wheal reaction [32]. The cellular origins of LTB_4 are not well defined. LTB_4 is a potent chemoattractant for both neutrophils and eosinophils in vitro and induces a tender reaction with prominent neutrophil infiltration at 6 hours after intradermal injection in humans [32]. In skin chamber studies, impressive accumulation of LTB_4 at allergic reaction sites has not been demonstrable [51].

PGD_2 is a prostaglandin released from human mast cells [34]. Intradermal injection of synthetic PGD_2 induces an immediate transient whealing reaction. It is currently unclear whether PGD_2 is released during immediate human allergic skin reactions. In one study [22] there was evidence of impressive fibrin deposition at 6–8 hours in late phase reactions but not in the immediate wheal and flare allergic reaction.

Indirect evidence for the role of different mediators in immediate allergic skin reactions may be found in studies of the possible modulation of such reactions by therapeutic agents. Cromolyn does not inhibit codeine-induced histamine release [54]. Antihistamines inhibit to varying degree the immediate wheal and flare response in such reactions. However, the inflammatory cell accumulation was not altered in such sites even when the whealing response was markedly suppressed by prior hydroxyzine treatment [3]. Conversely, when corticosteroids were administered, inflammatory cell infiltration was markedly reduced [47, 48] even though antigen-induced whealing responses were not altered significantly [46]. Neither cyclooxygenase inhibitors nor orally administered β_2-adrenergic agonists significantly affect the whealing response; however, topical terbutaline has been shown to inhibit both local histamine release and eosinophil accumulation in reaction sites [56]. Thus, these studies also support the impression that different mediators are responsible for different aspects of the allergic inflammatory response.

24.4 Conclusions

In the studies that we have reviewed above, it is clearly shown in humans that mast cell activation (of the skin or airways) can result in the release of mediators that can produce *inflammation,* i.e., increased vasodilation and vascular permeability with accumulation of fluid and inflammatory cells in the local tissues. Once inflammatory cells are present locally, the action of chemotactic factors upon these cells produces a metabolic burst of activity. In the case of neutrophils, this metabolic burst results in the production of arachidonic acid metabolites, (predominantly leukotriene B_4 and prostaglandins) and superoxide radicals and possibly other factors deleterious to the bronchial tissues. Since depletion of granulocytes reduces airway hyperresponsiveness in certain animal models, and since introduction of granulocytes into the lung increases irritability [37], it is felt that one or more of the products of activated neutrophils is responsible for this increased bronchomotor responsiveness. Furthermore, in animal models, arachidonic acid metabolites have been shown to enhance mast cell mediator release. Thus, inflammation is a two-edged sword. Mast cell activation can induce a local inflammatory response, which in turn can result in

- toxic effects on local tissue,
- bronchomotor hyperresponsiveness, and
- further mast cell mediator release.

It is also possible that a non-mast cell-mediated response can result in a local inflammatory cell accumulation, leading to bronchial hyperresponsiveness, mast cell mediator release and further inflammation. At the present time the occurrence of inflammation during immediate hypersensitivity responses in the lung, nose and skin is indisputable. Its role in the production of symptoms remains to be elucidated. However, perhaps the dramatic beneficial clinical effects of corticosteroids, whose action is predominantly *anti-inflammatory,* supports the important role of inflammation in the pathophysiology of asthma.

References

1. Adams GK, Newball HH, Lichtenstein LM (1982) Generation of leukotrienes by purified human mast cells. J Clin Invest 70:747–751
2. Atkins PC, Bedard RM, Zweiman B, Dyer J, Kaliner MA (1984) Increased antigen-induced local and systemic mediator release in rhinitis subjects with pulmonary symptoms in the pollen season. J Allergy Clin Immunol 73:341–347
3. Atkins PC, Green GR, Zweiman B (1973) Histologic studies of human eosinophil and mast cell responses to ragweed, compound 48/80 and histamine. J Allergy Clin Immunol 51:263–273
4. Atkins PC, Norman ME, Weiner H, Zweiman B (1977) Release of neutrophil chemotactic activity during immediate hypersensi-

tivity reactions in humans. Ann Intern Med 86:415–418
5. Atkins PC, Norman ME, Zweiman B (1978) Antigen-induced neutrophil chemotactic activity in man: Correlation with bronchospasm and inhibition by disodium cromoglycate. J Allergy Clin Immunol 62: 149–155
6. Atkins PC, Norman ME, Zweiman B, Rosenblum F (1979) Further characterization and biologic activity of ragweed antigen-induced neutrophil chemotactic activity in man. J Allergy Clin Immunol 64:251–258
7. Atkins PC, Rosenblum F, Dunsky EH, Coffey R, Zweiman B (1980) Comparison of plasma histamine and cyclic nucleotides after antigen and methacholine inhalation in man. J Allergy Clin Immunol 66:478–485
8. Atkins PC, Valenzano M, Zweiman B (1982) Plasma concentrations of histamine measured by radioenzymatic assay: effects of histamine incubations. J Allergy Clin Immunol 69:39–45
9. Atkins PC, Wasserman S (1983) Chemotactic mediators. Clin Rev Allergy 1:385–396
10. Barnes P, Fitzgerald G, Brown M, Dollery C (1980) Nocturnal asthma and changes in circulating epinephrine, histamine and corticosteroids. N Engl J Med 303:263–267
11. Bedard PM, Zweiman B, Atkins PC (1983) Antigen induced local mediator release and cellular inflammatory responses in atopic subjects. J Allergy Clin Immunol 71:394–398
12. Bhat KN, Arrayaue CM, Marney SR, Stevenson DD, Tan EM (1976) Plasma histamine changes during provoked bronchospasm in asthmatic patients. J Allergy Clin Immunol 58:647–656
13. Boulet L-P, Cartier A, Thomson NC, Roberts RS, Dolovich J, Hargreave FE (1983) Asthma and increases in non-allergic bronchial responsiveness from seasonal pollen exposure. J Allergy Clin Immunol 71:399–406
14. Brown MJ, Ind PW, Causon R, Lee TH (1982) A novel double isotope technique for the enzymatic assay of plasma histamine: application to estimation of mast cell activation by antigen challenge in asthmatics. J Allergy Clin Immunol 69:20–24
15. Bruce CA, Rosenthal RR, Lichtenstein LM, Norman PS (1974) Diagnostic tests in ragweed-allergic asthma. J Allergy Clin Immunol 53:230–239
16. Bruce CA, Rosenthal RR, Lichtenstein LM, Norman PS (1975) Quantitative inhalation bronchial challenge in ragweed hayfever patients: A comparison with ragweed allergic asthmatics. J Allergy Clin Immunol 56:331–337
17. Bryant DH, Kay AB (1977) Cutaneous eosinophil accumulation in atopic and nonatopic individuals: The effect of ECF-A tetrapeptide and histamine. Clin Allergy 7:211–218
18. Clark RAF, Gallin JI, Kaplan AD (1975) The selective activity of histamine. J Exp Med 142:1462–1476
19. Cockcroft DW, Cotton DJ, Mink JT (1979) Nonspecific bronchial hyperreactivity after exposure to Western Red Cedar. Am Rev Respir Dis 119:505–510
20. Cockcroft DW, Ruffin RE, Frith PA, Cartier A, Juniper EF, Dolovich J, Hargreave PE (1979) Determinants of allergen-induced asthma: Dose of allergen, circulating IgE antibody concentration and bronchial responsiveness to inhaled histamine. Am Rev Respir Dis 120:1053–1058
21. Creticos PS, Peters SP, Adkinson NF, Naclerio RM, Hayes EC, Norman PS, Lichtenstein LM (1984) Peptide leukotriene release after antigen challenge in patients sensitive to ragweed. N Engl J Med 310:1626–1630
22. deShazo RD, Levinson AI, Dvorak HF, Davis RW (1979) The late phase skin reaction: evidence for activation of the coagulation system in an IgE dependent reaction in man. J Immunol 122:692–698
23. Dorsch W, Ring J (1981) Induction of late cutaneous reactions by skin blister fluid from allergen tested and normal skin. J Allergy Clin Immunol 67:117–123
24. Drazen JM, Austen KF, Lewis RA, Clark DA, Goto G, Martat A, Corey EJ (1980) Comparative airway and vascular activities of leukotrienes C-1 and D in vivo and in vitro. Proc Natl Acad Sci USA 77:4354–4358
25. Eidinger D, Wilkinson R, Rose B (1964) A study of cellular responses in human reactions utilizing the skin window technique. J Allergy 35:77–85
26. Fowler JW, Lowell FC (1966) The accumulation of eosinophils as an allergic response to allergen applied to a denuded skin surface. J Allergy 37:19–28
27. Hogg JC (1983) Pathology of asthma. In: Middleton E Jr, Reed CE, Ellis EF (eds) Allergy, Principles and Practice, 2nd edn. Mosby, St. Louis, pp 833–842
28. Kaplan AP, Horakova A, Katz S (1978) Assessment of tissue fluid histamine levels in patients with urticaria. J Allergy Clin Immunol 61:350–358
29. Lee TH, Brown MJ, Nagy L, Causon R, Walport MJ, Kay AB (1982) Exercise-induced release of histamine and neutrophil chemotactic factor in atopic asthmatics. J Allergy Clin Immunol 70:73–81

30. Lee TH, Nagakura T, Cromwell O, Brown MJ, Causon R, Kay AB (1984) Neutrophil chemotactic activity and histamine in atopic and non-atopic subjects after exercise-induced asthma. Am Rev Respir Dis 129:409–412
31. Lee TH, Nagy L, Nagakura T, Walport MJ, Kay AB (1982) Identification and partial characterization of an exercise induced neutrophil chemotactic factor in bronchial asthma. J Clin Invest 69:889–899
32. Lewis RA, Soter NA, Corey EJ, Austen KF (1981) Local effects of synthetic leukotrienes on monkey and human skin. Clin Res 29:492A
33. Lichtenstein LM, Osler AG (1964) Studies on the mechanisms of hypersensitivity phenomenon. IX. Histamine release from human leukocyte by ragweed pollen antigen. J Exp Med 120:507–517
34. MacGlashan DW, Schleimer RP, Peters SP, Schulman ES, Adams GK, Newball HH, Lichtenstein LM (1982) Generation of leukotrienes by purified human mast cells. J Clin Invest 70:747–751
35. Martin GL, Atkins PC, Dunsky EH, Zweiman B (1980) Effects of theophylline terbutaline and prednisone on antigen-induced bronchospasm and mediator release. J Allergy Clin Immunol 66:204–212
36. Naclerio RM, Meier HL, Kagey-Sobotka A, Adkinson NF, Meyers DA, Norman PS, Lichtenstein LM (1983) Mediator release after nasal airway challenge with allergen. Am Rev Respir Dis 128:597–602
37. Nadel JA (1984) Inflammation and Asthma. J Allergy Clin Immunol 73:651–653
38. Nagakura T, Lee TH, Assaufi BK, Neuman-Taylor AJ, Dennison DM, Kay AB (1983) Neutrophil chemotactic factor in exercise and hyperventilation induced asthma. Am Rev Respir Dis 128:294–296
39. Nagy L (1981) The effect of disodium-cromoglycate on human serum neutrophil chemotactic activity in antigen induced bronchospasm. Allerg Immunol 27:48–52
40. Nagy L (1981) Serum neutrophil chemotactic activity and leukocyte count after house dust induced bronchospasm. Eur J Respir Dis 62:198–203
41. O'Driscoll BRC, Lee TH, Cromwell O, Kay AB (1983) Immunologic release of neutrophil chemotactic activity from human lung tissue. J Allergy Clin Immunol 72: 695–701
42. Oertel H, Kaliner M (1981) The biologic activity of mast cell granules. III. Purification of inflammatory factors of anaphylaxis (IF-A) responsible for causing late phase reactions. J Immunol 127:1398–1402
43. Papageorgiou N, Lee TH, Nagakura T, Gramwell O, Wraith DG, Kay AB (1983) Neutrophil chemotactic activity in milk induced asthma. J Allergy Clin Immunol 72:75–82
44. Proud D, Togias A, Naclerio RM, Crush SA, Norman PS, Lichtenstein LM (1983) Kinins are generated in vivo following nasal airway challenge of allergic individuals with allergen. J Clin Invest 72:1678–1685
45. Schenkel E, Atkins PC, Yost R, Zweiman B (1982) Antigen-induced neutrophil chemotactic activity from sensitized lung. J Allergy Clin Immunol 70:321–325
46. Simon RA, Stevenson DD, Arrayave CM, Tan EM (1977) The relationship of plasma histamine to the activity of bronchial asthma. J Allergy Clin Immunol 60:312–316
47. Slott RI, Zweiman B (1974) A controlled study of the effects of corticosteroids on the immediate hypersensitivity skin test response. J Allergy Clin Immunol 54:229–234
48. Slott RI, Zweiman B (1975) Histologic studies of human skin test responses to ragweed and compound 48/80. II. Effect of corticosteroid therapy. J Allergy Clin Immunol 55:232–240
49. Solley GO, Gleich GJ, Jordan RE, Schroeber AC (1977) Late cutaneous reactions due to IgE antibodies. Monogr Allergy 12:179–188
50. Talbot SF, Atkins PC, Valenzano M, Zweiman B (1984) Correlations of in vivo mediator release with late cutaneous allergic responses in humans. J Allergy Clin Immunol 74:819–826
51. Talbot SF, Atkins PC, Zweiman B, Goetzl E (1984) In vivo antigen induced release of leukotrienes in human skin. Clin Res 32:146A
52. Tennenbaum S, Oertel H, Henderson WR, Kaliner M (1980) The biologic activity of mast cell granules. I. Elicitation of inflammatory responses in rat skin. J Immunol 125:325–335
53. Ting S, Dunsky EH, Lavker RM, Zweiman B (1980) Patterns of mast cell alteration and in vivo mediator release in human allergic skin reactions. J Allergy Clin Immunol 66:417–423
54. Ting S, Reimann B, Zweiman B (1982) Cromolyn does not inhibit codeine induced histamine release in vivo. In: Kerr JW, Ganderton MA (eds) Proceedings of the XIth International Congress of Allergology and Clinical Immunology. Macmillan, London Basingstoke, p 402P
55. Ting S, Zweiman B, Lavker RM (1981) In vivo release of eosinophil chemoattractant activity in human allergic skin. J Immunol 127:557–560

56. Ting S, Zweiman B, Lavker R (1983) Terbutaline modulation of human allergic skin reactions. J Allergy Clin Immunol 71:437–441
57. Townley RG, Dennis M, Itkin IH (1965) Comparative action of acetylthetamethylcholine, histamine and pollen antigens in subjects with hayfever and patients with bronchial asthma. J Allergy 36:121–137
58. Turnbull LW, Evans DP, Kay AB (1977) Human eosinophils tetrapeptides (ECF-A) and histamine. Immunology 32:56–63
59. Venge P, Dahl R, Hakansson L, Petterson C (1982) Generation of heat labile chemotactic activity in blood after inhalation challenge and its relationship to neutrophil and monocyte/macrophage turnover and activity. Allergy 37:55–62
60. Weiner H, Atkins PC, Zweiman B, Altose M (1979) A prospective classification of the respiratory manifestations of pollen sensitivity. Ann Allergy 43:146–150
61. Zweiman B, Slott RI, Atkins PC (1976) Factors in the tissue eosinophil response in human immediate hypersensitivity reactions. Int Arch Allergy Appl Immunol 52:48–52

25. Late Phase Reactions

W. Dorsch

Late phase reactions (LPR) have been considered generally as Arthus phenomenon (type III allergy according to Coombs and Gell). IgE antibodies, however, are able to initiate not only immediate (WFR), but also late cutaneous reactions (LCR). Using the skin blister technique we could show LCR to be mediated by inflammatory mediators generated during the preceding WFR. Histamine, active kallikrein, leukotrienes, thromboxanes and platelet activating property were demonstrable in dual skin reactions. The concentration of these mediators in skin blister fluid was in part related to the time course of skin reactions. LCRs were diminished by eicosatetraynoic acid (not by indomethacin), by dazoxiben (thromboxane synthetase inhibitor) as well as by ethanolic onion extract. β-mimetics as salbutamol and anticholinergics as ipratropium bromide could reverse late bronchial reactions (LBR), besides disodium cromoglycate ethanolic onion extract could prevent LBR. Other authors found prostaglandin D_2 and chemotactic substances during LPRs as well as protective effects of corticosteroids, combined histamine H_1/H_2-receptor antagonists and tranexamic acid.

Two types of LPR have to be distinguished: type I and type III. The first is initiated by an IgE-dependent mast cell degranulation and maintained by a complex interaction of mediators and cells. It may represent a laboratory model of long-lasting asthmatic conditions.

25.1 History

Late phase reactions (LPRs) have been observed since the dawn of clinical allergy: In 1873 Blackley [13], who was, like many allergists, himself atopic (he suffered from hay fever), experienced nasal and bronchial discomfort lasting from several hours to 2–4 days after handling pollens. In 1921 Prausnitz and Küstner [104] undertook their famous "studies on hypersensitivity" and discovered the transferability by serum not only of immediate wheal and flare reactions (WFRs), but also of late cutaneous reactions (LCRs). LPRs were also observed by Cooke [23]. In 1952, Herxheimer [63] stressed the clinical importance of late bronchial reactions (LBRs), since this reaction pattern can be observed predominantly in patients with chronic bronchial asthma.

The pathogenesis of LPR was of minor interest until 1968, when Pepys and coworkers [99, 131] observed in patients with bronchopulmonary aspergillosis a close relationship between LCRs and/or LBRs on the one hand and serum precipitins against aspergilli on the other. In skin biopsies they found typical signs of an Arthus reaction: deposits of IgG, IgM, and C_3 as well as infiltrating neutrophil leukocytes. They concluded that LPRs generally represent a type III reaction according to the classification of Gell and Coombs [54]. Doubts regarding this pathogenetic concept arose when Booij-Noord et al [14] noted in 1971 that there are two types of LBR: LBRs after inhalation of house dust differ distinctly from exogenous allergic alveolitis (= hypersensitivity pneumonitis EAA) by virtue of the lack of fever, leukocytosis, and pulmonary infiltrates. This *late bronchial obstruction* (LBO) was reversed by corticosteroids (similar to EAA) and prevented by disodium cromoglycate (in contrast to EAA).

In the following years (1973–1976), Dolovich et al [27, 28], Solley et al [123], de Shazo et al [117], and Atkins et al [6] were able to show LCR to be mediated by IgE antibodies. A great number of investigations now focus on the pathogenesis of

LPRs and their pharmacological modulation. The central role of mast cell degranulation is generally accepted, while the importance of pro-inflammatory mediators – including chemotactic factors – and the role of infiltrating cells are subjects of controversy.

25.2 Definitions

The term *late phase reaction* describes the time course of an inflammatory response. It lasts longer than the immediate reaction, usually peaks between the 4th and 8th hour after allergen challenge, and subsides within 12–48 hours. This definition ("an inflammatory response lasting 2 hours to 2 days") abrogates consciously all pathophysiological interpretations because different mechanisms seem to be involved in the pathogenesis of LPR, some acting in combination.

25.2.1 Late Cutaneous Reaction

The intracutaneous injection of an antigen into the skin of sensitive individuals first provokes an immediate reaction: The wheal is sharply distinct from the surrounding flare (which is caused by an axon reflex [21]). Usually this WFR subsides within 90 min. Great wheals (more than 15 mm in diameter) enlarge continually. After 1 hour the border of the wheal becomes less distinct and merges with the flare zone. During the next 2–3 hours the lesion remains more or less unchanged. Thereafter a second phase of the reaction starts with mild pruritus. Depending on its intensity, the peak of the inflammatory reaction is reached between the 6th and the 12th hour. The fully developed LCR is characterized by edema, erythema, pruritus, tenderness, hyperalgesia, and hyperthermia. The site of the LCR is much more extensive than the preceding WFR, its border less well-defined. In some cases a *target lesion* similar to that seen in erythema multiforme may be observed. Thereafter the LCR subsides within hours – first the subjective complaints, then the erythema and edema. In rare cases residual petechiae persist for days [6, 27–29, 39, 57, 104, 117, 118, 123].

25.2.2 Late Nasal Reaction

Late phase reactions of the nose follow a time course similar to LCRs: The immediate reaction is characterized by itching, sneezing, rhinorrhea, and nasal congestion. These symptoms subside within 1 hour and peak again 4–12 hours later. During late nasal reactions (LNRs) itching and sneezing are less pronounced than nasal congestion. The obstruction of nasal airways can be estimated quantitatively by rhinomanometry [44, 66, 97, 109].

25.2.3 Late Bronchial Reaction

The immediate bronchial reaction peaks 15–20 min after allergen inhalation. After incomplete or complete recovery the airway resistance again increases, reaching a maximum between the 4th and 10th hour. In contrast to the immediate reaction, LBO is manifested predominantly in peripheral areas of the lung. Clinical symptoms and lung function studies make possible easy differentiation of LBO from EAA [14, 34, 110]. LBO must also be distinguished from changes in bronchial tonus due to circadian rhythm [55]. The pathogenesis of LBO will be outlined later; for EAA see reviews from other authors, e.g., Reed [108].

25.2.4 Frequency of Late Phase Reactions

Nearly all common antigens causing immediate reactions in sensitive individuals can initiate dual responses too, i.e., the combination of immediate and late phase reactions. The frequency varies from author to author and from antigen to antigen between 40% and 80%. LBO is observed most frequently after house dust or house dust mite inhalation challenges. There is great interindividual variance in the ratio between the intensity of immediate and late bronchial responses [34, 137]. In routine skin (prick) testing LCRs will seldom be observed, probably owing to the low antigen doses used (wheals with 8 mm or less in diameter are seldom followed by LCRs [27]). Increasing the allergen dose injected leads to wheals greater than 15 mm in diameter and causes LCRs in more than 90% [34, 120, 123]. As in the lung, there is no close relationship between the intensity of immediate and late reactions in the skin [34]. Depending on the sensitivity of the rhinomanometric method used, LNRs are observed in 3%–50% of positive nasal allergen challenges [45, 109].

25.3 Pathogenesis of LCRs

It is generally assumed that bronchial, nasal, and cutaneous LPRs are caused by similar or identical pathomechanisms. This hypothesis has not been proven in all its details. However, it can be stated that studies of LCRs yield valuable insights into the pathogenesis of LBO.

25.3.1 Trigger Mechanisms

Virtually all antigens capable of inducing WFRs can cause LCRs too. In most cases, but not all, the reaction is mediated by IgE antibodies. Besides specific immunological mechanisms there are nonspecific direct mast cell activating pathways for inducing a late phase reaction.

IgE

After the injection of antihuman IgE antibodies (*reverse anaphylaxis*) mast cell degranulation occurs in the skin of atopics and nonatopics, followed by WFR and LCR [27]. The Fc part of anti-IgE, which could fix complement and initiate an Arthus-like reaction [64, 65], is not responsible since the same phenomena are observed when only $F(ab)_2$ fragments of anti-IgE are used. Allergen-dependent LCRs as well as WFRs can be passively transferred with the serum of atopics into the skin of nonatopic human beings and primates [32, 95, 104]. Destruction of the heat-labile IgE antibodies by heating the serum (56 °C, 4 hours) abolished LCR and WFR in the host. Similarly, extraction of IgE from the graft serum by means of an anti-IgE immunoabsorbent abolishes the host's LCR and WFR after allergen testing. Finally, if the host's IgE receptors are well-occupied by myeloma IgE, serum from atopics can no longer sensitize this skin area to WFR or LCR after allergen injection [123].

IgE-independent Mechanisms

Late cutaneous reactions occur after intracutaneous testing with anti-IgG antibodies, anaphylatoxins, and *Staphylococcus aureus* protein A [126], too. All agents are capable of activating mast cells: Anaphylatoxins act directly, protein A and anti-IgG indirectly, e.g., by complement activation and generation of anaphylatoxins [22, 68]. It has to be kept in mind that IgG antibodies can initiate immediate reactions as well [18].

Mast Cell-derived Mediators

Late cutaneous reactions are often observed after the injection of compound 48/80 [29, 123, 129], a direct mast cell degranulator [96]. In rodents isolated mast cell granules have been shown to induce LCRs [66, 72, 73, 92, 93].

Exudate from Human Skin

Using the skin blister method [12, 39] interstitial fluid from allergen-tested skin was collected at various times after antigen challenge. Reinjection of this fluid caused LCRs similar to those observed after allergen injection. Possible antigen transfer from one skin site to the other was excluded: As shown in the passive cutaneous anaphylaxis in *Macaca fasciolaris,* there was no detectable antigen contamination of skin blister fluids. These fluids were also free of cellular elements. It was concluded that LCRs are caused by soluble mediators generated or released during the early phase of dual skin reactions [39]. When suction blisters were induced over normal skin, higher amounts (250 µl instead of 50 µl after allergen testing) of this skin blister fluid provoked LCRs after intracutaneous injection, too. The intensity and extent of these LCRs, however, were much less pronounced. This observation demonstrates that the exudation of plasma itself – as caused artificially by the generation of skin blisters and naturally during inflammation – generates mediators capable of inducing LCRs [39].

25.3.2 Role of Mediators

Various methods [12, 39, 45, 85, 128] have been used in order to demonstrate the release or generation of inflammatory mediators in the skin during allergic reactions. The suction blister method yields high amounts of mediators, but also causes a slight irritation of the skin [39].

Histamine

Histamine is released from mast cells and circulating basophil leukocytes [8]. In the skin, histamine release was demonstrated during the immediate reaction [45]. Using the skin blister technique [41], a second wave of histamine release from mast cells and/or infiltrating basophil leukocytes during LCR was demonstrable only in a few cases (without correlation to the intensity of the LCR). The skin chamber technique [128] showed histamine release prolonged for up to 4 hours in LCR. There was a close interrelationship between the amount of histamine and the intensity of LCR; control studies in isolated WFR, however, were not performed.

The injection of histamine never causes LCRs in normal or atopic persons; however, such reactions have been observed in patients with acute urticaria [65]. Even the combination of allergen and histamine in order to augment WFR to an extent usually followed by LCR did not alter the frequency of LCR [119]. Antihistamines, both of the histamine H_1- and the histamine H_2-receptor type, did not affect LCR when administered alone; their combination, however, totally abolished it [22]. The underlying mechanism is not clear. Interestingly, guinea pigs can be protected against allergen-induced bronchial asthma more effectively by combined H_1-H_2-antagonists than by H_1-blockers alone (see below) [38, 44].

Prostaglandin D_2

Mast cells [75], but not basophil leukocytes, generate prostaglandin D_2 (PGD_2). Maximal concentrations were observed in the skin 2 hours after allergen challenge in both isolated WFR and dual skin reactions. There was a close relationship between the amount of PGD_2 and the occurrence of LCR (as the authors pointed out, this may be interpreted solely as an epiphenomenon indicating strong mast cell activation [101]). Upon intracutaneous injection PGD_2 (0.5 μg) leads to isolated WFR (peak 30 min after injection). There are synergistic effects with other mediators, such as leukotrienes.

Leukotrienes (LTB_4, LTC_4, LTD_4)

Leukotrienes are formed by several cell types, including mast cells [100, 111, 135]. It seems of special interest that different types of granulocytes seem preferentially to generate different kinds of leukotrienes (e.g., eosinophils especially generate LTC_4 [135]).

The generation of immunoreactive leukotrienes (LTC_4/LTD_4), during the immediate phase of dual skin reactions could be demonstrated by RIA in skin blister fluids: There was a significant increase from 83 ± 13 pg/100 μl (control skin) to 220 ± 23 pg/100 μl (allergen or anti-IgE-tested skin) in 13 patients ($p < 0.001$). In this preliminary study neither the intensity of LCR nor that of WFR showed a correlation to the concentration of LTC_4/LTD_4 in the blister fluid. The generation of the leukotactic LTB_4 in LCR has not yet been demonstrated. However, the injection of LTB_4 (0.5 μg) into monkey or human skin is followed within 6 hours by infiltration of neutrophil granulocytes accompanied by tenderness and induration. All symptoms are augmented by the simultaneous administration of 0.5 μg PGD_2. LTD_4 (0.5 μg) leads to WFR with maximal intensity after 2 hours, followed by erythema lasting 6 hours [76]. The pathophysiological role of leukotrienes in LCR is underlined by the fact that neither acetylsalicylic acid [orally, 122] nor indomethacin [topically, 31] prevents LCR, whereas eicosatetraynoic acid does show an inhibitory effect (see below).

Thromboxanes

Thromboxanes (Tx) are not generated by mast cells [100] but by other cell types [114] such as fibroblasts [50] and platelets. In blister fluids from dual skin reactions TxB_2 was detected in progressively increasing concentrations following allergen injection [41]. The biological role of this mediator – which causes long-lasting bronchial asthma in experimental animals [127] – was examined using a selective thromboxane biosynthesis inhibitor [132]: Dazoxiben diminished LCR induced by reverse anaphylaxis in 13 out of 16 patients. However, as an undesired side effect, this agent increased immediate WFR [42].

Prostaglandins E and $F_{2\alpha}$

These *classical* prostaglandins cause long-lasting erythema when injected into human skin [25]. Their role in LCR is unknown. The relative amount of both PGE_2 and $PGF_{2\alpha}$ generated in the lung during experimental anaphylaxis regulates allergen tachyphylaxis in guinea pigs, i.e., there is a progressive decrease in allergen sensitivity during sequential allergen challenge [37].

Platelet Activation/Coagulation System

Besides thromboxanes other substances can activate platelets, e.g., thrombin or platelet activating factor (PAF) [10, 26]. PAF is released from several cell types, including mast cells [8, 124]. It has been shown to provoke LCR in human and monkey skin [3]. Thromboxanes are generated by aggregated platelets and thus further promote platelet aggregation. Indeed, in rabbit skin a biphasic accumulation of platelets was demonstrable after injection of compound 48/80 or anti-IgE: A first wave lasting 1 hour was followed by a second lasting at least 3 hours and exceeding the first by far [70]. IgE-dependent reactions in human lung (and probably also in skin) lead to the activation of Hageman factor and thereby the blood clotting system [89]. Fibrin deposits were often seen in LCR [119]. Platelet activating properties have been found in skin blister fluid from both allergen-tested and normal skin [41].

Kallikrein-Kinin System

Bioassay on the rat uterus demonstrated active kallikrein in skin blister fluid during WFR and LCR [41]. In human skin, kallikrein causes an LCR identical to that seen after compound 48/80 with respect to clinical symptoms and histological pattern [29]. Human leukocytes are known to release kallikrein in vitro by an IgE-dependent mechanism [90].

Conclusion: "A Complex Interaction of Mediators"

At least three mediator systems seem to be involved in the pathogenesis of LCR: arachidonic acid metabolites, kinins, and the coagulation system. It may be that the complement cascade is involved too [9, 11, 61]. It seems of special interest that LCRs are influenced by regulatory mechanisms leading to long-lasting refractory states: The "partial refractory state of LCR" (first described by Umemoto [115, 133]) can last up to 4 weeks. The underlying mechanism of this refractory state occurring after challenge with allergen, anti-IgE, kallikrein, or compound 48/80 [29] is not known; one might speculate that so-called inflamed tissue factors play some role [121]. An impaired repair mechanism may also be involved in the pathogenesis of LPRs [see 81].

25.3.3 Role of Infiltrating Cells

The chemotactic substances released from mast cells during anaphylaxis involve other cell types in the development of LCRs [57, 117, 118, 123, 140]. Eight hours after allergen injection there are perivascular infiltrates of lymphocytes (35%), monocytes/macrophages (10%), neutrophils (13%), eosinophils (35%), and basophils (3%). The pathogenetic role of these cells is not fully understood as yet, since 6 hours [119] or 24 hours [109] after allergen injection there is neither a qualitative nor a quantitative difference in cellular infiltrates between isolated WFR and dual skin reactions (in which WFRs of the same extent were followed by LCRs). However, observations in rodents that isolated peritoneal mast cell granules induce LCR [66, 74, 93, 129] support an important role of infiltrating cells in LCR. Neutrophil depletion by immunological [72] or chemical [73] procedures reduces the intensity of LCR. However, species differences have to be kept in mind: LTB_4, which is known to provoke clinical symptoms similar to LCR in human beings (see above), has recently been shown to play no role in LCR in the rat [69]. Basophils also have been considered important in the generation of LCRs [5]. Further arguments for an active role of infiltrating cells in LPRs are the biphasic course of mediator release and leukocyte activation during dual bronchial and nasal reactions (see below).

25.4 Pathogenesis of Late Nasal Reactions

Few data are available on this topic. It is most likely that late cutaneous, nasal, and bronchial reactions follow similar pathophysiological pathways. The same antigens which cause LCR by IgE-dependent mechanisms are capable of inducing late nasal reactions. However, passive transfer experiments – analogous to the Prausnitz-Küstner model in skin – were negative in the nasal system [47].

One observation seems to be of special interest: Histamine release into nasal secretions was observed throughout the whole immediate and late nasal reaction; by contrast PGD_2 release was seen only during the immediate reaction [87]. Since PGD_2 is generated only by mast cells and not by basophil leukocytes (in contrast to histamine, which is released by both cell types), it was concluded that late nasal reactions are caused by the infiltration of basophil leukocytes.

25.5 Pathogenesis of Late Bronchial Obstruction

25.5.1 Trigger Mechanisms

Late bronchial obstruction has been observed after the inhalation of nearly all common allergens known to induce immediate reactions. In most cases LBO is triggered by IgE-dependent mechanisms leading to mast cell degranulation. This may be concluded from indirect evidence: The titer of allergen-specific IgE but not IgG antibodies correlates with the frequency of LBO [35, 83]. If the immediate bronchial reaction is prevented by disodium cromoglycate, no LBO will be observed. DSCG given after antigen challenge will affect neither the immediate nor the late bronchial reaction [14].

Exercise-induced immediate asthmatic attacks are often followed by late reactions. The pathogenesis of exercise-induced asthma is not fully understood; according to several authors, however, mast cell degranulation seems to be involved.

25.5.2 Role of Inflammatory Mediators and Cells

During dual bronchial reactions a biphasic increase in neutrophil chemotactic activity was observed in the serum of allergen-challenged patients [88]. The same authors recently reported a biphasic increase in immunoreactive leukotrienes (LTB_4, LTC_4, LTD_4) during dual bronchial reactions in the serum of three patients after allergen inhalation [24]. They were also able to demonstrate biphasic activation of leukocytes in allergen-induced dual bronchial responses [46]. The origin of these mediators is not exactly known. They may be released by mast cells activated subsequently or, in analogy to late nasal reactions, by infiltrating cells. The pharmacological action of corticosteroids on LPR favors the latter hypothesis: Corticosteroids, while strongly inhibiting LPRs, do not affect immediate reactions [60]. As shown recently, corticosteroids inhibit the degranulation of basophils, but not that of mast cells [112, 113]. In addition to various other effects (e.g., blockade of phospholipase A_2 [52, 82]) they also depress chemotaxis [120, 136].

25.5.3 Role of Bronchial Hyperreactivity

Bronchial hyperreactivity to nonimmunological stimuli is often seen in patients with chronic asthma. For clinical purposes it is tested by inhalation of acetylcholine or histamine. Bronchial hyperreactivity to these agents is not a prerequisite for the occurrence of LBO [34]. LBOs, however, are followed by bronchial hyperreactivity lasting up to several weeks [20]. This important fact may contribute considerably to the progressive increase in bronchial symptoms after continuous antigen exposure [130].

25.6 Pharmacological Modulation of Late Phase Reactions

Late phase reactions may be considered as models of chronic asthmatic conditions [39, 57]. They are often observed in patients with chronic bronchial asthma [63, 137]; therefore the pharmacological inhibition of LPRs is of great clinical interest [20]. Table 25.1 summarizes the most important data available.

25.6.1 Corticosteroids

Corticosteroids, administered orally or topically, are most efficient in preventing or treating nasal [86, 91, 98], cutaneous [60, 103], and bronchial [14] LPRs. Interestingly, immediate reactions are not affected by these drugs [60].

25.6.2 Disodium Cromoglycate

Disodium cromoglycate (DSCG) can effectively prevent LBO (but not acute hypersensitivity pneumonitis) when it is inhaled prior to allergen [14]. When it is given after the allergen, DSCG has no effect. The dampening effect of this compound on bronchial hyperreactivity may be explained by its inhibitory effect on LBO [2]. As mentioned above, LBO causes bronchial hyperreactivity lasting up to several weeks. There are, however, also direct effects on bronchial irritant receptors [63].

25.6.3 β-adrenergic Agents

Late bronchial obstruction can be markedly reduced by the inhalation of β-mimetics such as salbutamol. This drug also reverses impairments of gas transfer during LBO [33, 48].

25.6.4 Anticholinergic Agents

Ipratropium bromide per inhalation has been shown to relieve airway resistance during LBO, thus indicating the involvement of cholinergic mechanisms in LBO [33, see also 52]. The efficacy of this drug, however, is much weaker than that of β-mimetics.

25.6.5 Antihistamines

As mentioned above, neither histamine H_1-nor histamine H_2-receptor antagonists administered orally affect LCRs when given alone. In combinations, however, they abolish LCRs totally [122]. Data on similar experiments on LNRs or LBRs are lacking. H_1-H_2-antagonism has been recommended for preventing pseudoallergic anaphy-

Table 25.1. Pharmacologic modulation of late phase reactions in the skin (LCRs) and the bronchial system (LBRs)

Agent	Action on	
	LCRs	LBRs
Corticosteroids	↓	↓
Disodium cromoglycate		↓
β-sympathicomimetics	↓	↓
Anticholinergics		↓
Ketotifen	↓	
Combined H_1-H_2-histamine receptor antagonists	↓	
Eicosatetraynoic acid (ETYA)	↓	
Acetylsalicylic acid	0	
Indomethacin	0 (erythema ↓)	
Dazoxiben (inhibitor of thromboxane biosynthesis)	↓ (immediate reaction ↑)	
Ethanolic onion extract	↓	
Tranexamic acid	↓	

lactoid [79, 140]. Studium on the effect of combined histamine antagonists on bronchial asthma in human beings will be of great interest [66], since experimental data from animals are promising [37, 38].

25.6.6 *Ketotifen*

Ketotifen, an orally active agent with mast cell stabilizing and antihistaminic properties, inhibits both WFRs and LCRs [1].

25.6.7 *Eicosatetraynoic acid*

Eicosatetraynoic acid (ETYA) applied topically blocks both the cyclooxygenase and the lipoxygenase pathway of arachidonic metabolism. Even high doses (1 mg) do not affect WFRs when injected simultaneously with rabbit antihuman IgE antibodies. The subsequent LCRs, however, are reduced (30% reduction at the 8th hour, $n=6$, $p<0.05$) [Dorsch et al, to be published]. In guinea pigs, inhalation of ETYA shows marked protective effects against allergen-induced bronchial obstruction [43].

25.6.8 *Acetylsalicylic Acid and Indomethacin*

Neither of these cyclooxygenase inhibitors (oral acetylsalicylic acid, topic indomethacin) altered edema formation or clinical symptoms during LCR [31, 122]. Only the intensity of the erythema was reduced by indomethacin [31], an agent known to diminish erythema in sunburn.

In single cases relief of LBO by cyclooxygenase inhibitors has been reported [49].

25.6.9 *Thromboxane Synthetase Inhibitors*

Dazoxiben (administered orally) is used in the treatment of vascular diseases [132]. This agent selectively inhibits thromboxane formation in, for example, human platelets while increasing serum levels of prostacyclin and prostaglandins. It depressed edema formation during LCR in 13 out of 16 cases after reverse anaphylaxis and compound 48/80 injection. It showed, however, undesired and potentially serious side effects by increasing immediate WFR [42].

25.6.10 *Onion Extracts*

Onion and garlic oils have been shown to inhibit both lipoxygenase and cyclooxygenase pathways of human platelets' arachidonic metabolism in vitro [134]. This biochemical activity may be responsible for the well-known antiaggregatory effects of onions. In a double-blind study on 12 volunteers marked suppressive effects of topically applied ethanolic onion extract upon LCR after reverse anaphylaxis were observed [40]. Oral onion treatment effectively protected guinea pigs against allergen-induced bronchial asthma. This observation led to the detection of antiasthmatic properties of mustard oils [30]. In the two patients as yet tested, oral onion treatment (2×100 ml extract $=2\times200$ g onions) depressed both immediate and late bronchial obstruction.

25.6.11 *Tranexamic Acid*

Tranexamic acid is well-known as an inhibitor of fibrinolysis. As shown recently, it depresses late cutaneous reactions [29].

25.7 Animal Models of LPR

25.7.1 *Skin Tests on Monkeys Using Patients' Serum*

The skin of primates can be passively sensitized with serum of atopic patients [95]. Intracutaneous injection of the proper antigen causes not only immediate but also late cutaneous reactions [32]. In most of the cases the sensitizing property of patients' serum is heat-labile, indicating that IgE antibodies are the active agents. In some cases, however, passive Arthus phenomena can be observed which are mediated by heat-stable antibodies.

25.7.2 *Skin Tests on Rats Using Isolated Mast Cell Granules*

The injection of anti-IgE or compound 48/80 into the skin of rats is followed by increased vascular permeability and perivascular cell infiltration. Polymorphonuclear leukocytes present 1–2 hours later are gradually replaced by mononuclear cells (predominantly macrophages) at 24 hours. The same symptoms occur after injection of mast cell granules isolated from rat peritoneal mast cells [67, 74, 129]. From these membrane-free granules a so-called inflammatory factor of anaphylaxis (IF-A) was isolated [93] and characterized in part as a polypeptide containing 12 amino acids (molecular weight 1,400). IF-A caused both early polymorphonuclear and late mononuclear cell infiltrations.

Immunologically or chemically induced neutropenia diminished LCRs in this animal model [72, 73]. Both corticosteroids and combined histamine H_1-H_2-receptor antagonists are inhibitory, as in human LCRs [71, 92].

25.7.3 Bronchial Provocation Test in Rabbits

If neonatal rabbits are immunized with *Alternaria tenuis* they produce only IgE antibodies to this antigen. By the age of 1 week they synthesize precipitating antibodies of various isotypes. IgE-sensitive animals react to inhalative allergen challenges with immediate and late bronchial obstruction. This biphasic pulmonary response can be passively transferred with IgE serum to nonimmunized animals. Transfusion of IgG serum to IgE animals diminishes their biphasic pulmonary response after *Alternaria* aerosol challenge. Especially the latter observation may be important for the understanding of the beneficial effects of specific hyposensitization [116].

25.8 Clinical Consequences

In the past, patients with LPRs were excluded from hyposensitization because these reactions were generally considered to be the Arthus phenomenon. In our opinion, IgE-dependent LPRs certainly are not a contraindication to hyposensitization. Recent studies have even shown that hyposensitization will ameliorate IgE-dependent LPR rather than the corresponding immediate reaction [78, 102]. In clinical practice, however, demonstration of the IgE dependency of a certain LPR may be difficult. When there is doubt, bronchial provocation tests should be performed. LBO can be differentiated from hypersensitivity pneumonitis by clinical symptoms (lack of crepitations, chills, fever, marked leukocytosis), lung function tests (bronchial obstruction instead of impaired gas transfer), and its response to drugs such as DSCG and β-mimetics. Measurements of complement factors in the serum are not useful [9]. During hyposensitization, allergen-specific IgG antibodies occur. They may cause adverse reactions, but hyposensitization can be continued if certain precautions are taken [19, see also 78, 116].

25.9 Summary and Conclusion

Late phase reactions have generally been considered as the Arthus phenomenon (type III allergy according to Coombs and Gell). IgE antibodies, however, are able to initiate not only immediate (WFR), but also late cutaneous reactions. Using the skin blister technique we could show LCRs to be mediated by inflammatory mediators generated during the preceding WFR. Histamine, active kallikrein, leukotrienes, thromboxanes, and platelet activating properties were demonstrable in dual skin reactions. The concentration of the mediators in skin blister fluid was in part related to the time course of skin reactions. LCRs were diminished by ETYA (but not by indomethacin), by dazoxiben (thromboxane synthetase inhibitor), and by ethanolic onion extract. β-mimetics such as salbutamol and anticholinergics such as ipratropium bromide were able to reverse LBRs, whereas disodium cromoglycate and ethanolic onion extract were able to prevent LBR. Other authors have found PGD_2 and chemotactic substances during LPRs, as well as protective effects of corticosteroids, combined histamine H_1-H_2-receptor antagonists, and tranexamic acid.

Two types of LPR have to be distinguished: type I and type III. Late phase reactions are caused by IgE antibodies in most of the cases. They are initiated by mast cell degranulation and maintained by a complex interaction of inflammatory mediators and cells. LPRs represent models of chronic asthmatic conditions. Studies on their pharmacological modulation may yield new insights in the pathophysiology and therapy of bronchial asthma.

References

1. Aas K (1979) Effects of ketotifen and clemastine on passive transfer of reaginic reaction. Allergy 34:121–124
2. Altounyan REG (1980) Review of clinical activity and mode of action of sodium cromoglycate. Clin Allergy [Suppl] 10: 481–489
3. Archer CB (1983) Early and late inflammatory effects of PAF-Acether in the skin of experimental animals and man. J Invest Dermatol 80:346 (abstract)
4. Arroyave GM, Stevenson DD, Vaughan JH, Tah EH (1977) Plasma complement changes during bronchospasm provoked in asthmatic patients. Clin Allergy 7:173–182
5. Askenase PW (1977) Role of basophils, mast cells and vasoamines in hypersensitivity reactions with a delayed time course. Prog Allergy 3:211–215
6. Atkins PC, Green GR, Zweiman B (1973) Histologic studies of human skin test responses to ragweed, compound 48/80 and histamine. J Allergy Clin Immunol 51: 263–273
7. Atkins PC, Norman M, Weiner H, Zweiman B (1976) Release of neutrophil chemotactic activity during immediate hypersensitivity reactions in humans. Ann Intern Med 86:415–418
8. Austen KF, Orange RP (1975) Bronchial asthma: The possible role of the chemical mediators of immediate hypersensitivity in the pathogenesis of subacute disease. Am Rev Respir Dis 112:423–451
9. Baur X, Dorsch W, Becker T (1980) Levels of complement factors in human serum during immediate and late asthmatic reactions and during acute hypersensitivity pneumonitis. Allergy 35:383–390
10. Benveniste J, le Couedie JP, Polansky J, Tence M (1977) Structural analysis of purified platelet-activating factor by lipases. Nature 269:170–171
11. Berrens L, van Rijswijk-Verbeck J (1973) Inactivation of complement (C3) in human serum by atopic allergens. Int Arch Allergy 45:30–39
12. Black AK, Greaves MW, Hensby CN, Plummer NA (1976) A new method of obtaining human skin inflammatory exudate for pharmacological analysis. Br J Pharmacol 58:317 (abstract)
13. Blackley CH (1873) Experimental researches in the causes and nature of catarrhus aestivus (hay fever or hay asthma). Baillière, Tindall and Cox, reprinted by Dawson's of Pail Mall, London, 1959, pp 77–81
14. Booij-Noord II, Orie NGM, de Vries K (1971) Immediate and late bronchial obstructive reactions to inhalation of house dust and protective effects of disodium cromoglycate and prednisolone. J Allergy Clin Immunol 43:344–354
15. Brady R, Glovsky M, Hugli T (1978) Complement (C) activation by house dust extract; Implications in immediate hypersensitivity. J Allergy Clin Immunol 61: 187–188
16. Brocklehurst WE (1971) Role of kinins and prostaglandins in inflammation. Proc R Soc Med 64:4–6
17. Brostoff J, Roitt IM (1969) Cell mediated (delayed) hypersensitivity in patients with summer hayfever. Lancet 2:1269–1272
18. Bryant DH, Burns MW, Lazarus L (1975) New type of allergic asthma due to IgG "reaginic" antibody. Br Med J 4:580 (abstract)
19. Busse WW, Storms WW, Flaherty DK, Crandall M, Reed CE (1976) Alternaria IgG precipitating an adverse reaction. J Allergy Clin Immunol 57:367–372
20. Cartier A, Thomson NC, Frith PA, Roberts R, Tech M, Hargreave FE (1982) Allergen-induced increase in bronchial responsiveness to histamine: relationship to the late asthmatic response and change in airway caliber. J Allergy Clin Immunol 70:170–177
21. Chapman LF (1977) Mechanism of the flare reactions in human skin. J Invest Dermatol 69:88–97
22. Cochrane CG, Dixon FJ (1976) Antigen-antibody complex induced disease. In: Miescher PA, Müller-Eberhard HJ (eds) Textbook of immunopathology. Grune & Stratton, New York, pp 137–156
23. Cooke RA (1922) Studies in specific hypersensitiveness IX. On the phenomenon of hyposensitization (the clinically lessened sensitiveness of allergy). J Immunol 7:219–227
24. Cromwell O, Shaw RJ, Durham SR, Kay AB (1984) Plasma LTB_4 concentrations during early and late phase antigen-induced asthmatic reactions. J Allergy Clin Immunol 73:147 (abstract)
25. Crunkhorn P, Willis AL (1971) Cutaneous reactions to intradermal prostaglandins. Br J Pharmacol 41:49–56

26. Demopoulos CA, Pinckard RN, Hanahan DJ (1976) Platelet activating factor. J Biol Chem 254:9355–9358
27. Dolovich J, Hargreave FE, Chalmers R, Shier KJ, Gauldie Bienenstock J (1973) Late cutaneous allergic responses in isolated IgE dependent reactions. J Allergy Clin Immunol 52:38–46
28. Dolovich J, Little DC (1972) Correlates of skin test reactions to *Bacillus subtilis* enzyme preparations. J Allergy Clin Immunol 49: 43–53
29. Dor PJ, Vervloet D, Sapene M, Andrac L, Bonerandi JJ, Charpin J (1983) Induction of late cutaneous reaction by kallikrein injection: comparison with allergic-like late response to compound 48/80. J Allergy Clin Immunol 4:363–370
30. Dorsch W, Adam O, Weber J, Ziegeltrum T (1985) Antiasthmatic effects of onion extracts – detection of benzyl- and other isothiocyanates (mustard oils) as antiasthmatic compounds of plant origin. Eur J Pediatr 141:264 (abstract), Eur J Pharmacol 107: 17–24
31. Dorsch W, Baur X (1980) Effect of topical indomethacin on allergen-induced dual skin reaction. Allergy 35:503–508
32. Dorsch W, Baur X, Becker TH (1979) Zur Pathogenese verzögerter Immunreaktionen beim Asthma bronchiale. Atemwegs Lungenerkrankungen 5:294–297
33. Dorsch W, Baur X, Emslander HP, Fruhmann G (1980) Zur Pathogenese und Therapie der verzögerten Bronchialobstruktion. Prax Pneumonol 34:461–468
34. Dorsch W, Baur X, Polke H (1980) Quantitative Beziehungen zwischen Hauttestreaktionen, allergenspezifischem Serum-IgE-Spiegel und bronchialer Reagibilität bei Patienten mit exogen allergischem Asthma bronchiale. Allergologie 3: 12–16
35. Dorsch W, Baur X, Vogelmeier C (1979) IgE- and IgG-RAST bei Asthma-Patienten mit verzögerten Testreaktionen. Ein Beitrag zur Pathogenese der verzögerten Immunantwort in der cutanen und bronchopulmonalen Allergiediagnostik. II. RAST-Symposium Köln, Berichtsband. Grosse, Berlin (1981), pp 138–143
36. Dorsch W, Hintschich C, Neuhauser J, Weber J (1985) Sequential histamine inhalations cause increased bronchial histamine reactivity in guinea pigs: Role of platelets, thromboxanes and prostacyclin. Naunyn-Schmiedebergs Arch Pharmacol 327:148–155
37. Dorsch W, Frey L, Müller W (1984) In vitro allergen tachyphylaxis of guinea pig lung is mediated by endogenous prostaglandin E biosynthesis. Naunyn-Schmiedebergs Arch Pharmacol 325:275–282
38. Dorsch W, Reimann HJ, Neuhauser J (1982) $Histamine_1$-$histamine_2$-antagonism: effect of combined clemastine and cimetidine pretreatment on allergen and histamine induced reactions of the guinea pig lung in vivo and in vitro. Agents Actions 12:113–118
39. Dorsch W, Ring J (1981) Induction of late cutaneous reactions by skin blister fluid from allergen tested and normal skin. J Allergy Clin Immunol 67:117–123
40. Dorsch W, Ring J (1984) Suppression of immediate and late anti-IgE-induced skin reactions by topically applied alcohol/onion extract. Allergy 39:43–49
41. Dorsch W, Ring J, Reimann H, Geiger R (1982) Mediator studies in skin blister fluid from patients which dual skin reactions. J Allergy Clin Immunol 70:236–244
41a. Dorsch W, Ring J, Strasser T, Weber PC (1985) Detection of immunoreactive leukotrienes (LTC_4/LTD_4) in skin blister fluid after allergen testing in patients with late cutaneous reactions. Arch Dermatol Res 277: 400–401
42. Dorsch W, Ring J, Melzer H (1983) A selective inhibitor of thromboxane biosynthesis enhances immediate and reduces late cutaneous allergic reactions in man. J Allergy Clin Immunol 72:168–173
43. Dorsch W, Waldherr U, Rosmanith J (1981) Continuous recording of intrapulmonary "compressed air" as a sensitive noninvasive method of measuring bronchial obstruction in guinea pigs. Pflügers Arch 391:236–241
44. Dvoracek JE, Yunginger JW, Kern EB, Hyatt RE, Gleich GJ (1984) Induction of nasal late-phase reactions by insufflation of ragweed-pollen extract. J Allergy Clin Immunol 73:363–368
45. Dunsky EH, Zweiman B (1978) The direct demonstration of histamine release in allergic reactions in the skin using a skin chamber technique. J Allergy Clin Immunol 62:127–130
46. Durham SR, Carrol M, Walsh G, Boghossian S, Kay AB (1984) Leucocyte activation during antigen-induced early and late-phase asthmatic reactions. J Allergy Clin Immunol 73:146 (abstract)
47. Edwards JH, Baker JR, Davies BH (1974) Precipitin test negative farmer's lung-activation of the alternative pathway of complement by mouldy hay dusts. Clin Allergy 4:379–388

48. Emslander HP, Dorsch W, Baur X (1979) Airway resistance and $C^{18}O$-gas transfer in the late reaction following inhalant challenge by allergen. International Congress on Respiratory Diseases, Basel, Switzerland, p 79
49. Fairfax AJ (1982) Inhibition of the late asthmatic response to house dust mite by nonsteroidal anti-inflammatory drugs. Prostaglandins Leukotrienes Med 8:239–248
50. Feinmark SJ, Bailey JM (1982) Lipid metabolism in cultured cells: activation of endogenous thromboxane A_2 synthesis in cultured lung fibroblasts. J Biol Chem 257: 2816–2821
51. Flower R (1978) Steroidal antiinflammatory drugs as inhibitors of phospholipase A_2. Adv Prostaglandin Thromboxane Leukotriene Res 3:103–107
52. Folco G, Omini C, Rossini G, Vigan'o T, Berti F (1982) Anticholinergic agents prevent guinea-pig airway constriction induced by histamine, bradykinine and leukotriene C_4: relationship to circulating TXA_2. Eur J Pharmacol 78:159–165
53. Geiger R (1985) The kallikrein-kinin systems. In: Türk VLJ (ed) Proteinases and their inhibitors. Mladinska Knjian – Pergamon, Ljubljana Oxford, pp 353–376
54. Gell PGH, Coombs RRA (1968) Clinical aspects of immunology, vol. 3. Blackwell, Oxford, p 3
55. Gervais R, Reinberg A, Gervais C, Smolensky M, de France O (1977) Twenty-four-hour rhythm in the bronchial hyperreactivity to house dust in asthmatics. J Allergy Clin Immunol 59:207–213
56. Gigli I (1976) Immunochemistry and immunobiology of the complement system. J Invest Dermatol 67:346–350
57. Gleich GJ (1982) The late phase of the immunoglobulin E-mediated reaction – a link between anaphylaxis and common allergic disease? J Allergy Clin Immunol 70:160–169
58. Gleich GJ, Muller SA (1980) Atopic dermatitis: a review with emphasis on pathogenesis. Clin Immunol 43:1316–1335
59. Goetzl EJ (1980) Occasional notes: mediators of immediate hypersensitivity derived from arachidonic acid. N Engl J Med 303:822–824
60. Gronneberg WE, Strandberg K, Stalenheim G, Zetterstrom O (1981) Effect in man of anti-allergic drugs on the immediate and late cutaneous allergic reaction induced by anti-IgE. Allergy 36:201–208
61. Grönneberg R (1984) Inhibition of the late phase reaction to antihuman IgE in man by oral tranexamic acid. Allergy 39:115–118
62. Harris MG (1981) Bronchial irritant receptors and a possible new action for cromolyn sodium. Ann Allergy 46:156–158
63. Herxheimer H (1952) The late bronchial reaction in induced asthma. Int Arch Allergy Appl Immunol 3:189–207
64. Ishizaka TCM, Sian K, Ishizaka K (1972) Complement fixation by aggregated IgE through alternate pathway. J Immunol 108: 848–851
65. Juhlin L, Michaelsson G (1969) Cutaneous reactions to kallikrein, bradykinin and histamine in healthy subjects and in patients with urticaria. Acta Derm Venerol 49:26–36
66. Kaliner M (1984) Hypotheses on the contribution of late phase allergic responses to the understanding and treatment of allergic diseases. J Allergy Clin Immunol 73:311–315
67. Kaliner M, Lemanske RF (1985) Inflammatory responses to mast cell granules. Fed Proc (in press)
68. Keller R (1968) On the role of secondary mast-cell damage and histamine-release in the course of immune reactions. In: Dusten K, Becker EL (eds) Biochemistry of acute allergic reactions. Blackwell, Oxford, pp 253–265
69. Kopp D, Esser B, Goetzl E, Lemanske R, Madison WI (1984) The role of leucotriene B_4 in rat cutaneous late phase reactions. J Allergy Clin Immunol 73:158 (abstract)
70. Kravis TC, Henson PM (1977) Accumulation of platelets at sites of antigen-antibody-mediated injury: a possible role for IgE antibodies and mast cells. J Immunol 118: 1559–1573
71. Lemanske RF, Barr L, Guthman DA, Kaliner M (1983) The biologic activity of mast cell granules. V. The effect of antihistamine treatment on rat cutaneous early late phase allergic reactions. J Allergy Clin Immunol 72:94–99
72. Lemanske RF, Guthman DA, Kaliner M (1983) The biologic activity of mast cell granules. VII. The effect of antineutrophil antibody induced neutropenia on rat cutaneous late phase reactions. J Immunol 131:929–933
73. Lemanske RF, Guthman DA, Oertel H, Barr L, Kaliner M (1983) The biologic activity of mast cell granules. The effect of vinblastine-induced neutropenia on rat cutaneous late phase reactions. J Immunol 6:2837–2842

74. Lemanske RF, Kaliner M (1982) Mast cell dependent late phase reactions. Clin Immunol Rev 1:547–580
75. Lewis RA, Holgate ST, Roberts LJ, Oates JA, Austen KF (1971) Preferential generation of prostaglandin D_2 by rat and human mast cells. In: Becker EL, Simon AJ, Austen KF (eds) Biochemistry of the acute allergic reaction. Blackwell, Oxford, pp 239–254
76. Lewis RA, Soter YA, Corey EJ, Austen KF (1981) Local effects of synthetic leukotrienes on monkey and human skin. Clin Res 29:492 (abstract)
77. Lichtenstein LA, Gillespie E (1973) Inhibition of histamine release by histamine controlled by H_2 receptors. Nature 244: 287–288
78. Lichtenstein LM, Valentine MD, Norman PS (1984) A reevaluation of immunotherapy for asthma. Am Rev Respir Dis 129: 657–659
79. Lorenz W, Doenicke A, Schoening B, Mamorski J, Weber D, Hinterlang E, Schwarz B, Neugebauer E (1980) H_1-H_2-receptor antagonists for premedication in anaesthesia and surgery. Agents Actions 10:114–124
80. Lotner GZ, Lynch JM, Betz SJ, Henson PM (1980) Human neutrophil-derived platelet activating factor. J Immunol 124:676–684
81. Mayno G (1964) Mechanism of abnormal vascular permeability in acute inflammation. In: Thomas L, Uhr J, Grant L (eds) Injury inflammation and immunity. Williams and Wilkins, Baltimore, pp 58–93
82. Marone G, Kagey-Sobotka A, Lichtenstein LM (1981) Possible role of phospholipase A_2 in triggering histamine secretion from human basophils in vitro. Clin Immunol Immunopathol 20:231–239
83. Metzger WJ, Dorminey HC, Robbins D, Richerson HB (1981) Late asthmatic responses during allergen bronchoprovocation. Correlation with specific IgE and symptoms. J Allergy Clin Immunol 67:11 (abstract)
84. Metzger WJ, Richerson HB, Kregel K, Barfknecht C, Moore K (1982) Late phase obstructive airways responses (LPR) in a rabbit model: physiology and anatomic findings. Am Rev Dis 125:62 (abstract)
85. Michel B, Russell TH, Winkelmann RK, Gleich GJ (1970) Release of kinins from site of wheal and flare allergic skin reactions. Int Arch Allergy 39:616–624
86. Mygind N, Johnson NJ, Thonsen J (1977) Intranasal allergen challenge during corticosteroid treatment. Clin Allergy 7:69–74
87. Naclerio R, Togias A, Proud D, Adkinson NF, Kagey-Sobotka A, Plaut M, Norman PS, Lichtenstein LM (1984) Inflammatory mediators in nasal secretions during early and late reactions. J Allergy Clin Immunol 73:148 (abstract)
88. Nagy L, Lee Th, Kay AB (1982) Neutrophil chemotactic activity in antigen-induced late asthmatic reactions. N Engl J Med 306: 497–501
89. Newball HH, Meier HL, Kaplan AP, Revak SD, Cochrane CG, Lichtenstein LM (1981) Activation of the Hageman factor dependent systems during IgE mediated reactions of the human lung. Int Arch Allergy Appl Immunol 66:165 (abstract)
90. Newball HH, Talamo RC, Lichtenstein LM (1975) Release of leucocyte kallikrein mediated by IgE. Nature 254:635–636
91. Norman PS (1983) Review of nasal therapy: update. J Allergy Clin Immunol 72: 421–429
92. Oertel H, Kaliner M (1981) The biologic activity of mast cell granules in rat skin. II. The effects of adrenocorticosteroids upon late phase inflammatory responses induced by mast cell granules. J Allergy Clin Immunol 68:238–245
93. Oertel H, Kaliner M (1981) The biologic activity of mast cell granules. III. Purification of inflammatory factors of anaphylaxis (IF-A) responsible for causing late phase reactions. J Immunol 1127:1398–1402
94. Parish PE (1970) Short-term anaphylactic IgG antibodies in human sera. Lancet 2:591 –592
95. Patterson R, Fink JN, Nishimura ET (1965) The passive transfer of immediate type hypersensitivity from man to other primates. J Clin Invest 44:140–148
96. Paton WDM (1951) Compound 48/80: A potent histamine liberator. Br J Pharmacol Chemother 6:499–508
97. Pelikan Z (1978) Late and delayed responses of the nasal mucosa to allergen challenge. Ann Allergy 41:37–47
98. Pelikan Z, Pelikan-Filipek M (1982) The effects of disodium cromoglycate and beclomethasone dipropionate on the immediate response of the nasal mucosa to allergen challenge. Ann Allergy 49:238– 292
99. Pepys J, Turner-Warwick M, Dawson PL, Hinson KFW (1968) Arthus (type III) skin test reactions in man. Clinical and immunopathological features. In: Excerpta Medica International Congress Series, Allergology, Proceedings of the Sixth Congress of the International Association of Allergology 162:221–235

100. Peters SP, MacGlashan DW, Schulman ES, Schleimer RP, Hayes EC, Rokach J, Adkinson NF, Lichtenstein LM (1984) Arachidonic acid metabolism in purified human mast cells. J Immunol 4: 1972–1979
101. Pienkowski M, Adkinson NF, Norman PS, Lichtenstein LM (1984) Mediators during cutaneous allergic immediate and late-phase reactions. J Allergy Clin Immunol 73: 147 (abstract)
102. Pienkowski M, Norman PS, Lichtenstein LM (in press) Suppression of late phase skin reaction in patients on immunotherapy with ragweed. Ann Allergy (abstract)
103. Poothullil J, Umemoto L, Dolovich J, Hargreave FE, Day RP (1976) Inhibition by prednisone of late cutaneous allergic responses induced by antiserum to human IgE. J Allergy Clin Immunol 57: 164–167
104. Prausnitz C, Küstner H (1921) Studien über die Überempfindlichkeit. Zentralbl Bakteriol 86: 160–169
105. Price JF, Hey EN, Soothill JF (1982) Antigen provocation to the skin, nose and lung in children with asthma; immediate and dual hypersensitivity reactions. Clin Exp Immunol 47: 587–594
106. Radermecker M, Maldague MP (1981) Depression of neutrophil chemotaxis in atopic individuals: an H_2 histamine receptor response. Int Arch Allergy Appl Immunol 65: 144–152
107. Ratnoff OD (1971) A tanglet web: the interdependence of mechanism of blood clotting fibrinolysis, immunity and inflammation. Thromb Diath Haemorrh [Suppl] 45: 109–129
108. Reed CHE (1974) Allergic mechanisms in extrinsic allergic alveolitis. In: Brent L, Holborow S (eds) Progress in immunology, vol. 4, part 2. North Holland, Amsterdam, pp 271–281
109. Richerson HB, Rajtora DW, Penik GD, Dick FR, Yoo TJ (1979) Cutaneous and nasal allergic responses in ragweed hay fever: lack of clinical and histopathologic correlations with late phase reactions. J Allergy Clin Immunol 64: 67–77
110. Ring J, Rothenberger KH, ClaußW (1985) Prevention of anaphylactoid reactions after radiographic contrast media infusion by combined histamine H_1- and H_2-receptor antagonists: results of a prospective controlled trial. Int Arch Allergy Appl Immunol 78: 9–14
111. Robertson DG, Kerigan AT, Hargreave FE, Chalmers K, Dolovich J (1974) Late asthmatic responses induced by ragween pollen allergen. J Allergy Clin Immunol 54: 244–254
112. Samuelsson B (1982) The leukotrienes: an introduction. In: Samuelsson B, Paoletti R (eds) Leukotrienes and other lipoxygenase products. Raven Press, New York, pp 1–17
113. Schleimer RP, MacGlashan DW, Gillespie E, Lichtenstein LM (1982) Inhibition of basophil histamine release by anti-inflammatory steroids. II. Studies on the mechanism of action. J Immunol 129: 1632–1635
114. Schleimer RP, Schulman ES, MacGlashan DW (1983) Effects of dexamethasone on mediator release from human lung fragments and purified human lung mast cells. J Clin Invest 71: 1830–1835
115. Schulman ES, Newball HH, Demers LM, Fitzpatrick FA, Adkinson NF (1981) Anaphylactic release of thromboxane A_2, prostaglandin D_2 and prostacyclin from human lung parenchyma. Am Rev Respir Dis 124: 402–406
116. Shaikh W, Umemoto L, Poothullil J, Hargreave FE, Dolovich J (1977) Relative refractory state for late cutaneous allergic response. J Allergy Clin Immunol 60: 242–246
117. Shampain MP, Behrens BL, Larsen GL, Henson PM (1982) An animal model of late pulmonary responses to *Alternaria* challenge. Am Rev Respir Dis 126: 493–498
118. de Shazo RD, Dvorak H, Davis R, Evans R (1978) The late phase skin reaction. J Allergy Clin Immunol 61: 186–202
119. de Shazo RD, Boehm TM, Kuman D (1982) Dermal hypersensitivity reactions to insulin: correlations of three patterns to their histopathology. J Allergy Clin Immunol 69: 229–237
120. de Shazo RD, Levinson AI, Dvorak HF, Davis RW (1979) The late phase skin reaction: evidence for activation of the coagulation system in an IgE-dependent reaction in man. J Immunol 122: 692–698
121. Shea C, Morse ED (1978) Inhibition of human neutrophil chemotaxis by corticosteroids. Ann Clin Lab Sci 8: 30–33
122. Smith MHJ, Ford-Hutchinson AW (1979) Inflamed tissue factors. In: Vane JR, Ferreira SH (eds) Antiinflammatory drugs. Springer, Berlin Heidelberg New York, pp 675–677 (Handbook of experimental pharmacology, vol. 50, part 2)
123. Smith JA, Mansfield LE, de Shazo RD, Nelson HS (1980) An evaluation of the pharmacologic inhibition of the immediate and late cutaneous reactions to allergen. J Allergy Clin Immunol 65: 185–222
124. Solley GO, Gleich GJ, Jordon RE, Schroeter AL (1976) The late phase of immediate wheal and flare skin reactions. J Clin Invest 58: 408–420

125. Soter NA, Austen KF (1976) The diversity of mast cell-derived mediators: implication for acute, subacute and chronic cutaneous inflammatory disorders. J Invest Dermatol 67:313–319
126. Staszewska-Barezak J, Vane JR (1975) The role of prostaglandins in the local control of circulation. Clin Exp Pharmacol Physiol 2: 71–78
127. Stalenheim G, Zetterström O (1979) Late cutaneous reactions without the participation of IgE. Monogr Allergy 14:264–267
128. Svensson J, Strandberg K, Turemo T, Hamberg M (1977) Thromboxane A_2: Effects on airway and vascular smooth muscle. Prostaglandins 14:425–436
129. Talbot S, Atkins P, Zweiman B (1984) Prolonged histamine release in cutaneous allergic reactions. J Allergy Clin Immunol 73:147 (abstract)
130. Tannenbaum S, Oertel H, Henderson W, Kaliner M (1980) The biologic activity of mast cell granules. I. Elicitation of inflammatory responses in rat skin. J Immunol 125:325–335
131. Tiffeneau R (1960) Über nicht kontinuierliche (Pollen) und kontinuierliche (Hausstaub) Allergeneffekte und deren Einfluß auf die bronchomotorische Erregbarkeit des Asthmatikers. Allergie Asthma 6:10–15
132. Turner-Warwick M (1978) Immunology of the lung. Edward Arnold, London, p 165
133. Tyler HM, Saxton CATD, Parry JM (1981) Administration to man of UK-37, 248-01, a selective inhibitor of thromboxane synthetase. Lancet 21:629–632
134. Umemoto L, Poothullil J, Dolovich KE, Hargreave AP, Day RP (1976) Factors which influence the late cutaneous allergic response (LCAR). J Allergy Clin Immunol 58:60
135. Vanderhoek JY, Makheja AN, Bailey JM (1980) Inhibition of fatty acid oxygenases by onion and garlic oils. Evidence for the mechanism by which these oils inhibit platelet aggregations. Biochem Pharmacol 29:3169–3173
136. Verhagen J, Bruynzeel PLB, Koedam JA, Wassink GA, de Boer M, Terpstra GK, Kreukniet J, Veldink GA, Vliegenthart JFG (1984) Specific leukotriene formation by purified human eosinophils and neutrophils. FEBS Lett 168:23–28
137. Ward PA (1966) The chemosuppression of chemotaxis. J Exp Med 124:124–209
138. Warner JA (1976) Significance of late reactions after bronchial challenge with house dust mite. Arch Dis Child 51:905–911
139. Williams TJ, Morley J (1973) Prostaglandins as potentiators of increased vascular permeability in inflammation. Nature 246:215–217
140. Zetterström O (1978) Dual skin test reactions and serum antibodies to subtilisin and *Aspergillus fumigatus* extracts. Clin Allergy 8:77–91

F. Bronchial Pathophysiology

26. Bronchi of Asthmatic Patients

Ph. Godard, Y. Maria, F. B. Michel

This work was supported in part by a grant from le Fonds Spécial du Comité National de Lutte contre les Maladies Respiratoires.

Bronchial asthma is mainly characterized by variable dyspnea due to the widespread narrowing of airways, varying in severity over short periods of time [3]; the airway obstruction is the consequence of a bronchospasm and also of bronchial inflammation.

Our knowledge of the bronchi of asthmatic patients owes much to the first descriptions made by Vallery-Radot, Dubois de Montreynaud and Lemoine [20]. Now, bronchofiberscopes are widely used and offer at least three advantages which justify a real "come back to the bronchi" as we suggested some years ago [9, 21]:

- good tolerance, and this point is very important, especially in asthmatic patients who have bronchial hyperreactivity;
- a better exploration of the bronchi, in the near future it should be interesting to explore the more peripheral bronchi by using the new fiberscopes which have a 1.8 mm diameter; and
- the procedure of bronchoalveolar lavage (BAL), to study the bronchoalveolar cells which are involved in the pathogenesis of bronchial asthma [2, 24].

We report herein the lessons we learned from our daily practice of bronchofiberscopy in asthmatic patients.

26.1 Endoscopic Aspects

More than 200 patients were studied during the last 18 months.

Normal appearance (20 to 30%): The appearance of the bronchi of the asthmatics who were examined was rarely normal, even though there was no recent history of an attack.

Chronic bronchitis (70 to 80%): Hypersecretion was almost always present; sometimes there were no clinical symptoms and, as suggested by Lemoine [20], the diagnosis we proposed was *latent chronic bronchitis.* The bronchial secretions were viscous, adherent to the bronchi and could form crescents which reduced the bronchial caliber.

Bronchoscopy enabled us to ascertain the lesional status (numerous and/or enlarged mucous gland, hyperemia), and was helpful in making the prognosis; moreover, for example, extensive changes in the mucosa were grounds for instituting a more vigorous treatment. The finding of a bronchial superinfection which was not clinically evident could indicate a deterioration which was usually ascribed to a failure of treatment or to desensitization.

Edema (40 to 50%): Edema of the proximal carinae was fairly common in allergic asthma; such a finding raised the suspicion of this etiology as was suggested by Dubois de Montreynaud [26].

Bronchial obstructions and stenosis: Mucous plugs were always present during status asthmaticus; they were very often observed in the BAL fluids, made up of dead cells, desquamated epithelial cells and eosinophils, and might have contributed to the airway obstruction.

In two cases of severe asthma in young subjects, an irreversible, quite complete stenosis of the apical bronchus of the right lower lobe was observed. The significance of such a finding remains uncertain.

The clinical, radiological and immunological picture of allergic bronchopulmonary aspergillosis is well-known. Bronchiectasis is a possible complication especially if the diagnosis and treatment are delayed. We have observed two bronchial mycelian tumors in one such case; they manifested the permanent bronchial parasitism which is a main feature of this disease.

Finally it was sometimes possible to observe a spontaneous bronchial collapse either in the main or in segmental bronchi (10 to 20% of cases); such a finding contributed to the diagnosis of a dynamic compression of the airways and led to the proposal of teaching correct breathing [25].

26.2 Cytological Aspects

Bronchoalveolar lavage (BAL) is a well-known procedure to obtain the so-called bronchoalveolar cells (BAC); a combination of clinical findings and BAL fluid results can lead to the diagnosis of some interstitial pneumonia [11]. To date BAL was counterindicated in airways' diseases.

However some evidence suggests that BAC could play an important role in the pathogenesis of bronchial asthma. Indeed the BAC of sensitized monkeys could induce asthma when they are injected into the trachea of an unsensitized syngeneic monkey [24]. Few mast cells are free in the bronchoalveolar lumen which could promote the inflammatory process which leads to the asthma attack [12].

Bronchoalveolar lavage: Bronchoscopy was performed with a flexible fiberoptic instrument (Olympus BF-B3), 15 min after premedication with chlorazepate 10 mg, atropine 0.25 mg, and local anesthesia with 5–10 ml of 1% lidocaine. BAL was performed by progressive instillation of 100 to 150 ml (or 200 to 400 ml in some patients) of 0.9% saline at room temperature into a subsegmental bronchus of the right middle lobe, followed by gentle aspiration as previously described [16].

Preparation of the bronchoalveolar cells (BAC): The fluid obtained from BAL was immediately filtered through a single layer of sterile gauze, then centrifugated at 500 g for 10 min. The BAC were then washed twice with Hank's balanced salt solution and counted in a hemocytometer. Differential counts of BAC were performed after cytocentrifugation on smears stained with Giemsa and toluidine blue.

Tolerance of BAL [22] (Figs. 26.1, 26.2): No complications were observed in normal volunteers. In asthmatic patients, no laryngeal spasm was noted; 20 mild asthmatic attacks were observed, always after the procedure, never during the 5 to 10 min of endoscopy and BAL, and for each one of them, theophylline by IV route was very efficient in a few minutes. In 6 patients we noted a slight rise in the temperature, never more than 38.5 °C, at the end of the day, which spontaneously resolved in each case.

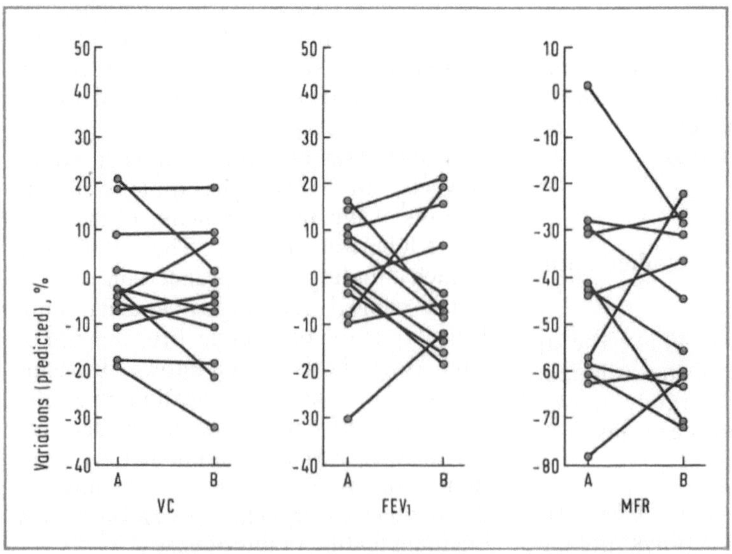

Fig. 26.1. Tolerance of BAL. Forced expiratory graphs have been recorded before and 2 hours after the end of the BAL

Local anesthesia [27] did not induce, on average, any deterioration of the spirometric parameters (i.e., a drop in the FEV_1 greater than 20%); in one patient a significant increase was noted in the FEV_1, +26%.

The repeated recording of spirometric values in some patients revealed an average decrease in FVC ($-22 \pm 5\%$), in the FEV_1 ($-21 \pm 5\%$) and in the MMEFR ($-17 \pm 5\%$) during the 15 to 30 min following the end of the BAL ($p < 0.01$). But at the end of the 120th min no difference was recordable.

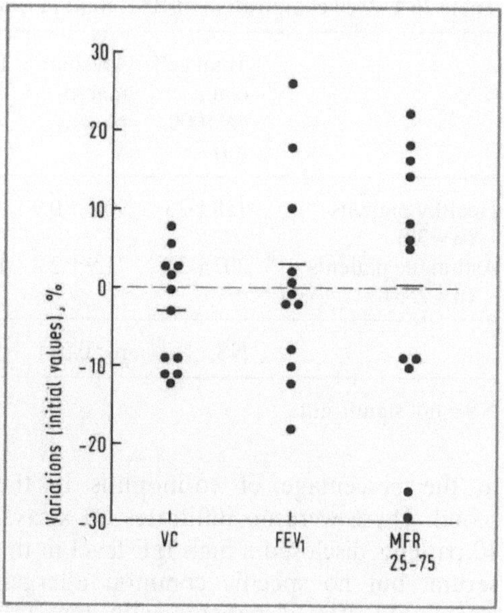

Fig. 26.2. Tolerance of local anesthesia

BAL fluid recovery (Fig. 26.3): Of the saline instillated into the bronchoalveolar lumen, 40 to 65% were recovered in normal volunteers. In asthmatic patients, the percentage of BAL fluid recovery was significantly decreased ($p < 0.01$). It ranged from 15 to 75% and averaged $30 \pm 4\%$ (mean + SD).

There was no correlation with the intensity of airway obstruction as assessed by either FEV_1, MMEFR or FEV_1/FVC.

On the other hand when the quantity of instillated saline was different, the percentage of fluid recovery was significantly different: $32.2 \pm 1.9\%$ (when 100 to 150 ml were instillated) versus $59.2 \pm 2.2\%$ (when 200 to 400 ml were instillated – $p < 0.01$).

In some patients the gentle aspiration of BAL fluid induced an almost complete collapse of the bronchus which was not predictable by any clinical or spirometric parameter.

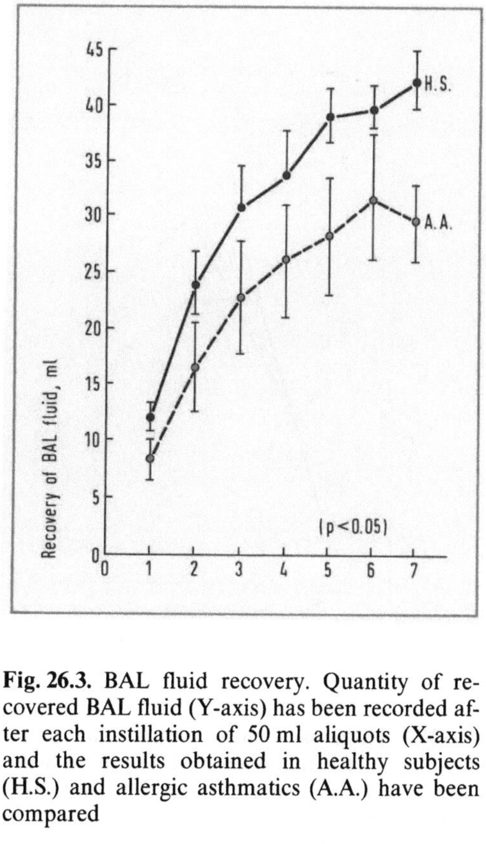

Fig. 26.3. BAL fluid recovery. Quantity of recovered BAL fluid (Y-axis) has been recorded after each instillation of 50 ml aliquots (X-axis) and the results obtained in healthy subjects (H.S.) and allergic asthmatics (A.A.) have been compared

Bronchoalveolar cell counts: The results are shown in Table 26.1; the cell yield per milliliter of recovered BAL fluid was statistically equivalent for the normal healthy subjects and the asthmatic patients as a whole, the differential cell counts were different, but important variations in these counts could be observed according to the patients (Table 26.1).

In asymptomatic asthmatic patients, the differential BAC count was for the most part quite normal; the percentage of eosinophils was always less than 6%.

Eosinophils [5–7] averaged $6.8 \pm 1.8\%$ and ranged from 0 to 90%. 17 patients had a percentage of eosinophils higher than 20%; the percentage of eosinophils in BAL fluid correlated to the total cell count and

Table 26.1. Cell composition of BAL fluid in asthmatic patients

	Total cell count (× 1000/ ml)	Alveolar macro-phages %	Lympho-cytes %	Neutro-phils %	Eosino-phils %	Mast cells %	Bronchial cells %
Healthy patients (n = 30)	158 ± 23	90.0 ± 0.9	8.7 ± 0.9	0.9 ± 0.1	0.2 ± 0.1	0.0 ± 0	0.1 ± 0.06
Asthmatic patients (n = 253)	207 ± 21	71.9 ± 2.3	15.3 ± 1.9	5.7 ± 1.4	6.8 ± 1.3	0.04 ± 0.02	0.4 ± 0.13
	NS	p < 0.001	p < 0.001	p < 0.001	p < 0.001	p < 0.05	NS

NS = not significant

to the percentage of eosinophils in the blood. There were no infiltrates on x-rays. 10 patients disclosed a high IgE level in the serum, but no specific common allergen was found. The 7 patients with low IgE level disclosed some interesting features: Their mean age was higher; they had a higher percentage of eosinophils; and they were corticosteroid-dependent (6 to 12 months follow-up).

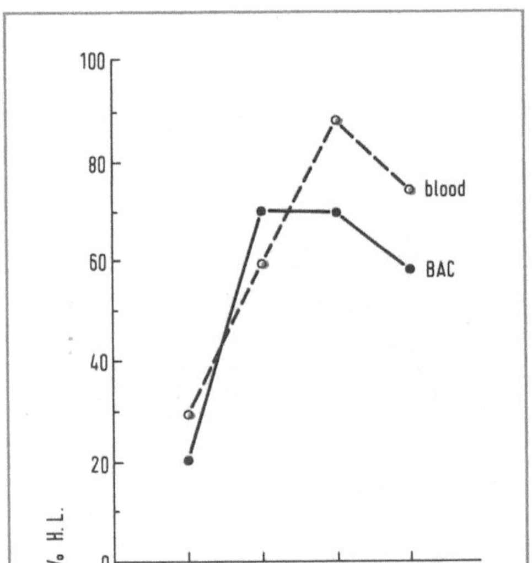

Fig. 26.4. Histamine release from the bronchoalveolar cells (obtained by BAL) in an asthmatic patient who was sensitized to mite (D. pteronyssinus)

Neutrophils averaged 5.7 ± 1.4%, but a high percentage of eosinophils did not correlate with an increased number of neutrophils. This high percentage was the consequence of bacterial infection in some patients.

Lymphocytes averaged 15.3 ± 1.9%. Some patients had a very high percentage of lymphocytes which ranged from 30 to 55% and averaged 40 ± 5%. These patients had no evidence of interstitial pneumonia [19]; we found high percentages of lymphocytes in BAL in patients with viral airway and/or pulmonary infection.

Mast cells (and to a lesser extent basophils) have been found in BAL fluids; after cytocentrifugation and toluidine blue staining, the percentage was always very low (less than 2%). However we have shown that the BAC were able to release histamine after specific challenge in vitro in patients with allergic bronchial asthma [12] (Fig. 26.4). We can conclude with Patterson et al that viable and immunoreactive mast cells are free in the bronchoalveolar lumen [24], they could be a starter for a cascade of events induced by a specific trigger, and the cascade of events probably includes the activation of the other BAC (mainly AM [1, 4, 10, 14, 17, 18]) and the release of chemical mediators which could amplify the reactions by recruitment of other inflammatory cells [13].

The bronchi of asthmatic patients [15, 23] have to be carefully examined not only by clinical, radiological and spirometric means but also by endoscopic means [8]. BAL is a good method for checking the cells which are involved in the pathogenesis.

References

1. Aubas P, Cosso B, Godard P, Michel FB, Clot J (1984) Decreased suppressor cell activity of alveolar macrophages in bronchial asthma. Am Rev Respir Dis 130:875–878
2. Aubas P, Godard P, Michel FB (1981) Contribution du lavage bronchiolo-alvéolaire à la connaissance de l'asthme. Allergol Immunopathol [Suppl IX]: 19–22
3. Charpin J (1973) Les faux asthmes. Quelques pièges de diagnostic différentiel. Rev Prat 23:319
4. Damon M, Chavis C, Godard P, Michel FB, Crastes de Paulet A (1983) Purification and mass spectrometry identification of leukotriene D4 synthetized by human alveolar macrophages. Biochem Biophys Res Commun 111:518–524
5. de Blic J, Dhont P, Scheinmann P, Pfister A, Paupe J, Delage C (1980) Intérêt diagnostic de l'éosinophilie des sécrétions bronchiques chez l'enfant. Nouv Presse Méd 9:3627
6. Dry J, Leynadier F, Aberaf M, Luce H, Pouillard J, Herman D (1978) Eosinophilie et fonction respiratoire chez l'asthmatique. Pathol Biol 26:489–494
7. Frigas E, Loegering DA, Solley GO, Farrow GM, Gleich GJ (1981) Elevated levels of the eosinophils granule major basic protein in the sputum of patients with bronchial asthma. Mayo Clin Proc 56:345–353
8. Godard P (1983) Chronic cough: bronchoscopy or pulmonary function testing? Am Rev Respir Dis 127:257
9. Godard P, Aubas P, Calvayrac P, Taib J, Michel FB (1981) Endoscopie et lavage bronchiolo-alvéolaire chez l'asthmatique allergique. Nouv Presse Méd 10:3141–3148
10. Godard P, Chaintreuil J, Damon M, Coupe M, Flandre O, Crastes de Paulet A, Michel FB (1982) Functional assessment of alveolar macrophages: comparison of cells from asthmatic and normal subjects. J Allergy Clin Immunol 70:88–93
11. Godard P, Clot J, Jonquet O, Bousquet J, Michel FB (1981) Lymphocyte sub-populations in bronchoalveolar lavages of patients with sarcoidosis and hypersensitivity pneumonitis. Chest 80:447–452
12. Godard P, Terral C, Michel FB (1982) Histamine release by bronchoalveolar cells of allergic asthmatic patients. Am Rev Respir Dis 125:75 (A)
13. Godard P, Clot J, Michel FB (1983) Inter-relations cellulaires et sécrétions des médiateurs de l'inflammation dans les espaces aériens distaux. Rev Fr Mal Respir 11: 275–284
14. Godard P, Damon M, Michel FB, Corey EJ, Austen KF, Lewis RA (1983) Leukotriene B4 production from human alveolar macrophages. Clin Res 31:548A
15. Helm WH, Banan KA, Mukerjie SC (1972) Bronchial lavage in asthma and bronchitis. Ann Allergy 30:518–523
16. Hunninghake GW, Godik JE, Kawanani O, Ferrand VJ, Crystal RG (1979) Inflammatory and immune processes in the human lung in health and disease. Evaluation by bronchoalveolar lavage. Am J Pathol 97:149–206
17. Joseph M, Tonnel AB, Capron A, Voisin C (1980) Enzyme release and superoxide anion production by human alveolar macrophages stimulated with IgE. Clin Exp Immunol 40:416–422
18. Joseph M, Tonnel AB, Capron A, Voisin C (1983) Involvement of Immunoglobulin E in the secretory processes of alveolar macrophages from asthmatic patients. J Clin Invest 71:221–230
19. Lawrence EC, Blaese M, Martin RR (1978) Immunoglobulin secreting cells in normal human bronchial lavage fluids. J Clin Invest 62:832–835
20. Lemoine JM (1966) Les aspects endoscopiques dans l'asthme des adultes. Bronches 16:93–105
21. Michel FB, Godard P (1982) Caractères endo-bronchiques et alvéolaires de l'asthme. Bull Acad Natl Med 166:1019–1024
22. Nakhesteen JA (1978) Bronchofiberscopy in asthmatics: a method for minimizing risk of complications. Respiration 36:112–116
23. Passy V, Esmshar C, Brothers M (1976) Bronchopulmonary lavage to remove pulmonary casts and plugs. Arch Otolaryngol 102:193–197
24. Patterson R, Susko IM, Harris KE (1978) The in vivo transfer of antigen-induced airway reactions by bronchial lumen cells. J Clin Invest 61:519–524
25. Touaty E, Karsenti P, Bussi S, Baldeyren P, Lochon B, Derenne JP, Fournier M, Pariente R (1980) Collapsus bronchique au cours des bronchopathies chroniques obstructives. Ann Med Interne 131:29–33
26. Vallery-Radot P, Halpern BN, Dubois de Montreynaud JM, Pean V (1950) Les bronches au cours de la crise d'asthme. Etude expérimentale, bronchoscopique et anatomopathologique. Presse Méd 58:661–664
27. Weiss EB, Patwardhan AV (1977) The response to lidocaine in bronchial asthma. Chest 72:429–438

27. The Site of Bronchial Obstruction in Asthma

Ch. Préfaut

As for the diagnosis, the function or even the therapy, the asthmatic's airways are often considered as a whole: It is a *bronchial* obstruction which is to be determined, induced or treated. It is implicitly making the assumption: that asthma is a disease affecting the entire airways uniformly, either in a critical, intercritical or in a complicated stage; and that therapies have the same effects on every bronchial level. For many years, this unique aspect of the asthmatic disease has been in opposition to various clinical, radiological, functional, therapeutic studies. Unfortunately, these studies are complex, their interpretation difficult and the site of bronchial obstruction cannot yet be localized precisely. Indeed we can only say that the obstruction probably occurs in the central or in the peripheral airways, knowing that the inner diameter of the peripheral airways is less than 2 mm (i.e., starting in the segmental bronchi).

In this paper, we shall first review the methods that have been used, then we shall consider the evolution of the concepts on the site of bronchial obstruction during the asthmatic disease and we shall try to point out the interest of these methods in the future.

27.1 Methods

27.1.1 Morphological Methods

They have been the first methods used. Indeed, from 1933 Christopherson [5] used bronchography in the asthmatic patients. More recently, Hungerfold et al [11] studied the thickness of the bronchial walls in seriously ill patients.

27.1.2 Common Tests of Lung Function

Most of the usual techniques of lung function give a general information on the site of bronchial obstruction.

The value of airway resistances (Raw) is primarily influenced (80%) by the size of the large airways in normal subjects. In patients, an important increase in this parameter is a good indicator of predominantly central obstruction.

It is more difficult to interpret, in terms of localization, a change in forced expiratory flows. According to Mead [19] it is generally stated that at high lung volumes large airways have the major influence, while the more the lung volume decreases the more important the influence of the peripheral airways becomes. Therefore, a decrease in flows at low lung volumes with normal flows at higher lung volumes very likely means that the obstruction is located in the small airways. Unfortunately, when flows decrease at high lung volumes they are usually abnormal at lower lung volumes. That means either the entire airways are obstructed or a central obstruction modifies the shape of the forced expiratory curve at lower lung volumes.

On a spirogram a decrease in the forced expiratory flow between 25 and 75% of the vital capacity (FEF_{25-75}) associated with a normal forced expiratory volume in one second (FEV_1) probably indicates a distal obstruction. In the same way considering flow volume curves, the small airways are mostly obstructed when there is a decrease in the maximal expiratory flows at 25% of vital capacity ($\dot{V}_{max_{25}}$) with normal flows at higher lung volumes.

Other parameters can indicate a peripheral obstruction. Frequency dependence of dynamic compliance is considered the most reliable test to reveal a distal obstruction, provided that the static compliance and the airway resistances are normal [31]. Under the same conditions, an increase in the closing volume would also reveal a peripheral obstruction [15]. It is interesting to note that an isolated hypoxia can reveal a shunt which is usually secondary to an obstruction in the small airways [13].

27.1.3 Density Dependence of Airflows

A more specifical method, comparing the maximal expiratory flow measured first in air and then in a helium (80%) oxygen (20%) mixture (HeO_2), has been described in 1972 by Despas et al [7]. This method was based on the theory of equal pressure point (EPP) by Mead et al [20] and on physical properties of gases. The main purpose of the thus measured *density dependence* of the flow volume curve was to study the relative contribution of peripheral versus central pressure loss along the airways.

In normal subjects, maximal flows increased with the HeO_2 mixture at high and medium lung volumes (density dependence) but not at low lung volumes, the response being expressed as the difference between the flows in HeO_2 and in air at 50% of the vital capacity ($\Delta\dot{V}_{max_{50}}$).

In obstructive patients two kinds of responses have been observed: There are the responders, who, like normal subjects, showed density dependence and the nonresponders who did not. For responders it has been suggested [7] that the major site of obstruction was, like for normal subjects, in the large airways. A nonresponse was explained by an upstream movement of EPP. Macklem et al [14] demonstrated by direct measurements, that in most cases of peripheral obstruction EPP moved upstream. Therefore, a nonresponse suggests that the major site of airway obstruction is in the small airways [7].

The study by Mink et al [21, 22] on canine lungs and aged human excised lungs revealed some discrepancies with the initial theory. They essentially observed that the geometry of airways was different in air and in HeO_2, partly explaining the density independence. They pointed out that their findings were consistent if the results were interpreted in terms of the wave-speed theory of flow limitation [6]. This theory is based both on the EPP theory [20] and on the flow limiting segment theory of Pride [27]. From their results they were able to explain the large interindividual variability of $\Delta\dot{V}_{max}$. For instance, normal subjects with large central airways will have large $\dot{V}_{max}$ and low $\Delta\dot{V}_{max}$ and vice versa. Although they agreed with the fact that $\Delta\dot{V}_{max}$ decreases with peripheral airways obstruction, Mink et al questioned the interpretation of $\Delta\dot{V}_{max}$ as an index of peripheral airway obstruction.

In 1982 Pedersen et al [23] performed in dogs similar experiments to those of Mink et al. They confirmed most of the results of Mink et al and proved the usefulness of the wave-speed theory. However, their interpretation differs since they conclude that decreases in density dependence mainly reflect increased frictional pressure losses in airways upstream of the EPP, therefore an obstruction in peripheral airways.

In 1983 the same group (Castile et al [3]) concluded that minimal density dependence always signifies the presence of air flow obstruction in the lung periphery although a high degree of density dependence does not rule out peripheral narrowing. However, these authors showed that a maximal density dependence with markedly reduced flow rates, strongly suggests predominant central obstruction.

Clearly, the interpretation of HeO_2 response is complex, primarily because of a misunderstanding of the determinants of maximum expiratory flow. Probably the most valuable information of this method could be obtained in longitudinal studies. To follow up, the HeO_2 responses could minimize interindividual variability like relating the density dependence before and after various stimuli. In transversal studies, interindividual variability of subjects probably complicates the interpretation and at least large series of studies are needed. A good alternative to this kind of study could be to measure the density dependence of airway resistances. The problem of forced expiration is thus eliminated and the different properties of gases in relation to the different sizes of airways are used [28].

27.1.4 Site of Bronchial Obstruction in Asthma

Morphological studies: In 1933, Christopherson [5] reported that in severe asthma the lipidol could not reach the bronchioles and they became opaque if the patient was examined during an intercritical stage. In 1948, Epstein et al [8] showed that an instillation of iodine oil at the carina level in asthmatic patients induced a bronchospasm oscillating between the main bronchi and their first subdivisions. More recently, Hungerford et al [11] reported that the thickness of the walls of the large bronchi was doubled in severe asthma and that the thickness of the walls of the small bronchi increased by less than 40%. Clearly, these morphological studies assume that the site of the obstruction is central in the asthmatic disease.

Lung function 1st period: The ulterior development of the tests of lung function has set the problem differently. In some patients a severe obstruction was observed; in others airway resistances and FEV_1 were normal whereas an isolated hypoxia [13], a frequency dependence of compliance [17] and a persistant decrease in FEF_{25-75} [26] were observed. The study of Weng and Levison [30] seems to summarize these different data. These authors have studied 30 patients just after an acute asthmatic attack and far away from one. The first data showed a large increase in airway resistances and a large decrease in FEV_1. Far from the acute attack the only damage was a decrease in FEF_{25-75}. At this time the different papers had mostly emphasized the peripheral obstruction and the sensibility of some parameters which could reveal a residual obstruction, whereas clinical examination and more classical tests were quite normal. Unfortunately, they do not seem to have considered the contradiction between the latest functional data suggesting a peripheral obstruction and the data obtained after the acute attack indicating a mainly central obstruction. Moreover, in 1969 McFadden and Lyons [16] tried to localize the site of bronchial obstruction. They followed up functional data in 4 asthmatic patients during the treatment of an acute attack. They concluded that during the acute attack the entire airways were affected, but mostly the peripheral airways, and that during the recovery only peripheral obstruction remained. From this period asthma was considered as a small airway disease.

Lung function 2nd period: This period starts with the work of Despas et al in 1972 [7]. The authors measured the density dependence of airflow in 25 asthmatic patients, most of them being symptomatic when studied. Among the 25 patients, 12 were responders indicating an obstruction in central airways, the others were nonresponders, i.e., with an obstruction in the small airways.

In 1975 Benatar et al [2] confirmed these data in 31 asthmatic patients. However they observed that ⅔ of the patients were responders. In 1976, Antic and Macklem [1] tried to determine the influence of clinical factors on the site and nature of airway obstruction in asthmatics with significant reversible airway obstruction, but free of acute symptoms. They observed that asthmatics without a history of smoking, chronic bronchitis or repeated respiratory infections had narrowing of the central airways. Therefore, Antic and Macklem concluded that, if there were no added clinical factors, the site of bronchial obstruction was mostly central during the asthmatic disease.

In 1979, Préfaut et al [24] studied the density dependence of airflow in 33 asthmatic children by analyzing more completely the relation between HeO_2 and air (three points of comparison instead of one). Their results suggested that when there was no history of recurrent infections, the site of obstruction in asthmatic children was mainly central. However, a coexisting peripheral obstruction could persist after recovery of the central component. For these authors, pure asthma is an obstructive disease of the entire airways, but the preferential site of obstruction depends on the stage of the disease. In the first stage, during an acute attack and its recovery, the obstruction is mainly central, but this component disappears first. Then in the second stage, i.e., far from the acute attack, the major site of obstruction is in the peripheral airways. This interpretation is consistent with the previous morphological or functional studies.

According to this interpretation, during induced bronchoconstriction, obstruction should affect the entire airways, but should be predominant in the central airways. An indirect argument favorable to this central predominance is that airway resistances are the parameter most often modified in response to the challenges [10, 32]. During inhalation challenge tests (red cedar, mites, gramineous pollens etc.) Chan-Yeung et al [4] and Terral et al [28] observed a predominantly central obstruction in terms of density dependence of airflow [4, 28] or total pulmonary resistances [28]. This observation is in accordance with the above hypothesis, but also with a probably preferential disparition of allergen particles in the large airways during inhalation tests. During induced bronchoconstriction by exercise, Chan-Yeung et al [4] observed that the obstruction mainly occurred in the central airways. However McFadden et al [18] found an increase in density dependence in some patients and a decrease in others suggesting that *exercise-induced asthma* probably involves different mechanisms than those of inhalation tests.

A direct confirmation of the above hypothesis implies longitudinal studies in asthmatic patients after an acute attack and during a long remission period which rarely occurs in severe asthma. Our group [unpublished data] conducted such a study in asthmatic children at an altitude which usually induces a longer remission. In 9 patients we observed that the obstruction was preferentially central near the attack but was mainly peripheral after a remission of 2 or 3 months. After 6 months, the obstruction had almost disappeared and the HeO_2 response was subnormal. These interesting findings must be interpreted with great care because the patients were observed at an altitude which can, per se, influence density dependence.

Now there still remains facts to show that asthma, at least allergic pure asthma, is an obstructive disease affecting the entire airways. During and near the acute attack period the obstruction is, probably, mainly central. Then, after a two or three months' remission and up to the complete recovery, the obstruction is, probably, mainly peripheral.

How can we interpret these phenomena on a physiopathological basis? The asthmatic disease is primarily due to three factors: spasm, edema and hypersecretion. Obviously they do not play the same role in the entire airways. The spasm could be predominant in the central airways and the edema in the peripheral airways. It is also clear that they do not occur or even disappear at the same time. The edema could occur after the spasm. Moreover, one can expect, that the therapies which have been used do not have the same efficacy on every factor. Many authors have studied the site of action of some bronchodilators [9, 12, 25, 29]. Although the results are often contradictory it would seem that the β_2-sympathomimetics had a greater effect on the small airways and the atropine on the entire airways or on the large bronchi.

In the future, it will be necessary to improve the methods in order to localize more precisely the main site of bronchial obstruction as it will also be necessary to determine whether the spasm, the edema and the hypersecretion are localized uniformly in the entire airways or not. These studies should contribute to a better therapy.

References

1. Antic R, Macklem PT (1976) The influence of clinical factors on site of airway obstruction in asthma. Am Rev Respir Dis 114:851–859
2. Benatar SR, Clark TJM, Cochrane GM (1975) Clinical relevance of the flow rate response to low density gas breathing in asthmatics. Am Rev Respir Dis 111:126–134
3. Castile RG, Pedersen OF, Drazen JM, Ingram RH Jr (1983) Density dependence of maximal flow in dogs with central and peripheral obstruction. J Appl Physiol 55: 717–725
4. Chan-Yeung M, Abboud R, Tsao MS, Maclean L (1976) Effect of helium on maximal expiratory flow in patients with asthma before and during induced bronchoconstriction. Am Rev Respir Dis 113:433–443
5. Christopherson JB (1933) Anatomy of chronic bronchitis and bronchial asthma as disclosed by lipidol examination. Am J Med Sci 186:504–509
6. Dawson SV, Elliott EA (1977) Wave-speed limitation on expiratory flow, a unifying concept. J Appl Physiol 43:498–515
7. Despas PJ, Leroux M, Macklem PT (1972) Site of airway obstruction in asthma as determined by measuring. Maximal expiratory flow breathing air and a helium oxygen mixture. J Clin Invest 51:3235–3243

8. Epstein BS, Sherman J, Walzer EE (1948) Bronchography in asthmatic patients with the aid of adrenalin. Radiology 50:96–97
9. Faimrster RD, Wilson AF (1980) Relationship between the site of airflow limitation and localisation of the bronchodilator response in asthma. Am Rev Respir Dis 122:27–32
10. Haydu SP, Empey DW, Hugues DTD (1974) Inhalation challenges tests in asthma: an assessment of spirometry, maximum expiratory flow rates and plethysmography in measuring the responses. Clin Allergy 4:371–378
11. Hungerford GD, Williams HBL, Gandevia B (1977) Bronchial walls in the radiological diagnosis of asthma. Br J Radiol 50:783–787
12. Ingram RH Jr, Wellman JJ, McFadden ER, Mead J (1977) Relative contribution of large and small airways to flow limitation in normal subjects before and after atropine and isoproterenol. J Clin Invest 59:696–703
13. Levigne G, Housley F, Macleod P, Macklem PT (1970) Gas exchange abnormalities in mild bronchitis and asymptomatic asthma. N Engl J Med 282:1277–1282
14. Macklem PT, Fraser RG, Brown WC (1965) Bronchial pressure measurements in emphysema and bronchitis. J Clin Invest 44:897–905
15. McCarthy DS, Spencer R, Green R, Milic-Emili J (1972) Measurement of "closing volume" as a simple and sensitive test for early detection of small airway disease. Am J Med 52:747–753
16. McFadden ER Jr, Lyons HA (1969) Serial studies of factors influencing airway dynamics during recovery from acute asthma attacks. J Appl Physiol 27:452–459
17. McFadden ER Jr, Lyons HA (1968) Airway resistance and uneven ventilation in bronchial asthma. J Appl Physiol 25:365–370
18. McFadden ER Jr, Ingram RH Jr, Haynes RL, Wellman JJ (1977) Predominant site of flow limitation and mechanisms of post exertional asthma. J Appl Physiol 42:746–752
19. Mead J (1979) Problems in interpreting common tests of pulmonary mechanical function. In: Macklem PT, Permutt SM, Lenfant C (eds) The lung in the transition between health and disease. Marcel Dekker, New York, pp 43–51
20. Mead J, Turner JM, Macklem PT, Little JB (1967) Significance of the relationship between lung recoil and maximum expiratory flow. J Appl Physiol 22:95–108
21. Mink SN, Wood LDH (1980) How does HeO_2 increase maximum expiratory flow in human lungs. J Clin Invest 66:720–729
22. Mink S, Ziesmann M, Wood LDH (1979) Mechanisms of increased maximum expiratory flow during HeO_2 breathing in dogs. J Appl Physiol 47:490–502
23. Pedersen OF, Castile RG, Drazen JM, Ingram RH Jr (1982) Density dependence of maximum expiratory flow in the dog. J Appl Physiol 53:397–404
24. Préfaut C, Lloret MC, Tronc JF, Michel FB, Chardon G (1979) Density dependence of the maximal expiratory flow volume curves in normal and asthmatic children. Scand J Respir Dis 60:109–118
25. Préfaut C, Lloret MC, Tronc JF, Michel FB, Chardon G (1977) Role des bronchodilatateurs sur la sensibilité à la densité gazeuse des débits maximaux. Bull Eur Physiopathol Respir 13:813–828
26. Préfaut C, Tournoux A, Michel FB, Bianchi M, Chardon G (1972) Debit maximum expiratoire 25–75% (DME 25–75). Son intérêt chez le sujet normal et chez l'asthmatique. Poumon Coeur 28:179–184
27. Pride NB, Permutt S, Riley RL, Bromberger-Barnea B (1967) Determinants of maximal expiratory flow from the lungs. J Appl Physiol 23:646–662
28. Terral C, Bourgouin-Karaouni D, Jonquet O, Godard P, Préfaut C (1983) Effets de l'hélium oxygène au cours des tests de provocation bronchique chez l'asthmatique. Bull Eur Physiopathol Respir 19:51–58
29. Wellman J, McFadden ER, Ingram RHJ (1976) Density dependence of maximal expiratory flow rates before and after bronchodilators in patients with obstructive airways disease. Clin Sci Mal Med 51:133–139
30. Weng TR, Levison H (1969) Pulmonary function in children with asthma at acute attack and symptom free status. Am Rev Respir Dis 99:719–728
31. Woollock AJ, Vincent MJ, Macklem PT (1969) Frequency dependence of compliance as a test for obstruction in the small airways. J Clin Invest 48:1097–1106
32. Yernault JC, Englert M, de Coster A (1973) Evaluation de l'action bronchoconstrictive de l'acetylcholine chez l'asthmatique. Respiration 30:260–269

28. Factors in Bronchial Hyperreactivity

H. A. Boushey

Supported in part by U.S. National Heart, Lung, and Blood Institute Program Project Grant HL-24136.

In patients with asthma, bronchospasm can be provoked by the inhalation of a wide variety of different agents [11]. These agents, which are sometimes called *inciters* of bronchospasm [31], include analogues of the parasympathetic neurotransmitter acetylcholine, chemical mediators of inflammation such as histamine, serotonin, prostaglandins, and leukotrienes, and agents that may occur in inhaled air such as fog (distilled water aerosol), sulfur dioxide, and particulate matter. Other agents appear important not so much because they trigger bronchoconstriction, but rather because they act as *inducers* of increased bronchomotor responsiveness [31]. Some agents appear to act both as *inciters* and as *inducers.* Inhalation of specific antigens, for example, may trigger both an immediate and a delayed asthmatic response; the delayed response is associated with an increase in bronchial reactivity that persists long after tests of airway caliber have returned to baseline [15]. It thus appears that the persistent, striking bronchial hyperreactivity of asthma may be the result of a kind of positive feedback loop, with the agents or events responsible for causing acute bronchospasm in reactive individuals also causing a further increase in reactivity. This accounts for the interest in defining the factors underlying both the acute and the delayed responses to inhaled materials, for a better understanding of the mechanisms of bronchial hyperreactivity may lead to the development of means of preventing or reversing asthma itself.

This review will focus first on the mechanisms of bronchomotor responsiveness, reviewing the possible sites of disturbance that could account for an exaggeration of responsiveness to *inciters* of bronchospasm such as inert carbon particles, distilled water aerosol, and sulfur dioxide. It will then turn to an analysis of the actions of ozone, a well-characterized *inducer* of bronchial hyperreactivity.

28.1 Mechanisms of Bronchial Responses

Rapid changes in airway caliber are caused by the contraction of bronchial smooth muscle, which in turn is caused by a change in the muscle's chemical environment, that is, by a local increase in chemicals causing constriction (*agonists*) or by a decrease in chemicals causing relaxation (*antagonists*). The list of agonists and antagonists grows ever longer as new derivatives of membrane phospholipids are identified and characterized, but it includes hormones that are released distantly and delivered to the airways via the bloodstream (e.g., epinephrine and norepinephrine), mediators released locally from inflammatory cells (e.g., histamine, prostaglandins, leukotrienes and platelet activating factor), and neurotransmitters released locally from specialized cells of the nervous system (e.g., acetylcholine, norepinephrine, and vasoactive intestinal peptide). Defining the mechanisms responsible for muscle contraction therefore involves identifying the causes of release of agonists or of an inhibition of release of antagonists into the muscle environment. Defining the mechanisms responsible for enhancement of the contractile response is more difficult, for such enhancement could result from a change in the function of contractile elements within the muscle as well as from changes in the local concentration of agonists or antagonists.

Whatever the level of responsiveness, it is clear that the tone of airway smooth muscle is not regulated by a single system but rather by a series of integrated systems. Studies of single systems taken in isolation have nevertheless been instructive, and in vitro studies of isolated smooth muscle, of mast cells, basophils, leukocytes and other cellular sources of inflammatory mediators, and of isolated components of the neural system, such as airway ganglia, have yielded important information. Interactions between systems have also been examined in vitro by studying the effect of the mediator of one system on the action of another. These studies have enabled the interpretation of studies of more complex systems, such as bronchial rings, strips of lung parenchyma, in situ preparations of trachealis muscle, anesthetized animals, and of both diseased and healthy human subjects.

28.1.1 Airway Smooth Muscle

The airways are supplied by nonstriated, smooth muscle. That smooth muscle can be activated by a variety of endogenous and exogenous agents, whereas striated muscle is exclusively responsive to cholinergic agonists, may help explain the diversity of stimuli that can provoke bronchoconstriction [80]. A variety of amines and peptides that bind to specific receptor sites are agonists of smooth muscle contraction [40]; their effect can be selectively blocked by specific antagonists. In muscle studied in vitro, for example, atropine blocks the response to acetylcholine but does not affect the response to histamine [79]. Smooth muscle contraction can also be provoked by nonspecific activation, as by potassium chloride or calcium ionophore. Whatever the stimulus, contraction appears to result from an increase in intracellular calcium and the interaction between calcium and the contractile proteins [40]. This may explain why *slow channel calcium antagonists,* such as nifedipine, are effective in inhibiting provoked bronchospasm [16]. Drugs that modify the biochemical steps linking the binding of ligand to the receptor and the contraction of myofibrils, such as those that act on the adenyl cyclase-CAMP system, are also effective inhibitors of muscle contraction.

Airway smooth muscle function is most directly studied in vitro, where the local concentration of agonists and the confounding influence of hormones, mediators, and neurotransmitters can be controlled. Studies of this type have shown that acetylcholine [4], histamine [26], prostaglandins [48], leukotrienes [25], thromboxane A_2 [82], and other peptides, amines, and products of the metabolism of membrane phospholipids are among the endogenous materials that directly provoke smooth muscle contraction.

But even in so simple a system as a strip of muscle in an organ bath, the response to an agonist is often not simply the function of activation of a single receptor. It may instead reflect the integrated response of stimulation of two (or possibly more) subtypes of receptors with opposing effects (e.g., H_1- and H_2-receptors for histamine). Furthermore, muscle contraction may cause the de novo synthesis and release of endogenous substances, such as prostaglandins, that they themselves alter the intensity of contraction. But even if all the determinants of in vitro responsiveness to an agent are well defined, the findings can be extrapolated to the in vivo function of airway smooth muscle only with great caution. Great differences in responsiveness to the same agonist can be shown, for example, not only in muscle obtained from different species [18] but also in muscle obtained from animals of the same species, but from different sites in the tracheobronchial tree [32].

Despite these difficulties, in vitro studies of tracheal and bronchial strips have been used to evaluate the hypothesis that exaggerated bronchomotor responsiveness results from an abnormality in muscle contractility. The results show little difference in the in vitro behavior of muscle obtained at thoracotomy from patients with a widely different responsiveness to inhaled materials in vivo [3, 86]. These results do not exclude the possibility that muscle contractility might be enhanced by a chemical removed in the process of preparing the muscle strips, but they make it seem unlikely that abnormal airway responsiveness results from a permanent, inherent difference in contractility. Heightened responsiveness may instead result from delivery to the muscle of excessive quantities of compounds provoking contraction or of insufficient quantities of compounds inhibiting contraction.

28.1.2 Mast Cells

Mast cells are found free in the bronchial lumen as well as in the bronchial mucosa, are well positioned to respond to inhaled materials [69, 84], and are a source of many chemicals that influence airway smooth muscle tone [76, 87]. Mast cells are recognized as primary mediators of immediate hypersensitivity reactions, in which the binding of antigen to IgE antibody on the cell surface leads to the extrusion of cell granules and the release of stored mediators (histamine, proteoglycans, and neutral proteases) and to the synthesis and release of other, highly potent inflammatory mediators derived from the metabolism of membrane phospholipids (prostaglandins, thromboxane, leukotriene and platelet activating factors) [68, 74]. The involvement of the mast cell is best established for airway responses to allergens, but it seems increasingly likely that the mast cell may be activated by nonspecific stimuli, such as sulfur dioxide or aerosols of hyper- or hypotonic solutions [37].

Because uncontaminated human lung mast cells are difficult to obtain, their function has been inferred from studies of rat peritoneal mast cells or circulating human basophils. Despite the potential differences between species and cell type and despite the recent discovery of heterogeneity in mast cells obtained from different sites in the same species [69], the model that has been developed from studies of these closely related cells is accepted as generally correct. It is clear that activated mast cells release many mediators that can provoke intense smooth muscle contraction. We are, in fact, faced with what has been termed "an embarrassment of riches" in deciding which mediator is most important, for with so many mediators capable of provoking bronchoconstriction, the system seems redundant [61]. Histamine, prostaglandins D_2 and $F_{2\alpha}$, thromboxane A_2, leukotrienes C_2 and D_2, and platelet activating factor (AGEPC) are only some of the potent agonists released from mast cells [42, 47, 58].

The release of these mediators can be shown with nonantigenic as well as antigenic challenge of mast cell preparations. Chymotrypsin and phospholipases, ionophores, radiocontrast media, opiates, and hypertonic solutions may all trigger mast cell degranulation [37, 87]. The involvement of mast cell degranulation in the bronchospastic responses of people with asthma is made to seem more likely by the findings that asthmatics have a greater number of mast cells in the bronchial lumen [84] and that the cells may have a heightened *releasability* [38].

The involvement of mast cells (or of other cells capable of synthesizing or storing mediators of immediate hypersensitivity) is most often tested by examining the effect of pretreatment with disodium cromoglycate, an agent thought to directly inhibit mast cell degranulation [23], or by analyzing circulating blood for the presence of chemicals thought to be specific for mast cells and basophils: histamine and neutrophil chemotactic factor [81, 88]. For some stimuli, such as exercise and inhalation of distilled water aerosol, both approaches have implicated involvement of mast cells, for the bronchomotor response can be blocked by cromolyn and is associated with an increase in arterial levels of histamine or neutrophil chemotactic factor [2, 57]. But even this apparently persuasive evidence is circumstantial. Cromolyn may have effects on airway nerves and smooth muscle [30], and mediators may be released from circulating basophils or other sites rather than from airway mast cells. Indeed, the bronchospastic response to eucapnic hyperpnea with cold, dry air is inhibitable by cromolyn, but is not associated with the rise in neutrophil chemotactic factor found with exercise [27]. It has yet to be directly proved that nonantigenic stimuli provoke the degranulation of airway mast cells in vivo, but such evidence may come with the application of bronchoscopic techniques for introducing material directly into the airways and for lavaging out a sample of airway secretions shortly thereafter.

28.1.3 Autonomic Nervous Systems

Another source of chemicals that influence airway smooth muscle tone are the autonomic systems supplying the airways, including the parasympathetic, sympathetic, and nonadrenergic inhibitory nervous systems. α-adrenergic and muscarinic agonists cause muscle contraction, whereas β-adrenergic agonists and activation of nonadrenergic inhibitory nerves cause relaxation. Thus, airway hyperreactivity could be due to an increase in the activity of the α-adrenergic or parasympathetic systems or to a decrease in the activity of the β-adrenergic or nonadrenergic inhibitory systems. Showing an exaggeration of activity in any one of these systems in subjects with bronchial hyperreactivity will not necessarily define the cause of the abnormality, however, for neural activity may well be altered by chemicals synthesized and released from cells not thought of as belonging to the nervous system.

Of the autonomic systems, the parasympathetic nervous system seems to play the dominant role in regulating airway caliber and in mediating acute bronchomotor responses in laboratory animals, and may play an important role in the bronchial hyperreactivity of asthma. The mediator for this system is acetylcholine [20, 65], and the distribution of narrowing of the tracheobronchial tree provoked by vagal stimulation is mirrored by the distribution of muscarinic receptors, with constriction greatest in central, conducting airways and least in peripheral airways [6, 59].

The involvement of parasympathetic nerves in airway responses in animals is shown by the effectiveness of vagal transection in blocking the bronchoconstriction provoked by inhaled or injected materials [28]. The involvement of a reflex is established by studies in which the site of delivery of the stimulus and the site of bronchoconstriction are separated. In cats, for example, bronchoconstriction is provoked by mechanical irritation or insufflation of sulfur dioxide into the larynx and can be blocked by interrupting conduction through the superior laryngeal nerves (afferent supply to the larynx) or through the vagus nerves (efferent supply to the airways) [12, 60].

Afferent receptors that may be responsible for initiating reflex responses are plentiful, for receptors supplied by both myelinated [36] and nonmyelinated [21] fibers have been described in the mucosa of the larynx, trachea, and bronchi. The conclusion that stimulation of any particular type of receptor provokes bronchoconstriction is inferential and is based on the observation that the agents that stimulate activity in the receptors also stimulate bronchoconstriction that is dependent on afferent and efferent neural pathways.

The possibility that an increase in parasympathetic activity could be responsible for the bronchial hyperreactivity of asthma is suggested by two facts: First, virtually all people with asthma demonstrate airway hyperreactivity to muscarinic agonists [24, 54], and second, airflow obstruction in asthmatic patients is partially reversed by muscarinic antagonists [46]. Proof of the involvement of parasympathetic reflexes in bronchomotor responses of humans with asthma has been difficult to establish, however, for responses to inhaled materials before and after transecting the vagi cannot ethically be compared. The approaches have therefore been indirect: One approach involves comparing responses before and after pharmacologic blockade of parasympathetic efferent pathways (e.g., with atropine or hexamethonium); another approach involves analyzing the concordance of the bronchoconstrictor response with a response known to be mediated by afferent nerves in the airways (e.g., cough).

Studies using the first approach have yielded conflicting results [39, 41, 45, 52, 62, 77], with some reporting that hexamethonium or atropine blocks responsiveness, and others reporting little effect. The difficulty with studies showing no effect is the absence of proof that the dose of antagonist given was adequate to block the effects of maximal parasympathetic efferent activity. In the absence of such proof, the persistence of a response despite treatment with an antagonist could be ascribed to persistence of parasympathetic activity.

One solution to this difficulty is to study the effects of a range of doses of a parasympathetic antagonist on the dose response curve to a given stimulus. If parasympathetic pathways uniquely mediate the response, then increasing doses of the antagonist should progressively inhibit the response. Since the quantity of acetylcholine that can be released from parasympathetic nerve endings must be finite, some dose of the antagonist should be sufficient to completely inhibit bronchoconstriction. If, on the other hand, nonparasympathetic mechanisms are also involved, administration of increasing doses of the antagonist should have only a limited effect that, once achieved, would not be increased by larger doses.

Tam et al used this approach in analyzing the effects of ipratropium bromide, a potent muscarinic antagonist, on the response to eucapnic hyperpnea with cold, dry air in asthmatic subjects [83]. Their results showed a progressive, dose-dependent inhibitory effect in only some of the subjects studied. In others, only a modest degree of inhibition could be obtained, and no greater inhibition was produced by delivery of higher doses of ipratropium bromide or by the addition of an intravenous dose of atropine sulfate (1.0 mg) to the highest inhaled dose of ipratropium bromide (200 μg). This lack of further inhibition despite increasing doses of a muscarinic antagonist suggests that parasympathetic mechanisms cannot entirely mediate the response, at least in some asthmatic subjects.

The second approach taken to analyze the concordance of bronchoconstriction and cough is the prototypic response to stimulation of afferent receptors in the respiratory tract. Empey and his colleagues used this approach in showing that the increase in bronchial reactivity caused by viral respiratory infections is associated with an increase in the sensitivity of cough receptors, as assessed by the concentration of aerosolized citric acid needed to provoke coughing [33].

But cough and bronchoconstriction are not invariably concordant in people with asthma, for while distilled water aerosol, an agent known to stimulate afferent receptors in the airway mucosa of laboratory animals [9, 13], indeed provokes both cough and bronchoconstriction in people with asthma [1], cough is abolished by pretreatment with lidocaine aerosol, and bronchoconstriction is unaffected [78]. The converse is true for the effects of cromolyn: Bronchoconstriction is inhibited, and cough is unaffected. Cough and bronchoconstriction can also be dissociated by changing the ion content of the inhaled solutions. Inhalation of an isotonic aerosol of sodium gluconate provokes cough but not bronchoconstriction [34].

These findings indicate that the same population of afferent receptors cannot be responsible for both the cough and the bronchoconstriction provoked by distilled water aerosol. If afferent nerves are involved at all in the bronchomotor response, they must differ from the receptors responsible for cough in location or in sensitivity to lidocaine and cromolyn. Another possibility is that while cough is mediated by afferent nerve activity, bronchoconstriction is provoked by other mechanisms, possibly including the action of chemical mediators released from mast cells [37]. Since the bronchoconstrictor response to distilled water aerosol is partially inhibitable by atropine [78], it may be that these mediators act not just on the muscle, but also on neural tissue as well.

The sympathetic nervous system appears less important than the parasympathetic system in determining smooth muscle tone. Histochemical and electron microscopic studies of human airways show that while sympathetic fibers directly innervate ganglia, blood vessels, and submucosal glands, they do not directly supply smooth muscle [71]. The anatomic evidence suggests, then, that the activity in sympathetic nerves may alter airway caliber indirectly, by altering perfusion or by altering transmission of neural activity through airway ganglia.

Physiologic studies seem to bear out this suggestion, for electrical stimulation of sympathetic nerves causes little change in airway caliber of anesthetized animals, unless bronchoconstriction is first produced by electrical stimulation of the vagi [14]. Stimulation of sympathetic nerves will then produce a weak, partial reversal of the airway narrowing. The possibility that sympathetic nerves may regulate activity in parasympathetic ganglia has lately been supported by the finding that norepinephrine inhibits cells in airway ganglia [5].

The sympathetic system's influence on airway caliber is not limited to the effects of neural activity, however, for airway smooth muscle is well equipped, with β- and α-adrenergic receptors, and responds to circulating epinephrine and norepinephrine, whether released from the adrenal glands or from sympathetic nerve endings just upstream. The density of adrenergic receptors is not uniform throughout the airways; in ferrets, β_2-receptors are present on the muscle of all generations of the airways, whereas the density of α_1-receptors increases strikingly from central to peripheral airways [6].

β-adrenergic agonists appear potent in causing smooth muscle relaxation [72], whereas α-adrenergic agonists are inconsistent in causing contraction. α-agonists have little effect on healthy airway smooth muscle but cause contraction of muscle obtained from people with respiratory disease and of muscle pretreated with endotoxin, potassium chloride, or histamine [53]. Similarly, α-agonists provoke bronchoconstriction in asthmatic subjects but have no effect in healthy subjects [67].

The involvement of these sympathetic mechanisms in bronchomotor responses has been studied by analyzing the effects of pretreatment with adrenergic agonists or antagonists. Because β-agonists are such potent inhibitors of smooth muscle contraction, the fact that they block bronchoconstriction only confirms that smooth muscle contraction is involved. It does not identify the cause of muscle contraction. A deficiency in β-activity seems unlikely as a fundamental cause of bronchial hyperreactivity, for treatment with β-blocking drugs does not alter airway responsiveness in healthy people [66]. The slight and variable effects of α-antagonists on airway responsiveness may have been due to other actions of the drugs used; some had antihistaminic and antimuscarinic effects, and most are likely to have altered vascular perfusion of the airway. In summary, an abnormality in the function of the sympathetic system cannot be dismissed as a contributing cause of abnormal responsiveness to physical agents, but it is far from established as the most important cause.

The airways are supplied by a third autonomic system, the nonadrenergic inhibitory system, whose action provokes relaxation of airway tone. Studies of the role of the system in regulating airway responses in vivo are based on the belief that vasoactive intestinal peptide (VIP) is the system's neurotransmitter. The results of these studies are provocative, for they show that inhaled VIP inhibits the bronchospastic effect of histamine [7, 22, 73]. A deficiency in the activity of the nonadrenergic noncholinergic system should therefore be added to the list of possible abnormalities in autonomic neural regulation that might underlie bronchial hyperreactivity.

In summary, autonomic nervous activity must certainly be considered a factor in bronchial reactivity, for the mechanisms for response to inhaled materials are well in place. Afferent receptors sensitive to a wide variety of inhaled materials line the respiratory tract, and efferent fibers supply the airway musculature. Interaction between different systems seems possible at many locations: at the muscle itself, at postganglionic nerve endings, and at airway ganglia. Other factors surely complicate the study of neural systems, for mediators released from mast cells and inflammatory cells may alter neural function. Inflammation has in fact already been shown to be associated with some forms of induced hyperreactivity of the airways, as is illustrated by the studies of ozone as an *inducer* of hyperresponsiveness.

28.2 Airway Inflammation

The hypothesis that hyperreactivity might be caused by airway inflammation derived from the observation that the stimuli that have been used to cause hyperreactivity experimentally can also cause airway inflammation. These stimuli include exposure to ozone [29, 44, 50, 56] or to allergen [10, 19, 70] and infection with respiratory viruses [33, 55]. Of these stimuli, ozone was the most appealing stimulus for study because it is easily generated and quantified and because it causes an increase in bronchomotor responsiveness in both animals and humans [44, 50, 56]. The increase in responsiveness has recently been shown to be accompanied by increases in the numbers of airway neutrophils recovered in bronchoalveolar lavage fluid, without significant changes in the numbers of macrophages, lymphocytes, or eosinophils [35, 75]. Tracheal biopsies show that the increase in neutrophils is most striking in the airway epithelium, implying that epithelial cells might generate chemotactic factors [51]. Subsequent studies have confirmed this implication, for isolated canine tracheal epithelial cells generate metabolites of the 5-lipoxygenase pathway from arachidonic acid [8, 49]. Some of the metabolites, such as leukotriene B_4, are potent neutrophil chemotaxins [43]. An important role for neutrophils is further implied by the effect of neutrophil depletion. In dogs made neutropenic, ozone exposure no longer increases airway reactivity [64]. It thus appears that while epithelial cell products may attract neutrophils to the airways, it may be products of the neutrophils that alter bronchomotor responsiveness. The identity of these mediators is uncertain, but they now seem most likely to be products of cyclooxygenation of arachidonic acid; pretreatment with indomethacin inhibits the change in responsiveness but not the influx of neutrophils caused by ozone in dogs [63].

Taken together, the results suggest that exposure to an inflammatory stimulus may lead to the development of hyperreactivity by the following sequence: first, the activation of airways epithelial cells to release lipoxygenase-derived chemotactic factors; second, the movement of neutrophils into the airway epithelium; and third, the release from activated neutrophils of prostaglandin or thromboxane that acts on smooth muscle or nerves to increase airways responsiveness.

Studies of ozone-induced changes in airway responsiveness, then, clearly indicate that inflammation may be another factor influencing bronchial reactivity. The unanswered question is whether the information obtained on ozone's effect is relevant to the hyperreactivity of asthma. Ozone-induced changes in reactivity certainly differ in duration. After ozone exposure, airway reactivity is increased only for a day or two, whereas the increase produced by antigen challenge often persists for weeks [19], the hyperreactivity associated with occupational asthma persists for months [17], and the hyperreactivity of common asthma persists for years [85]. It is possible that the striking increase in neutrophils and the activation of arachidonate metabolism that occurs after ozone exposure is specific to this stimulus, or may only mimic what occurs in the airways with exacerbations of asthma. They may not reflect the mechanisms responsible for sustained hyperreactivity associated with *stable* asthma. Indeed, bronchial lavage fluid obtained from asthmatic patients does not invariably reveal an abnormal number of neutrophils [84].

28.3 Conclusions

Bronchial hyperreactivity, an abnormality so characteristic of asthma that it is included in definitions of the disease, is thus seen to depend on complex interactions between cells. The immediate bronchospastic response depends on smooth muscle contraction, which in turn may be triggered by chemicals released from mast cells, basophils, platelets, leukocytes, or specialized cells of the nervous system. The mechanisms for this response seem to be in place in healthy people as well as in those with asthma. The cause of the increase in gain of the system remains undefined but seems to reflect an effect of inflammation. Defining the specific mediator(s) responsible and their sites of action may lead to the development of specific treatment that would reduce or eliminate asthmatic attack by reducing the responsiveness of the airways to the provocative antigens and agents that currently interfere with the asthmatic patient's enjoyment of life.

References

1. Allegra L, Bianco S (1980) Non-specific broncho-reactivity obtained with an ultrasonic aerosol of distilled water. Eur J Respir Dis [Suppl 106] 61:41–49

2. Anderson S, Torzillo P, Shaw RJ, Durham SR, Kay AB (1984) Possible participation of mediator (mast) cells in "fog"-induced asthma. J Allergy Clin Immunol 73:170 (abstract)
3. Armour CL, Lazar NM, Schellenberg RR, Taylor SM, Chan N, Hogg JC, Pare PD (1984) A comparison of in vivo and in vitro human airway reactivity to histamine. Am Rev Respir Dis 129:907–910
4. Arunlakshana O, Schild HO (1959) Some quantitative uses of drug antagonists. Br J Pharmacol 14:48–58
5. Baker DG, Basbaum CB, Herbert DA, Mitchell RA (1983) Transmission in airway ganglia: inhibition by norepinephrine. Neurosci Lett 41:139–143
6. Barnes PJ, Basbaum CB, Nadel JA (1983) Autoradiographic localization of autonomic receptors in airway smooth muscle: marked differences between large and small airways. Am Rev Respir Dis 127:758–762
7. Barnes PJ, Dixon CMS (1984) The effect of inhaled vasoactive intestinal peptide on bronchial reactivity to histamine in humans. Am Rev Respir Dis 130:162–166
8. Bigby TD, Goetzl EJ, Holtzman MJ (in press) Canine tracheal epithelial cells generate leukotriene B_4 in response to calcium ionophore. Clin Res (abstract)
9. Boggs DF, Bartlett D (1982) Chemical specificity of a laryngeal apneic reflex in puppies. J Appl Physiol 53:455–462
10. Boucher RC, Pare PD, Hogg JC (1979) Relationship between airway hyperreactivity and hyperpermeability in Ascaris-sensitive monkeys. J Allergy Clin Immunol 64:197–201
11. Boushey HA, Holtzman MJ, Sheller JR, Nadel JA (1980) State of the Art. Bronchial hyperreactivity. Am Rev Respir Dis 121:389–413
12. Boushey HA, Richardson PS, Widdicombe JG (1972) Reflex effects of laryngeal irritation on the pattern of breathing and total lung resistance. J Physiol (Lond) 224:501–513
13. Boushey HA, Richardson PS, Widdicombe JG, Wise JCM (1974) The response of laryngeal afferent fibers to mechanical and chemical stimuli. J Physiol (Lond) 240: 153–175
14. Cabezas GA, Graf PD, Nadel JA (1971) Sympathetic versus parasympathetic nervous regulation of airways in dogs. J Appl Physiol 31:651–655
15. Cartier A, Thomson NC, Frith PA, Roberts R, Hargreave FE (1982) Allergen-induced increase in bronchial responsiveness to histamine: relationship to the late asthmatic response and change in airway caliber. J Allergy Clin Immunol 70:170–177
16. Cerrina J, Denjean A, Alexandre G, Lockhart A, Duroux P (1981) Inhibition of exercise-induced asthma by a calcium antagonist, nifedipine. Am Rev Respir Dis 123:156–160
17. Chan-Yeung M, Lam S, Koerner S (1982) Clinical features and natural history of occupational asthma due to Western red cedar (Thuja plicata). Am J Med 72:411–415
18. Chand N (1980) Distribution and classification of airway histamine receptors. The physiologic significance of histamine H_2-receptors. Adv Pharmacol Chemother 17:103–131
19. Cockcroft DW, Ruffin RE, Dolovich J, Hargreave FE (1977) Allergen-induced increase in non-allergic bronchial reactivity. Clin Allergy 7:503–513
20. Colebatch HJH, Halmagyi DFJ (1963) Effect of vagotomy and vagal stimulation on lung mechanics and circulation. J Appl Physiol 18:881–887
21. Coleridge JCG, Coleridge HM (1984) Afferent vagal C fibre innervation of the lungs and airways and its functional significance. Rev Physiol Biochem Pharmacol 99:1–110
22. Cox CP, Lerner MR, Wells JH, Said SI (1983) Inhaled vasoactive intestinal peptide (VIP) prevents bronchoconstriction induced by inhaled histamine. Am Rev Respir Dis 127:249 (abstract)
23. Cox JSG (1967) Disodium cromoglycate (FPL 670) ("Intal"): a specific inhibitor of reaginic antibody-antigen mechanisms. Nature 216:1328–1329
24. Curry JJ (1946) The action of histamine on the respiratory tract in normal and asthmatic subjects. J Clin Invest 25:785–791
25. Dahlen S-E, Hedqvist P, Hammarstrom S, Samuelsson B (1980) Leukotrienes are potent constrictors of human bronchi. Nature 288:484–486
26. Dale HH, Laidlaw PP (1910) The physiological action of beta-imidazolylethylamine. J Physiol (Lond) 41:318–344
27. Deal EC, Wasserman SI, Soter NA, Ingram RH, McFadden ER (1980) Evaluation of role played by mediators of immediate hypersensitivity in exercise-induced asthma. J Clin Invest 65:659–665
28. DeKock MA, Nadel JA, Zwi S, Colebatch HJH, Olsen CR (1966) New method for perfusing bronchial arteries: histamine bronchoconstriction and apnea. J Appl Physiol 21:185–194
29. DiMeo MJ, Glenn MG, Holtzman MJ, Sheller JR, Nadel JA, Boushey HA (1981) Threshold concentration of ozone causing an

increase in bronchial reactivity in humans and adaptation with repeated exposures. Am Rev Respir Dis 124:245–248
30. Dixon M, Jackson DM, Richards IM (1980) The action of sodium cromoglycate on "C" fiber endings in the dog lung. Br J Pharmacol 70:11–13
31. Dolovich J, Hargreave F (1981) The asthma syndrome: inciters, inducers, and host characteristics. Thorax 36:641–644
32. Drazen JM, Schneider MW (1978) Comparative responses of tracheal spirals and parenchymal strips to histamine and carbachol in vitro. J Clin Invest 61:1441–1448
33. Empey DW, Laitinen LA, Jacobs L, Gold WM, Nadel JA (1976) Mechanisms of bronchial hyperreactivity in normal subjects following upper respiratory tract infection. Am Rev Respir Dis 113:131–139
34. Eschenbacher WL, Boushey HA, Sheppard D (1984) Alteration in osmolarity of inhaled aerosols cause bronchoconstriction and cough, but absence of a permeant anion causes cough alone. Am Rev Respir Dis 129:211–215
35. Fabbri LM, Aizawa H, Alpert SE, Walters EH, O'Byrne PM, Gold BD, Nadel JA, Holtzman MJ (1984) Airway hyperresponsiveness and changes in cell counts in bronchoalveolar lavage after ozone exposure in dogs. Am Rev Respir Dis 129:288–291
36. Fillenz M, Widdicombe JG (1972) Receptors of the lungs and airways. In: Neil E (ed) Handbook of Sensory Physiology. Springer, Berlin Heidelberg New York, pp 81–112
37. Findlay SR, Dvorak AM, Kagey-Sobotka A, Lichtenstein L (1981) Hyperosmolar triggering of histamine release from human basophils. J Clin Invest 67:1604–1613
38. Findlay SR, Lichtenstein LM (1980) Basophil "releasability" in patients with asthma. Am Rev Respir Dis 122:53–59
39. Fish JE, Rosenthal RR, Summer WR, Menkes H, Norman PS, Permutt S (1977) The effect of atropine on acute antigen-mediated airway constriction in subjects with allergic asthma. Am Rev Respir Dis 115:371–379
40. Fleisch JH (1980) Airway smooth muscle pharmacology: general principles. In: Hargreave FE (ed) Airway Reactivity. Astra Pharmaceuticals, Ontario
41. Godfrey S, Konig P (1976) Inhibition of exercise-induced asthma by different pharmacological pathways. Thorax 31:137–143
42. Goetzl EJ (1980) Mediators of immediate hypersensitivity derived from arachidonic acid. N Engl J Med 303:822–825
43. Goetzl EJ, Pickett WC (1980) The human PMN leukocyte chemotactic activity of complex hydroxy-eicosatetraenoic acids (HETEs). J Immunol 125:1789–1791
44. Golden JA, Nadel JA, Boushey HA (1978) Bronchial hyperirritability in healthy subjects after exposure to ozone. Am Rev Respir Dis 118:287–294
45. Griffin MP, Fung KF, Ingram RH Jr, McFadden ER Jr (1982) Dose-response effects of atropine on thermal stimulus-response relationships in asthma. J Appl Physiol 53:1576–1582
46. Gross NJ, Skorodin MS (1984) State of the Art. Anticholinergic, antimuscarinic bronchodilators. Am Rev Respir Dis 129:856–870
47. Halonen M, Palmer JD, Lohman IC, McManus LM, Pinckard RN (1980) Respiratory and circulatory alterations induced by acetyl glyceryl ether phosphorylcholine, a mediator of IgE anaphylaxis in the rabbit. Am Rev Respir Dis 122:915–924
48. Hamberg M, Hedqvist P, Strandberg K, Svensson J, Samuelsson J (1975) Prostaglandin endoperoxides. IV. Effects on smooth muscle. Life Sci 16:451–461
49. Holtzman MJ, Aizawa H, Nadel JA, Goetzl EJ (1983) Selective generation of leukotriene B_4 by tracheal epithelial cells from dogs. Biochem Biophys Res Commun 114:1071–1076
50. Holtzman MJ, Cunningham JH, Sheller JR, Irsigler GB, Nadel JA, Boushey HA (1979) Effect of ozone on bronchial reactivity in atopic and non-atopic subjects. Am Rev Respir Dis 120:1059–1067
51. Holtzman MJ, Fabbri LM, O'Byrne PM, Gold BD, Aizawa H, Walters EH, Alpert SE, Nadel JA (1983) Importance of airway inflammation for hyperresponsiveness induced by ozone in dogs. Am Rev Respir Dis 127:686–690
52. Holtzman MJ, Sheller JR, DiMeo M, Nadel JA, Boushey HA (1980) Effect of ganglionic blockade on bronchial reactivity in atopic subjects. Am Rev Respir Dis 122:17–25
53. Kneussl MP, Richardson JB (1978) Alpha-adrenergic receptors in human and canine tracheal and bronchial smooth muscle. J Appl Physiol 45:307–311
54. Laitinen LA (1974) Histamine and methacholine challenge in the testing of bronchial reactivity. Scand J Respir Dis [Suppl] 86:1–47
55. Laitinen LA, Empey DW, Poppius HA, Lemen RJ, Gold WM, Nadel JA (1976) Effects of intravenous histamine on static lung compliance and airway resistance in normal man. Am Rev Respir Dis 114:291–295
56. Lee L-Y, Bleecker ER, Nadel JA (1977) Effect of ozone on bronchomotor response to inhaled histamine aerosol in dogs. J Appl Physiol 43:626–631

57. Lee TH, Nagakura T, Cromwell O, Brown MJ, Causon R, Kay AB (1984) Neutrophil chemotactic activity and histamine in atopic and nonatopic subjects after exercise-induced asthma. Am Rev Respir Dis 129:409–412
58. Murphy RC, Hammarstrom S, Samuelsson B (1979) Leukotriene C: a slow-reacting substance from murine mastocytoma cells. Proc Natl Acad Sci USA 76:4275–4279
59. Nadel JA, Cabezas GA, Austin JHM (1971) In vivo roentgenographic examination of parasympathetic innervation of small airways: use of powdered tantalum and a fine focal spot x-ray tube. Invest Radiol 6:9–17
60. Nadel JA, Salem H, Tamplin B, Tokiwa Y (1965) Mechanism of bronchoconstriction during inhalation of sulfur dioxide. J Appl Physiol 20:164–167
61. Newball HH, Lichtenstein LM (1981) Mast cells and basophils, effector cells and inflammatory disorders in the lung. Thorax 36:721–725
62. O'Byrne PM, Thomson NC, Morris M, Roberts RS., Daniel EE, Hargreave FE (1983) The protective effect of inhaled chlorpheniramine and atropine on bronchoconstriction stimulated by airway cooling. Am Rev Respir Dis 128:611–617
63. O'Byrne PM, Walters EH, Aizawa H, Fabbri LM, Holtzman MJ, Nadel JA (1984) Indomethacin inhibits the airway hyperresponsiveness but not the neutrophil influx induced by ozone in dogs. Am Rev Respir Dis 130:220–224
64. O'Byrne PM, Walters EH, Gold BD, Aizawa HA, Fabbri LM, Alpert SE, Nadel JA, Holtzman MJ (1984) Neutrophil depletion inhibits airway hyperresponsiveness induced by ozone exposure. Am Rev Respir Dis 130:214–219
65. Olsen CR, Colebatch HJH, Mebel PE, Nadel JA, Staub NC (1965) Motor control of pulmonary airways studied by nerve stimulation. J Appl Physiol 20:202–208
66. Orehek J, Gayrard P, Grimaud C, Charpin J (1975) Effect of beta adrenergic blockade in bronchial sensitivity to inhaled acetylcholine in normal subjects. J Allergy Clin Immunol 55:164–169
67. Patel KR, Kerr JW (1973) The airways response to phenylephrine after blockade of alpha and beta receptors in extrinsic bronchial asthma. Clin Allergy 3:439–448
68. Paterson NAM, Wasserman SI, Said JW, Austen KF (1976) Release of chemical mediators from partially purified human lung mast cells. J Immunol 117:1356–1362
69. Patterson R, McKenna JM, Suszko IM, Solliday NH, Pruzansky JJ, Roberts M, Kehoe TJ (1977) Living histamine-containing cells from the bronchial lumens of humans. Description and comparison of histamine content with cells of rhesus monkeys. J Clin Invest 59:217–225
70. Popa V, Douglas JS, Bouhuys A (1973) Airway response to histamine, acetylcholine, and propranolol in anaphylactic hypersensitivity in guinea pigs. J Allergy Clin Immunol 51:344–356
71. Richardson JB (1979) State of the Art. Nerve supply to the lungs. Am Rev Respir Dis 119:785–802
72. Russell JA (1984) Differential inhibitory effect of isoproterenol on contractions of canine airways. J Appl Physiol 57:801–807
73. Said SI, Geumi A, Hara N (1982) Bronchodilator effect of VIP in vivo: protection against bronchoconstriction induced by histamine or prostaglandin $F_{2\alpha}$. In: Said SI (ed) Vasoactive Intestinal Peptide. Raven Press, New York, pp 185–191
74. Schwartz LB, Austen KF (1984) Structure and function of the chemical mediators of mast cells. Prog Allergy 34:271–299
75. Seltzer J, Geffroy B, Stulbarg M, Holtzman MJ, Nadel JA, Boushey HA Jr (1984) Association between airway inflammation and changes in bronchial reactivity induced by ozone exposure in human subjects. Am Rev Respir Dis 129:A262 (abstract)
76. Selye H (1965) The Mast Cell. Butterworths, Washington
77. Sheppard D, Epstein J, Holtzman MJ, Nadel JA, Boushey HA (1982) Dose-dependent inhibition of cold air-induced bronchoconstriction by atropine. J Appl Physiol 53:169–174
78. Sheppard D, Rizk N, Boushey HA, Bethel RA (1983) Mechanism of cough and bronchoconstriction induced by distilled water aerosol. Am Rev Respir Dis 127:691–694
79. Skoogh B-E, Nadel JA, Fabbri LM, Sheppard D, Holtzman MJ (1983) Antihistaminic versus anticholinergic effects of atropine on canine trachealis muscle. Am Rev Respir Dis 128:603–606
80. Somlyo AB, Somlyo AV (1970) Biophysics of smooth muscle excitation and contraction. In: Bouhuys A (ed) Airway Dynamics. Thomas, Springfield, pp 209–227
81. Soter NA, Wasserman SI, Austen KF, McFadden ER (1980) Release of mast-cell mediators and alterations in lung function in patients with cholinergic urticaria. N Engl J Med 302:604–608
82. Svensson J, Strandberg K, Tuvemo T, Hamberg M (1977) Thromboxane A_2: effects on airway and vascular smooth muscle. Prostaglandins 14:425–436

83. Tam E, Sheppard D, Epstein J, Ancic P, Boushey H (1983) Effect of increasing doses of ipratropium bromide on dose-response curve to isocapnic hyperventilation with cold air in asthmatic subjects. Am Rev Respir Dis 127:250 (abstract)
84. Tomioka M, Ida S, Shindoh Y, Ishihara T, Takishima T (1984) Mast cells in bronchoalveolar lumen of patients with bronchial asthma. Am Rev Respir Dis 129:1000–1005
85. Townley RG, Ryo UY, Kolotkin BM, Kang B (1975) Bronchial sensitivity to methacholine in current and former asthmatic and allergic rhinitis patients and control subjects. J Allergy Clin Immunol 56:429–442
86. Vincenc KS, Black JL, Yan K, Armour CL, Donnelly PD, Woolcock AJ (1983) Comparison of *in vivo* and *in vitro* responses to histamine in human airways. Am Rev Respir Dis 128:875–879
87. Wasserman SI (1980) The lung mast cell: its physiology and potential relevance to defense of the lung. Environ Health Perspect 35:153–164
88. Wasserman SI, Soter NA, Center DM, Austen KF (1977) Cold urticaria: recognition and characterization of a neutrophil chemotactic factor which appears in serum during experimental cold challenge. J Clin Invest 60:189–196

29. Bronchial Hyperreactivity: Autonomic Nervous System Abnormalities

M. A. Kaliner

Homeostasis is a complex, ever-changing state of internal balances between opposing influences maintaining a relatively steady, healthy state. Over the years, evidence, often contradictory, has been generated about the possible role of imbalances in the factors contributing to the maintenance of airway homeostasis (bronchodilation) in the asthmatic subject. Moreover, in addition to these inherent imbalances in homeostasis, the asthmatic airway is characteristically much more sensitive to multiple, often nonspecific, stimuli as compared to nonasthmatic subjects. Such nonspecific stimulation causes airway smooth muscle constriction that is usually unassociated with the other clinical signs and symptoms of asthma (e.g., mucus production, cough).

Our studies on the possible contributions of autonomic nervous system dysfunction in asthma, allergy, and cystic fibrosis have confirmed and substantiated the presence of an array of autonomic abnormalities. In this paper, we will try to summarize the role that autonomic nervous system dysfunction can contribute to airway hyperreactivity.

29.1 Evidence that β-adrenergic Hyporeactivity Exists

In 1968, Szentivanyi proposed the β-adrenergic blockade theory of asthma [1] as a unifying concept to partially explain many of the abnormalities seen in patients with asthma and, possibly, in other atopic diseases as well. The theory was advanced based on the observation that the injection of living or killed *Bordetella pertussis* organisms into certain strains of mice and rats modified the normal responses of these animals in such a way as to mimic many of the clinical abnormalities seen in asthmatic and allergic individuals. Animals so treated developed hypersensitivity to endogenously released or exogenously administered histamine, serotonin, bradykinin and acetylcholine; hypersensitivity to less specific stimuli such as cold, changes in atmospheric pressure, and respiratory irritants; enhanced antibody formation with reagin-like activity; and finally, marked eosinophilia. Moreover, associated with the development of these abnormalities was a concomitant reduction in the animals' sensitivity to catecholamines and, in some cases, even a reversal of normal adrenergic activity. These results were interpreted to suggest a relationship between autonomic nervous system dysfunction and the various physiologic and immunologic abnormalities seen in allergic patients. As a corollary conclusion, the data implied that a diminished responsiveness to β-adrenergic stimulation might potentiate impulse transmission or receptor stimulation along α-adrenergic or cholinergic pathways.

Since its inception, the β-adrenergic theory has been the subject of intense study by many investigators. Support for the theory has come from both *in vivo* and *in vitro* studies. Early support for Szentivanyi's β-adrenergic blockade theory of asthma came from *in vivo* observations [2–7] demonstrating a decreased rise in blood sugar, lactate, pyruvate, cyclic adenosine 3′,5′-monophosphate (CAMP), pulse pressure, and urine CAMP in response to β-adrenergic stimulation in allergic asthmatic patients compared to normal individuals. Makino and co-workers were able to demonstrate that the reduction in β-adrenergic responsiveness observed in their patient population correlated with the degree of bronchial responsiveness to acetylcholine [8]. Furthermore, the β-antagonist, propranolol, was found to cause acute bronchoconstriction in asthmatic subjects [9], whereas, in normal subjects, it had no effect on airway responses to histamine or cholinergic aerosol [10].

α-adrenergic agonists may produce bronchoconstriction in asthmatic patients, but not in normal subjects [11, 12], and *in vitro* studies have demonstrated α-adrenergic receptor-mediated constriction of bronchial smooth muscle from patients with increased airways resistance, but not from normal controls [13, 14]. In addition, allergic rhinitis patients are more sensitive to methacholine challenge after propranolol administration, as compared to normal subjects [10, 15]. These data point to a functional imbalance of the autonomic nervous system such that antigen-induced mast cell mediator release into the tracheobronchial tree might be able to cause bronchoconstriction that is unopposed by the normal β-adrenergic bronchodilating (homeostasis) mechanisms.

These *in vivo* observations were extended to *in vitro* studies employing circulating blood cells and radioligand binding techniques to measure β-receptor density and affinity. Since both human leukocytes and lung possess β_2-adrenergic receptors, leukocytes provide a readily accessible model for the study of β-adrenergic responsiveness in allergic and nonallergic subjects.

The results of investigations utilizing these methods have produced some interesting observations with unresolved problems. Some investigators have reported that asthmatic patients have a lower density of β-receptors on lymphocyte membranes [16, 17], and lymphocytes of asthmatics have been found to generate less CAMP in response to β-agonists [18]. When granulocytes from asthmatics are stimulated by β-adrenergic agonists, they do not respond with the same degree of inhibition of lysosomal enzyme release as do normal controls [19]. Although all these observations support the β-adrenergic theory of asthma, other investigators have found reduced leukocyte β-adrenergic responsiveness and decreased β-adrenergic receptor number only after continuous treatment with β-adrenergic agonists [20–23]. Most recently, Meurs and co-workers [24] have suggested that the reduced β-adrenergic function and receptor number found on lymphocytes from asthmatic subjects is not an intrinsic component of allergic bronchial asthma, but rather the consequence of the active disease state. These investigators found a reduction in β-adrenergic responsiveness and receptor density only after an allergen-induced asthmatic reaction. Thus, although the ability to study β-adrenergic receptor responsiveness and density on leukocytes is a convenient tool, the conclusions that one is able to draw from these investigations are still unclear.

We have studied atopic individuals using *in vivo* assessments of their autonomic nervous system responsiveness [25]. α- and β-adrenergic and cholinergic responsiveness was studied in four groups of subjects: allergic asthmatics; allergic rhinitics with no history of asthma; *preallergic* individuals who had no history of allergic diseases, but had positive skin tests to common allergens; and normal controls. Parallel studies were also performed with cystic fibrosis patients and their parents.

α-adrenergic responsiveness was ascertained by two methods, each measuring the concentration of the α-agonist phenylephrine needed to elicit a predetermined response. In one test, the concentration of topical phenylephrine that was needed to induce mydriasis of 0.5 mm or larger in the dark was ascertained. In the other, the concentration of intradermal phenylephrine that was needed to reduce cutaneous blood flow by 50% was measured. By both tests of α-adrenergic responsiveness, subjects with allergic asthma were singularly hyperresponsive to α-adrenergic stimuli, as compared to the other three groups [26].

Cholinergic responsiveness was assessed by measuring the concentration of the muscarinic cholinergic agonist, carbachol, needed to constrict pupils 1.0 mm or more [27]. Allergic subjects with asthma or rhinitis, as well as preallergic subjects were found to have increased sensitivity to cholinergic stimulation of pupillary constrictor muscles. Parenthetically, allergic subjects have also been noted to produce significantly more sweat in response to intradermal cholinergic stimulation of eccrine sweat glands, as compared with normal subjects [28]. Thus, both allergic and *preallergic* individuals appear to have increased cholinergic responsiveness.

Table 29.1. Summary of autonomic abnormalities identified by *in vivo* assessment. [Data summarized from 25]

	β-adrenergic responsiveness	Cholinergic responsiveness	α-adrenergic responsiveness
Allergic asthma	Reduced	Heightened	Heightened
Allergic rhinitis	Reduced	Heightened	Normal
Pre-allergy	Reduced	Heightened	Normal

Finally, β-adrenergic responsiveness was evaluated by determining the concentration of intravenous isoproterenol required to raise pulse pressure by 22 mmHg and to increase plasma CAMP levels by 50%. None of the subjects had taken β-agonists for at least 1 month before examination. The normal control subjects were significantly more sensitive to intravenously administered isoproterenol by both parameters than were the other three groups. There was no significant difference between the concentrations of isoproterenol required by the groups with allergic asthma, allergic rhinitis, and preallergy [7]. There are two major conclusions from these studies; first, intrinsic β-adrenergic hyporeactivity exists in asthmatic subjects unrelated to previous adrenergic drug administration; and second, a comparable degree of β-adrenergic hyporesponsiveness exists in nonasthmatic allergic subjects as well.

The results of these studies, summarized in Table 29.1, suggest the presence of close correlations between the different components of the autonomic nervous system. All allergic subjects show abnormal β-adrenergic hyporeactivity and cholinergic hypersensitivity, whereas only allergic asthmatics are associated with excessive α-adrenergic responsiveness.

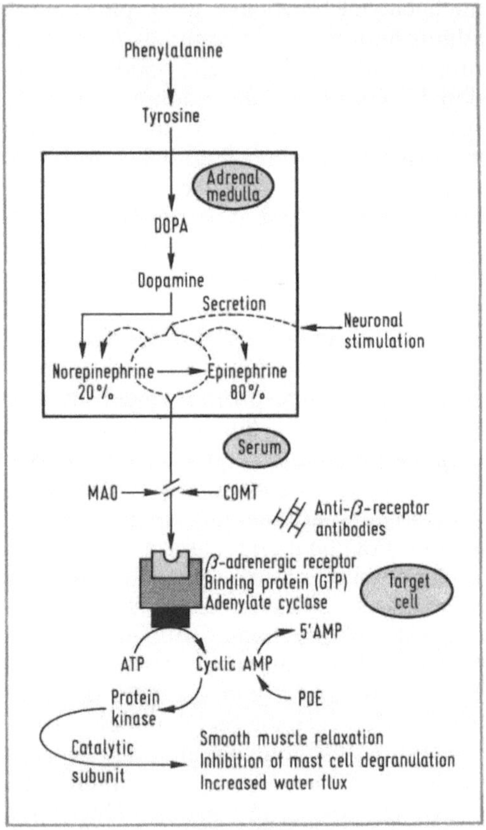

Fig. 29.1. Biochemical cascade involved in epinephrine synthesis, the enzymes capable of metabolizing epinephrine and the receptor-linked biochemical responses to epinephrine stimulation of membrane-bound receptors. Along the side of the figure are listed the possible sites which might affect β-adrenergic responses. Many of the possible influences on β-adrenergic responsiveness have not been studied as yet

29.2 Possible Mechanisms for β-adrenergic Hyporesponsiveness

β-adrenergic stimulation occurs when circulating epinephrine interacts with β-adrenergic receptors on cell surfaces. The steps involved in epinephrine synthesis, release, and receptor stimulation are summarized in Fig. 29.1. Epinephrine is predominantly found in the adrenal medulla

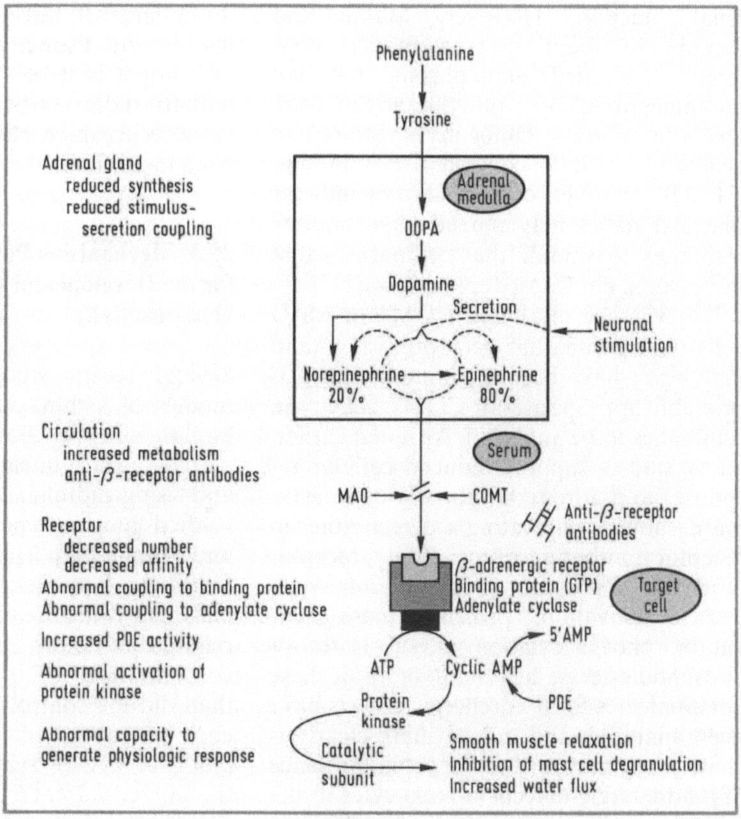

Fig. 29.2. Each step in the biochemical cascade involved in epinephrine synthesis, release, metabolism, and action could be altered so as to make a subject relatively hyporeactive. Potential sites of such alterations are listed along the left-hand portion of the figure and are detailed in the text

and is stored in chromaffin granules separately from its precursor molecule, norepinephrine. About 80% of the catecholamine content of the adrenal gland is epinephrine and 20% is norepinephrine. These catechols derive from phenylalanine, tyrosine, DOPA and dopamine. When the adrenal gland is stimulated by neuronal discharge through the splanchnic nerve fibers, adrenal discharge of chromaffin granules occurs releasing catecholamines into the circulation. Of the two enzymes usually implicated in the degradation of circulating catecholamines (COMT and MAO), COMT is the predominant metabolic factor in serum. Epinephrine acts by stimulating all adrenergic receptors that it encounters, although the mechanism of movement of epinephrine out of the circulation and into the tissue is unclear.

Epinephrine stimulates both β_1- and β_2- (as well as α-) adrenergic receptors leading to the coupling of a guanine nucleotide-binding protein which activates the enzyme, adenylate cyclase, which in turn generates CAMP from adenosine triphosphate (ATP). CAMP binds to the cyclic nucleotide-dependent protein kinase and cleaves from the protein kinase a catalytic subunit that induces phosphorylation of susceptable proteins. These actions lead to the final biochemical alterations reflected in epinephrine-induced responses, including increased cardiac output, increased systolic blood pressure, increased blood flow to muscles and the splanchnic circulation, hyperglycemia, lactic acidemia, bronchodilation, and inhibition of mast cell degranulation, among other actions.

Each step in Fig. 29.1 could conceivably be affected in order to influence β-adrenergic responsiveness. Details of such potential disturbances are summarized in Fig. 29.2. Analysis of urine catecholamines in subjects with asthma has usually been normal [29] indicating normal baseline adrenal function. However, Mathe and Knapp [30] found that asthmatics registered a blunted epinephrine, but not norepinephrine or vanillylmandelic acid, response to stress. Other investigators had generally failed to confirm these findings [31, 32]; however, current studies indicate that asthmatics may indeed have blunted responses to stimuli that ordinarily cause increases in circulatory epinephrine [32].

No evidence of altered COMT or MAO activity in asthma has been published (and may never have been examined), and it is probably appropriate for COMT activity in asthmatics to be analyzed. As noted earlier, many studies support reduced cellular responses to β-adrenergic stimulants in asthmatic subjects, indicating a defect either in receptor number, receptor affinity, receptor binding – protein coupling, adenylate cyclase activation, protein kinase activation, phosphorylation of substrates or phosphodiesterase activity. Not all of these potential sites for β-adrenergic defects have been analyzed, and indeed there clearly is controversy in regard to the actual presence of β-adrenergic defects in leukocytes in the first place. Nonetheless, Galant et al examined neutrophil sonicates for adenylate cyclase activity and membrane-rich neutrophil preparations for β-adrenergic receptors by radioligand methods and could detect no defect in either preparation [33, 34]. Moreover, while attention has focused upon leukocyte responsiveness, it is not clear whether β-adrenergic responsiveness of asthmatic airways *in vivo* is normal or not. An equal number of observations indicate no β-adrenergic impairment of bronchodilation to β-agonists [35, 36], as compared to studies suggesting reduced responses [37, 38]. A case in point is the simultaneous publication of two recent studies by the same investigators who, in one study, suggest that a small number of asthmatics (five) develop central airway β-adrenergic hyporeactivity while receiving inhaled salbutamol [39] while a parallel study by the same investigators failed to detect reduced airway responses in 11 asthmatics receiving oral terbutaline [40].

The weight of the data indicates the presence of reduced β-adrenergic responsiveness in the asthmatic (and perhaps in atopics in general), but it is impossible to localize the site distinctly. Thus, Figs. 29.1 and 29.2 might best be viewed as maps of potential studies rather than a biochemical cascade in which clear abnormalities have been identified.

29.3 Mechanisms Possibly Responsible for the Development of β-adrenergic Hyporeactivity

Several recent studies involving animal models of asthma may shed light on the human disease. Barnes and co-workers, employing a guinea pig model of asthma and using radioligand binding techniques, studied lung adrenergic receptor number and affinity [41]. These investigators found that lung homogenates of sensitized animals had twice the concentration of α_1-adrenergic receptors and a marginally lower concentration of β-adrenergic receptors than did the controls. No significant difference was observed in β-adrenergic stimulation of CAMP synthesis, suggesting that the altered adrenergic responses in asthma may be mediated by a reduction in the numbers of receptors rather than a biochemical defect. Mita and co-workers [42] extended Barnes' observation to include cholinergic receptors and found that the dose and route of antigen administered to guinea pigs affected the number of lung receptors. For instance, prolonged aerosol sensitization with low dose antigen selectively increased cholinergic receptor number while higher dose sensitization increased α-adrenergic receptor density, reduced β-adrenergic receptor number, and had no effect on cholinergic receptors.

Halonen and co-workers investigated the possibility that the development of an allergic immunologic response might affect autonomic responsiveness. The methods employed included immunizing rabbits with horseradish peroxidase (HRP) in a manner which elicits the selective generation of IgE-anti-HRP antibodies [43]. Autonomic responsiveness was assessed by measuring the pupillary responses of these rabbits to cholinergic and α-adrenergic agonists as compared to their littermates who were not immunized. The IgE-producing rabbits were significantly more sensitive to carbachol-induced miosis than were the controls [44, 45]. Conversely, both groups of rabbits responded equally to topical phenylephrine. Thus, rabbits that were immunized in a manner which selectively induces IgE production developed apparent cholinergic hyperresponsiveness combined with normal α-adrenergic responsiveness. This pattern of abnormal autonomic responses is reminiscent of that seen in nonasthmatic human atopics [25] (Table 29.1). These data suggest that stimulation of an immunologic response might in some manner affect autonomic responsiveness. Indeed, sensitization of sheep with horse plasma has been noted to affect lung parenchymal strip responsiveness to catecholamines [46]. Thus epinephrine and phenylephrine responses before sensitization were dilatory, and these responses become constrictory after sensitization. These data suggest that sensitization affects autonomic responsiveness, and these observations relate directly to the abnormalities noted in atopic humans.

Two of the possible explanations for these abnormal autonomic responses in animal models are, first, a change in receptor number as suggested by Barnes' et al and Mita's et al studies of guinea pig lung receptors [41, 42] and, second, the generation of β-adrenergic receptor antibodies which might prevent normal β-receptor stimulation and thus lead to unopposed α-adrenergic and cholinergic responsiveness. In order to investigate this latter possibility, Fraser and co-workers developed techniques to identify β_2-adrenergic receptor antibodies in plasma [47]. These antibodies were characterized by their ability to affect binding of ^{125}I-protein A to calf-lung membranes, inhibit β-adrenergic ligand binding to calf-lung β-adrenoceptors, and precipitate solubilized calf-lung β-adrenoceptors in an indirect immunoprecipitation assay. Using the previously outlined techniques to assess autonomic responsiveness *in vivo* [7, 26, 27], these investigators detected antibodies in atopic subjects, some of whom had asthma. Moreover, the presence of autoantibodies to β_2-receptors correlated with abnormal autonomic responsiveness characterized by α-adrenergic and cholinergic hyperresponsiveness and β-adrenergic hyposensitivity. However, β-receptor autoantibodies were found in a few normal subjects as well as atopics. These findings suggest that autoantibodies to β-adrenergic receptors may play a part in the development of autonomic abnormalities in a portion of subjects so affected; however, their presence is not restricted to atopic individuals.

29.4 Relationship Between Autonomic Abnormalities and Asthma

Whereas all the asthmatics we have studied have autonomic abnormalities, not all the subjects with autonomic abnormalities have airway hyperreactivity. Therefore, the presence of autonomic abnormalities is not sufficient to cause asthma. It is clear, however, that autonomic disturbances can uncover the asthmatic tendency. For instance, the infusion of histamine into normal subjects or mild asthmatics fails to cause bronchospasm [47, 48]. Prior treatment of normal subjects with propranolol, however, uncovers the bronchospastic nature of intravenous histamine and results in impressive airway obstruction [48]. In much the same way, propranolol treatment increases airway responsiveness to antigen challenge in allergic rhinitis subjects [49] and induces airway hyperreactivity in guinea pigs [50, 51]. These data indicate that autonomic abnormalities are not sufficient to cause asthma but may be a necessary component.

29.5 Conclusions

The precise contribution of autonomic nervous system abnormalities to various disease manifestations is as yet unclear. However, it is reasonable to suggest that three levels of response that are critical to the maintenance of homeostasis in asthma may be influenced (Table 29.2):

- Bronchial smooth muscle dilation in response to β-adrenergic stimulation would be reduced, while cholinergically and α-adrenergically mediated constriction would be augmented;

Table 29.2. The sites of action of autonomic agonists relevant to asthma

	β-adrenergic	α-adrenergic	Cholinergic
Agonist:	Isoproterenol	Phenylephrine	Carbamylcholine Methacholine
Bronchial smooth muscle	Dilator	Constrictor	Constrictor
Submucous gland	–	Stimulate	Stimulate
Mast cell degranulation	Inhibit	Enhance	Enhance
Measured responses in allergic asthma patients	Hyporesponsive	Hyperresponsive	Hyperresponsive

- mast cell mediator release, ordinarily suppressed by β-adrenergic stimulation, would be resistant to β-adrenergic agonists, while both cholinergic and α-adrenergic enhancement of mediator release might be exaggerated;
- increased mucus secretion in response to α-adrenergic and cholinergic stimulation would be augmented, while sodium and water fluxes into tracheobronchial secretions in response to β-adrenergic stimulation would be reduced.

Thus, subjects manifesting the pattern of altered autonomic responses seen in asthma would be primed for increased mast cell degranulation, bronchospasm, and increased mucus secretion. It is not clear how or why these autonomic defects develop, but Halonen and Kaliner's study suggests a relationship between immunoglobulin production and autonomic abnormalities [45], much as suggested by Szentivanyi originally [1]. Busse observed that viral infection affected β-adrenergic responses in asthmatics [19] while animal models indicate that certain viral infections facilitate IgE production [52]. Thus, the underlying defect could well be a genetic predisposition to atopy augmented by environmental exposure to antigens and infectious agents resulting in coupled autonomic derangements and IgE production.

References

1. Szentivanyi A (1968) The beta-adrenergic theory of the atopic abnormality in bronchial asthma. J Allergy 42:203–232
2. Middleton E Jr, Finke SR (1968) Metabolic response to epinephrine in asthma. J Allergy 42:288–299
3. Kirkpatrick CH, Keller C (1967) Impaired responsiveness to epinephrine in asthma. Am Rev Respir Dis 96:692–699
4. Lockey SD Jr, Glennon JA, Reed CE (1967) Comparison of some metabolic responses in normal and asthmatic subjects to epinephrine and glucagon. J Allergy 40:349–354
5. Grieco MH, Pierson RN Jr, Pi-Sunyer FX (1968) Comparison of the circulatory and metabolic effects of isoproterenol, epinephrine and methoxamine in normal and asthmatic subjects. Am J Med 44:863–872
6. Bernstein RA, Linarelli K, Facktor MA et al (1972) Decreased urinary adenosine 3′,5′-monophosphate (cyclic AMP) in asthmatics. J Lab Clin Med 80:772–779
7. Shelhamer JH, Metcalfe DD, Smith LJ, Kaliner M (1980) Abnormal beta-adrenergic responsiveness in allergic subjects: analysis of isoproterenol-induced cardiovascular and plasma cyclic adenosine monophosphate responses. J Allergy Clin Immunol 66:52–60
8. Makino S, Ouelette JJ, Reed CE, Fishel C (1970) Correlation between increased bronchial response to acetylcholine and diminished metabolic and eosinopenic responses to epinephrine in asthma. J Allergy 46:178–189
9. McNeill RS (1964) Effect of a beta-adrenergic blocking agent, propranolol, on asthmatics. Lancet 2:1101–1102
10. Zaid G, Beall GN (1966) Bronchial response to beta-adrenergic blockade. N Engl J Med 275:580–584
11. Anthracite RF, Vochon L, Knapp PH (1977) Alpha-adrenergic receptors in the human lung. Psychosom Med 33:481–489
12. Snashall PD, Boother FA, Sterling GM (1978) The effect of alpha-adrenergic receptor stimulation on the airways of normal and asthmatic man. Clin Sci Molec Med 54:283–289

13. Simonsson BG, Svedmyr N, Skoogh BE et al (1972) *In vivo* and *in vitro* studies on alpha-receptors in human airways. Potentiation with bacterial endotoxin. Scand J Respir Dis 53:227–236
14. Kneussl MP, Richardson JB (1978) Alpha-adrenergic receptors in human and canine tracheal and bronchial smooth muscle. J Appl Physiol 45:307–311
15. Townley RG (1980) Receptors and nonspecific bronchial reactivity. In: Kerr JW, Ganderton MA (eds) Proceedings of the XIth International Congress of Allergology and Clinical Immunology. Macmillan, London Basingstoke, pp 197–206
16. Kariman K (1980) Beta-adrenergic receptor binding in lymphocytes frcm patients with bronchial asthma. Lung 158:41–51
17. Brooks SM, McCowan K, Bernstein IL et al (1979) Relationship between numbers of beta-adrenergic receptors in lymphocytes and disease severity in asthma. J Allergy Clin Immunol 63:401–406
18. Parker CW, Smith JW (1973) Alterations in cyclic adenosine monophosphate metabolism in human bronchial asthma. I. Leukocyte responsiveness to beta-adrenergic agents. J Clin Invest 52:48–59
19. Busse WW (1977) Decreased granulocyte response to isoproterenol in asthma during upper respiratory infections. Am Rev Respir Dis 115:783–791
20. Conolly ME, Greenacre JK (1976) The lymphocyte beta-adrenoceptor in normal subjects and patients with bronchial asthma. The effect of different forms of treatment on receptor function. J Clin Invest 58:1307–1316
21. Morris HG, Rusnak SA, Barzens K (1977) Leukocyte cyclic adenosine monophosphate in asthmatic children. Effects of adrenergic therapy. Clin Pharmacol Ther 22:352–357
22. Galant SP, Duriseti L, Underwood S, Insel PA (1978) Decreased beta-adrenergic receptors on polymorphonuclear leukocytes after adrenergic therapy. N Engl J Med 229:933–936
23. Bruynzeel PLB, van den Berg W, Hamelink ML et al (1979) Desensitization of the beta-adrenergic receptor on leukocytes after long-term oral use of a beta-sympathicomimetic: its effect on the beta-adrenergic blockade hypothesis of Szentivanyi. Ann Allergy 43:105–109
24. Meurs H, Koeter GH, de Vries K, Kauffman HF (1982) The beta-adrenergic system and allergic bronchial asthma: changes in lymphocyte beta-adrenergic number and adenylate cyclase activity after an allergen-induced asthmatic attack. J Allergy Clin Immunol 70:272–280
25. Kaliner M, Shelhamer JH, Davis PB et al (1982) Autonomic nervous system abnormalities and allergy. Ann Intern Med 96:349–357
26. Henderson WR, Shelhamer JH, Reingold DB et al (1979) Alpha-adrenergic hyperresponsiveness in asthma, analysis of vascular and pupillary responses. N Engl J Med 300:642–647
27. Smith LJ, Shelhamer JH, Kaliner M (1980) The cholinergic nervous system and immediate hypersensitivity II. An analysis of pupillary responses. J Allergy Clin Immunol 66:374–378
28. Kaliner M (1976) The cholinergic nervous system and immediate hypersensitivity. I. Eccrine sweat responses in allergic patients. J Allergy Clin Immunol 58:308–315
29. Kolesov DV (1965) Excretion of free catecholamines with the urine during paroxysmal periods of bronchial asthma. Pediatriia 44, 1:56–60
30. Mathe AA, Knapp PH (1969) Decreased plasma free fatty acids and urinary epinephrine in bronchial asthma. N Engl J Med 281:234–238
31. Ouellette JJ, Chosy JJ, Reed CE (1967) Catecholamine excretion and bronchial response to methacholine after *Salmonella enteritides* endotoxin in a normal and an asthmatic subject. J Allergy 39:234–237
32. Barnes PJ (1983) Endogenous plasma adrenaline in asthma. Eur J Respir Dis 64:559–563
33. Galant SP, Allred S, Griffiths R (1980) Characterization of adenylate cyclase activity in asthmatic neutrophil sonicates. Am Rev Respir Dis 122:231–238
34. Galant SP, Duriseti L, Underwood S, Allred S, Insel PA (1980) Beta-adrenergic receptors of polymorphonuclear particulates in bronchial asthma. J Clin Invest 65:577–585
35. Wilson AF, Novey HS, Cloninger P, Davis J, White D (1976) Cardiopulmonary effects of long-term bronchodilator administration. J Allergy Clin Immunol 58:204–210
36. Larsson S, Svedmyr N, Thiringer G (1976) Lack of bronchial beta-adrenoceptor resistance in asthmatics during long-term treatment with terbutaline. J Allergy Clin Immunol 59:93–99
37. Nelson HS, Raine D, Doner HC, Posey WC (1977) Subsensitivity to the bronchodilator action of albuterol produced by chronic administration. Am Rev Respir Dis 116:871–878
38. Plummer AL (1978) Development of drug tolerance to beta$_2$-adrenergic agents in asthmatics. Chest 73 [Suppl]: 949–951
39. Conolly ME, Tashkin DP, Hui KK, Littner MR, Wolfe RN (1982) Selective subsensiti-

zation of beta-adrenergic receptors in central airways of asthmatics and normal subjects during long-term therapy with inhaled salbutamol. J Allergy Clin Immunol 70:423–431
40. Tashkin DP, Conolly ME, Deutsch RI, Hui KK, Littner M, Scarpace P, Abrass I (1982) Subsensitivity of beta-adrenoceptors in airways and lymphocytes of healthy and asthmatic subjects. Am Rev Respir Dis 125:185–193
41. Barnes PJ, Dollery CT, MacDermot J (1980) Increased pulmonary alpha-adrenergic and reduced beta-adrenergic receptors in experimental asthma. Nature 285:569–571
42. Mita H, Yui Y, Yasueda H, Shida T (1983) Changes of $alpha_1$ and beta-adrenergic and cholinergic muscarinic receptors in guinea pig lung sensitized with ovalbumin. Int Arch Allergy Appl Immunol 70:225–230
43. Pinckard RN, Halonen M, Meng AL (1972) Preferential expression of anti-bovine serum IgE homocytotropic antibody synthesis and anaphylactic sensitivity in the neonatal rabbit. J Allergy Clin Immunol 49:301–310
44. Halonen M, Kaliner M (1983) Determinants of autonomic abnormalities in atopy. In: Kerr JW, Ganderton MA (eds) Proceedings of the XIth International Congress of Allergology and Clinical Immunology. Macmillan, London Basingstoke, pp 193–196
45. Halonen M, Kaliner M (1984) Heightened cholinergic responsiveness in IgE-producing rabbits. Int J Immunopharmacol 6:351–356
46. Mirbahar KB, Eyre P (1982) Autocoid and autonomic reactivity of sheep lung parenchymal strip and its modification by antigenic sensitization. Int J Immunopharmacol 4:533–539
47. Fraser CM, Venter JC, Kaliner M (1981) Autonomic abnormalities and auto-antibodies to beta-adrenergic receptors. N Engl J Med 305:1165–1170
48. Ploy-Song-Sang Y, Corbin RP, Engel LA (1978) Effects of intravenous histamine on lung mechanics in man after beta-blockade. J Appl Physiol 44:690–695
49. Ouellette JJ, Reed CE (1967) The effect of partial beta adrenergic blockade on the bronchial response of hay fever subjects to ragweed aerosol. J Allergy 39:160–166
50. Bongrani S, Folco GC, Razzetti R, Schianterelli P (1983) B_2-adrenoceptor blockade is the basis of guinea pig bronchial hyper-responsiveness to leukotriene C4 and other agents. Br J Pharmacol 79:839–848
51. Ney UM (1983) Propranolol-induced airway hyperreactivity in guinea pigs. Br J Pharmacol 79:1003–1009
52. Katz DH (1978) The allergic phenotype: manifestation of "allergic breakthrough" and imbalance in normal "damping" of IgE antibody production. Immunol Rev 41:77–86

30. Bronchial Hyperresponsiveness and Asthma: Unanswered Questions

J. Orehek

Inhalation of pharmacological agents known to constrict isolated airways results in excessive airway narrowing in patients with asthma as compared to normal subjects (bronchial hyperresponsiveness = BH) [4, 23]. This feature was recognized more than 40 years ago and it has given birth to two commonly accepted concepts.

30.1 Concept 1: BH is an Important (Perhaps Essential) Determinant of Asthma

This concept stems from two undisputable facts: a) Airway smooth muscle spasm is an important feature of asthma (as the efficacy of dilator drugs testifies); b) endogenous smooth muscle constricting substances (e.g., histamine) are released in extrinsic and intrinsic asthma. Therefore it seems logical to assume that BH to constricting agents would facilitate bronchospasm and make it abnormally intense.

Such a cause-and-effect relationship between asthma and BH is suggested by several observations and some of them even support the idea that BH is a sine qua non of asthma.

- Pharmacological airway responsiveness of patients with allergic rhinitis, but without asthma, is less pronounced than that of patients with allergic asthma [25, 30, 31]. This suggests that rhinitic patients do not suffer from clinical bronchospasm despite the allergic release of endogenous constricting substances, because their airways are not hyperresponsive. Indeed, in experimental conditions, the severity of the bronchial reaction caused by inhalation of a given dose of allergen in sensitive patients is closely dependent on both the degree of allergy and of pharmacological responsiveness [7].
- When constricting pharmacological agents are administered to normal subjects, a measurable bronchospasm ensues. But, due to extrapulmonary effects, administration must be stopped before the bronchospasm so induced reaches a degree comparable to that spontaneously observed in asthma [34]. This suggests that hyperresponsiveness of airway smooth muscle is more important than hyperstimulation for determining clinically significant bronchospasm and that the bronchospasm of asthma may represent a greatly exaggerated response to a moderately increased stimulation.
- The degree of BH parallels the severity of asthma [15], increasing when asthma worsens and decreasing when it improves, as one would expect if the degree of responsiveness determined the symptoms.

These observations, however, are not irrefutable proofs.

- The lack of asthma in rhinitic patients could be explained if the allergic reaction were solely located in supraglottic airways or if these patients had a subglottic airway reaction different from that of allergic asthmatics. As it is likely that natural airborne allergens reach the subglottic airways of both rhinitic and asthmatic patients, it remains to be understood why the allergic reaction of subglottic airways should differ in these two categories of patients.
- The importance of BH as a determinant of the response to inhaled allergens [7] cannot be dismissed easily. However, it is noticeable that the antigen challenge was not natural, having been done with a liquid aerosol similar to that used for the pharmacological challenge. For this reason it is likely that the allergenic and pharmacological challenges stimulated

the same category of airways, which may not be the case when subjects are exposed to natural airborne allergens.
- It is possible that the inhalation of constricting agents by normal subjects does not duplicate the effects of constricting substances released locally, at the smooth muscle level.
- Parallel variation of BH and asthma symptoms does not necessarily imply a cause-and-effect relationship. If the same disorder (e.g., inflammation) caused both BH and asthma symptoms, fluctuations of this disorder would make variations of BH and asthma appear to be related.

There is another reason for questioning the importance of BH as a determinant of asthma. Traditionally BH has been assessed by forced expiratory volume in one second (FEV_1) measurement which requires a prior maximal inspiration. In this circumstance much of the observed difference between an asthmatic and a nonasthmatic population is attributable to different responses to maximal inspiration (dilatation more marked in nonasthmatics) rather than to true difference in pharmacological responsiveness [10, 22, 24]. In fact, when functional techniques not requiring a prior maximal inspiration were used to assess pharmacological responsiveness in asthmatic and rhinitic patients, the two groups overlapped [10].

Finally, it is intriguing that BH can be demonstrated in chronic bronchopulmonary diseases other than asthma: chronic bronchitis [1, 4, 17, 23, 26], cystic fibrosis [19], bronchiectasis [2, 32], byssinosis [14], anti-trypsin deficiency [13], tuberculosis [17], sarcoidosis [18], farmer's lung [18] and survivors of the adult respiratory distress syndrome [27]. Why then, if BH is a major determinant of the asthmatic syndrome, is such a syndrome not present in these diseases? Indeed β-adrenergic agonists are generally considered as having little therapeutic value in nonasthma respiratory diseases, suggesting that airway smooth muscle spasm is not a major feature of these diseases. One may therefore consider that BH only reflects the existence of bronchopulmonary lesions but does not play a role in their clinical expression.

In fact, two other hypotheses are conceivable. 1) The BHs of asthma and of nonasthma respiratory diseases correspond to two different mechanisms (e.g., nonmuscular mechanisms in the latter group, see below). Two observations support this hypothesis: BH is often less marked in nonasthma diseases than in asthma; a positive relationship between the degree of baseline airway obstruction and the degree of BH is usually present in nonasthma respiratory diseases whereas such a relationship is not always found in asthma. Incidentally, it is worth mentioning that BH could not be demonstrated in asthmatics entirely free from functional abnormalities, as assessed by the most sensitive tests at our disposal [5]. 2) BH of nonasthma diseases is not fundamentally different from that of asthma but its expression, both in the lab and clinically, is somewhat different. *In the lab,* the techniques used for exploring BH are still rudimental. The bronchopulmonary system is comparable to a black box [20] as we can only evaluate (at the mouth in both cases) the input (dose of pharmacological agent) and the output (change in some index of lung function). We know that the output results from complex events occurring inside the box but we cannot separate them. For example, it is not possible to assess possible longitudinal or regional differences in airway responsiveness. Thus, if BH is somewhat less marked in nonasthma diseases which preferentially or exclusively involve the peripheral airways (like sarcoidosis) as compared to asthma, such a difference may reflect not a true difference in response of diseased asthmatic and nonasthmatic airways, but our inability to selectively explore small airways reactivity. Because the pharmacological agents used for BH testing act on bronchial glands and because hypertrophy of these glands is a cardinal feature of chronic bronchitis, it is possible that hypersecretion biases the assessment of BH in such patients. A plateau response often occurs in patients with chronic bronchitis in spite of increasing doses of constricting agents [22]; such a plateau could be due to drug-induced hypersecretion that would dilute the constricting agent and prevent it from reaching the smooth muscle. *Clinically,* nonasthma diseases may lack bronchospasm despite BH because they possibly have specific pathologic features, not present in asthma, which modify the clinical expression of BH. Again, it may be important to consider factors such as lesion sites (peripheral vs diffuse) or hypersecretion. Alternatively, it is possible that the importance of bronchospasm in nonasthma diseases was underestimated because it was evaluated with β-adrenergic agonists, which may be less efficient than other classes of bronchodilators in these diseases [12].

30.2 Concept 2: Bronchial Hyperreactivity is the Consequence of Abnormal Airway Smooth Muscle Functioning

Because the pharmacological agents used to assess BH are known constrictors of airway smooth muscle it seems logical to assume that any exaggerated response (airway obstruction) occurring after the inhalation of such agents results from an exaggerated response of the airway smooth muscle. Abnormalities of airway smooth muscle have been postulated in asthma, either intrinsic (e.g., single unit behavior) or extrinsic to the muscle (e.g., increased parasympathetic activity). In fact, BH could exist even if the response of muscular cells to constricting agents were normal and without assuming smooth muscle hypertrophy. Isolated bronchi of patients demonstrating BH in vivo are not hyperreactive [33]. This suggests that the disorder creating in vivo hyperreactivity is either extrinsic to the muscle or nonmuscular. Increased epithelial permeability could create in vivo BH since the pharmacological agent would, in this situation, reach more easily and in greater amount the smooth muscle located beneath the epithelium. Such BH would probably have little relevance to the clinical situation as it is likely that, in pathological conditions, the smooth muscle constricting mediators are released inside the bronchial wall and do not have to cross the epithelial barrier. This, however, does not apply to mediators released from mast cells situated inside the bronchial lumen. Epithelial permeability is not increased in common asthma [9]. But increased epithelial permeability may play a role in special situations. In animals, allergen challenge increases both pharmacological reactivity and epithelial permeability of the airways [3]. Such a mechanism could thus explain the increase in reactivity observed in man after provoked [6] or natural [29] exposure to airborne allergens.

Increased thickness of airway mucosa (and/or submucosa) is another possible cause of BH in vivo despite normal smooth muscle response in vitro [21]. Such a thickening is indeed present in asthmatic airways [11].

Since several mechanisms can create BH it is possible that several types of BH exist. We are unable at present to separate them. But such a possibility raises an important question: How can the validity of animal models of BH be judged? In dogs, airway inflammation seems responsible for ozone-induced BH [16]. In man, it is likely that the increase in BH occurring after exposure to allergens, is also related to inflammation since it is prevented by corticosteroids [29]. As a rule, however, BH of common asthma is not influenced by corticosteroids [8, 28, 31]. Thus, inflammation may not be the cause of BH in common asthma and the dog model of ozone-induced BH may be inadequate. By the way, the lack of action of corticosteroids on BH may be regarded as a further argument against concept 1, since corticosteroids are very effective in controlling asthma; if they do so without modifying BH it is unlikely that BH is important for determining asthma.

30.3 Conclusions

Concept 1 leads us to think that understanding the mechanism of BH is essential for understanding asthma. This hope has greatly stimulated the research on BH in recent years. But the results may be disappointing if BH is not a major determinant of asthma, but only a stigma of bronchopulmonary disease.

Concept 2 should not mask the possibility that the mechanisms of BH are multiple and, as a consequence, that experimentally induced BH may not duplicate spontaneously occurring BH.

References

1. Bahous J, Cartier A, Quinet G, Pineau L, Malo JL (1984) Non allergic bronchial hyperexcitability in chronic bronchitis. Am Rev Respir Dis 129:216–220
2. Bahous J, Cartier A, Pineau L, Bernard C, Ghezzo H, Martin RR, Malo JL (1984) Pulmonary function tests and airway responsiveness to methacholine in chronic bronchiectasis of the adult. Bull Eur Physiopathol Respir 20:375–380
3. Boucher RC, Paré PD, Hogg JC (1979) Relationship between airway hyperreactivity and hyperpermeability in ascaris-sensitive monkeys. J Allergy Clin Immunol 64:197–201
4. Boushey HA, Holtzman MJ, Sheller JR, Nadel JA (1980) Bronchial hyperreactivity (State of the Art). Am Rev Respir Dis 121:389–413
5. Brown R, Ingram RH, Wellman JJ, McFadden ER (1977) Effects of intravenous histamine on pulmonary mechanics in nonasthmatic and asthmatic subjects. J Appl Physiol 42:221–227
6. Cartier A, Thomson NC, Frith PA, Roberts R, Tech M, Hargreave FE (1982) Allergen-induced increase in bronchial responsiveness to histamine = relationship to the late asthmatic response and change in airway caliber. J Allergy Clin Immunol 70:170–177
7. Cockcroft DW, Ruffin RE, Frith PA, Cartier A, Juniper EF, Dolovich J, Hargreave FE (1979) Determinants of allergen-induced asthma: dose of allergen, circulating IgE antibody concentration and bronchial responsiveness to inhaled histamine. Am Rev Respir Dis 120:1053–1058
8. Easton JG (1981) Effect of an inhaled corticosteroid on methacholine airway reactivity. J Allergy Clin Immunol 67:388–390
9. Elwood RK, Kennedy S, Belzerg A, Hogg JC, Paré PD (1983) Respiratory mucosal permeability in asthma. Am Rev Respir Dis 128:523–527
10. Fish JE, Ankin MG, Kelly JF, Peterman VI (1981) Regulation of bronchomotor tone by lung inflation in asthmatic and non-asthmatic subjects. J Appl Physiol 50:1079–1086
11. Fleury J, Bernaudin JF, Ehouman A, Pinchon MC, Bignon J (1982) Histopathologie des bronches de l'asthmatique. In: Michel FB (ed) Bronches de l'asthmatique. Masson, Paris, pp 14–19
12. Gross NJ, Skorodin MS (1984) Role of the parasympathetic system in airway obstruction due to emphysema. N Engl J Med 311:421–425
13. Groth S, Lindell SE, Kabiraj MU, Bülow K, Arborelius M, Simonsson BG (1984) Bronchial reactivity and small airway dysfunction in subjects with intermediate alpha$_1$-antitrypsin deficiency. Bull Eur Physiopathol Respir 20:279–284
14. Haglind P, Bake B, Belin L (1983) Is mild byssinosis associated with small airways disease? Eur J Respir Dis 64:449–459
15. Hargreave FE, Juniper EF, Ryan G, Dolovich M, Cartier A, Frith PA, Newhouse MT (1980) Clinical significance of non specific airway hyperreactivity. In: Hargreave FE (ed) Airway reactivity. Astra Pharmaceuticals, Mississauga, pp 216–221
16. Holtzman MJ, Fabbri LM, O'Byrne PM, Gold BD, Aizawa H, Walters EH, Alpert SE, Nadel JA (1983) Importance of airway inflammation for hyperresponsiveness induced by ozone. Am Rev Respir Dis 127:686–690
17. Laitinen LA (1974) Histamine and metacholine challenge in the testing of bronchial reactivity. Scand J Respir Dis [Suppl] 86:48
18. Laitinen LA, Haahtela T, Kava T, Laitinen A (1983) Non-specific bronchial reactivity and ultrastructure of the airway epithelium in patients with sarcoidosis and allergic alveolitis. Eur J Respir Dis 64 [Suppl 131]:267 283
19. Mitchell I, Corey M, Woenne R (1978) Bronchial hyperreactivity in cystic fibrosis and asthma. J Pediatr 93:744–748
20. Orehek J (1980) Airway response to inhaled bronchoconstrictor drugs: clinical measurement and standardization. In: Hargreave FE (ed) Airway reactivity. Astra Pharmaceuticals, Mississauga, pp 201–209
21. Orehek J (1983) The concept of airway sensitivity and reactivity. Eur J Respir Dis 64 [Suppl 131]:27–48
22. Orehek J (1983) Pharmacologic airway hyperreactivity. In: Serafini I, Errigo E (eds) Proceedings of the XIIth Congress of the European Academy of Allergology and Clinical Immunology. O.I.C. Medical, Firenze, pp 177–182
23. Orehek J, Gayrard P (1976) Les tests de provocation bronchique non-spécifiques dans l'asthme. Bull Eur Physiopathol Respir 12:565–598
24. Orehek J, Nicoli MM, Delpierre S, Beaupré A (1981) Influence of the previous deep inspiration on the spirometric measurement of provoked bronchoconstriction in asthma. Am Rev Respir Dis 123:269–272
25. Permutt S, Rosenthal RR, Norman PS, Menkes HA (1977) Bronchial challenge in ragweed sensitive patients. In: Lichtenstein LM, Austen KF (eds) Asthma. Academic Press, New York, pp 265–281

26. Ramsdell JW, Nachtwey FJ, Moser KM (1982) Bronchial hyperreactivity in chronic obstructive bronchitis. Am Rev Respir Dis 126:829–832
27. Simpson DL, Goodman M, Spector SL, Petty TL (1978) Long-term follow-up and bronchial reactivity testing in survivors of the adult respiratory distress syndrome. Am Rev Respir Dis 117:449–454
28. Spector SL, Farr RS (1975) A comparison of methacholine and histamine inhalations in asthmatics. J Allergy Clin Immunol 56:308–316
29. Sotomayor H, Badier M, Vervloet D, Orehek J (1984) Seasonal increase of carbachol airway responsiveness in patients allergic to grass pollen: reversal by corticosteroids. Am Rev Respir Dis 130:56–58
30. Stevens WJ, Vermeire PA (1980) Bronchial responsiveness to histamine and allergen in patients with asthma. Eur J Respir Dis 61:203–210
31. Tiffeneau R (1957) Examen pulmonaire de l'asthmatique. Masson, Paris, p 245
32. Varpela E, Laitinen LA, Kestinen H, Korhola O (1978) Asthma, allergy and bronchial hyperreactivity to histamine in patients with bronchiectasis. Clin Allergy 8:273–280
33. Vincenc KS, Black JL, Yan K, Armour CL, Donnelly PM, Woolcock AJ (1983) Comparison of in vivo and in vitro responses to histamine in human airways. Am Rev Respir Dis 128:875–879
34. Woolcock AJ, Salome CM, Yan K (1984) The shape of the dose-response curve to histamine in asthmatic and normal subjects. Am Rev Respir Dis 130:71–75

G. Asthma due to Allergy Occupation, Food and Drugs

31. Preparation and Stability of Pollen Extracts

H. Baer, M. C. Anderson

Recent developments in allergy have created the potential for a better understanding of the importance of the quality of pollen extracts. New biochemical and immunological techniques, coupled with the refinement of existing procedures are providing new information regarding extraction and storage conditions. These techniques supply the means to evaluate and monitor the effects of various extraction procedures and storage conditions, in order to determine optimal conditions for producing and storing extracts that contain relevant allergens in measurable quantities.

31.1 Extraction Methodology

The quality of a pollen extract is significantly affected by extraction conditions such as time, temperature, and extraction media. The process of extraction should be optimized to produce an extract that has multiple antigens and allergens. Extraction processes that favor the extraction of individual components or small groups of proteins may distort the profile of allergenicity as determined by skin testing or direct RAST. Enzymatic and thermal degradation may be a factor in extraction procedures that are conducted for extended time periods. Extraction buffers that are conducive to enzymatic activity may accelerate degradation, and extraction temperatures between 25 and 30 °C may affect allergens that are heat-labile. Antigens that are altered during extraction, due to thermal or enzymatic degradation, may make it difficult to evaluate the relative potency and allergenic activity of an extract.

Isoelectric focusing may be utilized to evaluate qualitatively the product that results from various extraction methods. Quantitative measurements of the effects of changes in extraction methods as they affect extract potency may be obtained using specific antigen analysis. RAST inhibition assays and quantitative skin tests.

Each variable in an extraction procedure must be examined for the effect that this factor has on the allergenic properties of the extract. Fig. 31.1 illustrates the effects of time, temperature and extraction media on the IEF patterns and the antigen E content when the same lot of short ragweed pollen is subjected to various extraction conditions.

31.2 Extract Stability

In vitro methods: There are a number of studies on the stability of allergenic extracts. Most of the data was obtained using concentrated solutions since one of the characteristics of in vitro tests is that they are much less sensitive than in vivo tests.

The majority of the published stability studies have been carried out with short ragweed pollen extracts using the antigen E content as the measure of the extract's stability. One study showed that, when stored continuously at 4–8 °C, 73% of the antigen E was measurable after 9 months and 45% after 18 months. After storage at 24 °C, 80% was detectable after 1 week, but after storage at 35 °C for the same interval, less than 3% was left [1]. In another study, after 8 months of storage at 4 °C or after 2 months at 24 °C, about one half of the antigen E remained in the extracts [2]. A third study showed that when stored at 5 °C about one half of the antigen E was lost in a year [3].

A more detailed study, using kinetics of the decay of antigen E, indicated that at 4 °C, less than one half of the antigen E would be lost in 3 to 4 months and at 35 °C one half would be lost in 5–10 days. This study also demonstrated that the phenol preservative increased the rate of antigen E

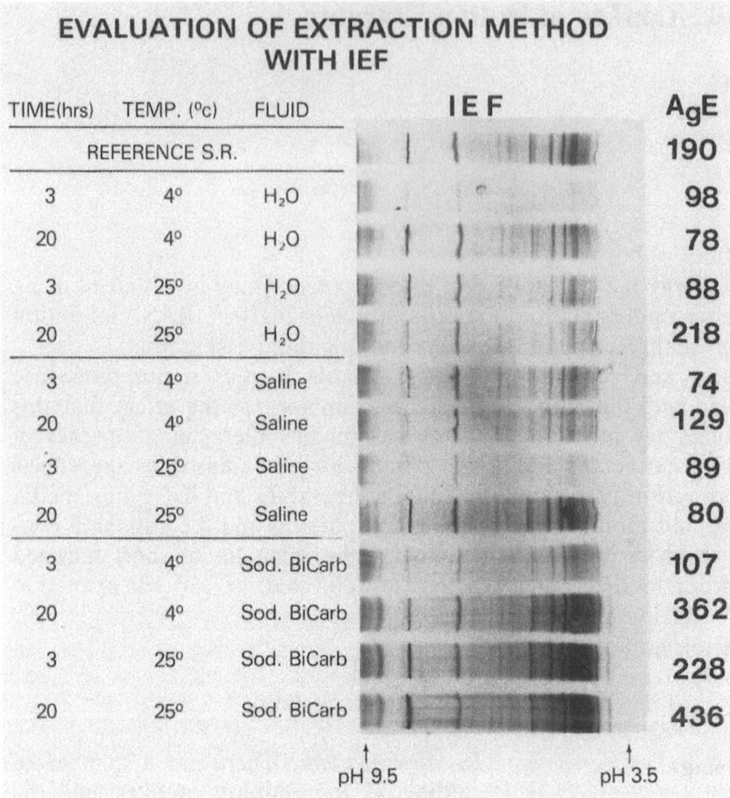

Fig. 31.1. Isoelectric focusing patterns and antigen E content of short ragweed pollen extract produced by different extraction conditions. Saline = 0.9% NaCl without additives; Sod. BiCarb = 0.1 M sodium bicarbonate. Antigen E is expressed in units/ml

decay and that in 50% glycerol, the rate of decay was so slow that it could not be accurately measured at temperatures ranging from 4 °C to 35 °C [2, 4].

The above studies are in general agreement that concentrated extracts stored in buffer containing phenol preservative start to lose measurable amounts of antigen E after a few months even at refrigerator temperatures and lose about one half of their activity between 8 months and a year. They also demonstrated that storage in 50% glycerol markedly reduced the loss of measurable antigen E even after one year.

A study of a timothy grass pollen extract using RAST inhibition indicated that about one half of the activity was lost when the extract was stored for 2 months at 10 °C, 5 days at 20 °C, and 1 day at 30 °C [5]. Another study using a timothy grass pollen extract showed that when RAST was used to measure the rate of decay, there was no measurable activity lost after 3 months of storage at 4 °C in buffer containing phenol. At 22 °C, 84% of the activity was left at 2 months, and 67% at 3 months. When the extract was stored at 35 °C, only 57% of the original activity remained after 1 week, 33% after 1 month, and 15% after 2 months. IEF patterns as well as crossed immuno- and crossed radioimmunoelectrophoretic patterns showed changes that paralleled the RAST activity [6].

In vivo tests: One of the most important findings resulting from careful skin testing is that there are allergic individuals who have skin reactivity to extracts that have been subjected to elevated temperatures, or other conditions that result in the degradation of proteins [7]. The presence of stable allergens has been shown for extracts of short ragweed and birch pollens, cockroach, cottonseed and cat extracts and honeybee venom [8]. For example, a short ragweed pollen extract that is maintained

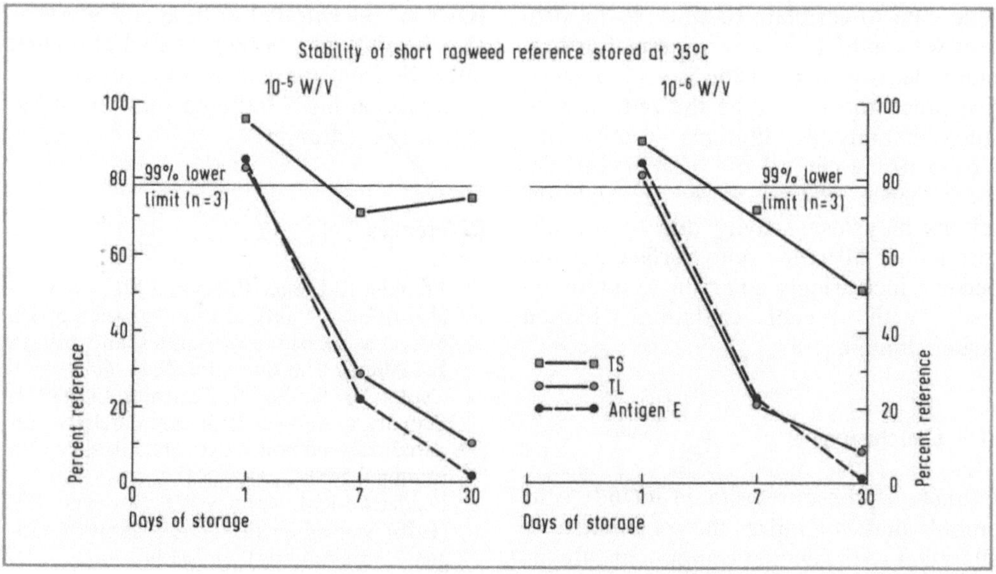

Fig. 31.2. Effect of patient sensitivity to thermostable (TS) and thermolabile (TL) ragweed allergens on stability of short ragweed reference stored at 35 °C. Patients sensitive to thermostable ragweed allergens react to short ragweed 1 : 100 wt/v and boiled short ragweed 1 : 40 wt/v with E 40 mm by puncture. Patients reactive to thermolabile ragweed allergens did not react to boiled ragweed but did react to short ragweed 1 : 100 wt/v. Diluent used was phosphate-buffered saline with 0.03% human serum albumin. AgE was determined on the 1 : 10 wt/v short ragweed reference stored at 35 °C for the time periods specified. [From 8]

at 24 °C for one week showed a reduction in skin reactivity in 2 of 9 individuals. Extracts stored at 35 °C had a loss in skin reactivity in 8 of 10 individuals [1]. In another study, a boiled short ragweed pollen extract appeared to have no loss in skin reactivity in some allergic individuals, some loss in others, and was nonreactive in another group [7]. In this study, it was possible to identify at least one heat-labile allergen, antigen E, and at least one heat-stable antigen, Ra5. There are undoubtedly other heat-labile and heat-stable allergens in this extract, however, the skin reactivity of the boiled extract showed a statistically significant correlation with the titer of anti-Ra5 in the sera of the individuals tested. The concentration of allergen Ra5 in short ragweed pollen extracts is about 0.1% of the total protein content, but this allergen is clearly important for skin test reactivity in some allergic individuals.

Because of the presence of both heat-stable and heat-labile allergens, it is unusual for any extract to lose all of its skin reactivity when the extract is subjected to adverse or extended storage conditions. A long-term study of a short ragweed pollen extract stored at 4–8 °C showed that the extract retained 16% of its original reactivity after 2 years of storage, 4.5% after 6 years, and 1.2% after 10 years [9].

The effect of patient selection on stability studies that employ skin testing has been demonstrated very dramatically as shown in Fig. 31.2. Patients who were reactive to thermostable (TS) ragweed allergens, showed very little loss in skin reactivity to an extract stored at 35 °C, while patients reactive to thermolabile (TL) ragweed allergens showed a dramatic loss in skin reactivity which closely paralleled the loss of antigen E [8].

The use of skin testing for stability studies is very important since there is very little data to correlate stability by in vitro tests with stability by in vivo tests. Furthermore, because skin testing is such a sensitive procedure it may be the only way to study stability at dilutions usually employed in the clinical use of allergenic extracts. Since extracts stored at high dilutions may lose activity due to the absorption of allergens onto surfaces, it has become increasingly common to dilute extracts with diluent containing human serum albumin [10].

31.3 Conclusions

Extraction procedures should include conditions that minimize the possibility of alteration of the extract components. Regulation of extraction temperature and time, and the selection of extracting fluid should be determined by the results of appropriate tests.

The above data demonstrate that extracts in phenol-buffered solutions maintained continuously at 4–8 °C are stable for 8–12 months, but that an increase in temperature to 22–24 °C causes degradation to become noticeable in 1 week to 1 month. At 35 °C, one half of the activity is lost in a few days. The data also show that there are some components of extracts that are more stable than others at elevated temperatures. Stability studies carried out in humans using quantitative skin test methods should preferably include patients who are skin-reactive to the thermolabile components of an extract.

The use of 50% glycerol results in a great increase in stability of pollen extracts. The use of a human serum albumin diluent is now being used in some extracts to prevent losses due to absorption of the allergens onto vial surfaces.

This information can be put to practical use by maintaining extracts at low temperatures at all times, and by storing extracts in concentrated form in 50% glycerol. Dilute solutions can be prepared at regular intervals from the concentrates in glycerol preferably using a buffered solution of human serum albumin.

References

1. Franklin RM, Baer H, Hooton ML, Brown H (1976) The stability of short ragweed pollen extract as measured by skin test and antigen E. J Allergy Clin Immunol 58:51–60
2. Center JG, Shuller N, Zeleznick LD (1974) Stability of antigen E in commercially prepared ragweed pollen extracts. J Allergy Clin Immunol 54:305–310
3. Peddecord KM, Northey WT, Goodman DH (1976) Studies on the deterioration of antigen E in extracts of *Ambrosia elatior.* J Allergy Clin Immunol 57:56–61
4. Hiatt CW, Baer H, Hooton ML (1977) Kinetics of thermal decay of antigen E from short ragweed pollen. J Biol Stand 5:39–44
5. Nielsen L, Lowenstein H, Weeke B (1974) Quantitative immunoelectrophoresis used in the analysis of the antigens in timothy (*Phleum pratense*) pollen extract. Acta Allergologica 29:385–401
6. Anderson MC, Baer H (1982) Antigenic and allergenic changes during storage of a pollen extract. J Allergy Clin Immunol 69:3–10
7. Baer H, Anderson MC, Hale R, Gleich GJ (1980) The heat stability of short ragweed pollen extract and the importance of individual allergens in skin reactivity. J Allergy Clin Immunol 66:281–285
8. Turkeltaub PC, Rastogi SC, Baer H, Anderson MC, Norman PS (1982) A standardized quantitative skin-test assay of allergen potency and stability: Studies of the allergen dose-response curve and effect of wheal, erythema and patient selection on assay results. J Allergy Clin Immunol 70:343–352
9. Arbesman CE, Eagle H (1939) The thermolability of ragweed pollen extract and its corresponding reagin. J Allergy 11:18–26
10. Norman PS, Marsh DG (1978) Human serum albumin and Tween 80 as stabilizers of allergen solutions. J Allergy Clin Immunol 62:314–319

32. Allergen Standardization *

R. A. Goldstein

In 1911 Noon [1] and Freeman [2] demonstrated that sterile extracts of pollen could be used for skin testing and that repeated injections improved the clinical tolerance of sensitive subjects following natural exposure. Subsequent clinical experience extended these observations to a variety of allergic disorders including asthma; a host of other environmental agents such as molds, animal hairs, danders and various dusts were extracted and used for testing and treatment. In fact, over 1,500 substances which are extracted and licensed as allergenic extracts have been reviewed by the USA Food and Drug Administration (FDA) Panel on Review of Allergenic Extracts [3] which aimed to determine which extracts were safe and effective and which were not. This Panel recognized that testing and treatment of allergic patients was performed with chemically crude preparations. The reason for this is that nearly all allergens in common use are prepared from naturally occurring source materials and contain nonallergenic components which do not appear to interfere with diagnostic or therapeutic efficacy. To date very few allergens have been isolated in a relatively pure state and removal of all impurities would be difficult, costly and perhaps unnecessary.

In other words, by their very nature allergenic extracts are unlike typical drugs or other chemically pure substances. The FDA Panel recognized this problem and presumably made pragmatic judgements concerning diagnostic and therapeutic efficacy based upon available data. A summary of their judgement in 1981 showed that 353 of 1,519 extracts used for diagnosis and 4 of 1,662 used for immunotherapy were deemed safe and effective [4]. The reason for these initial recommendations appeared related to the lack of well-controlled clinical studies which specifically assessed each material. Thus, many extracts were placed in a category where data appeared insufficient, despite the fact that empirical clinical data appeared supportive. It should be mentioned, in this regard that in those instances where relatively purified allergens have been examined, carefully controlled studies have, in fact, confirmed earlier clinical impressions and purified allergens have thus provided the means to develop more sensitive assays and more efficacious regimens for treatment. By accepting empirical data this Panel reevaluated their recommendations in 1983 and found that 1,069 of 1,385 extracts for diagnosis and 636 of 1,530 for treatment were considered to be safe and effective [5].

32.1 State of the Art

The difficulties confronting the FDA Panel reflect the basic problems confronting allergists and their patients; lack of standardized allergenic extracts combined with lack of sufficiently broad-based clinical trials using identical materials has impeded widespread acceptance of common clinical conclusions. It is especially disconcerting that uncertainty exists at a time when the scientific methods for answering many of these questions are at hand. In 1978 deWeck [6] stressed the need for international cooperative efforts in the field of allergen standardization and noted that the creation of a single international group in which representation from allergists, scientists dealing with allergen chemistry, manufacturers and control authorities should be a prerequisite to achieving concrete results

* The views expressed are those of the author and not the official views of either NIAID or IUIS

Table 32.1. Goals of IUIS allergen standardization subcommittee

1. Generate and make available to investigators, manufacturers and control authorities allergen reference preparations (with assigned arbitrary international units), standard and reagents.
2. Develop and publicize, on the basis of the appropriate collaborative trials, tests enabling assessment of:
   a) allergenic activity,
   b) composition and content of important allergenic molecules.
3. Provide an international collaborative framework for immunochemical allergen research.

in that field. In 1981 under the auspices of IUIS and the World Health Organization (WHO), the Allergen Standardization Subcommittee reconvened and set forth a series of goals (Table 32.1) [7, 8].

This group set out to consolidate prior national and international efforts and, for the first time, provide international reference preparations and standards which would meet stringent WHO requirements for acceptance and distribution worldwide [9]. By 1984 one of the initial goals was accomplished in that standards of extracts for short ragweed (*Ambrosia elatior*), timothy grass (*Phleum pratense*) and mite (*Dermatophagoides pteronyssinus*) were made available (National Institute for Biological Standards and Control, Holly Hill, Hampstead, London NW3 6RB, United Kingdom). In addition, work is nearing completion on standards of extracts for *Alternaria alternata,* Bermuda grass (*Dactylon cynadon*), birch (*Betula verrucosa*), cat and dog.

It should be emphasized that these standards are intended to provide high quality, broadly representative, and clinically useful materials. They were not intended to be either the most chemically pure or perfect materials. Used appropriately, they should provide the researcher, the clinician, the manufacturer and the control authorities with the necessary tools for comparative and collaborative studies. Their potential value and role, therefore, should be in providing the allergology community with an appropriate study tool and not in dictating the composition of allergenic extracts forever more.

32.2 Rationale for Future Efforts

Modern science has finally caught up with empirical clinical findings. Lichtenstein et al [10] have summarized the current rationale that immunotherapy in the management of bronchial asthma may not only ablate allergic reactions, but also diminish nonspecific bronchial hyperreactivity. They argue that an appropriate model for the study of asthma should focus not on the immediate response, which may after all be episodic, but rather on the late response which may be more likely responsible for subacute and chronic asthma. Data from antigen-provoked bronchoprovocation showing that the biphasic appearance of mast cell mediators in venous blood correlates with the early and late bronchospastic responses [11] combined with data showing that blocking IgG antibody production can ablate the late reaction [12] provides significant additional rationale for dissecting immune and physiological responses in asthmatic patients in relation to immunotherapy. The application of the modern technology of bronchoalveolar lavage in patients with asthma, which has demonstrated that direct application of antigen to the airways of allergic individuals can faithfully reproduce local and systemic airways constriction [13, 14], provides further rationale as well as an improved method to study the immunopathogenesis of asthma.

What Lichtenstein and co-workers emphasize however, is that when studying specific immune mechanisms and specific immune responses in treated patients, the allergenic extract utilized must, of necessity, be well-characterized, relatively pure, widely accepted and available – in other words – *standardized.* Furthermore, the use of standards permits improved decisions regarding appropriate immunizing dose, duration of therapeutic trial, and accurate *in vitro* measurements of results. It is not surprising that without available standards for allergenic extracts, few clinical trials have been accomplished confirming or denying the role of immunotherapy in treatment of asthma.

32.3 Conclusions

Progress toward our understanding of the role of allergens in the immunopathogenesis of asthma and the role of immunotherapy in management has been impeded, in part, because asthma is a disease state lacking a precise definition and also because we have lacked the critical tools necessary to accomplish the task. Within the past 5 years major advances have occurred in asthma research, most of which are discussed in other sections of this text, which now permit critical studies to be accomplished. One of the previous major obstacles, lack of standardized allergenic extracts, has now been partly overcome.

Individual and institutional efforts in the field of allergen standardization have been ongoing and productive for many years. NIAID convened a committee in 1959 which led to the research and development program which eventually led to the characterization of antigen E in ragweed. National control authorities including the National Institute for Biological Standards and Control (NIBSC) in the United Kingdom, the Food and Drug Administration of the Bureau of Biologics in the United States, the Nordic Council on Medicines, and others have all provided individual initiatives. In France the creation of the Groupe d'Etudes Français pour la Standardization des Allergènes (GEFSA) and in Germany, the series of Paul-Erlich Seminars have all made important contributions toward improved international cooperation and collaboration toward developing allergen standards. Without the above mentioned foundation of knowledge and goodwill, the IUIS Subcommittee on Allergen Standardization could not have succeeded.

Since 1981 three allergenic extracts have been accepted as WHO International Reference Standards and significant progress has been achieved on five more. The research community in allergology in 1985 has thus been provided with the essential tools to accomplish studies concerned with the immunopathogenesis of asthma that, for the first time, should clarify unequivocally the role of allergy in etiology and pathogenesis and the role of immunotherapy in management.

Acknowledgement: I wish to acknowledge the help and collaboration of Sylvia Cunningham, Research Resources Section, National Institute of Allergy and Infectious Diseases.

References

1. Noon L (1911) Prophylactic inoculation against hay fever. Lancet I: 1572–1573
2. Freeman J (1911) Further observations on the treatment of hay fever by hypodermic inoculations of pollen vaccine. Lancet II: 814–817
3. National Technical Information Service, U.S. Department of Commerce (1981) Panel on review of allergenic extracts final report, March 13, 1981. Accession Number PB81–182115
4. Sisk C (1983) Allergenic extracts-regulatory activities in the USA. In: Brede HD, Göing H, Schaeffer M (eds) Second International Paul-Erlich Seminar. Gustav Fischer, Stuttgart New York, pp 13–21
5. Schaeffer M, Sisk C (1984) Allergenic extracts: A review of their safety and efficacy. Ann Allergy 52:2
6. deWeck AL (1980) Statement on behalf of the International Union of Immunological Societies (IUIS) and International Congress of Allergology and Clinical Immunology (IAACI). In: Brede HD, Göing H (eds) Regulatory control and standardization of allergenic extracts. First International Paul-Erlich Seminar, Heft 75. Gustav Fischer, Stuttgart New York
7. International Union of Immunologic Societies Allergen Standardization Subcommittee. Scientific and Administrative Report 1980–1982. Available upon request from Dr. Goldstein, NIAID, Bethesda, MD, USA
8. Lowenstein H (1983) Report on behalf of the International Union of Immunological Societies (IUIS) Allergen Standardization Subcommittee. In: Brede HD, Göing H, Schaeffer M (eds) Regulatory Control and Standardization of Allergenic Extracts. Second International Paul-Erlich Seminar. Gustav Fischer, Stuttgart New York, pp 41–58
9. Guidelines for the preparation and establishment of reference materials and reference reagents for biological substances; WHO Technical Report Series, 1978, No. 626

10. Lichtenstein LM, Valentine MD, Norman PS (1984) A re-evaluation of immunotherapy for asthma. Am Rev Respir Dis 129:657–659
11. Nagy L, Lee TH, Kay AB (1982) Neutrophil chemotactic activity in antigen-induced late asthmatic reactions. N Engl J Med 306:497–501
12. Behrens BL, Marsh WR, Henson PM, Larsen GL (1983) Passive transfer of the late pulmonary response in an animal model: relationship of immunologic status to pulmonary physiologic changes. Am Rev Respir Dis 127:65
13. Godard P, Aubas P, Calvayrac P et al (1981) Endoscopie et lavage bronchiolo-alvéolaire chez l'asthmatique. Nouv Presse Méd 10:3131–3138
14. Rankin JA, Snyder PE, Schachter EN, Matthay RA (1984) Bronchoalveolar lavage: Its safety in subjects with mild asthma. Chest 85:723–728

33. Allergen Avoidance

D. Vervloet, A. Arnaud

Allergen avoidance may be a specific form of therapy. If a patient is shown to be sensitive to an antigen its removal from the environment may result in marked diminution of symptoms. Recently it was shown that prolonged allergen avoidance also decreased nonspecific bronchial reactivity [11, 14]. These results show that it is profitable to review allergens which can be eliminated or decreased and the techniques used for environmental control.

33.1 Mites and House Dust Avoidance

The discovery of mites led to an increased interest in dust avoidance since it was demonstrated that, in the world, the most common allergen associated with asthma is the dust mite, *Dermatophagoides pteronyssinus* with antigen P_1 as a major allergen.

Vacuum cleaning of mattress surfaces or bedrooms produced conflicting results in available literature. In two uncontrolled studies, vacuum cleaning was shown to decrease the mite concentration. In contrast, Arlian et al [1] found that repeated vacuum cleaning of mattresses, furniture, living rooms and bedrooms had no effect on mite numbers. Korsgaard [6] showed that only a limited amount of dust is removed when vacuuming the mattress surface once. On the other hand, Sarsfield et al [15] in an uncontrolled study, reported good clinical results by the drastic cleaning of bedrooms; the advice often given to patients to clean their bedrooms more carefully was found to have little or no effect on symptoms, mite numbers or allergen levels [3]. Mites and mite allergens can be present throughout a house and there is no evidence that allergen exposure in the bedroom only has any special significance.

Changes in ecological conditions have also been suggested as making a difference to the control of mites. Recently Korsgaard [7] confirmed that the seasonal variation in the occurrence of house dust mites was associated with the seasonal variation in indoor humidity and that the concentration of house dust mites in different homes during the same season is associated with differences in indoor humidity. Because of this it was suggested by the author that in a temperate climate, avoidance measures against house dust mites should be supplemented at least by a drying out period in the winter. Other changes in ecological conditions such as covering mattresses with plastic sheeting, heating blankets in the oven, reduction of moisture contents with silicagel or the use of fungistat such as nipagin or natamycine were proposed. However while these measures can decrease mite concentrations, no study has yet been done on their clinical efficacy.

The use of acaricides to control house dust mites has also been considered. Leysen et al who studied thirty pesticides against Dermatophagoides pteronyssinus obtained complete satisfaction only with lindane, but its toxicity prohibits its use in a patient's house [8]. Paragerm, a nontoxic bactericidal and fungicidal spray, killed cultures of dermatophagoides in experimental conditions and also when sprayed on the patients' mattresses [13]. Recently, Acardust, a product of synergized synthetic pyrethrinoid could demonstrate an adulticide and larvicide activity with good clinical tolerance [4]. Reduction of house dust mite allergen levels was also demonstrated by the use of another acaricide, pirimiphos methyl [9].

Change in climate or location is rarely indicated, but can be beneficial. Dutch authors [17] working at Davos in the Swiss Alps pointed out that house dust mites decrease in number with altitude. In a recent study [18] 42 children with asthma and al-

Table 33.1. House dust mites on the plain and at higher altitudes. [From 18]

	Positive samples			Total no. of samples each season[b]
	No. of positive samples	% positive[a]	Mites (mean no. ± SEM per 100 mg of house dust)[a]	
Plain				
0–300 m	62	80	88±6	77
Altitude				
900–1100 m	26	40	7±1	67
1200–1350 m	12	14	4	84
1400–1600 m	3	6	2	52
1600–3170 m	0	0	0	15
Total	41			218

[a] Significant decrease at high altitude ($p \leq 0.05$)
[b] Each sample comes from a different mattress studied at each season of the year

lergy to mites were sent away for a 9-months period at a high altitude. An improvement was observed in the first week and maintained during the entire stay. In this case, the improvement might be explained by the removal of antigenic stimulation, as shown by the decrease in the number of mites (Table 33.1) and in the specific IgE antibodies at higher altitude.

While at the moment, it seems very difficult to control totally the number of house dust mites we must persevere in this direction.

Recently, Platts-Mills et al [14] showed the decrease of non specific bronchial reactivity to histamine in asthmatic children allergic to Dermatophagoides pteronyssinus after prolonged allergen avoidance in modified hospital rooms (240 ng antigen P_1/g house dust in the hospital for 13,000 ng/g in the house). Murray and Fergusson [9] also suggested that the vigorous cleaning of bedrooms of dust allergic asthmatic children can lead to reduced bronchial reactivity. In this work, vacuum cleaning was associated with changes in ecological conditions (zippered vinyl covers and the following instructions: launder the curtains, wash blankets and mattress pads, clean drawers and closets, clean floors, remove toys, heat rooms etc.).

Thus it is possible to achieve some good clinical results if advice for mite control is given firmly and followed through. A simple technique recently described [19] based on the detection of guanine level in the house dust could be a useful aid in house dust mite allergen management in homes of allergic patients.

33.2 Avoidance of Other More Frequently Inhalant Allergens

Typical examples of allergic asthma due to inhalant allergens other than house dust mites are asthma due to household pets or to feather pillows. In these cases, etiologic diagnosis is of great value since no drug therapy or specific desensitization can completely resolve respiratory symptoms. Murray et al [10] found that children are more often allergic to cats than dogs and suggested increased intimacy of exposure to cats as one reason for the difference. The authors concluded that it may therefore be preferable for an atopic child to have a dog rather than a cat. However, although many allergists suggest that all furred and feathered pets should be avoided in homes of atopic children, there are at least as many doctors who disagree. In the work of Kjellman and Petterson [5] even frequent information from Health Services exerted little influence on asthmatic children keeping furred pets: 57% of asthmatic children, without allergy to danders, owned indoor furred pets as did 30% of asthmatic children with allergy to danders. The authors felt that the emotional conflict was sometimes so difficult and the mechanisms of repression so strong that is was almost impossible to persuade some families to get rid of their pets, although extensive general information programs and cleaning recommendations were given at individual consultations.

Environmental control of pollens and fungi is much more difficult to manage. While few years ago the question of the existence of extrinsic asthma, especially due to ragweed pollen, was asked, it is now recognized that bronchial hyperreactivity which increases during the pollen season responds well to corticosteroids [16]. Although the eviction of pollen seems reasonable in the prevention of asthma it is, however, very difficult to realize. Some advice can be given, i.e., cut down a tree near the house which is responsible for pollen asthma, shut windows, avoid walking in the country during the pollen season. Air conditioning and particulate matter control are also proposed with varying efficacy. Mold growth control can only be suggested for allergy to indoor molds. Dehumidifiers and room ventilators have proven useful. Occasionally the use of a fungicide may be desirable, but problems of toxicity are difficult to resolve.

33.3 Avoidance of Food and Drug Allergens

As with conjunctivitis and upper respiratory symptoms of rhinitis, asthma may be related to food hypersensitivity reactions, however, the true prevalence is probably small and confined to early childhood. Most cases of food allergen-induced asthma are related to cow milk sensitivity. In this case when breast feeding is not possible, a milk-free formula may be used. Furthermore, although more carefully conducted prospective studies are needed, the evidence of a number of investigators suggests that the substitution of cow's milk with soy formula or breast milk in early infancy can result in a delayed or lowered incidence of allergic diseases [2].

A subset of asthmatics has reported the development of wheezing after ingesting food chemically preserved with sodium metabisulfite and related compounds such as sulfur dioxide, and sulfites. Common offenders such as salads, sausages or drinks (wines, soft drinks etc.) must be avoided especially in restaurants. Similar, but delayed, induction of wheezing by asthmatics ingesting monosodium L-glutamate, an additive common in Chinese food has recently been described. In rare cases, azo dyes, particularly tartrazine yellow and possibly benzoate preservatives have been implicated in triggering symptoms in a subset of asthmatics. If diagnosis is made such additives must be discarded.

Drug asthma needs to be diagnosed. The most known example is aspirin-induced asthma. Patients intolerant to aspirin must avoid all nonsteroidal analgesics. However, in such patients relief of respiratory symptoms is generally incomplete, even after avoidance. Allergic asthma to other drugs such as penicillin or other antibiotics results from occupational airborne exposure and disappears after avoidance of the allergens.

33.4 Prevention of Occupational Asthma

Prevention must be the prime objective in the management of occupational asthma. This can be achieved in part by reducing the levels of exposure to potentially harmful industrial materials. For example, in the case of alcalase, a proteolytic enzyme prepared from bacillus subtilis, substantial improvements in the manufacturing process were made to reduce the levels of alcalase in the air and protect factory workers making detergents containing alcalase [12]. Avoidance of allergens such as western red cedar, colophony fumes, isocyanates led to clinical improvement, and/or a decrease in bronchial reactivity.

Environmental control may be a very efficacious, specific form of therapy in allergic asthma, however, we cannot forget that complete allergen avoidance is often impossible and that environmental control also concerns irritants (including i.e., air pollution, cigarette smoke), aggressive management of infection, physical measures (i.e., physical education, general exercise) and psychological management.

References

1. Arlian LG, Bernstein IL, Gallagher JS (1982) The prevalence of house dust mites, Dermatophagoides spp. and associated environmental conditions in homes in Ohio. J Allergy Clin Immunol 69, 6:527–532
2. Bjorksten B (1983) Does breast-feeding prevent the development of allergy? Immunology Today 4, 8:215–217
3. Burr ML, Neale E, Dean BV, Verrier-Jones ER (1980) Effect of a change to mite-free bedding on children with mite-sensitive asthma: a controlled trial. Thorax 35:513–514
4. Jean-Pastor MJ, Vervloet D, Thibaudon M, Belaube P (1986) Destruction des acariens de la poussière de maison: efficacité et tolérance d'un nouvel acaricide en aerosol. Rev Fr Allergol 26, 3:125–129
5. Kjellman B, Petterson R (1983) The problem of furred pets in childhood atopic disease. Failure of an information program. Allergy 38:65–73
6. Korsgaard J (1983) Preventive measures in mite asthma. A controlled trial. Allergy 38:93–102
7. Korsgaard J (1983) House-dust mites and absolute indoor humidity. Allergy 38:85–92
8. Leysen MT, Reybrouck G, van de Voorde H (1974) Susceptibility of the house dust mite to pesticides and disinfectants. Acta Allergologica 29:455–461
9. Mitchell EB, Wilkins S, McCallum D, Platts-Mills TAE (1985) Reduction of house dust mite allergen levels in the home: use of the acaricide pirimiphos methyl. Clin Allergy 15:235–240
10. Murray AB, Ferguson AC, Morrison BJ (1983) The frequency and severity of cat allergy vs. dog allergy in atopic children. J Allergy Clin Immunol 72:145–149
11. Murray AB, Ferguson AC (1983) Dust-free bedrooms in the treatment of asthmatic children with house dust or house dust mite allergy: a controlled trial. Pediatrics 71, 3: 418–422
12. Newhouse ML, Tagg B, Pocock SJ (1970) An epidemiological study of workers producing enzyme washing powders. Lancet 4:689–693
13. Penaud A, Nourrit J, Timon-David P, Charpin J (1977) Results of a controlled trial of the acaricide Paragerm on Dermatophagoides spp. in dwelling houses. Clin Allergy 7:49–53
14. Platts-Mills TAE, Tovey ER, Mitchell EB, Mozarro H, Nock P, Wilkins SR (1982) Reversal of bronchial hyperreactivity during prolonged allergen avoidance. Lancet II:675–678
15. Sarsfield JK, Gowland G, Toy R, Norman ALE (1974) Mite sensitive asthma of childhood: trial of avoidance measures. Arch Dis Child 49:716–721
16. Sotomayor H, Badier M, Vervloet D, Orehek J (1984) Seasonal increase of carbachol airway responsiveness in patients allergic to grass pollen. Reversal by corticosteroids. Am Rev Respir Dis 130:56–58
17. Spieksma FTM, Zuidema P, Leupen MJ (1971) High altitude and house dust mites. Br Med J 1:82
18. Vervloet D, Penaud A, Razzouk H, Senft M, Arnaud A, Boutin C, Charpin J (1982) Altitude and house dust mites. J Allergy Clin Immunol 69, 3:290–296
19. van Bronswijk J, Bischoff E, Schirmacher W, Berreno L, Schober G (1986) A rapid house dust allergen test: Preliminary results. J Med Entomol 23, 2:217–218

34. Allergens Inducing Asthma (Introduction)

In 1873 Charles Blackley, an allergic physician, discovered that pollens could cause hay fever and trigger asthma. Performing most of his experiments on himself, he saved pollens from the flowering season and sniffed them during the winter, producing the typical symptoms of *summer catarrh,* including asthma. During the twenties and thirties, the concept of allergy was broadened and it was shown that epithelia and molds were inducing allergic reactions and asthma. About the same time Storm van Leeuwen reported that when he moved patients with asthma from the climate of Holland to the mountains of Switzerland, many subjects did not present symptoms anymore. However he did not find the reason for these therapeutic benefits. House dust was supposed to elicit asthma during the eighteenth century but, although mites were suspected to be allergenic in 1920, it was not until 1964 that Voorhorst and Spieksma confirmed the role of *Dermatophagoides pteronyssinus* as the most important allergen in house dust.

In 1986, most of the aeroallergens have been disclosed, but many questions remain unanswered. What are the major and minor allergenic constituants of allergens? Why do pollens, some mold species and mite feces, having a diameter of over 20 μm, cause a bronchial allergic reaction, when it is known that most particles over 5 μm cannot reach the bronchial tree? What are the doses of allergens required to elicit asthma? Is allergic asthma associated with neurogenic mechanisms? In the following chapters some of these questions will be discussed showing that allergens represent a significant cause of asthma.

34.1 Pollen-induced Asthma

J. Bousquet, P. Cour, F. B. Michel

Pollens contain the male germ cells of plants necessary for fertilization. Pollen grains are spheroid, ovoid or ellipsoid in shape and may have smooth, reticulated, spiculated or sculptured surfaces. These surface characteristics are used for identifying pollen grains in atmospheric surveys. They usually range in size from 10 to 100 μm (Fig. 34.1). The dispersion of pollens is directly related to their allergenic potency. The most primitive pollination is the dispersion of pollen grains by the wind and, since it is not efficient, this method must be compensated by the release of large amounts of pollens. With a few notable exceptions all wind-pollinated (anemophilous) pollens are allergenic. Other methods of pollination include insect

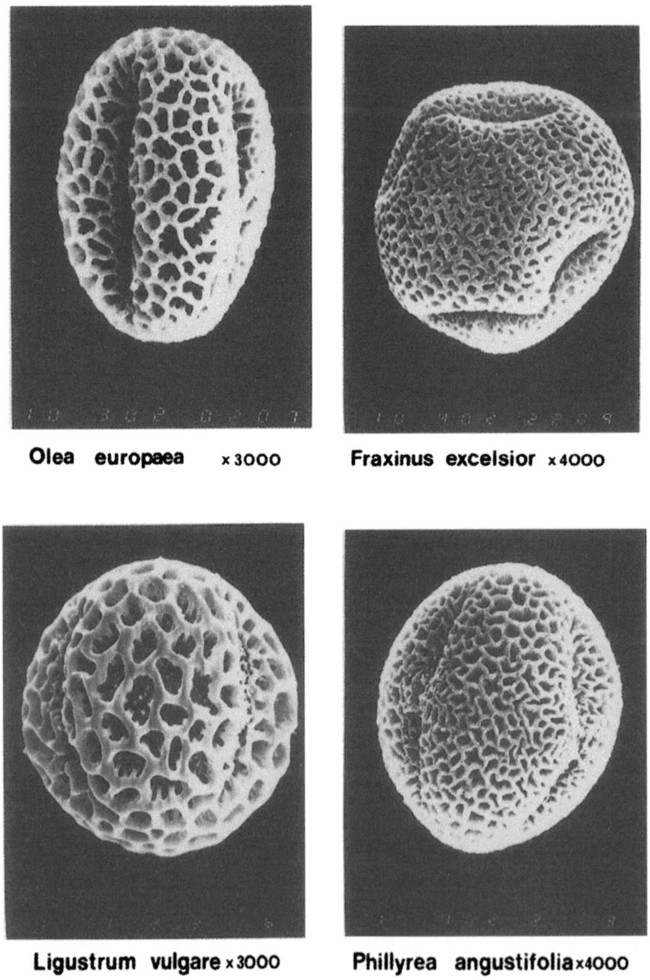

Fig. 34.1. Morphology of pollen grains by scanning electron microscopy

pollination (entomophilous) or pollination by water or other animals. These pollens are less allergenic since they are released in much smaller quantities in the atmosphere. Some pollens are both anemo- and entomophilous and can be allergenic [22] and, occupational allergy to entomophilous pollens is not rare [6]. Wind-pollinated flowers can be distinguished from insect-pollinated ones by the lack of qualities attractive to insects, such as colour, perfume and nectar. In general the flowers involved in the production of allergy are not the beautiful conspicuous flowers; those that release most pollens are dull and unattractive. This is the reason for the poor allergenicity of honey [4].

34.1.1 Atmospheric Distribution of Pollens

Dispersion of pollens: Pollen concentration of the atmosphere depends on the vegetation and the climate of a given area and substantial differences have been observed. Pollens become airborne when they fall into the airstream or are scoured by turbulent eddies. Pollen prevalence in a given area reflects the strength and vicinity of upwind sources and the activity of crosswinds both vertical and horizontal [36]. Mature pollens are released from dehiscent anthers in clumps. Release of these clumps occurs usually during a diurnal period and depends on a temperature rise and reduction of relative humidity. Although pollen emission, dispersion and transport are due to complex weather patterns, the level of airborne pollens is mostly increased by warm, dry and clear conditions and falls during cold or humid periods.

Climatic conditions effect the flowering of plants. In many cases, this depends on cumulated temperatures reached after the vegetative rest. Since both parameters are species-specific the variable occurrence of the pollen season can be understood especially for winter and early spring pollinating plants (Fig. 34.2). For other species such as some western ragweed, the flowers always bloom at the same time in the year since they need a specific amount of light.

Pollen sampling: Several methods are currently used for sampling airborne pollens [10, 23, 32, 38].

- The gravimetric method is based on the gravity of pollens and the most widely used device was proposed by Durham. This technique suffers from many disadvantages and is now being replaced by better ones.
- Suction traps such as the Burkard trap, a form of the automatic spore trap designed by Hirst [17] is a volumetric technique. Air is drawn into the sampler and the airborne particles impinge onto sampling slides covered by an adhesive substance. The deposition of particles depends on their aerodynamic mean diameter and it is not uniform.
- Rotating arm impactors are popular in America. Narrow cylinders, ribbons and adhesive-coated filaments intercept particles from moving airstream with high efficiency. Rotorod, rotoslide or flyshield rotobar samplers [38] are generally recommended for short period sampling for up to two hours. To prevent overloading efficiently, intermittent rotoslides were introduced.
- A filter trap made from orientable vertical gauze layers dipped into silicone oil was proposed by Cour et al [12, 13] (Fig. 34.3). The pollens are caught in the silicone and examined after dissolution of the gauze by acidic solutions and acetolysis. From 1,000 to 10,000 grains are counted for each analysis and the data obtained are directly fed into a computer. The very high efficiency of this device was shown when side-by-side comparisons were made with other pollen traps and from the prediction of crops [11].
- All these devices indicate a mean count either daily or weekly. However, the exact amount of pollens inhaled by each individual patient is only estimated. Individual pollen collectors have therefore been proposed but their exact accuracy is not yet fully evaluated [21].

Pollen calendars: Pollen calendars have been proposed by many investigators and the results are mostly expressed in number

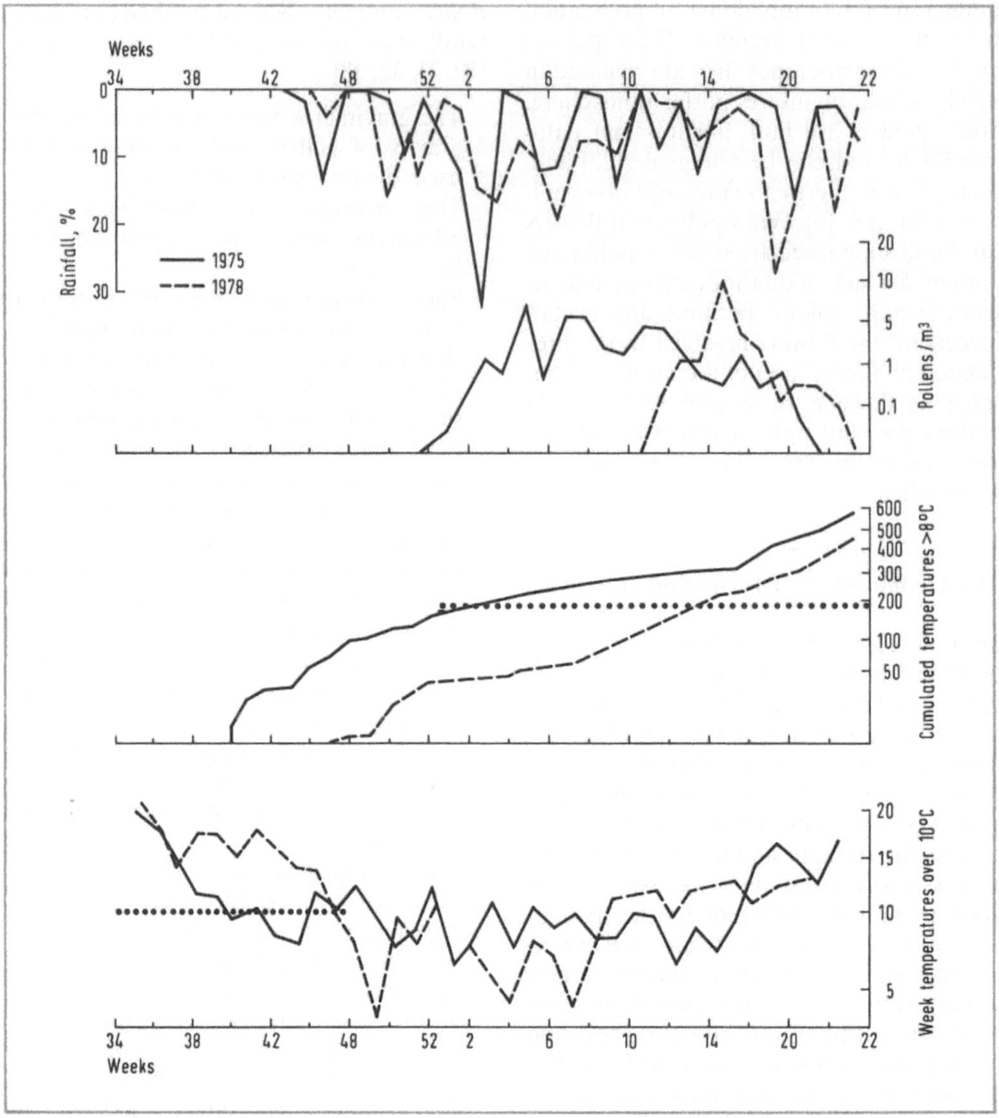

Fig. 34.2. Pollination of *Phyllirea angustifolia* (Oleaceae) in 1975 and 1978. The vegetative rest starts when weekly temperatures are under 10 °C. The flowers bloom when the cumulated temperatures, after the vegetative rest, are 200 °C. The rainfall explains the modulation of temperature gains

of grains per volume of air. However, the size and the shape of pollen grains differ widely and it may be better to give the results in weight per volume of air (Fig. 34.4) [5]. In the future, immunochemical methods will be available to give the results in amounts of allergens inhaled by the patients [1, 44].

Pollen calendars show the distribution of pollens in the atmosphere over a period of time (Fig. 34.5) and are extremely useful to the allergist. It is also interesting to determine the variation of the pollen rain in a cross section (Fig. 34.6) [12, 13]. The differences observed between many locations explain the variation in the mean sen-

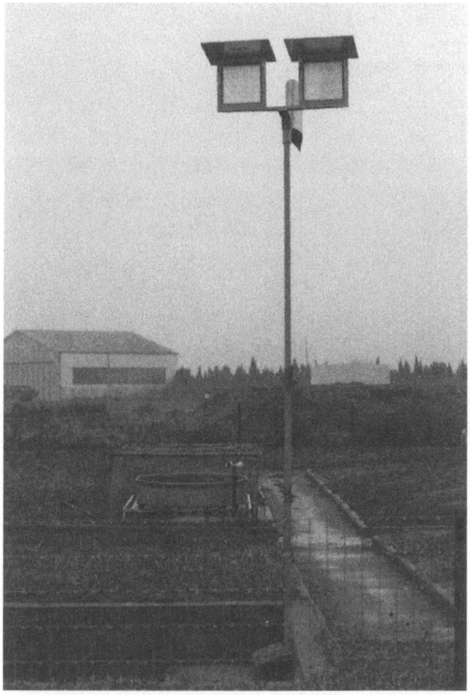

Fig. 34.3. Pollen sampler made from a filter trap. [From 12, 13]

sitivities of the patients since they are exposed to different amounts of allergens. The protocols of specific immunotherapy should be adapted to pollen calendars.

Pollen seasons: Pollens are emitted when flowers bloom. Their maximal release in most countries of the northern hemisphere ranges from the late spring to the fall. Among the most allergenic pollens are grasses. In the United States and in some parts of Europe ragweed pollens are the cause of a major pollinosis and the classical ragweed season is characteristic in the months of September and October. However, during the winter and early spring some species are relevant in terms of pollinosis. In the Mediterranean area cypress, ash and Phillyrea are often involved in pollinosis [30].

34.1.2 Allergenic Pollens

With a few notable exceptions, all pollens found in the ambiant air are potentially allergenic [22]. The major exception is the

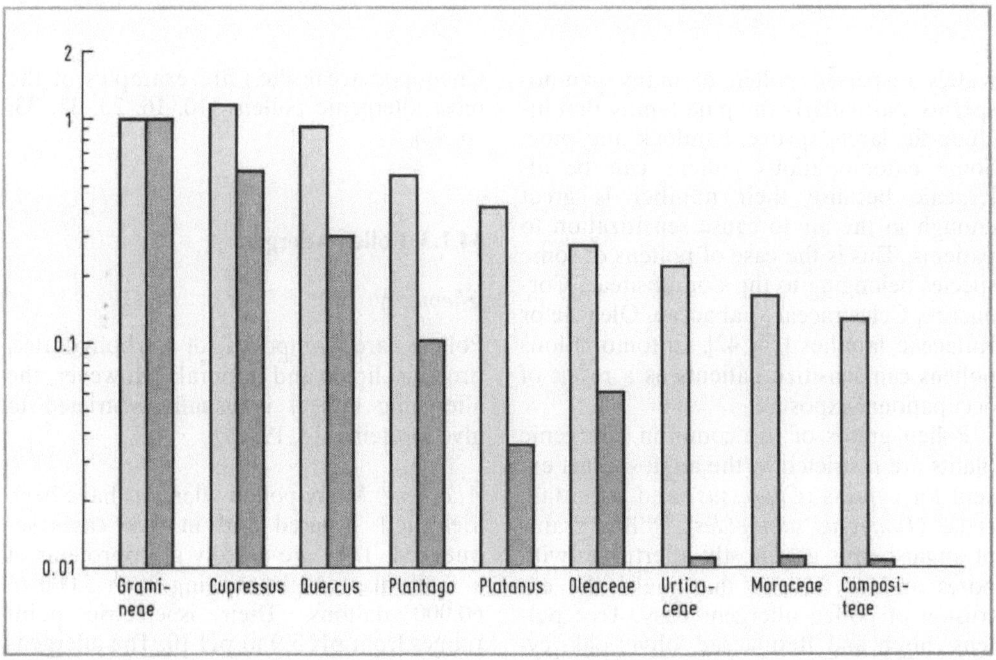

Fig. 34.4. Comparison of the number of pollen grains present in the atmosphere of Montpellier with the amount of grains inhaled by the patients. A ratio of 1 is given for grass pollens. Mean annual counts are indicated. [From 5]

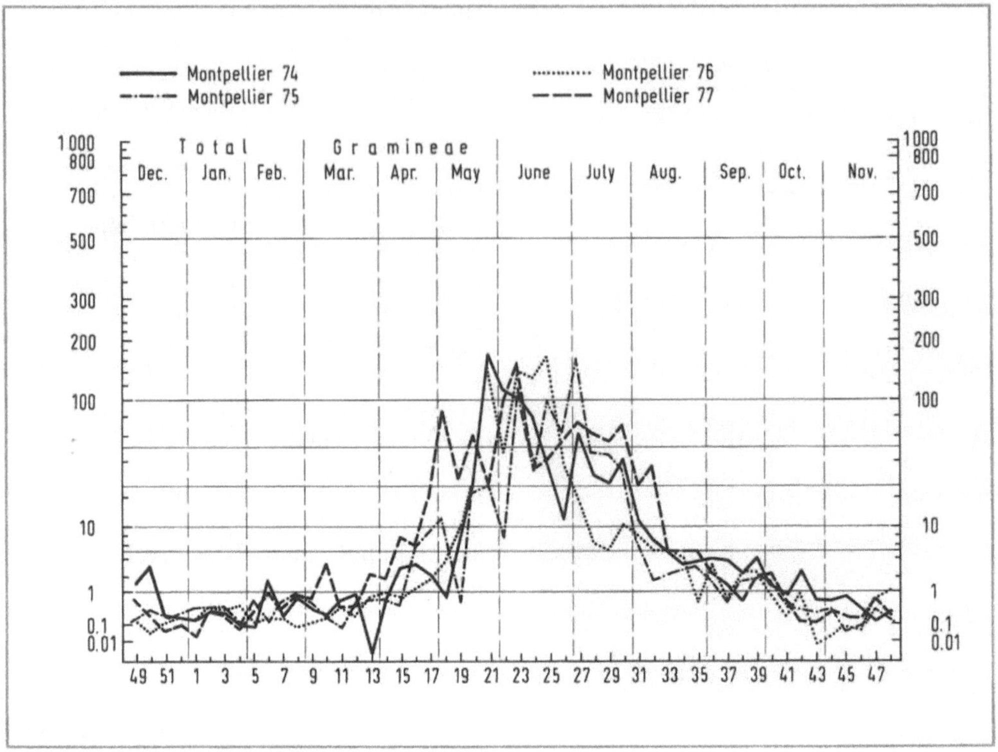

Fig. 34.5. Pollen calendar of grass pollens in Montpellier. [From 13]

widely dispersed pollen of many gymnosperms, particularly the pine family that include fir, larch, spruce, hemlock and pine. Some entomophilous pollens can be allergenic because their number is great enough in the air to cause sensitization to patients. This is the case of pollens of some species belonging to the Compositeae, Cornaceae, Celastraceae, Fabaceae, Oleacae or Rutaceae families [24, 42]. Entomophilous pollens can sensitize patients as a result of occupational exposure.

Pollen grains of the common allergenic plants are restricted to the angiosperms except for cypress (*Cupressus*) and mountain cedar (*Juniperus sabinoides*). Pollen grains of angiosperms are mostly aperturate with pores and/or furrows that make the extrusion of pollen allergens easy. Tree pollens (birch and Betulaceae, olive, oak, cypress, plane etc.), grass and weed pollens (ragweeds, *Parietaria* – restricted to the Mediterranean area –, Compositeae, Chenopodiaceae etc.) are examples of the most allergenic pollens [10, 16, 23, 31, 33, 36, 42].

34.1.3 Pollen Allergens

Chemistry

Pollens are composed of carbohydrates, proteins, lipids and minerals. However, the allergenic moiety is usually restricted to glycoproteins [18, 19, 39].

Allergens: Many pollen allergens have been identified, isolated and in rare cases sequenced. They are usually glycoproteins of a molecular weight ranging from 5,000 to 60,000 daltons. Their isoelectric point ranges from pH 3.9 to pH 10. The allergens are classified as major or minor according to the percentage of patients allergic to the whole pollen who are effectively sensitized

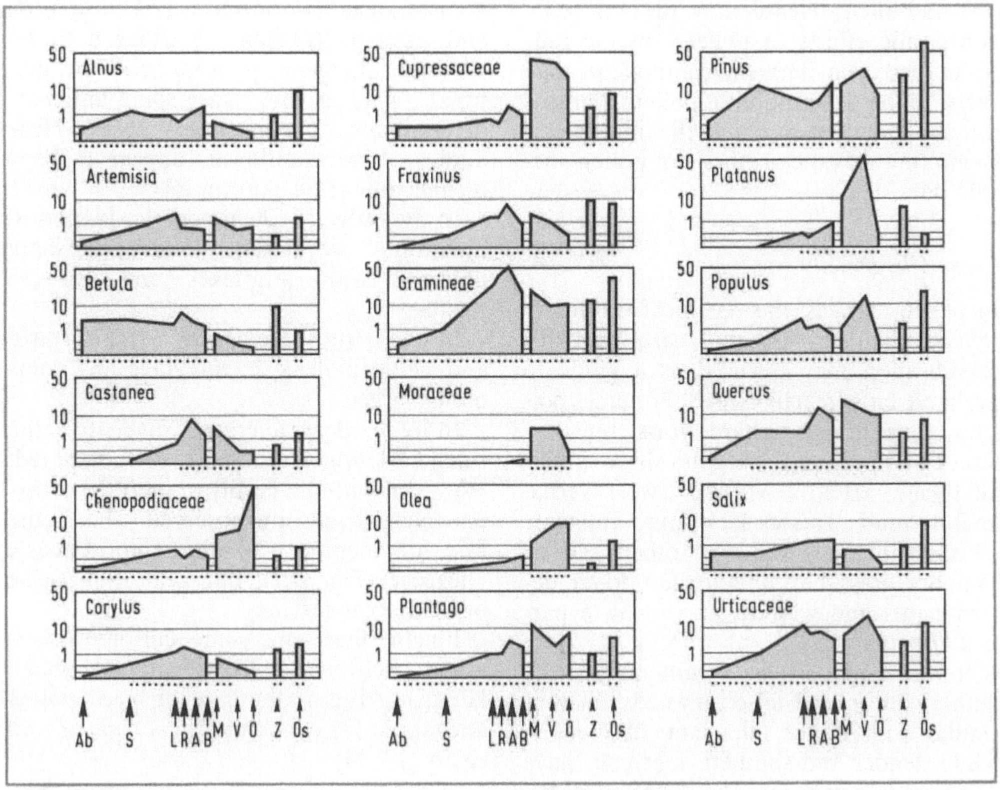

Fig. 34.6. Interregional variations of common allergenic pollens in Europe. Atlantic transect: Ab = Abisko (Northern Sweden), S = Stockholm (Sweden), L = Lille (France), R = Rouen (France), A = Angers (France), B = Bordeaux (France). Mediterranean transect: M = Montpellier (France), V = Valencia (Spain), O = Oran (Algeria). Mountain area: Z = Zurich (Swiss Alps), Os = Osseja (French Pyrenees). [From 12, 13]

to the given purified allergen. However, the definition of major and minor allergens varies according to authors. Marsh [28] proposed that the term *major allergen* should be restricted to a highly purified allergen "to which over 90% of clinically specifically allergic individuals react appreciably in high allergen dilutions". In Scandinavia, major allergens are those "to which 50% of the patients allergic to the allergen source in question react and to which 25% bind strongly" [26].

Most isolated allergens have been shown to exist in multiple molecular forms that exhibit slight physicochemical differences but have indistinguishable allergenic properties. Such allergens have been termed isoallergens.

The most extensively studied pollen is short ragweed (*Ambrosia artemisifolia*). In short ragweed pollen crossed immunoelectrophoresis studies [25] revealed the presence of 52 different antigens [27]. It was subsequently possible to identify by means of crossed radioimmunoelectrophoresis nine important allergens: antigens E, K and Ra 6. Antigen Ra 5 was found to be a minor but potent allergen.

Nonallergenic components: Pollens contain a wide variety of nonallergenic components which are under investigation since some may be allergenic (i.e., enzymes) [9] and others were shown to stimulate lymphocytes (lectins). Moreover hemolysins are present in large amounts

[15] and their release may explain some nonspecific effects of pollens on the mucosa. These nonallergenic components may enhance the penetration of pollen allergens through the mucosa or help the immune response towards the synthesis of pollen-specific IgE.

Cross Allergenicity

In pollen extracts, the botanical taxonomy reflects phylogeny in most cases and this classification may be used as a guide to probable cross reactivity [41]. For grass pollens, June grass, orchard grass, meadow fescue and perennial rye grass share similar allergenic patterns whereas sweet vernal and Bermuda grasses lack some antigenic determinants possessed by other grasses. Timothy grass has unique additional determinants and western grasses have particular patterns [7].

In the Compositeae family [20] short, giant, western and false ragweeds are very similar with minor allergenic differences, while slender and southern ragweeds have some distinct patterns. The members of the Anthemideae (wormwood and mugwort) and Astereae (goldenrod) tribes have no common allergenic patterns with the ragweeds, whereas they share some antigenic determinants. The members of the Heliantheae tribe (sunflower) appear to have distinct allergenic patterns [6].

In the order of Chenopodiales [41], most amaranths are closely related and share antigens with atriplexes and Russian thistle.

In the Urticaceae family [8] *Parietaria* and nettle pollens do not have any common allergen.

In tree pollens, allergenic diversity is the rule [7, 41] when all families are compared. However, within a family or an order cross-reactive patterns are observed. This is the case of members of the Cupressaceae, Oleaceae (Fig. 34.7), Fagaceae, Salicaceae or Betulaceae families.

Finally there are some curious associations between pollens and nonpollen allergens. This is the case of birch pollen and apple [2] or Compositeae pollen and celery [14, 34].

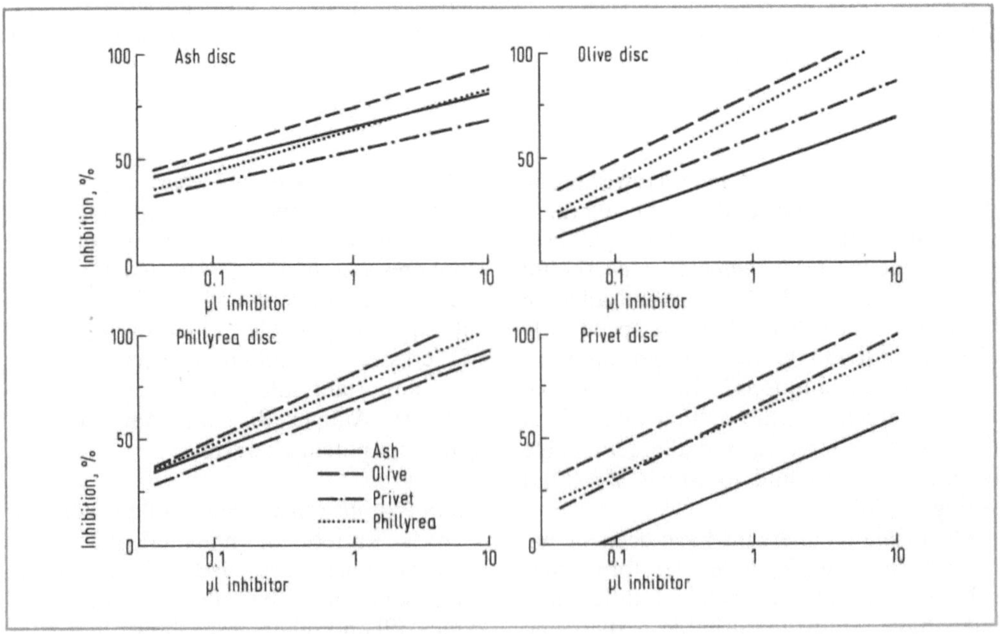

Fig. 34.7. Cross-allergenicity between different Oleaceae pollens demonstrated by means of RAST inhibition

Release of Pollen Allergens

The allergenic importance of each of the pollen allergens depends on many factors and is a function of their immunogenicity and concentration in the pollen. Other functions include the genetic capacity of the host to recognize the antigen as forming and to synthetize IgE antibodies [28], and to release pollen allergens when the grain impinges on a mucosal surface [3, 7, 29]. The rate of release of different ragweed pollen allergens was shown to differ and the so-called major allergen antigen E is released slowly (Fig. 34.8). The major plane tree pollen antigen (P) is also released at a relatively slow rate. These observations provoke a reevaluation of the role of the different allergenic components of each individual pollen since the symptoms induced by pollen grains appear immediately after the impingement of the grains on the mucosal surfaces.

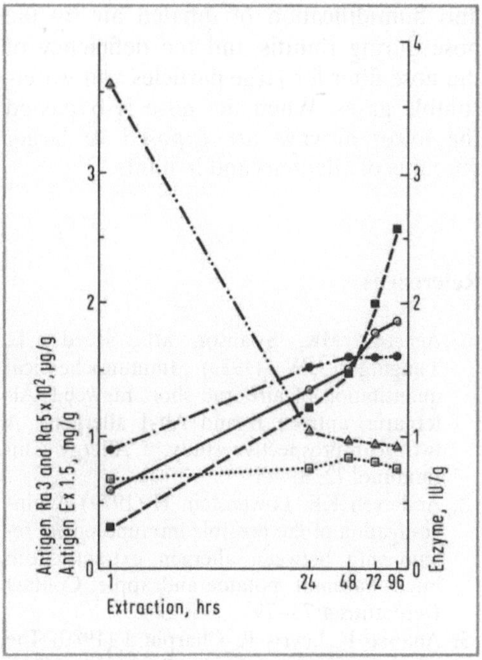

Fig. 34.8. Release of *Ambrosia eliator* pollen antigens according to the time of incubation. [From 7]

34.1.4 Pollen-induced Asthma

Penetration of pollen grains and pollen allergens into the respiratory tract: Pollen grains can penetrate through the deep lung [32, 35] but it is not known whether these grains can elicit bronchial responsiveness. Although intact grains are assumed to be the primary carriers of pollen allergens, specific immunoreactive components have been found to be present in submicronic particle-free atmospheric droplets [37]. These particles can easily reach the deep lung but many questions remain to be answered. The relative contribution of small aerosol-associated fractions to the total pollen allergen burden remains to be established. The origin of these fractions is still uncertain and overall pollen-induced symptoms are extremely important when the air is dry and hot. An alternative to this hypothesis can therefore be put forward. When pollen grains impinge on the nasal mucosa they are humidified and the humid air inhaled may carry pollen allergens into the small airways leading to asthma. This may be the reason for the onset of asthma during the peak of the pollen season.

Nonallergenic mechanisms: Nonallergenic mechanisms may also explain pollen-induced asthma. The upper airways can contribute to lower airway obstruction probably through reflex mechanisms. Several recent investigations suggest that many patients suffering from allergic rhinitis demonstrate evidence of physiological peripheral or central airways obstruction which may occur spontaneously during symptomatic stages or in response to the inhalation of a cholinergic agent. Moreover, in patients with asthma or rhinitis who are allergic to ragweed, a specific bronchial challenge can elicit a bronchoconstriction with asthmatics having the greater responsiveness. It appears therefore that rhinitis can elicit a nonspecific bronchial hyperreactivity. A nasobronchial or orobronchial reflex blocked by anticholinergic drugs may exist in asthma [40, 43].

Other nasobronchial relationships may be involved in the occurrence of bronchial obstruction during a pollen-induced rhinitis. These include the impaired heating and humidification of inhaled air by the nose during rhinitis and the deficiency of the nose filter for large particles and water-soluble gases. When the nose is bypassed the lower airways are exposed to larger amounts of allergens and irritants.

References

1. Agarwal MK, Swanson MC, Reed CE, Yunginger JW (1983) Immunochemical quantitation of airborne short ragweed, Alternaria, antigen E and Alt-1 allergens. A two year prospective study. J Allergy Clin Immunol 72:40–45
2. Andersen KE, Løwenstein H (1979) An investigation of the possible immunological relationship between allergen extracts from birch, hazelnut, potatoe and apple. Contact Dermatitis 4:73–79
3. Anfosso F, Leyris R, Charpin J (1980) The allergen of plane-tree pollen. Characterization of a major allergen. Allergy 8:196–198
4. Bousquet J, Campos J, Michel FB (1984) Food intolerance to honey. Allergy 39:73–75
5. Bousquet J, Cour P, Guérin B, Michel FB (1984) Allergy in the mediterranean area. I. Pollens counts and pollinosis of Montpellier. Clin Allergy 14:249–258
6. Bousquet J, Dhivert H, Clauzel AM, Hewitt B (1985) Occupational allergy to sunflower pollen. J Allergy Clin Immunol 75:70–74
7. Bousquet J, Guérin B, Furic R, Michel FB (1983) Standardization of allergen extract. In: Spector S (ed) Provocative testing. CRC Press, Boca Raton, pp 45–95
8. Bousquet J, Guérin B, Lim P, Hewitt B, Dhivert H, Michel FB (1986) Cross allergenicity between Parietaria and Urtica Pollens. Clin Allergy 16:57–64
9. Cooke RA (1918) Active immunization in hay fever. NY Med J 107:577
10. Charpin J, Surinyach R (1974) Atlas of European allergenic pollens. Sandoz, Basel
11. Cour P, Bousquet J (1981) Crop prediction using pollen count. Span 24:83–87
12. Cour P, Seignalet C, Cambon J, Guérin B, Mayrand L, Nilsson S, Michel FB (1981) Inter-regional studies of pollen incidence from Lapland to North Africa. The 1st International Conference on Aerobiology. E. Schmidt, Berlin, pp 61–80
13. Cour P, Bousquet J, Cambon G, Nilsson S, Michel FB (in press) Inter-regional variations of common allergenic pollens in Europe using a filter trap. Clin Allergy
14. Déchamp C, Michel J, Deviller P, Perrin LF (1984) Choc anaphylactique au céleri et sensibilisation à l'armoise. Allergie croisée ou allergie concomitante? Presse Méd 13:871–874
15. Freed DJL, Buckley CH, Tsivion Y, Sharon N, Katz DH (1983) Non-allergic haemolysins in grass pollens and house dust mites. Allergy 38:477–486
16. Halse RR (1984) Nomenclature of allergenic plants. Ann Allergy 53:291–310
17. Hirst JM (1952) An automatic volumetric spore trap. Ann Appl Biol 39:257
18. King TP (1976) Chemical and biological properties of some atopic allergens. Adv Immunol 23:77–105
19. Knox RB, Heslop Harrison J (1971) Pollen-wall proteins: localization of antigenic and allergenic proteins in the pollen-grain walls of Ambrosia spp. (ragweeds). Cytobios 4:49–54
20. Leiferman KM, Gleich GJ (1976) The cross reactivity of IgE antibodies with pollen allergens. I. Analyses of various species of grass pollens. J Allergy Clin Immunol 58: 129–139
21. Leuschner RM, Boehm G (1978) Investigations with the "Individual pollen collector" and the Burkard trap with reference to hay fever patients. Clin Allergy 8:589–594
22. Lewis WH (1978) Pollen structure and development. Their role in allergic reactions. Trans Am Soc Ophthalmol Laryngol Allergy 18:137–143
23. Lewis WH, Vinay P, Zenger VE (1982) Airborne and allergenic pollens of North America. Johns Hopkins University Press, Baltimore
24. Lewis WH, Vinay O (1979) North American pollinosis due to insect-pollinated plants. Ann Allergy 42:309–318
25. Lowenstein H (1978) Quantitative immunoelectrophoretic methods as a tool for the analysis and isolation of allergens. Prog Allergy 25:1–65
26. Lowenstein H, King TP, Goodfriend L, Hussain R, Roebber M, Marsh DG (1982) Antigens of Ambrosia eliator (short ragweed) pollen. II. Immunochemical identification of known antigens by quantitative immunoelectrophoresis. J Immunol 127:637–642
27. Lowenstein H, Marsh DG (1981) Antigens of Ambrosia eliator (short ragweed) pollen. I. Crossed immunoelectrophoretic analyses. J Immunol 126:943–950
28. Marsh DG (1975) Allergens and the genetics of allergy in the antigens. Academic Press, New York, p 271
29. Marsh DG, Belin L, Bruce A, Lichtenstein LM, Hussain R (1981) Rapidly released

allergens from short ragweed pollen. I. Kinetics of release of known allergens in relation to biologic activity. J Allergy Clin Immunol 67:206–216
30. Michel FB, Dhivert H, Marty JP, Cour P, Alquie MC, Guérin B (1978) Pollinoses hivernales. Rev Fr Allergol 18:83–89
31. Michel FB, Cour P, Quet L, Marty JP (1976) Qualitative and quantitative comparison of pollen calendars for plain and mountain areas. Clin Allergy 6:383–388
32. Michel FB, Marty JP, Quet L, Cour P (1977) Penetration of inhaled pollen into respiratory tractus. Am Rev Respir Dis 119: 609–616
33. Nilsson S, Praglowski J, Nilsson L (1977) Atlas of airborne pollen grains and spores in Northern Europe. Natur Och Kultur, Stockholm
34. Pauli G, Peltre G, Bessot JC, Braun PA, David B (1984) Allergy to celery root coincident with mugwort sensitivity. J Allergy Clin Immunol 73:114
35. Soler M, Le Bouffant L, Charpin J (1982) Retention of pollen grains in the human lung. Allergy 37:373–376
36. Solomon WR, Burge HA, Muilemberf ML (1983) Antigen carriage by atmospheric aerosol. I. Ragweed pollen determinants in smaller micronic fractions. J Allergy Clin Immunol 72:443–447
37. Bousquet J, Cour P, Michel FB (in press) Pollen allergens are also found in submicronic soluble particles. Ann Allergy
38. Solomon WR, Mathews KP (1983) Aerobiology and inhalant allergens. In: Middleton E Jr, Reed CE, Ellis EF (eds) Allergy – Principles and Practice, 2nd edn. Mosby, St. Louis, pp 1143–1202
39. Stanley RG, Linskens HF (1975) Pollen, Biology, Biochemistry, Management. Springer, Berlin Heidelberg New York
40. Townley RG (1984) Allergic rhinitis and airway reactivity to mediators. In: Settipane GA (ed) Rhinitis. The New England and Regional Allergy Proceedings, Providence, Rhode Island, pp 75–85
41. Weber RW (1981) Cross reactivity among pollens. Ann Allergy 46:208–214
42. Wodehouse RP (1971) Hay fever plants, 2nd edn. Hafner, New York
43. Yan K, Salone C (1984) The response of the airways to nasal stimulation in asthmatic with rhinitis. Eur J Respir Dis 64 [Suppl 128]: 105–108
44. Déchamp C, Cour P, Bousquet J, Marsh DG (1986) Relationship between atmospheric level of *Amb a I* (AgE) and short ragweed pollen grains in Central France. J Allergy Clin Immunol 77:199

34.2 Mite Allergens

G. Pauli, J. C. Bessot

Mites represent the most important atmospheric allergen. In 1928, Dekker [13] was the first to notice the relationship between the onset of asthma in some patients and the occurrence of mites in house dust. Thirty-six years later, following the collaborative studies of Voorhorst et al [52], Spieksma et al [42] and Fain [15] the role of pyroglyphid mites, particularly those of the genus Dermatophagoides, was clearly established in the etiology of some respiratory allergic diseases.

34.2.1 Taxonomy

Mites are members of the Arthropoda subkingdom and of the Arachnida class. The order of Acarideae includes several families but three of them have a particular importance in respiratory allergic diseases: Pyroglyphidae, Acaridae or Tyroglyphidae and Glycyphagidae. Among the Pyrogliphidae, three species are widely spread in house dust: Dermatophagoides pteronyssinus (the most prevalent mite species in Europe; Fig. 34.9), Dermatophagoides farinae (species often proliferating in the USA and Japan) and Euroglyphus maynei (more often found in the mountains). Acarus siro and Tyrophagus putrescentiae are members of the Acaridae family whereas Lepidoglyphus destructor and Glycyphagus domesticus belong to the Glycyphagidae family.

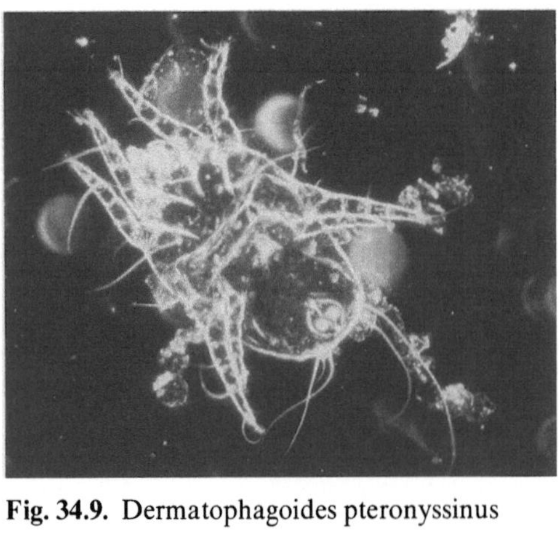

Fig. 34.9. Dermatophagoides pteronyssinus

34.2.2 Morphology

Adult pyroglyphid mites have a globular body with a joined abdomen and cephalothorax (idiosome) and four pairs of articulated legs bearing pili, claws or suckers. Their size ranges from 170 to 500 microns. The gnathosome is clearly visible and bears a mouth and annexes. The cuticle is smooth, striped or covered with small spicules. Female mites are usually bigger than males.

34.2.3 Biology and Ecology

The lifespan of adult mites ranges from 8 to 13 weeks. They mate once or twice in their life. The female mite lays about 20 to 50 eggs. Eggs change into larvae and successively into protonymph and tritonymph. This transformation lasts 20 to 26 days. Under unfavorable conditions, there is an intermediate development stage between proto- and tritonymph: hypope or deuteronymph.

House dust mites feed essentially on human or animal skin scales, or other keratinized debris (i.e., nails, dander, feathers). 250 mg of human skin scales are sufficient to feed several thousand mites for a period of three months, and a human adult sheds 70 to 140 mg of skin scales every day. Optimal growth conditions are a temperature of 25 °C at 80% relative humidity. These biological conditions explain why mattresses are the most favorable environment for the development and multiplication of mites. However, mites are also found in floor cracks, furniture or clothes. The mite life cycle fluctuates with the degree of hygrometry of the ambient air. In temperate zones, their number is maximal at the end of the summer or at the beginning of the autumn. Their number decreases during the winter due to a lowered humidity induced by heating. Climatic conditions in the mountains are not favorable for the growth of mites owing to dry, cold weather and ultraviolet radiations. The prevalence of mites in mountain house dust is lower [43, 50]. The characteristics of dwellings are of relevant importance and there is a close relationship between the hygrometric degree in a house and the number of house dust mites. Recent data have focused attention on the necessity to build houses correctly in order to reduce the relative indoor humidity.

The importance of storage mites in the etiology of respiratory allergy has certainly been underestimated [5, 11, 17]. They have common feeding properties since their essential nutriment comes from stored foods such as grain, flour, hay or straw. Their optimal growth conditions require higher temperatures than house dust mites (25–37 °C) and a relative humidity ranging from 80 to 100%. Main species are Acarus siro found in flour, certain cheese, whole grains, hay and animal litters. Lepidoglyphus destructor is mainly present in grain elevators; Tyrophagus putrescentiae, relevant in tropical areas and contaminates a large number of storage products rich in lipids and proteins even in temperate zones; Glycyphagus domesticus feeds on molds and animal or vegetal debris and is particularly resistant to variations of temperature and humidity. These species of storage mites can be found among house dust.

34.2.4 Allergens

Each mite species possess private allergens, but also share common allergens or epitopes with other mite species. Cross-reactive patterns between species follow their phylogeny. Recently developed immunochemical techniques (CIE, CLIE, CRIE) have shown that the antigenic properties of mites are a result of the combination of several distinct antigens. The immunization of rabbits with mites showed that more than 50 different antigens can be detected [21]. In humans, two major allergens have been isolated from Dermatophagoides pteronyssinus (Dpt). Chapman et al [9] have characterized antigen P_1, glycoprotein of a molecular weight of 24,000 daltons which was found to be identical to antigens Dp_{42} purified by Lind et al [24], Dp_7 [22] and Dp_{12} [45]. Allergen Dp_4 is another major allergen identified by Le Mao et al [22]. Table 34.1 indicates identical allergens identified by different groups from Dpt and Dermatophagoides farinae (Df). Other antigens of Dpt that were initially identified in animals may be minor allergens in humans [21]. A complete cross reactivity was demonstrated between two major allergens of Dpt and Df (Dp_1 and Df MB_7). Minor allergens may also be shared in common by different mite species: Antigen Dp MB_4, minor allergen of Dpt is also an

Table 34.1. Allergenic identity between major allergens from D. pteronyssinus and D. farinae

Major d. pteronyssinus allergens		Major d. farinae allergens
	Complete identity	
1 AG P_1 ou Dp_1 (Chapman and Platts-Mills) [9]	↔	1 Df_{11} (Le Mao et al) [22]
Dp_{42} (Lind et al) [24, 25]		Df MB_7 (Lind) [25]
Dp_{12} (Stewart) [45]		
Dp_7 (Le Mao et al) [22]		
2 Dp_4 (Le Mao et al) [22]		2 Df_6 (Le Mao et al) [22]
		Df MB_6 (Lind) [25]

allergen of Acarus siro, Lepidoglyphus destructor and Tyrophagus putrescentiae [25]. Other studies have confirmed the presence of common antigens in different mite species. There exists a common antigen between Df and Tyrophagus putrescentiae [3] and, in polymerized form, a Df allergen may be common to eight other mite species [12].

34.2.5 Demonstration of the Allergenic Role of Mites

Studies on the immunogenicity of mites have been performed in animals in whom precipitating antibodies have been initially measured by immunodiffusion techniques [1]. In humans, the allergenicity of mites was confirmed by in vivo and in vitro tests. Skin tests with Dpt extracts elicit typical reactions and their kinetics are compatible with an anaphylactic reaction. Bronchial provocation tests with Dpt extracts often induce immediate-type bronchial obstruction as well as nonimmediate reactions [4, 28]. Dpt-specific IgE was demonstrated in numerous investigations [6, 29, 44]. The levels of Dpt-specific IgE were found to vary with time in a given allergic subject [28] and a slow decline was observed in patients living for long periods in the mountains [50].

Mite-induced asthma, previously known as house dust-induced asthma, has some particular clinical features: asthma occurring at home, asthma or rhinitis attacks induced on some occasions by household activities, disappearance of asthma attacks in hospital, reappearance of attacks when the subjects return home after a temporary absence (i.e., holidays, climatic cure etc.) and renewed outbreak of attacks in one particular house. Mite-induced asthma persists all year round but may be seasonally worse. The symptom fluctuations reflect, with a certain time lapse, the variations in the relative humidity in homes; these variations being related to local, annual climatic conditions.

Mite allergens are borne in atmospheric particles present in suspension in the home environment [47]. Tovey et al [48] demonstrated that the amount of antigen P_1 was dependent on house activities. Antigen P_1 was mainly identified in mite feces, small particles having a mean size of 20 microns [48], in which the antigen P_1 concentration was very high (0.1 ng/particle). Swanson and Reed [46] have also confirmed the presence of Df allergens in suspension inside houses.

The effects of the control of the environment have been objectively measured in two recent studies [26, 33]. Murray and Ferguson [26] noted a significant improvement in the symptoms of ten children who each had a bedroom in which mite concentrations were low, when compared with the symptoms of ten asthmatic children who were left in their usual environment. As has been shown for other allergens, the nonspecific bronchial hyperreactivity (BHR) was decreased after prolonged mite eviction. Platts-Mills and co-workers demonstrated that nine Dpt-allergic asthmatics sleeping in mite-free rooms (in hospital) had a reduced BHR after several weeks. However, all studies investigating the respiratory benefits of mite eviction are not conclusive [7, 8, 37]. These discrepancies may be related to the difficulties of significantly eliminating mites.

34.2.6 Treatment of Mite Allergy

Preventive measures attempt to modify the ecological conditions that are favorable to the development and multiplication of pyroglyphid mites: regular cleaning of beds and houses and reduction of the relative indoor humidity. However, there is no general consensus on the efficiency of the former measures. For some authors [10, 18, 32, 35, 38], the number of mites was reduced after beds and/or other parts of the bedroom had been vacuumed, whereas others did not observe any difference [2, 7, 19, 49].

Other prophylactic measures attempt to reduce the relative indoor humidity and the house temperature. A relative humidity under 60% is the most efficient measure to reduce the proliferation of mites [20, 41, 49].

There is at present no chemical procedure that totally eradicates mites. As early as 1974, Leysen et al [23] showed that lindane was the only pesticide to destroy mites efficiently, however, owing to its toxicity it could not be used inside houses. A complex solution of balsam oils and different antiseptics (benzoic acid, salol, thymol, terpineol, phenyl alcohols etc.) used as a bactericidic agent was also found to be an efficient acaricide [32]. Another original method attempts to reduce some mold species that are an essential nutriment of mites [39] by means of fungicides such as natamycine [36]. However, the best prophylactic measure is probably a stay at high altitude. The efficacy of specific immunotherapy with mite extracts is variably appreciated. Some placebo-controlled studies have found a protective effect [14, 31, 34, 40]. Others did not disclose any benefit in treated patients [16, 27]. Owing to the perennial symptomatology of mite-induced asthma, the benefits of specific immunotherapy should be objectively evaluated by a prolonged follow-up of the patients by means of symptom-medication scores and serial pulmonary function tests, since these parameters cannot easily be compared with the allergenic content of the atmosphere.

It is now accepted that mites have a predominant, but not exclusive role in the allergenicity of house dust [30, 51]. Other allergens from animal (cat dander or hair, cockroaches etc.) or vegetal origin (molds etc.) can be responsible for the allergenic activity of house dust in one third of the patients. However, the discovery of the role of Dermatophagoides was a major clue in the understanding of house dust allergy.

References

1. Araujo-Fontaine A, Miltgen B, Mollet B, Pauli G, Rombourg H, Basset A (1974) Contribution à l'étude du rôle allergisant des acariens de la poussière: étude immunologique des sérums des malades et des sérums des lapins hyperimmunisés. Rev Fr Allergol 2:91–96
2. Arlian LG, Bernstein IL, Gallagher JS (1982) The prevalence of house dust mites, Dermatophagoides spp. and associated environmental conditions in homes in Ohio. J Allergy Clin Immunol 69, 6:527–532
3. Arlian LG, Geis DP, Vyszenski-Moher DL, Bernstein IL, Gallagher JS (1984) Cross antigenic and allergenic properties of the house dust mite Dermatophagoides farinae and the storage mite Tyrophagus putrescentiae. J Allergy Clin Immunol 74:172–179
4. Bachoffen H, Scherrer M, Trautlein F, Wyss F (1967) Ist das Hausstaubasthma ein Milbenasthma? Plethysmographische Untersuchungen vor und nach Asthmaprovokation mit Milbenextrakt. Dtsch Med Wochenschr 92:1597–1602
5. Blainey AD, Ollier S, Davies RJ (1983) Occupational respiratory disease in grain workers. Folia Allergol Immunol Clinica 30 [Suppl 115]
6. Bryant DH, Burns ME, Lazarus L (1975) The correlation between skin tests, bronchial provocation tests and the serum level of IgE specific for common allergens in patients with asthma. Clin Allergy 5:145–157
7. Burr ML, Dean BV, Merrett TG, Neale E, Leger AS, Verrier-Jones ER (1980) Effects of anti mite measures on children with mite sensitive asthma. A controlled trial. Thorax 35:506–512
8. Burr ML, Neale E, Dean BV, Verrier-Jones ER (1980) Effect of a change to mite-free bedding on children with mite-sensitive asthma: a controlled trial. Thorax 35:513–514
9. Chapman MD, Platts-Mills TAE (1980) Purification and characterization of the major allergen from Dermatophagoides pteronyssinus – antigen P1. J Immunol 125:587–592
10. Cunnington AM, Gregory PH (1968) Mites in bedroom air. Nature 217:1271–1272
11. Cuthbert OD, Brostoff J, Wraith DG, Brighton WD (1979) "Barn allergy": asthma and rhinitis due to storage mites. Clin Allergy 9:229–236
12. Dandeu JP, Rabillon J, David B (1984) Immunochemical and physicochemical studies of an allergenic glycoprotein present in nine different mite species. J Allergy Clin Immunol 73:119 (abstract)
13. Dekker H (1928) Asthma und Milben. MMW 75:515–516
14. d'Souza MF, Pepys J, Wells ID, Tai E, Palmer F, Overell BG, McGrath IT, Megson M (1973) Hyposensitization with Dermatophagoides pteronyssinus in house dust allergy: a controlled study of clinical and immunological effects. Clin Allergy 3:177
15. Fain A (1966) Allergies respiratoires produites par un acarien (Dermatophagoides pteronyssinus) vivant dans les poussières des habitations. Bull Mem Acad R Med Belg 6:479–500
16. Gaddie J, Skinner C, Palmer KNV (1976) Hyposensitization with house dust mite vaccine in bronchial asthma. Br Med J 2:561

17. Hillerdal G, Zetterström O, Johansson SGO, Engström B, Wiren A (1982) Mites living in hay: an important allergen source? Allergy 37:475–479
18. Hughes AM, Maunsell K (1973) A study of a population of house dust mite in its natural environment. Clin Allergy 3:127–131
19. Korsgaard J (1982) Preventive measures in house dust allergy. Am Rev Respir Dis 125: 80–84
20. Korsgaard J (1983) House dust mites and absolute indoor humidity. Allergy 38:85–92
21. Krilis S, Baldo BA, Basten A (1984) Antigens and allergens from the common house dust mite Dermatophagoides pteronyssinus. II. Identification of the major IgE-binding antigens by crossed radioimmunoelectrophoresis. J Allergy Clin Immunol 74:142–146
22. Le Mao J, Dandeu JP, Rabillon J, Lux M, David B (1983) Comparison of antigenic and allergenic composition of two partially purified extracts from Dermatophagoides farinae and Dermatophagoides pteronyssinus mite cultures. J Allergy Clin Immunol 71:588
23. Leysen MT, Reybrouck G, van de Voorde H (1974) Susceptibility of the house dust mite to pesticides and disinfectants. Acta Allergologica 29:455–461
24. Lind P, Korsgaard J, Löwenstein H (1979) Detection and quantitation of Dermatophagoides antigens in house dust by immunochemical techniques. Allergy 34:319
25. Lind P (1982) Identification of allergens in Dermatophagoides pteronyssinus and their identity to allergens in D. farinae. Allergy 37 [Suppl 1]:20 (abstract)
26. Murray AB, Ferguson AC (1983) Dust-free bedrooms in the treatment of asthmatic children with house dust or house dust mite allergy: a controlled trial. Pediatrics 71:418–422
27. Newton DAG, Maberley DJ, Wilson R (1978) House dust mite hyposensitization. Br J Dis Chest 72:21
28. Pauli G, Bessot JC, Guisard G, Roegel E, Oudet P (1972) Importance clinique des acariens chez les asthmatiques allergiques à la poussière domestique. Résultats des tests de provocation ventilatoire. Rev Fr Allergol 12:141–153
29. Pauli G, Bessot JC, Thierry R, Lamensans A (1977) Correlation between skin tests, inhalation tests and specific IgE in a study of 120 subjects allergic to house dust and Dermatophagoides pteronyssinus. Clin Allergy 7:337–346
30. Pauli G, Bessot JC, Hirth C, Thierry R (1979) Dissociation of house dust allergies. A comparison between skin tests, inhalation tests, specific IgE, and basophil histamine release measurements. J Allergy Clin Immunol 63:245
31. Pauli G, Bessot JC, Bigot H, Delaume G, Hordle DA, Hirth C, Thierry R (1984) Clinical and immunological evaluation of tyrosine-adsorbed Dermatophagoides pteronyssinus extract: a double-blind placebo-controlled trial. J Allergy Clin Immunol 74:524–535
32. Penaud A, Nourrit J, Timon-David P, Charpin J (1977) Results of a controlled trial of the acaricide Paragerm on Dermatophagoides spp. in dwelling houses. Clin Allergy 7:49–53
33. Platts-Mills TAE, Tovey ER, Mitchell EB, Moszoro H, Nock P, Wilkins SR (1982) Reduction of bronchial hyperreactivity during prolonged allergen avoidance. Lancet 25:675–678
34. Price JF, Warner JO, Hey EN, Turner MW, Soothill JF (1984) A controlled trial of hyposensitization with adsorbed tyrosine Dermatophagoides pteronyssinus antigen in childhood asthma: in vivo aspects. Clin Allergy 14:209–219
35. Rao VRM, Dean BV, Seaton A, Williams DA (1975) A comparison of mite populations in mattress dust from hospital and from private houses in Cardiff, Wales. Clin Allergy 5:209
36. de Saint-Georges-Gridelet D (1981) Mise au point d'une stratégie de contrôle de l'acarien des poussières (Dermatophagoides pteronyssinus) par utilisation d'un fongicide. Acta Oecologica Oecol Applic 2:117–126
37. Sarsfield JK, Gowland G, Toy R, Norman ALE (1974) Mite-sensitive asthma of childhood. Trial of avoidance measures. Arch Dis Child 49:716–721
38. Sesay HR, Dobson RM (1972) Studies on the mite fauna of house dust in Scotland with special reference to that of bedding. Acarologia 14:384–392
39. Sinha RN, Bronswijk JEMJ, Wallace HAH (1970) House dust allergy, mites and their fungal associations. Can Med Assoc J 103:300–301
40. Smith AP (1971) Hyposensitization with Dermatophagoides pteronyssinus antigen: trial in asthma induced house dust. Br Med J 4:204
41. Solomon ME (1961) Mites in houses, shops and other occupied buildings. The Sanitarian 69:291
42. Spieksma FTM, Spieksma-Boezeman MIA (1967) The mite fauna of house dust with particular reference to the house dust mite Dermatophagoides pteronyssinus (Trouessart, 1897) (Psoroptidae: sarcoptiformes). Acarologia 9:226–241

43. Spieksma FTM, Zuidema P, Leupen MJ (1970) High altitude and house dust mites. Br Med J 1:82–84
44. Stenius B, Wide L (1969) Reaginic antibody (IgE), skin and provocation tests to Dermatophagoides culinae and house dust in respiratory allergy. Lancet II:455–458
45. Stewart GA (1982) The isolation and characterization of the allergen Dpt 12 from Dermatophagoides pteronyssinus by chromatofocusing. Int Arch Allergy Appl Immunol 69:224–230
46. Swanson MC, Reed CE (1984) Quantitation and particle size distribution of indoor aeroallergens. J Allergy Clin Immunol 73:156 (abstract)
47. Tovey ER, Chapman MD, Platts-Mills TAE (1981) Mites faeces are the major source of house dust allergens. Nature 289:592
48. Tovey ER, Chapman MD, Wells CW, Platts-Mills TAE (1981) The distribution of dust mite allergen in the houses of patients with asthma. Am Rev Respir Dis 124:630–635
49. van Bronswijk JEMH (1984) Neues zur Ökologie der Wohnungsmilben. Allergologie 11:438–445
50. Vervloet D, Penaud A, Razzouk H, Senft M, Arnaud A, Boutin C, Charpin J (1982) Altitude and house dust mites. J Allergy Clin Immunol 69:290–296
51. Virchow CHR, Roth A, Moller E (1976) IgE antibodies to house dust, mite animal allergens, and moulds in house dust hypersensitivity. Clin Allergy 6:147
52. Voorhorst R, Spieksma-Boezeman MIA, Spieksma FTM (1964) Is a mite (Dermatophagoides spp.) the producer of the house dust allergen? Allergie und Asthma 10:329–334

34.3 Molds

M. Lopez, J. E. Salvaggio

The Eumycetes or true fungi, are members of the phylum Thallophyta, i.e., plants that lack definite roots, stems, or leaf structures. Most taxonomists, however, place them in a kingdom distinct from both plants and animals, although the presence of cell walls reflects a closer association with plants. Unlike algae, they do not contain chlorophyll. They may function as either obligate or facultative parasites, but are unable to synthesize their own food and depend on other organisms for nutrients.

It has long been established that fungal spores are present in the atmosphere in high concentration, considerably in excess of pollen grains. For example, Cladosporium spores can outnumber pollen grains by a ratio of 1,000 to 1. The sources of atmospheric fungal spores include, dying vegetation, leaves, stems, foliage, and branches of living plants as well as large macroscopic fungi such as the mushroom family.

The major classes of fungi that predominantly contribute to the airborne spore load and are considered important in allergy are discussed below (see also Table 34.2).

Table 34.2. Classification of Eumycetes

Phylum Thallophyta
Major classes that contribute to airborne spore load:

1. Phycomycetes
   - Rhizopus
   - Mucor
2. Ascomycetes
   - Saccharomycetaceae
     - Saccharomyces
   - Torulaceae
     - Rhodotorula
   - Chaetomiaceae
     - Chaetomium
3. Basidiomycetes
4. Fungi Imperfecti orders:
   1. Dematiaceae
      - Alternaria
      - Curvularia
      - Spondilocladium
      - Helminthosporium
      - Cladosporium
      - Stemphylium
      - Nigrospora
      - Pullularia
   2. Moniliaceae
      - Aspergillus
      - Botrytis
      - Gliocladium
      - Monilia
      - Mycogone
      - Penicillium
      - Paecilomyces
   3. Spaeriodiaceae
      - Phoma
   4. Tuberculariaceae
      - Fusarium

Class Phycomycetes

Of this class, the subclass Oomycetes is of little allergenic importance. A second subclass, the Zygomycetes, which includes the common sugar and bread molds and contains the important genera Rhizopus and Mucor, is clinically important. Many species of this class are prominent in soil, composts, and food residues.

Class Ascomycetes

Ascomycetes reproduce sexually by cytoplasmic fusion followed by formation of an ascus or sack in which sexual spores (ascospores) develop without any permanent wall attachment. They reproduce asexually forming conidia, either by budding, fragmentation or formation of special hyphae (Conidiophores). The black molds, yeasts, blue molds, and cup fungi are important groups of this class. Saccharomyces, a yeast, and Chaetomium are members among this class that are known to produce allergic respiratory symptoms in humans.

Class Basidiomycetes

These are the club fungi, so-called because after mycelial growth, a fruiting body is formed and club-shaped structures called basidia develop where basidiospores are produced. The Basidiomycetes reproduce asexually by means of conidia and fragmentation of hyphae. Sexual reproduction occurs by means of cytoplasmic fusion, formation of the fruiting bodies, and development of basidia. This class comprises many diverse forms, including puffballs, common rusts and smuts, mushrooms, and mirror yeasts. The great majority of Basidiomycetes, like most Ascomycetes, do not grow on common laboratory media. They feed on decaying organic matter and wood or exist as parasites of cereal grains, other plants, and trees. Abundant small, spiny smut teliospores and rust urediospores are often quite prominent in the atmosphere and may be discharged in bursts during times of high humidity. Although little is known about the relationship between basidiospores and asthma at present, they have recently been shown to be allergenic in humans and immunogenic in the rabbit [5]. Awareness of the potential importance of basidiospores as aeroallergens should become more apparent in the future, especially in view of their high atmospheric concentrations during the summer and fall months.

Class Deuteromycetes, or Fungi Imperfecti

This class is the largest and most diverse and contains most of the fungi allergenic for humans. In this class, sexual reproduction is extremely rare and the means of common asexual reproduction is by conidia. Their nutrition is either by parasitic means on plants and occasionally animals, or saprobic on decaying organic matter. Three orders are commonly distinguished: Spaeropsidales, of which the genus Phoma is a common allergenic mold; Melanoconiales, which contains important plant pathogens but no known human aeroallergens; and Moniales, which contains three families accounting for a large number of the fungi causing allergic respiratory disease in humans.

Atmospheric Concentration

The air spore content comes mainly from species highly adapted towards using wind energy for their dispersal. Wind dispersal of spores has three principle stages: (i) spore liberation, (ii) dispersion and (iii) deposition. The particular species and concentration represented in the air at a given time depends on temperature, degree of precipitation, prevailing winds, seasonal climatologic factors, circadian patterns of sunlight and darkness, availability of substrates, and degree of both substrate and atmospheric moisture. For example, the vegetative hyphae of most fungi grow best between 18° and 32 °C, whereas other thermotolerant fungi, such as several of the Aspergillus species, grow over a wide temperature range and certain thermophilic forms grow best between 65° and 75 °C. The growth and dispersal of some spores such as basidiospores is also markedly affected by atmospheric moisture. These spores are propelled into the atmosphere by a process dependent on the presence of free water, and they increase markedly in concentration during periods of rainfall and dampness. Conversely, spores of other fungi such as Cladosporium, Alternaria and Helminthosporium are blown free by wind and this type of *dry spore* increases in concentration with diminishing humidity and increased air flow. These species are often abundant during the midday period of maximal sunlight. Fungi also readily invade and propagate inside homes, and spores from these sources are often a source of perennial allergic symptoms. Areas of mold growth in the interior of homes are frequently noted, particularly growth of certain Deuteromycete species such as Penicillium and Aspergillus. Many specific interior areas are known to be prime sites for domestic mold growth. Among these are garbage containers, food storage areas, upholstery, wallpaper, areas of increased moisture such as shower curtains, window moldings, portable window units and damp basements. Emissions from cold mist vaporizers, in which high levels of fungal particles are present, have been implicated in production of asthma in mold-sensitive patients [10].

Sampling for airborne fungal spores is important for several reasons. It can establish airborne spore loads for different environments and it can aid in disease diagnosis since spore prevalence and composition may suggest the appropriate fungal extracts for skin testing and/or provocative inhalation challenge testing. Sampling may indirectly aid in the evaluation of the effectiveness of eliminating allergen sources, particularly with regard to indoor spore concentrations. The availability of data on spore counts may also allow correlation between airborne spore loads, climatologic variables, and sudden increases in asthma in particular geographic, occupational, or environmental settings. Such comparisons have been particularly useful in studying certain forms of epidemic asthma, such as New Orleans asthma [7–9].

Airborne surveys have been performed in many areas throughout the world. In a study by Gregory and Hirst [3] the mean spore concentrations between June and October was 125,000 spores/m^3. The most common spore type was Cladosporium, which accounted for 47% of the total; Basidiospores were the second most common with 31% and Alternaria amounted to 2% of the catch. In contrast, pollen made up 1% of the total count. Atmospheric mold counts in Canada by Collins-Williams and Beit [2] reported Alternaria, Cladosporium and yeasts as the most numerous molds, with a peak season between the middle of July and October. Basidiomycetes were quite prominent in July and August. In the United States several studies have shown that Cladosporium, Alternaria, and Basidiospores are the most common atmospheric spores [1, 4]. The indoor pattern of fungal spores, which is important to mold sensitive patients, reflects the outdoor spore composition plus an independent intrinsic fungal flora dominated by small spored deuteromycetes, including Penicillium, Aspergillus Rhizopus, Mucor and yeasts [11].

Seasonal Patterns

A defined *season* for molds often does not exist because of their universal presence in the atmosphere and their marked adaptability to environmental conditions. Outdoor levels range from peaks in late summer and fall to very low concentrations during periods of snow cover. In the Gulf South area of the USA, many ascospores and spores of the Fungi Imperfecti appear during the initial warming periods in early spring [8]. After this initial peak they persist throughout the summer months, often with a second peak during the fall months, followed by slight diminution during the cooler months of December and January. Basidiospores are also present throughout the year, with peaks during the humid, moist, late summer and early fall months. In the Great Lake areas, various ascospores appear during early spring and disappear by midsummer, whereas others persist throughout the growing season. Mold-sensitive patients have perennial symptoms often with exacerbations during the midsummer and fall season. In areas with cold winters significant relief of symptoms occurs after the first snowfall.

Clinical Relevance of Molds in Asthma

The role of fungi in asthma has long been considered established, based on anecdotal evidence. Although positive immediate and delayed skin reactivity is obtained with crude extracts of many fungal species, the clinical relevance of the reactivity is often uncertain. Since most atopic individuals demonstrate broad patterns of wheal and flare skin reactivity to multiple pollen, fungal, animal dander, and house dust allergens, the contribution of fungal allergens to the production of symptoms in any given patient is often difficult to assess. This is due to many factors, including 1) the choice and method of preparing fungal extracts for skin testing and provocative challenge which varies markedly among investigators; 2) the quality and potency of mold allergenic extracts is often poor and variable; 3) relatively few organisms have been studied in detail and many common fungi still need initial clinical evaluation and testing;

4) a single, well-defined, *mold season* usually does not occur, making it especially difficult to select a study population with unique seasonal mold allergy.

The following are the most commonly incriminated allergenic fungal species:

1. Cladosporium. The most widely distributed fungi, often reaching atmospheric concentrations up to 5,000 spores per m^3.
2. Alternaria. Known to be highly allergenic based on wheal and flare skin reactivity. A specific allergen (Alternaria 1) has been isolated and characterized.
3. Aspergillus. Widely distributed in outdoor as well as indoor environments. Aspergillus fumigatus is the etiologic agent of allergic bronchopulmonary aspergillosis.
4. Helminthosporium. Often gives rates of wheal and flare skin reactivity equal to those elicited by Alternaria.
5. Epicoccum. Prevalent in temperate regions, especially grassland and agricultural areas. In certain surveys it has been, along with Cladosporium and Alternaria, the most important source of spores isolated from the atmosphere.
6. Fusarium, Penicillium and Geotrichum.
7. Several of the Zygomycetes, such as Rhizopus and Mucor; these are often abundant in damp basement areas.
8. Several members of the Ascomycetes, airborne concentrations which often reach several thousand per m^3 of air.
9. Many of the Basidiomycetes, which are being found with increasing prevalence in the atmosphere in worldwide studies.

In general, since there is no clear mold season, the diagnosis of mold allergy is based on the identification of sensitivity by skin test, RAST and inhalation challenge [6].

References

1. Blatt H (1962) Microbiology of Allergy. Ann Allergy 20:263–281
2. Collins-Williams C, Beit CH (1955) Atmospheric mold counts in Toronto, Canada. J Allergy 26:468–470
3. Gregory P, Hirst J (1957) The summer airspora at Rothasmsted. J Gen Microbiol 17: 135–152
4. Long DL, Kranner CL (1972) Airspore of two contrasting ecological sites in Kansas. J Allergy 49:255–266
5. Lopez J, Salvaggio J, Butcher B (1976) Allergenicity and immunogenicity of basidiomycetes. J Allergy Clin Immunol 57:480
6. Salvaggio J, Aukrust L (1981) Mold induced asthma. J Allergy Clin Immunol 68:327–335
7. Salvaggio J, Hasselblad V, Seabury J et al (1970) New Orleans asthma. II. Relationship of climatologic and seasonal factors to outbreaks. J Allergy 45:257–265
8. Salvaggio J, Seabury J (1971) New Orleans asthma. IV. Semiquantitative airborne spore sampling, 1967 and 1968. J Allergy 48:82–105
9. Salvaggio J, Seabury J, Schoenhardt E (1971) New Orleans asthma. V. Relationship between Charity Hospital asthma admission rates, semiquantitative pollen, fungal spore counts and total particulate aerometric sampling data. J Allergy 48:96–114
10. Solomon W (1974) Fungus aerosols arising from cold-mist vaporizers. J Allergy Clin Immunol 54:222–228
11. Solomon WR (1976) A volumetric study of winter fungus prevalence in the air of midwestern homes. J Allergy 57:46–55

34.4 Allergy to Domestic Animals

B. Guérin, J. Bousquet

Man lives in close contact with animals either in occupational settings or in the home environment. Domestic animals are a principal source of perennial allergens. Immediately after the mites, cat or dog dander represent a major allergen of house dust [9, 10, 15, 28, 29].

Allergen standardization is especially important in animal allergy since major allergens of some species have been recognized and isolated, and the tissue origin of allergenic components has been isolated. The improvements made in the past 10 years have made it possible (i) to better diagnose animal-allergic patients, (ii) to propose efficient specific immunotherapy and (iii) to attempt to find preventive measures in occupational allergy to animals. Moreover, it has been widely shown that animal allergens do not only derive from danders or pelts. It seems, then, appropriate to use the term "allergy to animals".

34.4.1 Importance of Allergy to Animals

The high frequency of allergies to animals can be easily explained by the importance of the animal population in the west (Table 34.3). The sensitization of patients is greater when the contact with animals occurs early in life, since there is an increased susceptibility of infants to be sensitized [16].

Table 34.3. Domestic animal population in some western countries

Country	Dogs	Cats
USA	37	25
France	8	7
United Kingdom	5	4
Germany (FRG)	3	3.5
Italy	4	7
Benelux	2	2

The records of numbers (expressed in millions) or animals have been obtained from the animal food industry

The prevalence of allergy to animals is difficult to establish in the home environment. In a recent study it was observed that in school children 5.3% were asthmatic and the prevalence rate of animal allergy was as high as 57% with childhood asthma and 30% with rhinitis [17]. There is more significant professional allergy among animal handlers (Table 34.4). In the case of animals that are raised on farms it is more difficult to establish statistics. The incidence seems to be less, except in conditions of intensive animal raising. These conditions resemble those found in animal laboratories (i.e., chicken and turkeys) [21].

To summarize, allergy to domestic animals clearly forms distinguished entities, even though their clinical manifestations are similar. They comprise a true allergy in atopic subjects and a professional allergy found both in atopic and normal subjects, as though the illness had different genetic controls.

The sensitization of patients to animal proteins is usually accomplished in a few months (for small mammals such as guinea pigs), to a couple of years (for cat proteins) or, a few years (for dog allergens) as a mean. Rhinitis often appears earlier than asthma and represents a major warning [31]. The duration of sensitization varies with the intensity of the exposure to animal proteins and is dominated by the ecology i.e., the man-animal relationship.

34.4.2 Diversity and Multiplicity of Animal Allergen Sources

Allergenic materials from animals derive from a wide variety of tissues including the coat (cat fur [11] and dog hair), the squamae (danders), the entire skin, serum, urine, feces, saliva and sweat (Table 34.5). This long list includes badly defined raw materials some of which are similar to others such as squamae, epidermal debris and skin and this probably explains the frequent discussions between specialists on the relative importance and relationships of one or other allergens which are found in variable amounts in different locations. It also includes products that are essentially different, such as tissues, secretions and excrements, that perhaps may contain somatic antigens, but may also contain a mixture of somatic and metabolic antigens.

34.4.3 Allergy to Cats

Cat allergen 1 (cat 1) is considered to be the cat's major allergen [13, 25]. It is found in most tissues and organs of the cat that have been studied [1, 6, 14, 26]. Saliva, sweat and sebaceous glands are particularly rich in cat 1. It is composed of a glycoprotein with a molecular weight of about 35,000 daltons, without a doubt made from two subunits with a molecular weight of 1,000 daltons, not linked to sulfhydryl bounds occurring in the form of three isoallergens with a pH between 3.5 and 4.1 [1, 26]. Other cat allergens have been isolated, but albumin sensitizing more than 10% of all persons allergic to cat is the main one. This allergen cross-reacts with dog albumin (Table 34.5).

The elucidation of the allergens and their origin have made it possible to improve the quality of extracts used for both diagnosis [4] and treatment. It is therefore possible to perform specific immunotherapy efficiently [27].

34.4.4 Allergy to Dogs

Dog allergens are not yet totally known. Some, like albumin and immunoglobulins are derived from serum, but others are de-

Table 34.4. Prevalence of laboratory animal allergy in animal workers. [Adapted from 9]

	% symptoms due to LAA	% with asthma
Beeson et al [2]	22	5
Cockroft et al [7]	27	11
Davies and McCardle [8]	19	3
Gross [12]	15	7.5
Lutsky et al [21]	27	11
Dewdney [9]	22	4
Schumacher et al [32]	32	
Dewdney [9]	30	8

LAA = laboratory animal allergy

Table 34.5. Allergen sources from animals

	Epithelia	Serum	Urine	Saliva	Feces	Sweat	Cross-reactivities
Cat	+	+	+	+			Dog albumin, horse
Dog	+	+	?	+			Cat, dog
Mouse	+	+	+	?	?		Guinea pig (weak), rat
Rat	+	+	+	+	+		Mouse
Guinea pig	+	?	+	?	?		Mouse, horse (weak)
Horse	+	+	+			+	Cat, dog, cow, guinea pig
Cow	+	+	+	+			Goat

Cross-reactivities are indicated in this table, but only some of the allergens of a given species cross-react with some allergens of another species indicating that cross-reactivities are not mandatory but only possible among different species

Table 34.6. Clinical and immunological features of laboratory animal allergy. [Adapted from 9]

	Asthma	Conjunctivitis, rhinitis	Contact urticaria	Dermatoses
Association with atopy	Strong	Weak	Variable	Weak
Prick tests	Positive	+ or –	+ or – ?	Usually –
Specific IgE (RAST)	Positive	+ or –	+ or –	Usually –
Irritative activity	Moderate to important	Usually strong	Weak	Strong

rived from salivary origin [19, 22, 34]. The specificities between the breed that are considered by some authors to be important [20] seem to Wuttrich et al and Brant and Yman [5, 38] to be of minor importance, although quantitative differences may be present [3].

34.4.5 Allergy to Laboratory Animals

Allergens derived from small mammals such as rats, mice, guinea pigs or rabbits have been extensively studied in the past years. In rats, Longbottom and Walls [18, 35, 36] studied the origin of allergenic proteins. It appears that the proteinuric urine of male rats and, to a lesser extent, of female rats [18, 23, 36] is a major source of allergenic materials. A prealbumin and an α-2 euglobulin were found to be the major allergens of urine. However, fur, danders, saliva, feces and rat serum are also allergenic [35, 36]. Rat albumin is another allergen present in some of these materials. Rat bedding and diet do not appear to be a major allergen source. Cross-reactive proteins between rat and other small mammals are not important [18]. Proteins derived from other small mammals are less well characterized, but urine appears to be of major importance [23, 32, 33] as well as serum [37].

Laboratory animals can cause asthma by their allergenic proteins and by eliciting a nonspecific bronchial hyperreactivity, since the atmosphere of the room is highly irritative [24]. However, many asthmatic patients have a positive skin test and specific IgE antibodies against animal proteins (Table 34.6).

The diagnosis of laboratory animal allergy has greatly improved with allergen standardization. Since male animals are more allergenic than females it is possible to reduce the sensitization of exposed individuals and the symptoms of allergic subjects. It is now possible to quantitate the amount of rat allergens present in rat rooms and by efficient ventilation to reduce the allergen content of the atmosphere. These methods may, in the future, be very useful to decrease the prevalence of occupational allergy to animals.

34.4.6 Other Mammals

Horses are often highly allergenic. More than 15 allergens have been identified, but the major ones are found in serum (albumin), urine, sweat and danders [19]. Crossed allergenicity was observed between cat, dog, guinea pig and horse albumin.

Numerous allergens have been characterized from cows [30] but none of them seems to be a major allergen. Cow's milk allergic patients can usually eat cow's meat since β-lactoglobulin, the major cow's milk allergen is not found in cow's meat.

Recent knowledge on animal allergens represents one of the major advances in allergology in the past ten years. Although removal of animals has long been considered the only ethical therapeutic procedure, at least for domestic-type allergies, a better characterization of allergenic materials derived from animals has made it possible to achieve efficient immunotherapy or to better understand preventive measures.

References

1. Anderson MC, Baer H (1981) Allergenically active components of cat allergen extracts. J Immunol 127:972–975
2. Beeson MF, Dewdney JM, Edwards RG, Lee D, Orr RG (1983) Prevalence and diagnosis of laboratory animal allergy. Clin Allergy 13:433–442
3. Blands J, Lowenstein H, Weeke B (1977) Characterization of extract of dog hair and dandruff from six different dog breeds by quantitative immunoelectrophoresis. Identification of allergens by crossed radioimmunoelectrophoresis (CRIE). Acta Allergologica 32:147–169
4. Bousquet J, Guérin B, Michel FB (in press) Allergie aux animaux. Rev Fr Mal Respir
5. Brandt R, Yman L (1980) Dog dander allergens. Int Arch Allergy Appl Immunol 61:361–370
6. Brown PR, Leitermann K, Ohman JL (1984) Distribution of cat allergen 1 in cat tissues and fluids. Int Arch Allergy Appl Immunol 74:67–70
7. Cockroft A, Edwards J, McCarthy P, Andersson N (1981) Allergy in laboratory animal workers. Lancet I:827–830
8. Davies GE, McCardle LA (1981) Allergy to laboratory animals: a survey by questionnaire. Int Arch Allergy Appl Immunol 64:302–307
9. Dewdney JM (1981) Allergy induced by exposure to animals. J R Soc Med 74:928–932
10. Dewdney JM (1984) Animals in the aetiology of asthma. J R Soc Med 77:629–631
11. Didierlaurent A, Foglietti MJ, Guérin B, Hewitt BE, Percheron F (1984) Comparative study on cat allergens from fur and saliva. Int Arch Allergy Appl Immunol 73:27–31
12. Gross NJ (1980) Allergy to laboratory animals: epidemiologic, clinical and physiologic aspects, and a trial of cromolyn and its management. J Allergy Clin Immunol 66:158–165
13. Guérin B, Hewitt B (1981) A comparative study of allergen extracts from cat fur, cat pelt and cat saliva. Ann Allergy 46:127–131
14. Guérin B, Hewitt B (1981) The effect of commonly used extracting media on the allergenic composition of cat fur extract. Ann Allergy 47:166–170
15. Guérin B, Hewitt B, Wüthrich B (1981) Poussière de Maison. Activité corrélée de trois types d'extraits de poussière par rapport aux extraits d'acariens, fourrure de chat et squames humaines. Rev Fr Allergol 21:217–220
16. Haahtela T, Heiskala M, Suoniemi I (1980) Allergic disorders and immediate skin test reactivity in Finnish adolescents. Allergy 35:433–441
17. Kjellman B, Pettersson R (1983) The problem of furred pets in childhood atopic disease. Allergy 38:65–73
18. Longbottom JL (1983) Characterization of allergies from the urines of experimental animals. In: Kerr JW, Ganderton MA (eds) Proceedings of the XIth International Congress of Allergology and Clinical Immunology. Macmillan, London, pp 525–529
19. Lowenstein H (1983) Domestic animal allergens. In: Kerr JW, Ganderton MA (eds) Proceedings of the XIth Congress of Allergology and Clinical Immunology. Macmillan, London, pp 543–548
20. Lutsky I, Fink JN, Arkins JA, Hoffman F, Morouse M (1980) Skin test reactivity to dog-derived antigens. Clin Allergy 10:331–340
21. Lutsky I, Teichtahl H, Bar-Sela S (1984) Occupational asthma due to poultry mites. J Allergy Clin Immunol 73:56–60
22. Moore LS, Hyde JS (1980) Blood-specific dog hypersensitivity in humans. J Allergy Clin Immunol 66:198–203
23. Newman Taylor AJ, Longbottom JL, Pepys J (1977) Respiratory allergy to urine proteins of rats and mice. Lancet II:847–849
24. Newman Taylor AJ, Myers JR, Longbottom JL, Spackman D, Slovak AJM (1981) Immunological differences between asthma and other allergic reactions in laboratory animal workers. Thorax 36:229
25. Ohman JL Jr (1983) Human allergic responses to the domestic cat. In: Kerr JW, Ganderton MA (eds) Proceedings of the XIth Congress of Allergology and Clinical Immunology. Macmillan, London, pp 453–458
26. Ohman JL, Baer H, Anderson MC, Leiterman K, Brown P (1983) Surface washes of living cats: an improved method of obtaining clinically relevant allergen. J Allergy Clin Immunol 72:288–293
27. Ohman JL Jr, Findlay SR, Leiterman KM (1984) Immunotherapy in cat-induced asthma. Double-blind trial with evaluation of in vivo and in vitro responses. J Allergy Clin Immunol 74:230–239
28. Panel of Review of Allergenic Extracts (1981) Bureau of Biologics, Food and Drug Administration, Bethesda
29. Pauli C, Bessot JC, Hirth C, Thierry R (1979) Dissociation of house dust allergies. A comparison between skin tests, inhalation tests, specific IgE and basophil histamine release measurements. J Allergy Clin Immunol 63:245–252

30. Prahl P, Sondergaard I (1982) Allergen content in aqueous and hydrophobic extracts from cow hair and dander. Allergy 37:279–283
31. Rudolph R (1983) Frequency of animal sensitization. In: Kerr JW, Ganderton MA (eds) Proceedings of the XIth International Congress of Allergology and Clinical Immunology. Macmillan, London, pp 438–444
32. Schumacher MJ, Tait BD, Holmes MC (1981) Allergy to murine antigens in a biological research institute. J Allergy Clin Immunol 68:310–318
33. Siraganian RP, Sandberg AL (1979) Characterization of mouse allergens. J Allergy Clin Immunol 63:435–442
34. Viander M, Valovirta E, Vanto T, Koivikko A (1983) Cross-reactivity of cat and dog allergen extracts. RAST-inhibition studies with special reference to the allergenic activity in saliva and urine. Int Arch Allergy Appl Immunol 71:252–260
35. Walls AF, Longbottom JL (1983) Quantitative immunoelectrophoretic analysis of rat allergen extracts. I. Characterisation of fur, urine, saliva and other rat-derived materials. Allergy 38:419–431
36. Walls AF, Longbottom JL (1985) Comparison of rat fur, urine, saliva, and other rat allergen extracts by skin testing, RAST and RAST inhibition. J Allergy Clin Immunol 75:242–251
37. Wahn U, Peters T, Siraganian RP (1983) Studies on the allergenic significance and structure of rat serum albumin. J Immunol 125:1244
38. Wüthrich B, Guérin B, Hewitt B (in press) Cross-allergenicity between extracts of hair from different dog breeds and cat hair. Clin Allergy

35. Agricultural Asthma

J. Bousquet, A. Vergnenègre

Asthma is a common disease both in urban and rural areas and agricultural activities represent an important source of occupational asthma. However, the definitions of rural and agricultural are of relevant importance before the examination of agricultural asthma (Table 35.1).

Table 35.1. Definitions of rural and agricultural asthma

Rural asthma: Asthma found in persons living in the country, stationed or employed in country districts.
Agricultural asthma: Occupational asthma found in persons working in agriculture, or in the food processing industry.
Rural asthma includes agricultural asthma

Occupational asthma was first reported in the eighteenth century by Ramazzini who noted attacks of dyspnea upon the inhalation of organic dusts in sifters and millers, thus describing the first cases of agricultural asthma. However, among occupational causes of allergy or asthma, those occurring in agricultural settings or in food processing industries are usually less well recognized than others for many reasons. 1) Polluted urban areas are considered to be major environments favoring the onset of allergic diseases, whereas the rural environment appears to be less allergenic. Pollution certainly increases the incidence of chronic obstructive lung diseases and nonallergic asthma, but there is no definite data showing that it increases the prevalence of allergy. On the other hand, people living in rural areas are exposed to a wide variety of allergenic and irritative substances present in greater amounts than in the cities. Some are found in both environments (i.e., pollens, molds) but others are strictly related to agriculture. 2) Rural and agricultural allergens are usually poorly defined even though they affect a large number of exposed individuals. Conversely, allergy to some small molecular weight components affects a smaller number of subjects, but has been extensively investigated since it represents a useful model to investigate mechanisms underlying allergy. 3) Working conditions often differ between agricultural settings and industrial settings. In the former, in many parts of the world, individuals work alone or in small groups and often do not report their disorders since they may lose working days that are essential to their income. 4) Finally, the financial power of industry is much greater than that of agriculture and unions have more influence in industry. Moreover, occupational diseases lead to absenteeism. These combined influences have resulted in the recognition of occupational diseases better and more efficiently in industry than in agriculture. Accordingly, more efforts have been made in an attempt to prevent occupational diseases in the former environment.

Some other difficulties are encountered in the recognition of agricultural asthma. Agricultural development has led to the introduction of increasing numbers of new potentially asthmogenic materials, many of them being used both in industry and agriculture. Moreover, there are considerable differences and allergenic potentialities between modern and industrialized agriculture found in many, but not all developed countries, and antique and traditional agriculture often present in developing countries.

35.1 Prevalence

The prevalence of asthma or respiratory allergy is always difficult to determine and this is especially true for the rural or the agricultural environment. However, comparisons between rural and urban areas have shown that respiratory disorders are more frequent in the former as well as mortality due to respiratory causes. In some studies of occupational asthma 72% of the cases were observed in agricultural settings. The incidence of asthma in some well-known agricultural environments varies widely but it is accepted that 20 to 30% of bakers develop symptoms related to the flour they inhale. The incidence of byssinosis varies widely according to the type of cotton used and the preventive measures applied in the cotton industry. In developed countries it ranges between 20 and 80%, but is significantly lower (15 to 25%) in air-conditioned factories [92]. On the other hand, in some Egyptian villages almost all the workers are affected.

35.2 Pathophysiological Mechanisms

The pathogenesis of most forms of agricultural asthma is still speculative since a large percentage of workers are exposed to many harmful materials and those working outdoors are also faced with nonspecific factors, such as pollution, sun, rain etc. leading to the association of many mechanisms [18].

Immunological mechanisms have been widely studied and IgE-mediated allergic reactions rank first among the possible causes of agricultural asthma. Patients can be sensitized either by agriculture-specific allergens, i.e., animal danders, insect debris, grain, storage mites, vegetal matter, or occupational materials not restricted to agriculture such as small molecular weight haptens (antibiotics, plastic compounds, tropolone) and allergens that are not specific to occupational diseases, i.e., pollens and molds. However, as a rule in allergy, only a variable fraction of subjects developing an IgE immune response will present symptoms. Short-term sensitizing antibodies may be involved in agricultural asthma but their demonstration is not yet complete. Other types of immunological reactions are less common in agricultural asthma but many subjects can have both asthma and alveolitis because the same inhalant can lead to the generation of precipitins and IgE antibodies or, more frequently, because the inhalation of various materials can elicit different immune responses. This is the case of many dairy farmers in France who are often allergic to animal danders or storage mites (IgE-mediated asthma) and to Thermoactinomycetes (extrinsic alveolitis). The nonspecific activation of the complement cascade does not seem to be important in asthma but may be a relevant mechanism in extrinsic alveolitis.

Nonimmunological mechanisms are often involved either alone or in combination with allergic reactions. High concentrations of irritant gases and vapors or dusts can lead to nonspecific bronchial hyperreactivity or to more severe damage of the bronchi or alveoli. These irritative mechanisms are often of relevant importance in agriculture since in many small-sized farms there is no protection for the workers. Some substances are capable of directly activating mast cells, as is the case for cotton, [12] or have more complex pharmacological mechanisms such as a partial β-blockage or anticholinesterase activity by isocyanates. Finally, the autonomic nervous system can be modified by some chemicals (pesticides) which elicit asthma [72].

Immunological and nonimmunological properties of inhaled materials cannot explain totally the onset, the course and the outcome of agricultural asthma. Most offending compounds elicit bronchial inflammation leading to nonspecific bronchial hyperreactivity in nonatopic subjects or aggravate it in atopics. In the model of western red cedar it was observed [48] that most subjects presenting occupational asthma had a nonspecific bronchial hyperreactivity. When they were removed from the risk the sensitivity of the bronchi could return to baseline values when asthma was not too severe. On the other hand, in most severe and some mild asthmatics, the nonspecific bronchial hyperreactivity was unchanged after removal from work and in some instances eventually, gradually increased. In some severe asthmatics these mechanisms induced severe chronic bronchitis.

Many factors can modulate the onset and course of agricultural asthma. Atopic patients are more prone to develop an IgE-mediated allergy. Smoking increases significantly the onset and severity of chronic bronchitis. The duration of exposure, type of inhaled particles and association of risk factors (extrinsic and intrinsic) are also of relevant importance.

35.3 Causes of Agricultural Asthma

35.3.1 Mites

House dust mites and agricultur-specific mites (Table 35.2) can sensitize subjects. In many parts of the world, farm houses favor house dust mite growth more than urban dwellings because they are often more humid, older and built with traditional materials. Mite species vary according to the country.

Farmers can be affected by agricultural mites which are often found in stored grain or hay [1, 27, 36, 39, 62], in cheese [61], among animal danders and feathers [54, 55] or parasiting crops [58]. They are highly allergenic and many workers, especially atopics, are affected. In a recent Finnish study [83] it was shown that asthma among dairy farmers is more often due to storage mites than to cow's dander.

35.3.2 Animal Allergens

Mammals: Dog and cat dander allergy is not restricted to the urban environment and some allergens and irritants are almost exclusively found in agricultural settings (Table 35.3). Allergens of mammal origin are found in many tissues varying with different species. Pelt, saliva, urine, serum and eventually feces often contain allergens. Allergens of many species have been individualized and found in some instances to be cross-reactive. This explains why some patients allergic to a specific animal immediately develop asthma when exposed for the first time to another animal. These findings should also be taken into consideration when allergic workers are relocated.

Cow allergens usually derive from saliva, serum and urine [71]. Their physicochemical structure is partially elucidated. The incidence of asthma in exposed subjects varies with the type of farming; being relatively lower in industrialized farms than in traditional ones. Allergy to cow should not

Table 35.2. Allergenic mites

	House dust	Grain	Other origins
Pyroglyphid mites			
Dermatophagoides pteronyssinus	< 2000 m		
Dermatophagoides farinae	< 2000 m		
Euroglyphus longior, manei	+ to + + +[a]		
Leptidoglyphus destructor	+	+ + +	
Glycyphagus domesticus	+	+ + +	
Nonpyroglyphid mites			
Acarus siro		+ + +	Cheese
Acarus farris		+ + +	
Tyrophagus putrescentiae		+ + +	
Tarsonemus floricus	+	+ +	
Cheyletys erudicus		+	
Tydeus sp.		+	
Aleurobius farinae			Cheese
Chortoglyphus sp.		+	
Panonychus ulmi			Apple trees, vineyards
Ornithonyssus sylvarium			Poultry
Tyrophagus siro, putrescentiae			Cheese

[a] Prevalence of E. manei over 2000 m and in very damp and hot areas

Table 35.3. Origin of allergens derived from animal sources and cross-reactivities

	Serum albumin	Other serum proteins	Urine	Feces	Danders	Saliva	Cross-reactivities
Cat	+	+	+		?	Cat 1	Dog, cow, horse
Dog	+	+			?	+	Cat, horse
Cow		Ig, +	+		?	+	Goat, horse
Horse	+	+	+		?		Cow, cat, dog, guinea pig
Laboratory animals		+	+ + +	+	?	+	

be confused with immediate-type hypersensitivity towards other allergenic substances inhaled by farmers.

Sheep wool does not appear to be highly allergenic but many species of mites including *Dermatophagoides spp.* may colonize it.

Pig urine was found to be allergenic [37] but in another study it was observed that many pig farmers developed asthmatic attacks in barns due to a high content of irritants, rather than to an allergic reaction [43, 57].

Horse dander and serum are highly potent allergens but the incidence of horse allergy in developed countries is changing since most allergic patients are veterinary surgeons and riders. In developing countries horses are still largely used in agriculture. Cross-reactive antigens with ponies and donkeys have been observed. Moreover, horse dander is usually contaminated by mites [52], molds [16, 35] and bacteria that may also be allergenic.

Rabbits and small mammals are potent allergens through highly proteinuric urine of male animals and their danders. Rabbits, bred on many farms, and other small mammals can be allergenic either, directly, in the course of breeding as laboratory animals [49] or, indirectly, since they may contaminate storehouses and grains. Rat bites can cause anaphylaxis.

Birds: Birds are potent sensitizers but they usually cause a type III extrinsic alveolitis by their droppings. They are more rarely involved in IgE-mediated asthma by their feathers, poultry mites, other poultry allergens or substances used in poultry farming [4, 8, 54, 55, 78].

Insects: Insect debris is allergenic but only when it is present in large amounts. In some damp and hot areas such as the Midwest of the United States, the prevalence of allergy to cockroach antigens was found to be greater than that to ragweed. Many other species of Lepidoptera are also allergenic. These insects are found in house dust but seem to be predominant in low income areas and in rural dwellings, especially in developing countries.

Other insects are more related to agriculture. Antigenic substances from the silkworm moth cause IgE-mediated asthma in sericulture. Locusts, crickets, moths are widely used in laboratories to test the efficiency of various pesticides and insecticides. They are often involved in IgE-mediated asthma that is more common in atopic subjects [45]. Other insects are parasites of vine and were found in some cases to be allergenic [cochenial and endemis: 56, personal data].

Crustaceans: Crustaceans are known to elicit food allergy in some atopic individuals. However, they are also involved in occupational allergy (i.e., crab processing industry [19], preparation of dried daphnies or allergy to sea squirt body fluids in workers gathering oysters and pearls).

Fish: Fish antigens are sensitizers not only when they are eaten but also through inhalation in a fish processing factory [personal data]. Moreover, fish guano is widely used as a fertilizer and may cause asthma by poorly defined mechanisms.

Beekeeping: Beekeepers represent a high allergic risk group [14] and many of them

Table 35.4. Molds of allergenic importance found in agriculture

Fungi Imperfecti	*Alternaria*	Extremely common saprophyte frequently found in grain, tomatoes, potatoes, hay, colza; allergenically related to *Stemphylium & Phoma*
	Aspergillus	More than 300 species widely spread; frequently found in grain and hay
	Fusarium	Common soil fungus often found among tomatoes, cotton, banana, melon, celery, cabbagge, pea and barley (brewery)
	Epicoccum	Present in fruits and corn
	Stemphylium	Tomatoes, fruits and vegetables
	Trichoderma	Most widespread soil fungus; commonly found on fallen timber and paper; tulip bulbs frequently contaminated
Ascomycetes	*Chaetomium*	Textile and mushroom cultures
	Didymella	Abundant in some parts of the world in barley and wheat
Hyphomycetes	*Botrytis*	Parasite on a wide variety of plants and on soft fruits; under moist conditions, bean, lettuce, tomatoes, onions and strawberries; parasite of vineyards
	Paecilomyces	Wood trimmer's disease; humidifier's disease
	Penicillium	Most common fungus, saprophytic on decaying vegetation, or agent of decomposition on grains and many foods including citrus and blue cheese making
Phycomycetes	*Mucor*	"Sugar fungus" often present in canned foods especially if it contains glucides, i.e., fruit juice, jam and in cheese making
	Rhizopus	Closely related botanically to *Mucor* it is most important during storage, transfer and marketing of corn, peanuts, cherry, strawberries, sweet potatoes, peaches etc.
Basidiomycetes	*Ustilago*	"Smuts" present on grasses and grains

develop anaphylactic symptoms when stung by honey bees or vespids. However, they may also develop asthma upon the inhalation of bee hive's dust.

35.3.3 Molds

Mold spores are allergenic and lead to an IgE-mediated asthma. Due to their small size they can reach the deep lung and cause a type III extrinsic alveolitis or can grow in the bronchial wall leading to a destructive pulmonary disease such as bronchopulmonary aspergillosis. It appears that mold-induced asthma is equally prevalent in both urban or rural environments whereas extrinsic alveolitis is more frequently found in rural areas owing to agricultural distribution [62, 74] (Table 35.4).

Indoor mold spores: Farmhouses are usually more humid than urban dwellings and crops may be stored in the farmhouse or used as food.

Mold growth on crops: The presence of fungi as saprobes and/or parasites on vegetation has been well documented. Spore dispersion is affected by climatologic conditions when the crops are not yet harvested or by the relative indoor humidity when crops are stored [77]. The species of molds parasitizing crops is directly related to the type of crop [3]. Most of these species are found in significant amounts in the atmosphere in many locations throughout the world.

Grain molds are among the major agricultural molds (Table 35.5). They grow either on plants in the fields or on grain when it is stored [21, 22, 29, 30, 38, 53, 84]. Atmospheric molds are often found in huge amounts but the species and quantities of molds vary widely with the area, weather

Table 35.5. The microflora of grain dust. (From Lacey, J.: Academic Press, New York 1983)

Wheat	*Aspergillus glaucus* *Penicillium chrysogenum* *Penicillium oxalicum* *Mucor racemosus* *Rhizopus nigricans*
Barley	*Aspergillus fumigatus* *Aspergillus repens* *Aspergillus glucus* *Aspergillus flavus* *Penicillium chrysogenum* *Penicillium oxalicum* *Mucor racemosus* *Mucor sp.* *Rhizopus sp.*
Oat	*Aspergillus flavus* *Penicillium nigricans* *Penicillium oxalicum* *Mucor sp.* *Rhizopus nigricans*

conditions and season of year. *Cladosporium* is often found after the crop has been harvested, *Aspergillus* and *Actinomycetes* during storage. However, some molds are specifically related to certain occupations: *Verticilium necanii, Nocladium album, Paecilomyces farinosus* and *basilosporus* are commonly released during reaping and *Septoria nodatum* during threshing [28]. These molds can cause asthma in patients working in a large variety of occupations not always related to agriculture. They can sensitize farmers, subjects working in grain elevators or those, such as bakers, who use grains during their work.

Molds often contaminate woods and leaves. Wood cutting exposes a person to *Cladosporium, Epicoccum, Stemphylium, Botrytis, Chaetomium* and *Fusarium* found on leaves or to *Penicillium glaucum* and *candium* present near the roots of trees.

Fruits and vegetables are also a common source of molds [77] (Table 35.4). *Botrytis* is a common vine mold and can lead to occupational allergy [15, Bourgeois, unpublished data].

Molds used in the food processing industry: Many mold species are used to process cheese. *Penicillium* is widely used in the making of different blue cheeses and an IgE-mediated allergy has been described in Roquefort cheese makers [Bousquet et al, unpublished results]. Other species are used to process other cheeses and found to causa asthma (i.e., *Endothia parasitica*).

Yeasts are widely used in the food processing industry and allergy to *Saccharomyces cerevisiae* or *minor* is not uncommon. *Candida tropicalis* was shown to sensitize subjects preparing alimentary proteins from oil [23]. *Paecilomyces varioti,* used to prepare animal feed was shown to cause an IgE-mediated allergy in many workers [63].

Basidiospores: Some superior fungi are grown in semi-industrial plants and occupational allergy to spores of *Pleurotus* or other superior fungi is well-known to cause asthma or extrinsic allergic alveolitis [46, 51, 64, 81, 91].

35.3.4 Compounds Derived from Other Vegetal Matter

Many products deriving from vegetal matter are allergenic or elicit asthma through irritant and/or pharmacologic mechanisms either directly or indirectly by their contaminants.

Grain, flour and cereals: Grain flour is highly allergenic and used as food for animals or by bakers [5, 6, 29, 87]. Grain allergens have been widely studied and it was observed that most cereals have cross-reacting antigens and that some grass pollens also share common allergens with cereals [6]. These cross-reactive patterns explain some associations (Table 35.6). However, grain may also induce nonspecific bronchial hyperreactivity [60] or non-IgE-mediated immune mechanisms [65].

Moreover, grains are contaminated by insects (*Ephestia,* flies, mosquitos), flour parasites (*Climex lectuaris*), molds, grain weevils or storage mites.

Occupational allergy to pollen grains: Individuals living in rural areas are more exposed to common anemophilous pollens than those living in urban zones. In addition, some entomophilous or amphiphilous pollens can be allergenic. Occupational diseases have been described with sunflower

Table 35.6. Relationships between the common cereals and preparations used in manufacturing. [From 6]

Subfamily	Tribe	Genus and species	Common name
Festucoideae	Triticeae	*Triticum aestivum*	Wheat bread
		Triticum durum	Durum wheat
		Tricosecale Wittmark	Triticale
		Secale cereale	Rye cereal
		Hordeum distichon	Barley
	Festuceae	*Lolium sp.*	Rye grass
	Aveneae	*Avena sativa*	Oat
		Phleum pratense	Timothy grass
Oryzeae	Oryzeae	*Oriza sativa*	Rice
Panicoideae	Tripsaceae	*Zea mays*	Maize (corn)
	Andropogonaleae	*Sorghum bicolor*	Sorghum
		Sorghum halepense	Johnson grass

Usually closely botanically related species are cross-reactive whereas more distantly related species are less cross-reactive; Gramineae family

Table 35.7. Main wood dust eliciting asthma

Common names	Genus and species	Causative chemical substance
Gymnospermae		
Californian red wood	*Sequioa sempervirens*	
Western red cedar	*Thuja plicata*	Plicatic acid (tropolone)
Arbor vitae	*Thuja standishi*	Tropolone
Deodar	*Cedrus lebani*	
Angiospermae		
Iroko	*Chlorophora exselsa*	Chlorophorine (oxystilbene)
Knysma boxwood	*Gonomi kamassi*	Puebrachamine (?) (alcaloid)
Obeche	*Triphochiton scleroxylans*	
Central American walnut	*Juglans nigra*	Xanthoquinone
Ramin	*Gonystylis bancanus*	
Teak	*Tectora grandis*	
Okume	*Ancoumea klaineana*	
Munigna	*Pterocarpus indicus*	Pterostilbene
Oak(s)	*Quercus sp.*	
Mahogany	*Khaya swietenia*	Anthrolecol (?)
Cocobolo	*Dalbergia retusa*	Quinone
African zebrawood	*Microberlinia brazzavillensis*	
Soapbark	*Quillaja saponaria*	Quillaine (saponin)
Amiengre	*Tanganyika amingre*	

[13], strawberry, freezia, paprika [86], pear [82] or colza pollens [24].

Wood dust: Toxic woods are usually involved in contact dermatitis or as irritants inducing ENT symptoms. However, true asthma is not uncommon and can be due to several possible mechanisms (Table 35.7) [11, 17, 20, 38, 40, 41, 44, 69, 79, 88, 89]: direct irritative mechanism of wood dust on hyperreactive airways; irritation or pharmacological effects of quinons, tropolons, alcaloids or tannins; IgE-mediated allergy by wood antigens and haptens such as plicatic acid in western red cedar asthma (in wood dust asthma such allergic mechanisms are not very common); and irritative or allergenic effects of contaminants present in natural processed woods such as formaldehyde, isocyanates, anhydrides, dyes, glues, preservatives, resins, molds etc.

Cotton: Reversible airways obstruction has been shown to be a characteristic finding of early byssinosis. Symptoms such as cough, dyspnea and chest tightness often occur on the first day of the work week [12] and subside as the week continues. As the disease progresses, respiratory symptoms get worse and persist throughout the week. At a later stage of the disease, both obstructive and restrictive lung function abnormalities are observed, the more common pattern being obstructive [76].

The underlying mechanisms of byssinosis are still poorly understood and the natural constituents of the cotton plant or contaminants have been implicated. Immune mechanisms have been widely sought but only recently specific IgE against cotton dust and contaminating molds have been detected in patients suffering from byssinosis [66]. Extracts from cotton bracts are able to elicit a bronchoconstrictive response when inhaled by normal individuals, demonstrating a direct effect of cotton dust. This effect may be related to the histamine releasing activity of cotton dust or to its content in vasoactive amines. Finally, cotton dust contains a large amount of bacterial toxins that were shown to induce bronchoconstriction in humans [75].

Beans, oilseeds: Oilseeds, especially castor beans [3, 50], are highly allergenic and often cause asthma or other allergic reactions in subjects who come in direct contact with the allergic risk and in indirect contact, such as those living in the vicinity of a castor bean factory or the family members of subjects handling such allergens. The risk of sensitization is so high that castor bean is no longer used as food for animals in many countries.

Green coffee beans are also allergenic [67] and irritative leading to many asthmatic reactions in exposed individuals. One of the allergens present in coffee beans may be identical to some major components of castor beans [50].

Miscellaneous plant matters: Many other plant matters have been incriminated in asthma, acting either as an allergen or by means of other mechanisms. These include garlic dust [25, 31], tobacco leaves but not tobacco smoke [34], coriander [80], paprika dust [86], tea dust [85] or alfalfa flour [26]. Most of these agents induce asthma among farmers or in food processing and tobacco industries.

35.3.5 Chemicals

The list of chemicals used in agriculture is increasing in number and many can elicit asthma by all possible mechanisms.

Chemicals specifically used in agriculture: Farmers use a vast number of pesticides, insecticides, fungicides and chemically produced fertilizers [42, 56, 59, 62] that can act as an allergen or elicit pharmacological and neurological mechanisms such as the anticholinesterase activity of organophosphorus compounds [10, 73]. Other important chemicals involved are pyrethrins used in the disinfection of stables or hen houses. Pentachlorophenol is used as a wood preservative and in potato farming. Wine growers use a series of harmful chemicals among which $CuSO_4$ was recognized to induce asthma or extrinsic allergic alveolitis with a relatively high incidence. However, most harmful chemicals are not, at present, recognized as asthma inducers.

Chemicals not restricted to agriculture: Many small molecular weight chemicals used in industry were shown to cause agricultural asthma [7, 32]. Isocyanates and derivatives, plastic constituants, polyvinylchloride are among those most often involved.

Dyes and preservatives are universally employed in the food processing industry. Although the vast majority of asthmatic reactions are due to an idiosyncratic mechanism it has been shown [2] that dyes can mount an IgE-mediated immune response.

35.3.6 Foods for Animals

The list of foods used in agriculture that induce asthma is extensive. However some are more frequently involved.

Poultry farmers [90]: Grain flour is one of the major foods used to feed poultry. It appears that farmers who prepare their own grain-based foods develop more frequently an IgE-mediated hypersensitivity than those using industrially prepared ones, since the amount of grain dust inhaled is far greater during grain processing [Bousquet et al, unpublished data]. Amprolium chloride is a food preservative eliciting asthma.

Dairy farmers: Many foods used to feed cattle are highly allergenic and certain foods have been forbidden in some countries (i.e., castor bean-derived foods). Allergenic foods include grain flour [62], soybean [47], lactoserum [63], fish guanos and peanut seed.

Fish breeding: Daphnies (Crustaceae) used to feed fish are allergenic [62].

Additives and drugs used in foods: Antibiotics [62, 68] such as β-lactams (other than penicillin) that have been withdrawn, macrolides and tetracyclins are the most common antibiotics mixed with foods and can sensitize many farmers or veterinary surgeons.

Anthelmintics prepared from piperazine [70] can cause asthma through the nonspecific activation of mast cells and its cholinergic properties. Asthma in susceptible individuals appears rapidly and its course is usually severe. Anticoccidians based on amprolium chloride or nitrofurane, whose allergenic component is furfurol, are also asthma elicitors.

35.3.7 Other Compounds

Enzymes: Proteolytic or glycolytic enzymes are used in the food processing industry [9, 33]. Papain and pineapple bromelin are chiefly used while *Bacillus subtilis* protease or flaviostase are only occasionally used.

References

1. Aghan M, Gnanasakthy A (1981) A cluster analysis of the effects of storage mites as allergens in relation to certain occupations and living conditions. Clin Allergy 11:499–504
2. Alanko K, Keskinen H, Bjorskten F, Oganen S (1978) Immediate type hypersensitivity to reactive dyes. Clin Allergy 8:25–31
3. Amma MKP, Dani H, Sareen K (1977) Inflammatory response of *Ricinus communis* meal allergen. Indian J Exp Biol 15:277–279
4. Andersen P, Schonheyder H (1984) Antibodies to hen and duck antigens in poultry workers. Clin Allergy 14:421–428
5. Baldo BA, Krilis S, Wrigley W (1980) Hypersensitivity to inhaled flour allergens. Allergy 35:45–56
6. Baldo B, Sutton R, Wrigley C (1982) Grass allergens with particular reference to cereals. Prog Allergy 30:1–66
7. Bardana EJ, Anderson CJ, Andrasch RM (1980) Meatwrapper's asthma: clinical and pathogenic observations. In: Frazier CA (ed) Occupational asthma. Van Nostrand Reinhold, New York, pp 14–32
8. Bar Sela S, Teichtahl H, Lutsky I (1984) Occupational asthma in poultry workers. J Allergy Clin Immunol 73:271–275
9. Baur X, Fruhmann G (1979) Papain induced asthma: diagnosis by skin test, RAST and bronchial provocation test. Clin Allergy 9:75–82
10. Becker FL, Koza FP, Sigman M (1978) Organophosphorus inhibition of lysosomal enzyme secretion from polymorphonuclear leucocytes. Evidence of a lack of a requirement for esterase activation. Immunology 35:373–379
11. Belin L (1980) Clinical and immunological data on wood trimmer's disease in Sweden. Eur J Respir Dis 61 [Suppl 107]: 169–176
12. Bouhuys A, Wolfson RL, Hozner DW, Brain JB (1969) Byssinosis in cotton textile workers. Ann Intern Med 71:257–269
13. Bousquet J, Dhivert J, Clauzel AM, Hewitt B, Michel FB (1985) Occupational allergy to sunflower pollen. J Allergy Clin Immunol 75:70–74
14. Bousquet J, Ménardo JL, Michel FB (1982) Allergy in beekeepers. Allergol Immunopathol 10:395–398
15. Brégevin B (1974) Les allergènes de la vigne et du vin. Ouest Med 27:1649–1656
16. Burge HA, Solomon WR, Williams P (1979) Fungus exposure risks associated with animal care units. J Allergy Clin Immunol 64:29–31
17. Bush RK, Yunginger JW, Reed CE (1978) Asthma due to African Zebrawood (*Microberlinia*) dust. Am Rev Respir Dis 177:601–603
18. Butcher BT (1980) Approaches to the understanding of mechanisms in occupational

asthma. Eur J Respir Dis 61 [Suppl 107]: 183–191
19. Cartier A, Lafrance M, Dineau L, Dubois JY, Malo JL, Forest F (1983) Occupational asthma in crab processing workers. J Allergy Clin Immunol 71:159–165
20. Chan-Yeung M, Abbound R (1976) Occupational asthma due to California redwood (*Sequioa sempervirens*) dusts. Am Rev Respir Dis 114:1027–1033
21. Chan-Yeung M, Ashley MJ, Grzybowski S (1978) Grain dust and lungs. Can Med Assoc J 118:1271–1274
22. Chan-Yeung M, Schulzer M, MacLean L, Dormen E, Grzybowski S (1980) Epidemiologic health survey of grain elevator workers in British Columbia. Am Rev Respir Dis 121:329–338
23. Cornillon J, Touraine JL, Bernard JP, Le Sterlin P, Touraine R (1976) Manifestations asthmatiques chez des ouvriers préparant des protéines alimentaires dérivées du pétrole. Rev Fr Allergol 16:7–23
24. Couturier P, Coste P, Mallea M, Soler M (1977) Allergie aux pollens de colza. A propos de 2 observations dans la même fratrie. Rev Fr Allergol 17:51–52
25. Couturier P, Bousquet J (1982) Occupational allergy to inhalation of garlic dust. J Allergy Clin Immunol 70:145
26. Couturier P, Héritier JA, Marinier R (1984) Allergie immédiate à la farine de luzerne. Un nouvel allergène du milieu rural et de l'industrie agro-alimentaire. Rev Fr Allergol 24:157–159
27. Cuthbert OD (1981) The incidence and causative factors of atopic asthma and rhinitis in an Orkney farming community. Clin Allergy 11:217–225
28. Darke CS, Knowelden J, Lacey J, Milfordward A (1976) Respiratory disease of workers harvesting grain. Thorax 31:294–302
29. Dopico GA, Reddan W, Flaherty D, Tsiatis A, Peters ME, Rao P, Rankin J (1977) Respiratory abnormalities among grain handlers. A clinical physiological and immunological study. Am Rev Respir Dis 115:915–922
30. Dosman JA, Cotton DJ (1980) Occupational pulmonary disease: focus on grain dust and health, vol. 1. Academic Press, New York
31. Falleroni AE, Zeiss R, Levitz D (1981) Occupational asthma secondary to inhalation of garlic dust. J Allergy Clin Immunol 68:156–160
32. Fawcett IW (1980) Asthma caused by fumes from Pine Resin and Epoxy Resin systems. In: Frazier CA (ed) Occupational Asthma. Van Nostrand Reinhold, New York, pp 283–295
33. Flindt MLH (1978) Respiratory hazards from papain. Lancet I:430–432
34. Gleich GJ, Welsh PW, Yunginger JW, Hyatt RE, Catlett JB (1980) Allergy to tobacco: an occupational hazard. N Engl J Med 302:617–619
35. Gravesen S, Lowenstein H, Weeke B (1978) Demonstration, isolation and identification of culturable microfungi and bacteria in horse hair and dandruff. Immunochemical comparison with allergenic components. Allergy 33:89–92
36. Green WF, Woolcock AJ (1978) *Tyrophagus putrescentiae:* an allergenically important mite. Clin Allergy 8:135–144
37. Harries HG, Cromwell O (1982) Occupational asthma caused by allergy to pig's urine. Br Med J 284:867
38. Hendrick DJ, Butcher BT, Connolly MJ (1984) Occupational asthma due to allergens of organic origin. Clin Immunol Allergy 4:37–54
39. Hillerdal G, Zetterström O, Johansson SGO, Engström B, Wiren A (1982) Mites living in hay: an important allergen source. Allergy 37:475–479
40. Hinojosa M, Moneo I, Dominguez J, Delgado E, Losada E, Alcover R (1984) Asthma caused by African Maple (*Triplochiton scleroxylon*) wood dust. J Allergy Clin Immunol 74:782–786
41. Howie AD, Boyd G, Moran F (1976) Pulmonary hypersensitivity to rainim (*Gomystylus baucanus*). Thorax 31:585–587
42. Kahn E (1976) Pesticide related illness in California farm workers. J Occup Med 18:683–693
43. Karr RM, Lehrer SB, Butcher BT, Salvaggio JE (1978) Coffee worker's asthma, a clinical appraisal using the radio-allergo sorbent test. J Allergy Clin Immunol 62:143–148
44. Greenberg M (1972) Respiratory symptoms following brief exposure to Cedar of Lebanon (*Cedra lebani*) dust. Clin Allergy 2:219–225
45. Kino T, Oshima S (1980) Allergy to insects in Japan: The reaginic sensitivity to silkworm moth in patients with bronchial asthma. J Allergy Clin Immunol 64:131–138
46. Kondo O (1969) A case of *Cortinellus shutake* spore asthma. Jpn J Allergy 18:81
47. Kuissu S, Lenz D, Bessot JC, Pauli G (1980) Rhinite allergique professionnelle par exposition à la poudre de soja. Rev Fr Allergol 2:75–77
48. Lam S, Tan F, Chan H, Chan-Yeung M (1983) Relationship between types of asthmatic reaction, non specific bronchial reactivity and specific IgE antibodies in patients with red cedar asthma. J Allergy Clin Immunol 72:134–139

49. Lee D, Edwards RG, Beeson MF, Dewdney JM (1982) Development and use of radio-immuno-assays for the detection of human IgG antibodies to laboratory animal urinary proteins. Int Arch Allergy Appl Immunol 69:363–367
50. Lehrer SB, Taylor J, Salvaggio JE (1981) Castor bean allergens: evidence for distinct heat labile and stable entities. Int Arch Allergy Appl Immunol 65:69–75
51. Lopez M, Salvaggio JE, Butcher B (1976) Allergenicity and immunogenicity of Basidiomycetes. J Allergy Clin Immunol 57:480–488
52. Lowenstein H (1978) Characterization and chemical modification of isolated allergens from horse hair and dandruff. Int Arch Allergy Appl Immunol 57:349–357
53. Lunn JA, Hughes DTD (1967) Pulmonary hypersensitivity to the grain weevil. Br J Ind Med 24:158–161
54. Lutsky I, Bar Sela S (1982) Northern fowl mite (*Ornithonyssus sylviarium*) in occupational asthma of poultry workers. Lancet II:874–945
55. Lutsky I, Teichal H, Bar Sela S (1984) Occupational asthma to poultry mites. J Allergy Clin Immunol 73:56–60
56. Mallet JR, Boroas J, Enjalbert M, Teisier J, Freour P (1975) Allergies rencontrées chez les viticulteurs. Bordeaux Med 8:815–820
57. Matson SC, Swanson MC, Reed CE, Yunginger JW (1983) IgE and IgG immune mechanisms do not mediate occupation related respiratory or systemic symptoms in hog farmers. J Allergy Clin Immunol 72:299–304
58. Michel FB, Guin JJ, Seignalet C, Rambier A, Marty JC, Caula F, Laveil G (1977) Allergie à *Panonychus ulmi*. Rev Fr Allergol 17:93–97
59. Miller M (1982) Pesticide poisoning. JNE 8:288–294
60. Mink JT, Gerrard JW, Cockcroft DW, Cotton DJ, Dosman JA (1980) Increased bronchial reactivity to inhaled histamine in non smoking grain workers with normal lung function. Chest 77:28–31
61. Molina C, Tourreau A, Aïache JM, Brun J, Jeanneret A, Roche A (1977) Manifestations allergiques chez les fromagers: étude clinique épidémiologique et immunologique. Rev Fr Allergol 17:235–245
62. Molina C, Cheminat JC (1980) Allergies en milieu rural. In: Charpin J (ed) Allergologie. Flammarion, Paris, pp 678–689
63. Moneret-Vautrin DA, Pupil P, Courtine D, Grilliat JP (1984) Asthme professionnel aux protéines du lactosérum. Rev Fr Allergol 24:93–95
64. Noster U, Schulz KH, Hausen BM (1978) Immunofluorescence test in the diagnosis of mushroom worker's lung. Dtsch Med Wochenschr 103:655–657
65. Olenchock SA (1979) Immunological studies of grain dust. J Environ Pathol Toxicol 2:9–22
66. O'Neil CE, Reed MA, Aukrust L, Butcher BT (1983) Studies on the antigenic composition of aqueous cotton dust extracts. Int Arch Allergy Appl Immunol 72:294–298
67. Osterman K, Zetterström O, Johansson GO (1982) Coffee worker's allergy. Allergy 37:313–322
68. Paggario PL, Loi AM, Toma G (1979) Bronchial asthma and dermatitis due to spiramycine in a chick breeder. Clin Allergy 9:571–574
69. Paggario PL, Cantalupi R, Filieri M, Loi AM, Parlanti A, Toma G, Bashieri L (1981) Bronchial asthma due to inhaled wood dust: *Tanganyika Amingre.* Clin Allergy 11:605–610
70. Pepys J, Pickering CAC, Loudon HWG (1972) Asthma due to inhaled chemical agents – piperazine hydrochloride. Clin Allergy 2:189–196
71. Prahl P, Nexo E (1982) Human serum IgE against two major allergens from cow hair and dander. Allergy 37:49–54
72. Quigley C, Fuller RW, Dixon CMS, Barnes PJ (1985) Inhaled acetylcholinesterase inhibitors cause dose-related bronchoconstriction in asthmatic and normal subjects. Am Rev Respir Dis 131:A283
73. Raghuprasad PK, Brooks SM, Litwin A, Commander JJE, Berstein IL, Gallagher J (1980) Quillaja bark (soapbark) induced asthma. J Allergy Clin Immunol 65:285–287
74. Roby R, Sneller MR (1979) Incidence of fungal spores at the homes of allergic patients in an agricultural community. Correlation of skin tests with mold frequency. Ann Allergy 43:286–288
75. Rylander R (1981) Bacterial toxins and etiology of byssinosis. Chest 79 [Suppl]:345–375
76. Schacter EN, Maunder LR, Beck GJ (1984) The pattern of lung function abnormalities in cotton textile workers. Am Rev Respir Dis 129:523–527
77. Sneller MR (1984) Mould allergy and climate conditions. In: Al Doory Y, Domson JF (eds) Mould allergy. Lea and Febiger, Philadelphia, pp 244–266
78. So SY, Lam K, Yu D (1981) Colophony induced asthma in a poultry vender. Clin Allergy 11:395–399
79. Sosman AJ (1982) Wood dust asthma. In: Kerr JW, Ganderton MA (eds) The proceed-

ings of the XIth International Congress of Allergology and Clinical Immunology. Macmillan, Oxford, pp 419–421
80. Suhonen R, Keskinen H, Bjorksten F, Vaheri E, Zitting A (1979) Allergy to coriander: a case report. Allergy 34:327–330
81. Symington IS, Kerr JW, MacLean DA (1981) Type I allergy in mushroom soup processors. Clin Allergy 11:43–49
82. Teranishi H, Kasuya M, Aoshima K, Kato T, Ikarashi T (1980) An epidemiological survey of pollinosis among pear farmers. Sangyo Igaku: 465–470
83. Terho EO, Husman K, Vohlonen I, Rautalahti M, Tukiainen H (1985) Allergy to storages mites or cow dander as a cause of rhinitis among Finnish dairy farmer. Allergy 40:23–26
84. Tse KS, Craven N, Cherniack RM (1980) Allergy to saprophytic fungi in grain workers. In: Dosman JA, Cotton DJ (eds) Occupational Pulmonary Disease: focus on grain dust and health. Academic Press, New York, pp 335–347
85. Uragoda CG (1980) Respiratory disease in tea workers in Sri Lanka. Thorax 35:114–117
86. van Toorenenbergen AW, Dieges PH (1984) Occupational allergy in horticulture: demonstration of immediate type allergic reactivity to Freesia and paprika plants. Int Arch Allergy Appl Immunol 75:44–47
87. Warren CPW (1977) Lung disease in farmers. Can Med Assoc J 116:391–394
88. Wilhemsson B, Jernudd Y, Ripe E, Holmberg K (1984) Nasal hypersensitivity in wood furniture workers. An allergological and immunological investigation with special reference to mould and wood. Allergy 39:586–595
89. Woods B, Calnan CN (1976) Toxic woods. Br J Dermatol 95 [Suppl 13]: 1–97
90. Wuthe H, Bergmann K, Vogel J (1981) Frequency of lung function disturbancy and immunological status of industrial poultry workers. Eur J Respir Dis 113 [Suppl 62]: 38–39
91. Yin, Kaisheng, Wang, Kaiping, Yang, Zu, Zhang (1983) Allergy caused by inhaling *Pleurotus* spores. Clin J Tuberc Respir Dis 6:142–145
92. Zuskin E, Valic F, Kanceljak B (1981) Immunological and respiratory changes in coffee workers. Thorax 36:9–13

36. Investigation of Occupational Asthma due to Low Molecular Weight Agents

J.-L. Malo, A. Cartier

High molecular weight, mainly proteinic, materials derived from animal or plant constituants have, for a long time, been recognized in the etiology of occupational asthma (OA). Ramazzini [1] studied such an occupational hazard in grain handlers and provided the first description of OA. The development of new synthetic materials of low molecular weight in the chemical and pharmaceutical industries has been responsible for the onset of numerous types of OA. The first report of OA due to such a synthetic low molecular weight product, namely toluene diisocyanate, is attributed to Fuchs and Valade [2].

36.1 Etiologic Agents

In Table 36.1 are listed some etiologic low molecular weight agents with the occupations and possible mechanisms reported to be responsible for OA. This list is not exhaustive as new agents are constantly being described.

Although the relative importance of each agent may vary by country (viz., occupational asthma in British Columbia, Canada, due to western red cedar), isocyanates are by far the most common agents inducing OA in industrial countries, as they are incorporated in numerous products (paints, plastics, foams, molds). Although toluene diisocyanate was the type most frequently used in the past, other isocyanates (hexamethylene diisocyanate – HDI, diphenylmethane diisocyanate – MDI, naphthalene diisocyanate – NDI, polyphenyl isocyanate, papa-iso) are now more commonly used, although more than one type of isocyanates can be found in the work place. Also, it is known that isocyanates cause cross-reactive bronchial reactions in many instances [3, 4].

36.2 Mechanisms

Immunological mechanisms have been elicited for some of the products. For example, increased levels of specific IgE antibodies have been detected in subjects with occupational asthma to red cedar [5], tetrachlorophthalic anhydride [6] and azo dyes [7]. Although specific IgE [8, 9] and IgG [10, 11] antibodies have been identified in a few cases of OA due to isocyanates, this does not seem to be the mechanism involved in other individuals [12]. It has also been postulated that isocyanates can cause asthma by blocking β-adrenoreceptor activity [13].

36.3 Investigation

A summary of the proposed investigation of OA is shown in Table 36.2.

36.3.1 Questionnaire

The typical symptomatic presentation of OA is that exhibited by a subject whose asthma is present only at work and improves on weekends and holidays. However, this classical pattern may be absent for several reasons. It is to be remembered that asthmatic subjects may complain only of coughing [14]. The presence of a so-called late asthmatic reaction can mean that the asthma may be present after the end of a workshift and even several days and nights after a single exposure to the responsible agent [15, 16]. This is linked with the increase in nonallergic bronchial hyperexcitability following exposure to the agents [4, 17]. Finally, after prolonged exposure, asthma can persist and remain severe even after a subject is removed from his working environment [18–20]. Any subject with asthma should thus be questioned

Table 36.1. Occupational asthma due to low molecular weight agents

Products	Specific agents	Occupations	Mechanisms[a]	References
Acids derived from wood dust	Plicatic acid (red cedar)	Carpenters, wood workers	Specific antibodies, complement activation	[30, 31, 5]
	Abietic and primaric acids (colophony)	Electronic workers	Unknown	[30, 31]
	Other woods	Wood workers	Unknown	[30, 31]
Anhydrides	Phthalic, trimellitic hexahydrophthalic	Epoxy resin handlers, plastic workers, meat wrappers (PVC)	Specific antibodies	[30, 31, 6]
Antibiotics and drugs	Ampicillin, penicillin, spiramycin, metamucil	Pharmaceutical employees, hospital staff	Unknown	[30, 31]
Dyes	Various	Chemical workers	Specific antibodies	[7]
	Carmine	Chemical workers, cosmetic handlers	Unknown	[32]
Isocyanates	Toluene diisocyanate (TDI), diphenylmethane diisocyanate (MDI), hexamethylene diisocyanate (HDI), others	Painters, plastic, foam and mold producers	Specific antibodies, β-adrenoreceptor blockers	[30, 31]
Metal salts	Platinum	Platinum refiners	Specific antibodies	[30, 31]
	Nickel	Metal platers	Specific antibodies	[30, 31, 33]
	Chromium	Chrome platers	Unknown	[30, 31]
Others	Aminoethylethanolamine	Solderers (fluxes)	Unknown	[30, 31]
	Formalin	Various	Unknown	[30, 31]
	Persulfates	Beauty parlor operators	Unknown	[30, 31]

[a] Mechanism elicited in some but not every individual

Table 36.2. Investigation of occupational asthma

- History
- Working environment
- Skin tests (routine; specific products)
- Blood sample (WBC; serum stored)

Subject still at work	*Subject no longer at work*
• FEV_1–FVC	• FEV_1–FVC
• Response to bronchodilator	• Response to bronchodilator
• PC_{20} (if $FEV_1 > 1.5$ l)	• PC_{20} (if $FEV_1 > 1.5$ l)
PEFR monitoring	PEFR monitoring
PC_{20} at the end of working period	PC_{20}
Removal from work	Return to work
PEFR monitoring	PEFR monitoring
PC_{20} at the end of period off work	PC_{20} at the end of working period
Specific inhalation challenges	*Specific inhalation challenges*

FEV_1 = forced expiratory volume in one second; FVC = forced vital capacity; PC_{20} = concentration of histamine/methacholine causing a 20% fall in FEV_1; PEFR = peak expiratory flow rate; WBC = white blood count

about his present and past working environment.

A thorough investigation of the list of products in the working environment should be obtained. This is complicated by the fact that employers and employees are often not aware of the exact nature of the product present at work. Also, products are referred to as brand names or code numbers. Only a patient and thorough enquiry will reveal the nature of the products. Finally, one will have problems in convincing industrial hygienists that the amount of a product is not of critical importance in the enquiry. One should persuade them that tiny amounts of an agent may elicit significant reactions in sensitized individuals and that so-called threshold limit values (TLV) are not usually relevant.

36.3.2 Skin Tests

Whereas atopic history and the presence of one or more positive immediate skin reactions may predispose to OA, most of the cases of OA due to low molecular weight products will occur in nonatopic individuals. Assessment of these individuals with skin tests to a routine battery of common inhaled allergens is thus of limited use. Skin tests with the majority of low molecular weight products, except in the case of platinum salts, nickel and antibiotics, cannot be performed due to nonspecific irritation.

36.3.3 White Blood Count and Immunological Tests

As mentioned above, even if specific antibodies have been demonstrated in some individuals with OA to certain low molecular weight agents, these antibodies are not always present and may be present in some asymptomatic exposed individuals. Finally, coupling of the product to a matrix for antibody determination is often complex and the test is only available in specialized centers. Determination of significant eosinophilia may orient towards an asthmatic problem at work as opposed to nonspecific chronic obstructive lung diseases.

36.3.4 Spirometry and Airway Excitability

Documentation of airway obstruction with partial or complete reversibility after the administration of a bronchodilator may suggest asthma. Even without such a documentation, demonstration of airway hyperresponsiveness to nonallergic agents (histamine, acetylcholine derivatives, exer-

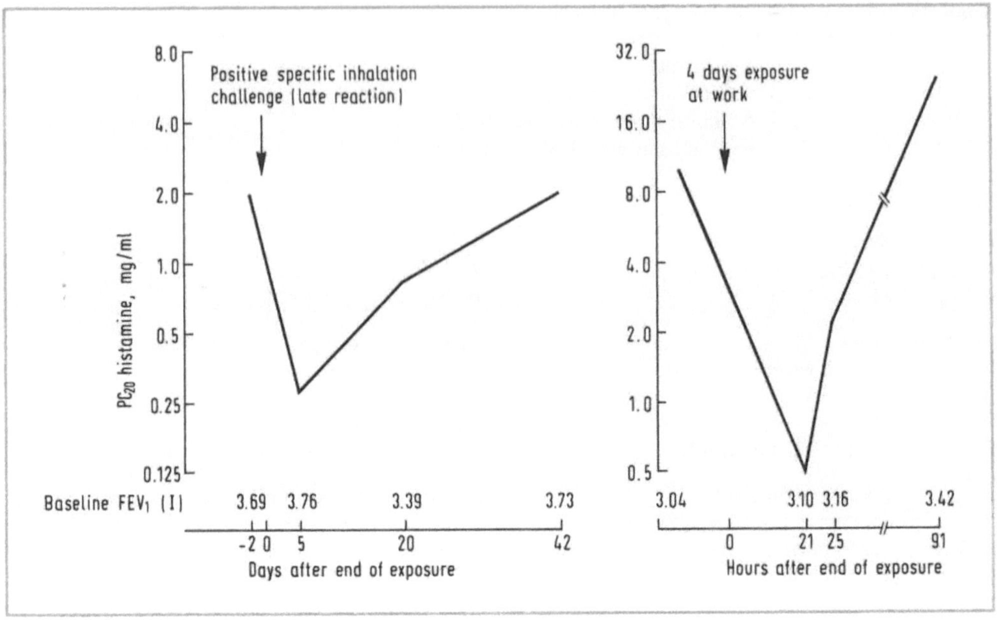

Fig. 36.1. *Left panel:* slow return of PC_{20} histamine (see text for definition) on the ordinate to the prespecific inhalation challenge result 42 days (abscissa) after end of exposure. *Right panel:* rapid return of PC_{20} results to baseline value 91 hours after the exposure. Baseline FEV_1 at the time of each histamine inhalation test is shown

cise, cold air) can orient towards an asthmatic problem. Indeed, most subjects with OA will show increased bronchial responsiveness even if they are removed from work for months and even years [18–20]. Persistence of bronchial hyperexcitability for weeks after a single exposure to a sensitizing agent has been documented (Fig. 36.1, left panel). However, in few circumstances, increased bronchial excitability can last for hours only and can disappear within one or two days after the end of exposure (Fig. 36.1, right panel).

36.3.5 Serial Functional Assessments of Airway Obstruction and Hyperexcitability

As asthma is a fluctuating condition, documentation of OA can be made by serial assessments of peak expiratory flow rates (PEFR). This is now possible as simple, inexpensive and reliable devices are available [21]. The results of such a monitoring in the investigation of OA were originally described by Burge and colleagues [22, 23]. There is a good correlation (specificity and sensitivity) between the results of PEFR and specific inhalation challenges (see below). Subjects should be asked to record their values at least four times a day, ideally every 2 hours and whenever they become symptomatic of asthma. This monitoring should be done before, during and after work. It should be performed on weekends and, if necessary, as weekends are not always sufficient for recovery, for one or two weeks off work. Positive recordings are recognized on the grounds of greater fluctuations (Fig. 36.2, upper panel) or progressive lowering of values and recovery after a period off work (Fig. 36.2, lower panel).

As monitoring of PEFR is effort-dependent and needs good collaboration by the subject, it has also been suggested to perform such a monitoring with serial assessments of airway hyperexcitability [24, 25]. Indeed, even if PEFR monitoring can help in the diagnosis of OA, one may criticize the information obtained on the grounds that the data can be falsified, as there is no supervision of the subject every

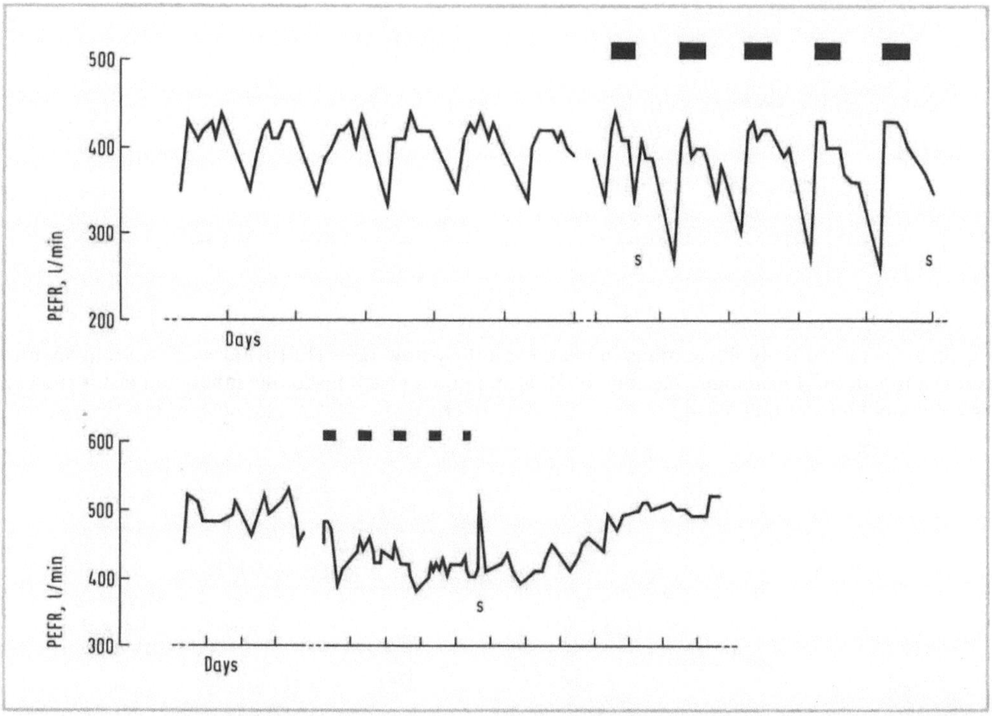

Fig. 36.2. *Upper panel:* increased daily fluctuations in peak expiratory flow rates (PEFR) after days at work (rectangles). *Lower panel:* progressive lowering of PEFR at work with recovery after leaving work. s = salbutamol inhalation (200 μg)

time he does the test. Furthermore, on occasion, such monitoring may not distinguish between an irritant and a specific or antigenic mechanism in the etiology of OA (Fig. 36.3). An example of the dual use of PEFR monitoring and airway responsiveness to histamine in confirming OA is shown in Fig. 36.4. When such changes are documented, one can suspect a late or dual asthmatic reaction at work, as such changes have been elicited after similar reactions to natural products [26]. Such a monitoring is important when the nature of the product at work is unknown and if specific inhalation challenges (see below) are impossible for various reasons.

36.3.6 *Specific Inhalation Challenges*

These tests have originally been proposed by Pepys et al in the assessment of OA [27]. Although the confirmation of OA can be obtained with PEFR monitoring and changes in airway responsiveness to histamine, specific inhalation challenges, when feasible, are still the gold standard to which PEFR monitoring and airway hyperexcitability should be compared. These tests should be performed in a hospital laboratory where the personnel is familiar with such procedures and where there are facilities to reverse acute bronchoconstriction. Although there is no standardization of such tests, progressive daily increase in the duration of exposure should be proposed. Duration of initial exposure should be guided by the clinical history, baseline spirometry and the level of nonallergic bronchial excitability. Monitoring of spirometry (preferably FEV_1, alone or with more sensitive tests) should be done before, every 10–15 min following exposure in the first hour, and then hourly up to 8 hours. At that time, if no significant changes (< 20% changes in FEV_1) in spirometry are documented, assessment of the level of

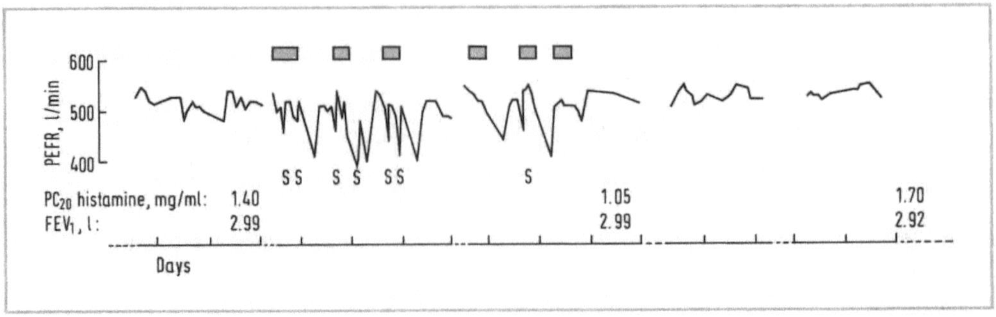

Fig. 36.3. Increased daily fluctuations in peak expiratory flow rates (PEFR) at work without significant changes in PC_{20} histamine. Baseline FEV_1 at the time of each histamine inhalation test is shown. s = salbutamol inhalation (200 μg)

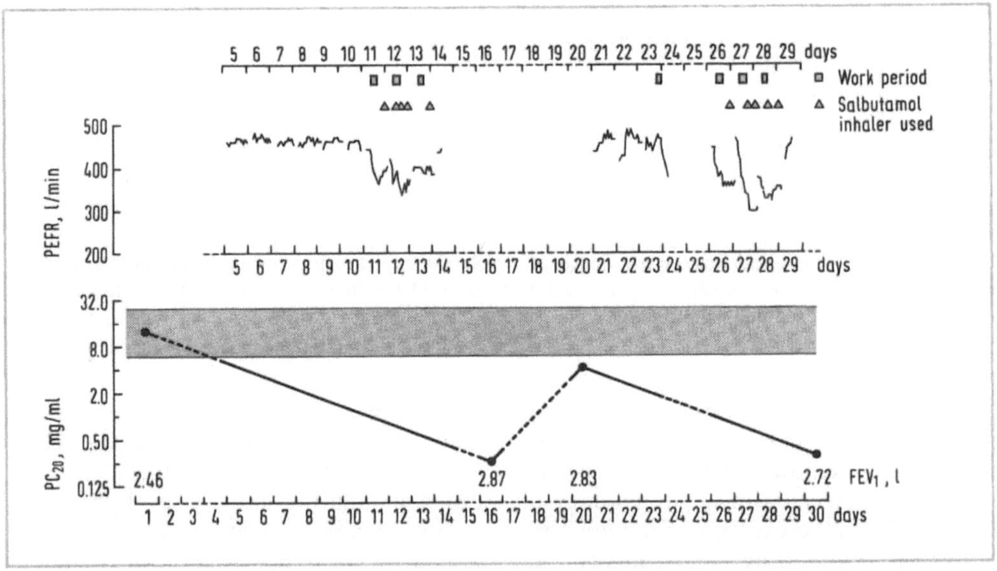

Fig. 36.4. Variations of peak expiratory flow rates (PEFR) and PC_{20} histamine on the upper and lower panels, respectively. Time (days) is shown on the abscissa. Work period and the use of salbutamol inhaler are indicated on top. The two horizontal interrupted lines represent the limits of a single 2-fold concentration variation in PC_{20} of day 1, which is the accepted reproducibility range of the test. (From [25], by kind permission of Blackwell Scientific Publications Ltd)

bronchial hyperexcitability should be carried out. Indeed, if changes in the latter are seen, longer exposure to the offending agent should be considered in the laboratory or at work. On occasion, changes in airway hyperexcitability can precede changes in airway caliber [28]. Oral temperature and white blood count should also be monitored before and after the challenges. Finally, when the individual has been away from work for long intervals, desensitization might have occurred and longer periods of exposure can be necessary before eliciting the reaction [29].

On occasion, specific inhalation challenges cannot be performed in a hospital laboratory due to the complexity of the work. In these cases, they can be carried out in the work place under medical supervision.

36.3.7 Follow-up of Affected Individuals

It would seem logical to assume that affected workers could get rid of the their asthmatic symptoms, airway obstruction and hyperexcitability after removal from work. Although this occurs, it does not seem to be the rule. Asthmatic symptoms can persist and require the use of bronchodilators and even corticosteroids on a PRN or continuous basis [18–20]. Moreover, even when asymptomatic, the majority of affected workers still show some degree of nonallergic bronchial hyperexcitability [20].

Acknowledgements: The authors thank the physicians of the Commission de la Santé et de la Sécurité du Travail du Québec for referring subjects for expertise. They also thank Lyette Rochon for her secretarial assistance and Patricia Hudson for reviewing the manuscript.

References

1. Ramazzini B (1700) De Morbis Artificum. Cited in: Gandevia B (1970) Occupational asthma. Med J Aust 2:332–335
2. Fuchs S, Valade P (1951) Etude clinique et expérimentale sur quelques cas d'intoxication par le Desmodur T (diisocyanate de toluène). Arch Mal Profess 12:191–196
3. O'Brien IM, Harries MG, Burge PS, Pepys J (1979) Toluene diisocyanate-induced asthma. I. Reactions to TDI, MDI, HDI and histamine. Clin Allergy 9:1–6
4. Malo JL, Ouimet G, Cartier A, Levitz D, Zeiss CR (1983) Combined alveolitis and asthma due to hexamethylene diisocyanate (HDI), with demonstration of crossed respiratory and immunologic reactivities to diphenylmethane diisocyanate (MDI). J Allergy Clin Immunol 72:413–419
5. Tse KS, Chan H, Chan-Yeung M (1982) Specific IgE antibodies in workers with occupational asthma due to western red cedar. Clin Allergy 12:249–258
6. Howe W, Venables KM, Topping MD, Dally MB, Hawkins R, Law SL, Newman Taylor AJ (1983) Tetracholorophthalic anhydride asthma: evidence for specific IgE antibody. J Allergy Clin Immunol 71:5–11
7. Alanko K, Keskinen H, Bjorksten F, Ojanen S (1978) Immediate-type hypersensitivity to reactive dyes. Clin Allergy 8:25–31
8. Butcher BT, O'Neil CE, Reed MA, Salvaggio JE (1980) Radioallergosorbent testing of toluene diisocyanate-reactive individuals using p-tolyl isocyanate antigen. J Allergy Clin Immunol 66:213–216
9. Baur X (1983) Immunologic cross-reactivity between different albumin-bound isocyanates. J Allergy Clin Immunol 71:197–205
10. Zeiss CR, Kanellakes TM, Bellone JD, Levitz D, Pruzansky JJ, Patterson R (1980) Immunoglobulin E-mediated asthma and hypersensitivity pneumonitis with precipitating anti-hapten antibodies due to diphenylmethane diisocyanate (MDI) exposure. J Allergy Clin Immunol 65:346–352
11. Malo JL, Zeiss CR (1982) Occupational hypersensitivity pneumonitis after exposure to diphenylmethane diisocyanate. Am Rev Respir Dis 125:113–116
12. Danks JM, Cromwell O, Buckingham JA, Newman-Taylor AJ, Davies RJ (1981) Toluene-diisocyanate induced asthma: evaluation of antibodies in the serum of affected workers against a tolyl mono-isocyanate protein conjugate. Clin Allergy 11:161–168
13. Davies RJ, Butcher BT, O'Neil CE, Salvaggio JE (1977) The in vitro effect of toluene diisocyanate on lymphocyte cyclic adenosine monophosphate production by isoproterenol, prostaglandin, and histamine. J Allergy Clin Immunol 60:223–229
14. Corrao WM, Braman SS, Irwin RS (1979) Chronic cough as the sole presenting manifestation of bronchial asthma. N Engl J Med 300:633–637
15. Siracusa A, Curradi F, Abbritti G (1978) Recurrent nocturnal asthma due to tolylene diisocyanate: a case report. Clin Allergy 8: 195–201
16. Newman Taylor AJ, Davies RJ, Hendrick DJ, Pepys J (1979) Recurrent nocturnal asthmatic reactions to bronchial provocation tests. Clin Allergy 9:213–219
17. Cockcroft DW, Cotton DJ, Mink JT (1979) Nonspecific bronchial hyperreactivity after exposure to western red cedar. Am Rev Respir Dis 119:505–510
18. Chan-Yeung M, Lam S, Koener S (1982) Clinical features and natural history of occupational asthma due to western red cedar (*Thuja plicata*). Am J Med 72:411–415
19. Burge PS (1982) Occupational asthma in electronics workers caused by colophony fumes: follow-up of affected workers. Thorax 37:348–353
20. Hudson P, Pineau L, Cartier A, Malo JL (1984) Follow-up of occupational asthma due to various agents. J Allergy Clin Immunol 73:174 (abstract)
21. Perks WH, Tams IP, Thompson DA, Prowse K (1979) An evaluation of the mini-Wright peak flow meter. Thorax 34:79–81

22. Burge PS, O'Brien IM, Harries MG (1979) Peak flow rate records in the diagnosis of occupational asthma due to colophony. Thorax 34:308–316
23. Burge PS, O'Brien IM, Harries MG (1979) Peak flow rate records in the diagnosis of occupational asthma due to isocyanates. Thorax 34:317–322
24. Cockcroft DW, Cartier A, Jones G, Tarlo SM, Dolovich J, Hargreave FE (1980) Asthma caused by occupational exposure to a furan-based binder system. J Allergy Clin Immunol 66:458–463
25. Cartier A, Pineau L, Malo JL (1984) Monitoring of maximum expiratory flow rates and histamine inhalation tests in the investigation of occupational asthma. Clin Allergy 14:193–196
26. Boulet LP, Cartier A, Thomson NC, Roberts RS, Dolovich J, Hargreave FE (1983) Asthma and increases in nonallergic bronchial responsiveness from seasonal pollen exposure. J Allergy Clin Immunol 71:399–406
27. Pepys J, Hutchcroft BJ (1975) Bronchial provocation tests in etiologic diagnosis and analysis of asthma. Am Rev Respir Dis 112:829–859
28. Cartier A, Pineau L, Malo JL (in press) Investigation of occupational asthma: Changes in non-specific airway responsiveness to histamine preceding fluctuations in bronchomotor tone. J Allergy Clin Immunol
29. Cartier A, Malo JL, Forest F, Lafrance M, Pineau L, St. Aubin JJ, Dubois JY (1984) Occupational asthma in snow-crab processing workers. J Allergy Clin Immunol 74: 261–269
30. Parkes WR (1982) Occupational asthma (including Byssinosis) In: Parkes WR (ed) Occupational Lung Disorders. 2nd edn. Butterworth, London, pp 415–453
31. Bernstein IL (1981) Occupational asthma. Clin Chest Med 2:255–272
32. Burge PS, O'Brien IM, Harries MG, Pepys J (1979) Occupational asthma due to inhaled carmine. Clin Allergy 9:185–189
33. Malo JL, Cartier A, Doepner M, Nieboer E, Evans S, Dolovich J (1982) Occupational asthma caused by nickel sulfate. J Allergy Clin Immunol 69:55–59

37. Occupational Asthma

R. J. Davies, A. D. Blainey

Airflow obstruction resulting from occupational exposure has been recognized for some time, but the importance of this form of asthma has been much more widely realized in recent years. Occupational asthma is potentially preventable, and the identification of the diverse industrial agents causing this disease may contribute to a reduction in morbidity from asthma. Furthermore the disease often occurs in individuals previously unaffected by asthma, and the study of occupational asthma may provide valuable insight into the mechanisms underlying sensitization to inhaled agents.

37.1 Prevalence

More than 200 inhaled agents have now been reported to cause occupational asthma but estimates of prevalence vary widely between industries and countries. In part this reflects the difficulties of recording the prevalence of a variable disease such as asthma where objective diagnosis requires multiple measurements over a period of time. Estimates of prevalence based on a single criterion, such as a history of wheezing, or a single lung function test, can be very misleading. The introduction of new techniques for the detection of asthmatic individuals, such as the measurement of bronchial hyperreactivity to inhaled methacholine, or ambulatory peak flow recordings, may well allow more precise epidemiological studies to be undertaken in different industries.

Existing estimates from Japan suggest that as many as 15% of all male asthmatics may have an occupational etiology, and in the USA about 2% of all asthmatic individuals have work-related symptoms. Recent information from Finland, where occupational asthma is a notifiable disease and where all new cases are recorded, has shown that the annual incidence of occupational asthma is approximately 70 per million of the economically active population. These records also show that the most common cause of occupational asthma in Finland is grain and flour, followed by isocyanates [1]. There appears to have been an increase in the number of cases reported in the last five years, but clearly this could reflect improvements in case detection rather than indicating a true increase.

Estimates vary widely from industry to industry; about 5% of workers in the plastic's industry exposed to toluene diisocyanate develop asthma due to that agent, whereas in a recent survey of grain handlers in the UK about 11% were thought to have work-related asthma. Prevalence surveys in occupational respiratory disease may give falsely low estimates because affected workers leave the industry early. Studies on retired hemp workers in a Spanish village, for example, revealed a much higher prevalence of respiratory symptoms than in matched control subjects who had worked in other industries.

Even within an industry, reliable prevalence rates are difficult to obtain. Exposure levels to a single agent may be different, and certain individuals may have enhanced susceptibility to the development of occupational asthma. Careful prospective studies are clearly required in different industries to define exactly what proportion of the exposed population is likely to develop occupational asthma. There is little doubt, however, that occupational asthma – a preventable disease affecting fit, working people – is a disease of major social and economic importance. This fact has indeed been recognized by the legislature of several countries. In France, W. Germany and most recently the United Kingdom occupational asthma is recognized as one of the diseases for which compensation is considered appropriate.

37.2 Predisposing Factors

In general, occupational asthma has the features of allergic disease. There is a latent period between first exposure and the onset of disease, only a small proportion of those exposed are affected, and attacks in those susceptible occur at concentrations of the provoking agent much less than that required to produce symptoms in the nonaffected population.

Occupational allergens of organic origin are usually macromolecules of similar complexity to commonly encountered domestic allergens such as the P_1 antigen of the house dust mite. It might therefore be expected that, as with allergy to domestic inhaled allergens, atopic subjects might be more susceptible to the development of occupational asthma due to these agents. This has indeed been demonstrated in some industries, such as the manufacture of biological detergents. In many industries, however, there appears to be no relationship between the development of respiratory symptoms and atopic status. There are several possible explanations for this. Firstly, atopic subjects may develop symptoms more rapidly (as has been shown in the platinum industry) and leave the industry, leaving an apparent excess of nonatopic subjects as a survivor population. Alternatively, as with TDI, mechanisms other than type I hyperreactivity may be involved. Other factors may further enhance the susceptibility of atopic subjects. Recent work has shown that in some industries, such as grain workers, cigarette smoking is itself associated with work-related respiratory symptoms. It is possible that smoking and atopy may interact to make occupational asthma more likely. In workers exposed to TCPA, it has been shown that specific IgE to TCPA was highest in those who smoked, and that atopy and current cigarette smoking interacted significantly to produce the highest levels of specific IgE [2]. In a recently studied group of prawn peelers a similar relationship was found between smoking, atopy and specific IgE.

The mechanisms underlying a possible smoking/atopy interaction in the pathogenesis of occupational asthma are so far unclear. In extrinsic allergic alveolitis (which may often have an occupational etiology) there is an inverse relationship between smoking and the development of disease; smoking farm workers appear to be less susceptible to the development of bronchoalveolitis. Total serum-IgE, on the other hand, is known to be higher in smokers than in nonsmokers, and there is no evidence that this reflects a specific allergic response to tobacco products [3]. Cigarette smoking can increase both pulmonary epithelial permeability to high molecular weight compounds, as well as produce a degree of bronchial hyperreactivity (though not as severe as that found in asthma). Allergen exposure in established asthmatics has also been shown to produce increased bronchial epithelial permeability, and the work of Hargreave and colleagues has shown that late asthmatic reactions are followed by increased bronchial reactivity to histamine [4]. Airways hyperreactivity is characteristic of occupational asthma as of asthma in general, and it is possible that factors which contribute to increased bronchial reactivity may enhance the immunologic response to allergen and therefore increase susceptibility to allergic disease. Few existing studies have reported on the relationship between smoking, allergic responses, airway hyperreactivity and symptoms in an occupational group, and clearly these factors need to be examined systematically in future studies.

Atmospheric pollutants such as ozone and sulfur dioxide are also known to cause increases in bronchial epithelial permeability and hyperreactivity, but the role of these agents in contributing to occupational asthma has been neglected so far and little is known.

37.3 Pathogenic Mechanisms

Many of the agents causing occupational asthma are also irritant to the respiratory tract in high concentrations and can cause respiratory symptoms through a vagally mediated reflex. Irritant mechanisms alone do not account for most cases of occupational asthma, as the few individuals of a workforce who are usually affected, develop symptoms at much lower concentrations than those associated with irritant responses. It is unlikely that the simple interaction of irritant substances with airway hyperreactivity is sufficient to account for most cases of occupational asthma, since some studies have shown that individuals with greatly enhanced bronchial hyperreactivity and significant occupational exposure still have no specifically work-related respiratory symptoms [5].

Irritant responses usually follow immediately on exposure to an occupational agent, but many individuals with occupational asthma have delayed responses typical of allergic asthma. The role of IgE and mast cells in the pathogenesis of asthma is now well documented but the involvement of specific IgE in many types of occupational asthma is controversial. For some agents, such as urinary proteins of small mammals which are responsible for occupational asthma in some laboratory workers, there is good evidence for IgE-mediated mechanisms. Atopic individuals are preferentially affected, skin tests with urine extracts are positive in most affected individuals, and specific IgE to these proteins may be demonstrated in the serum [6]. In asthma due to western red cedar specific IgE was found in the serum of only 40% of exposed individuals and antibody levels did not correlate with the airway response to plicatic acid [7]. In other industries specific IgE has never been convincingly demonstrated in a significant proportion of affected workers' serum, and, in these, it may be that other mechanisms are involved. TDI, itself for example, can reduce the CAMP response to isoprenaline, at least in human lymphocytes [8].

The role of the mast cell in the pathogenesis of allergic respiratory disease has become much clearer in recent years following the identification of the inflammatory mediators derived from these cells. Sensitive methods are now available for the detection of histamine in plasma and neutrophil chemotactic activity (NCA) can be measured in serum, but there are few examples of the application of such measurements to subjects with occupational asthma. In our laboratory we have demonstrated significant rises in neutrophil chemotactic activity (NCA) in plasma after challenge with a variety of occupational agents, including persulfate salts in asthmatic hairdressers [5]. In these patients, in whom specific IgE has not been demonstrated, such experiments provide some evidence in favor of mast cell involvement, and indeed persulfate salts have been shown to release histamine directly from rat and guinea pig mast cells. Whether such mechanisms play a significant role in asthma due to other occupational agents has not yet been demonstrated.

37.4 The Classification and Diagnosis of Occupational Asthma

The list of agents reported to cause occupational asthma (Table 37.1) is already lengthy, and new agents are frequently being reported. It is clear that there is considerable diversity in sensitivity agents, ranging from low molecular weight vapours to complex macromolecules.

The diagnosis of occupational asthma requires the demonstration of asthma in an individual as well as the identification of the etiological agent. The symptoms of occupational asthma are identical to those of asthma from any cause, but an occupational etiology may not be readily apparent. A late reaction to the agent may mean that symptoms do not start until the patient has left work, and symptoms may occur on successive nights extending over a weekend or short holiday without continuing exposure to the occupational agent. Conversely, symptoms suggestive of asthma may arise as an irritant response to an occupational agent in normal subjects, and may not be associated with objective proof of asthma.

There is usually a latent period between first exposure and the onset of symptoms, but this can greatly vary ranging from a few weeks to several years. An occupational cause should not be rejected merely because the patient has been in contact with an industrial agent for some years. Some patients in the platinum industry developed symptoms as long as 10 years after their first exposure to platinum.

Table 37.1. Agents causing occupational asthma

Low molecular weight	
Metals	– Chrome, platinum, nickels, cobalt, vanadium
Chemicals	– Formalin, phthalic anhydride, ethylene diamine isocyanates, dyes, bleaches, colophony
Drugs	– Penicillins, tetracycline, cephalosporins, cimetidine, methyldopa
Biological products	
Animal, bird and fish products	– Animal danders and urinary proteins, prawns, sea squirt
Insects	– Storage mites, locust, cockroach, grain weevil, silkworm
Foods	– Soybeans, green coffee beans, castor beans, vegetable gums, grain, flour
Wood dusts	– Western red cedar, iroko, oak, mahogany, California redwood, African zebrawood
Enzymes	– Proteolytic enzymes, enzymes of Bacillus subtilis (in detergents)

Occupational asthma may arise in those living or working in the vicinity of a factory where sensitizing material is produced or handled. Outbreaks of asthma at the University of Minnesota were shown to be related to high levels of dust blown by the prevailing wind from nearby grain mills [9]. Small quantities of industrial material may be brought home on skin, hair or clothing and give rise to continuing symptoms in those affected. Many cases of occupational asthma will only be diagnosed if the possibility is first considered and then carefully sought by close questioning, not only about the patient's occupation but also about nearby industries and the patient's leisure activities.

Definitive diagnosis of occupational asthma requires the demonstration of the objective signs of airways obstruction in relation to an occupational agent. Isolated measurements of simple lung function may not be adequate in this respect, as they may be normal in patients with variable airways obstruction. Even measurements timed in relation to a working shift may be misleading, because the circadian variation in airway caliber may obscure work-related changes and because of the existence of late asthmatic reactions which will not be detected by measurements made only at the workplace. The introduction of portable peak flowmeters has provided a significant advance in the diagnosis of occupational asthma. Peak flow recordings made at least in 2-hourly intervals at and away from work over a 3–4 week period will provide clear evidence of work-related airflow obstruction in at least some of those affected [10]. However, therapy with inhaled corticosteroids or cromoglycate may make these patterns undetectable, and the regular recordings of peak flow rates over this pattern is a demanding protocol for working individuals to follow. In our experience, peak flow measurement is of much less value in epidemiological surveys for this reason.

Bronchial hyperreactivity to inhaled pharmacological agents or cold air is almost always associated with asthma and is significantly greater in more severe asthma than in other causes of airflow obstruction. This technique can be used to distinguish asthmatic from nonasthmatic individuals and can provide a rapid and reproducible diagnostic test for asthma. It is of particular value in distinguishing subjects with nonspecific irritant symptoms from those with asthma, and recent work has demonstrated its usefulness in the epidemiological investigation of occupational asthma [11].

In certain circumstances the identification of a specific etiological agent may be straightforward. Where a patient develops symptoms as a result of exposure to a single agent known to cause occupational asthma, and objective proof of asthma is obtained, no further investigation is usually required. Where there is exposure to multiple potential sensitizing agents – as for example in the grain industry where not only grain itself but many of its insect contaminants are known to cause asthma – or where the occupational agent has not been previously recognized to cause asthma, specific bronchial provocation testing may be of value. Occupational-type bronchial provocation testing attempts to reproduce working conditions within the laboratory and the effects of a large number of dusts, gases and fumes may be assessed in this way. Such provocation tests may show an immediate reaction (Fig. 37.1), occurring within minutes of exposure and lasting up to one hour, or a late reaction, with falls in expiratory flow rates 2–8 hours after exposure (Fig. 37.2). Dual reactions are frequently seen, combining the features of both early and late reactions (Fig. 37.3). In some individuals a single exposure to an occupational agent can result in recurrent attacks of asthma over the following days – recurrent nocturnal reactions (Fig. 37.4).

Bronchial provocation testing with occupational materials can provide a specific diagnosis of occupational asthma, but is not without its disadvantages. Challenge testing with occupational materials can be hazardous as some patients are very sensitive to occupational materials and react to low doses. Furthermore the circumstances of the test are very difficult to standardize; with few exceptions it is extremely difficult to measure the dose of occupational material inhaled by the patient. This had led some to argue that bronchial provocation testing should not be performed routinely in the investigation of occupational asthma. The uncertainty associated with a clinical diagnosis of occupational asthma may nevertheless make specific challenge essential, particularly if a major environmental change is contemplated. Occupational-type bronchial provocation testing is also of value in the diagnosis of previously unrecognized causes of occupational asthma, and may also be useful when it is necessary to determine the precise agent causing the disease in an industrial environment where

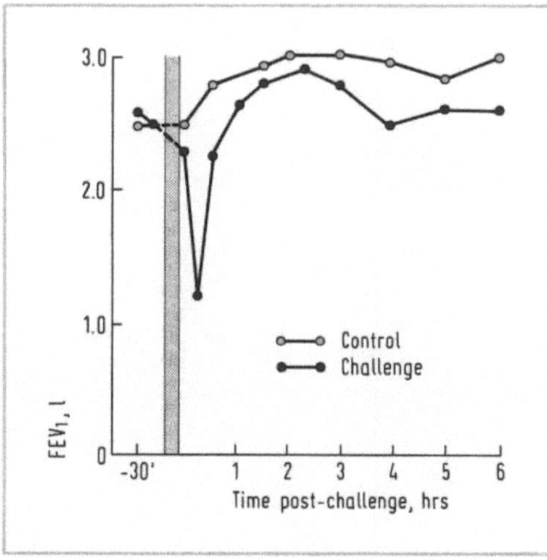

Fig. 37.1. Immediate reaction to bronchial provocation testing with colophony

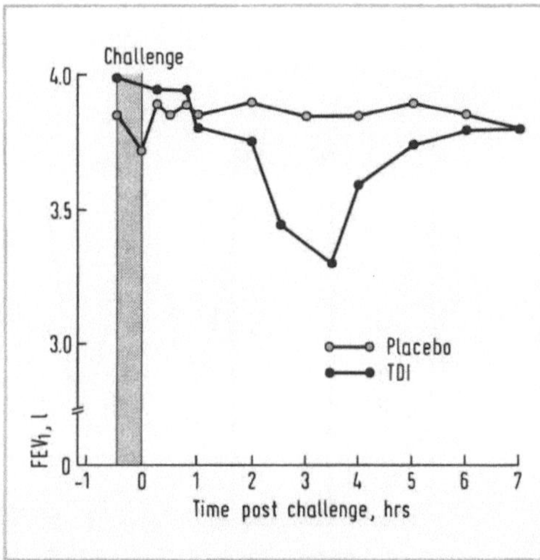

Fig. 37.2. Late reaction to bronchial provocation testing with toluene diisocyanate

the individual or workforce is exposed to more than one known sensitizing agent.

Skin prick tests with occupational materials are often negative in individuals with occupational asthma, and as with non-occupational asthma, the relationship between skin prick tests and disease is often not close. In many industries a significant number of affected individuals have negative skin prick tests or specific IgE. In

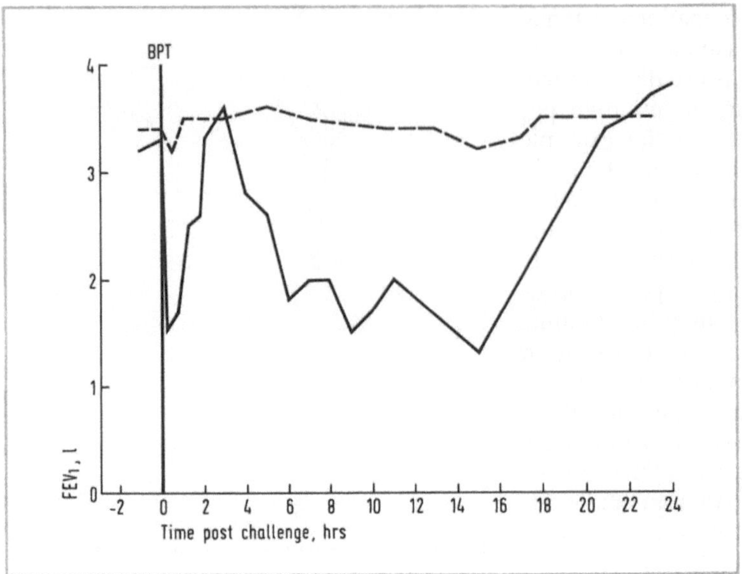

Fig. 37.3. Dual (immediate and late) reaction to bronchial provocation testing with flour

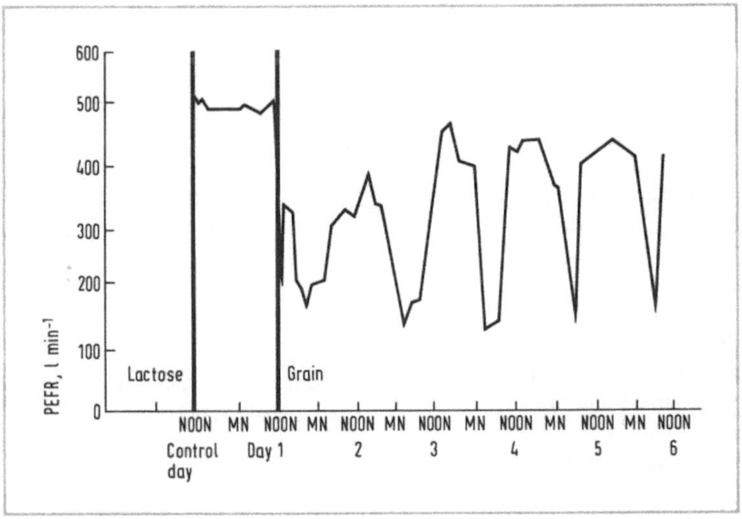

Fig. 37.4. Recurrent nocturnal reactions following bronchial provocation with grain dust

others a positive skin prick test to an occupational allergen may not be associated with the presence of disease. Few longitudinal studies relating skin tests to the development of disease exist, but it is clear that in most industries skin prick tests or specific IgE cannot be used alone to detect affected individuals. A positive skin test or specific IgE does not necessarily imply disease and neither does a negative test exclude it.

37.5 Prevention of Occupational Asthma

The primary objective in the management of occupational asthma must be its prevention. It is not enough to identify a new cause of occupational asthma. The prevalence of disease among those exposed must also be clearly established, and predisposing factors must equally be unequivocally identified. Little is known about the mechanisms of sensitization to occupational materials. This is partly due to the lack of information relating industrial exposure levels to disease. Detailed prospective studies relating personal exposure to the incidence of clinical disease are required to define this process more clearly.

Although there is little direct evidence in support, it would seem reasonable to keep occupational exposure to irritant or potentially allergenic substances to a minimum. This approach often requires considerable expenditure on the protection of the individual worker. The cheapest systems such as simple filter-type face masks are of little value in preventing disease in those already sensitized, and are often ignored by the workforce. Positive pressure air hoods and helmet respirators can be very effective in protecting against the harmful affects of organic and inorganic dusts, and may be of particular value in protecting those at greatest risk. The identification of individual risk factors is of great importance in the prevention of occupational asthma. In some industries there is little doubt that atopic subjects are at greater risk [12] and, as such, have often been excluded from direct contact with certain occupational allergens. The frequency of atopy in the working population – as much as 40% in some surveys – means that preventing atopic individuals from working with sensitizing agents often excludes a large number of individuals who will never develop disease. Indeed it has been calculated that in order to prevent one case of laboratory animal allergy, six healthy atopic workers would have to be excluded – and, even so, disease would still occur in 2% of the remainder [13]. It is clear that further prospective studies are required in many industries to identify the interaction between predisposing features such as smoking, atopy and bronchial hyperreactivity in order to quantify the risks of the development of disease for an individual.

37.6 Management of Occupational Asthma

It is essential that those affected by occupational asthma should be removed from contact with the relevant material. This may be achieved by transferring the individual to another part of the workplace, though affected workers who react to very low concentrations may still have symptoms and it may be necessary to terminate employment. Follow-up studies in patients with asthma due to western red cedar have shown that over half of those affected had persisting symptoms and airway hyperreactivity despite withdrawal from exposure, and that persistence of symptoms was associated with prolonged exposure to the occupational allergen [14]. Patients who develop symptoms as a result of exposure to occupational agents should be unequivocally advised to avoid further exposure.

In those who are unable to follow this advice, other forms of therapy may be considered. Asthma of occupational origin responds to therapy in a similar fashion to that resulting from other causes. Bronchial challenge with occupational agents has demonstrated the effectiveness of cromoglycate and steroids in preventing immediate and late asthmatic reactions [15], but if an affected worker does remain exposed to an occupational allergen, careful long-term observation with repeated tests of lung function (and possibly bronchial hyperreactivity) are essential. The possible risks of such a course of action will require a full explanation to the patient at an early stage.

References

1. Keskinen H (1983) Epidemiology of occupational lung disease: Asthma and allergic alveolitis. In: Kerr JW, Ganderton MA (eds) Proceedings of the XIth International Congress of Allergology and Clinical Immunology. Macmillan, London
2. Venables KM, Topping MD, Howe W, Luczynska CM, Hawkins R, Newman-Taylor AJ (1985) Interaction of smoking and atopy in producing specific IgE antibody against a hapten protein conjugate. Br Med J 290:201–204
3. Burrows B, Halonen M, Barbee RA, Lebowitz MD (1981) The relationship of serum immunoglobulin E to cigarette smoking. Am Rev Respir Dis 124:523–525
4. Cockcroft DW, Ruffin RE, Dolovich J, Hargreave FE (1977) Allergen-induced increase in non-allergic bronchial reactivity. Clin Allergy 7:503–513

5. Blainey AD, Ollier S, Cundell D, Smith RE, Davies RJ (1985) Occupational asthma in a hairdressing salon. Thorax 41:42–50
6. Newman-Taylor AJ, Longbottom J, Pepys J (1977) Respiratory allergy to the urinary proteins of rats and mice. Lancet II:847–849
7. Chan-Yeung M (1982) Immunologic and non-immunologic mechanisms in asthma due to western red cedar. J Allergy Clin Immunol 70:32–37
8. Davies RJ, Butcher BJ, O'Neill CE, Salvaggio JE (1977) The *in vitro* effect of toluene diisocyanate on lymphocyte and cyclic adenosine monophosphate production by isoproterenol, prostaglandin and histamine. A possible mode of action. J Allergy Clin Immunol 60:223–229
9. Cowan DW, Thompson HJ, Paulus HJ, Mielke PW (1963) Bronchial asthma associated with air pollutants from the grain industry. J Air Pollut Control Assoc 13:546
10. Burge PS, O'Brien M, Harries MG (1979) Peak flow records in the diagnosis of asthma due to colophony. Thorax 34:308–316
11. Blainey AD, Coe MJS, Ollier S, Davies RJ (1983) Methacholine provocation tests in grainworkers. Thorax 38:220
12. Pepys J, Wells ID, d'Souza ME, Greenberg M (1973) Clinical and immunological responses to enzymes of *Bacillus subtilis* in factory workers and consumers. Clin Allergy 3:143–160
13. Burge PS, Pickering CAC (1982) Prevention and management of small mammal allergy. Clin Allergy 12:427
14. Chan-Yeung M, Lam S, Koener S (1982) Clinical features and natural history of occupational asthma due to western red cedar (*Thuja plicata*). Am J Med 72:411–415
15. Pepys J, Davies RJ, Breslin ABX, Hendrick DJ, Hutchcroft BJ (1974) The effects of inhaled beclomethasone dipropionate (Becotide) and sodium cromoglycate on asthmatic responses to provocation tests. Clin Allergy 4:13–24

38. Food-related Asthma

D. A. Moneret-Vautrin

The relationship between asthma and food remains a controversial area owing to the complexity of the involved mechanisms. However, a rational approach to the diagnosis, based on recently clarified facts, is now available and enables some definite observations [1, 13].

Among the numerous clinical disorders in food allergy (FA), asthma was observed in 25% of our 188 cases [12]. Four clinical aspects can be described.

The acute wheezing, in atopic patients allergic to inhalant and food allergens occurred after handling or breathing fish, raw potatoes, wheat flour, or other foods which the patient was sensitive to.

Occupational asthma to food proteins included the ingestion of milk by workers in the dairy industry, of bread by bakers sensitized to flour and of soya nuts and green peas, by workers in the industry of oilcakes for cattle. These patients also presented an asthma attack upon the inhalation of the offending allergen. The allergens from animal origin might be much more aggressive, since the prevalence of asthma to snow-crab has been evaluated at 15.7% [5].

More recently rare cases of exercise-induced food anaphylaxis have been published [21].

On the other hand, the real importance of food antigens and food additives in chronic asthma is not clear [11]. It accounted for 40% of asthma in children and 20% of asthma in adults, according to Rowe [20], 5% and 3.6% respectively, according to Ganderton [8], 8.45% in asthmatic children, according to Oehling [15], 4% to 5.8% of adult asthmatics [4, 13].

Numerous mechanisms, partially depending on the substances, may be considered. The IgE-dependent FA is frequent in children (15% of the cases) and less frequent in adults (5% of the cases). The most common foods to produce wheezing are milk, egg, fish, soy and peanut (Tables 38.1 and 38.2); a few others, such as celery, carrot, potato, hazel nuts, apple and other fruits, have been confirmed in patients allergic to pollens [2, 6, 19]. However, all foods may elicit asthma [17].

Table 38.1. Major antigenic proteins in foods from vegetal origin, fruit and vegetables

Food	Allergens	Molecular weight	Thermo-stability	Other characteristics
Peanut	α-arachin	180,000–330,000	Yes	22 allergens in crude extract
	Conarachin I	140,000–295,000	Yes	10 in roasted peanuts
	con A-reactive glyco-protein	–	Yes	
Tomato	Glycoprotein	20,000– 30,000	Yes	
Soybean	Globulin 25	–	Yes	
	Kunithz inhibition	–	Yes	
Wheat	Globulins		Yes	Food allergy
	Albumins		No	Bakers' asthma
	Starches		Yes	
	Gliadine		Yes	Coeliac disease

Table 38.2. Major allergenic proteins in foods from animal origin

Food	Allergens	Molecular weight	Thermo-stability	Other characteristics
Milk	β-lactoglobulin	18,000–31,000	Yes	Products of digestion retain allergenic activity
	α-lactalbumin	16,000	No	
	Casein	20,000–24,000	Yes	
	Serum albumin	69,000	No	Four Ig-binding sites
Egg	Ovomucoide	27,000–31,000	Yes	186 amino acids sequence 69–130 thought to be allergenic
	Ovotransferrin		–	
	Ovalbumin		No	
	Lysozyme	14,500	Yes	129 amino acids
Fish (cod)	Allergen M (parvalbumin)	12,000	Yes	113 amino acids Peptide 13–32: haptenic determinant Peptides 33–44, 65–74, 88–96: Ig-binding sites
Shellfish	First protein	38,000	Yes	
	Second protein	21,000	Yes	

Adverse reactions to food additives, such as sodium metabisulfite and sodium benzoate, which are preservatives, or tartrazine and other dyes, occur in 11% of asthmatic patients [7, 10]. Sodium glutamate has been recently shown to elicit asthma. Some substances, such as sodium metabisulfite, act predominantly through a cholinergic mechanism by triggering the irritant receptors of the bronchial epithelium [22]. Others, such as sodium glutamate, enhance the synthesis of acetylcholine. Sodium benzoate, butylhydroxytoluene and tartrazine, act upon the cyclooxygenase, thus interfering with the normal balance between prostaglandins and leukotrienes. The bronchial spasm is then induced by SRS-A. Another possibility is an alteration in the bronchial reactivity to histamine induced by tartrazine [10]. Intolerance to alcohol may be linked to several mechanisms: intolerance to sodium metabisulfite or benzoate, allergy to grapes or to alcohol [12]. Lastly, nonimmunological release of NCF-A could explain some wheezing reactions to foods [18].

38.1 Suspicion of Food Intolerance in Asthma

(supported by ten facts)

- Atopy, when proven, points to a virtual food allergy, because food antigens are present as early as birth and can stimulate specific IgE while the protective intestinal IgA is not yet produced [12].
- A past history of FA evokes a present one, because multiple food allergies are usual (more than 60% of our cases [12]).
- The diurnal or postprandial rhythm of breathlessness points towards a FA when vagal asthma due to a gastroesophageal reflux is eliminated, but wheezing persists throughout the day [13, 14].
- The combination of symptoms involving other organs with asthma is very suggestive. The symptoms are rhinitis, nasal polyposis, urticaria, eczema, mouth ulcers, conjunctivitis, arthralgias, digestive troubles such as gastric pain or diarrhea and cystalgias without infection, bedwetting in children [24]. They are reported in 65% to 72% of cases [13, 24].
- Asthma without any proof of allergy to inhalants must not be classified as *in-*

trinsic asthma as long as a FA has not been investigated. Moreover, patients with intrinsic asthma have often rhinitis, or nasal polyposis, and intolerance to aspirin and nonsteroidal anti-inflammatory drugs. Additives in food and drugs are mostly responsible for transient exacerbations of asthma. Avoidance of these results in a marked improvement, and enables the steroids to be diminished. Wraith expresses the same opinion, contrary to Bock's [3, 22].

- Cross-reactive antigens are shared by mugwort pollens and celery or carrots [2, 19]. Birch pollen-allergic subjects are often sensitive to a wide variety of fruits and vegetables (apples, pears, plums, strawberries, celery, carrot, fennel, potatoes etc.) Crossed reactivities between grass pollens and wheat or other cereals are less common.
- The persistant inhalation of food proteins sets up a risk of subsequent allergic reactions to the same proteins when ingested.
- The excessive consumption of foods enhances the risk of sensitization, whether it concerns a person, or affects national habits. This fact explains why milk, egg and azoic dyes are the chief culprits in children. Soy is frequently incriminated in Japan, as are peanuts, in the USA [3].
- The common dislike for a food may reveal a latent digestive allergy and should be taken into consideration when examining the asthmatic patient.
- Intolerance to additives and potential adverse reactions to contaminants, such as penicillin, or dietetic substances, such as ammonium benzoic sulfimide, should be observed in well-developed countries.

38.2 Diagnosis of Food Allergy in Asthma

The diagnosis of food allergy in asthma varies according to different authors, but can be summarized (Fig. 38.1).

It should be pointed out that a thorough history often suggests a FA, but rarely makes possible the diagnosis of a specific food allergy [13, 24].

As far as IgE-dependent FA is concerned, a preliminary screening by skin tests is easily performed, not expensive and reasonably reliable. Pricks are specific but rarely positive, and intradermal tests are needed, though the specificity is feeble [4]. The suspicion of specific IgE should then be confirmed by RAST, HBDT, or histamine release [3, 11, 12]. If positive, these tests should be followed with challenges either by inhalation or, more commonly, by oral route with native foods, or with dried extracts in opaque capsules, making possible double-blind challenges [3, 9, 11]. The use of both tests (inhalation or oral route) is recommended, since the significance is different: A positive inhalation test evidences the local sensitization of bronchial mucosal mast cells. A positive oral challenge gives clear indication that food may be incriminated in the course of asthma [13]. Questionable challenges need to be repeated after about two weeks of avoidance [12]. The latter challenge performs an antigenic clearance and the organism is made more susceptible to the offending food.

In the case of persistent asthma, with negative skin tests to foods, the question of late onset FA is raised. According to Wraith the elimination of a food for several days is advisable, with serial measures of breathing tests (peak flow rate tests). A diagnosis trial is then realized by reintroducing the food, with or without oral sodium cromoglycate [24].

Whatever method is employed, it should include a careful study of the dietary record. This involves the labeling of foods and shows currently consumed additives which need to be tested.

When both methods fail, the introduction of a synthetic food (Vivonex) along with the successive reintroduction of the suspected foods can be tested.

38.3 Treatment

The treatment of FA undoubtedly lies in the strict avoidance of the offending foodstuff, or a diet free of additives [7]. Drugs which decrease the intestinal permeability by reducing histamine release from the mucosal mast cells, such as oral disodium cromoglycate and ketotifen, give favorable results and may be prescribed for a limited

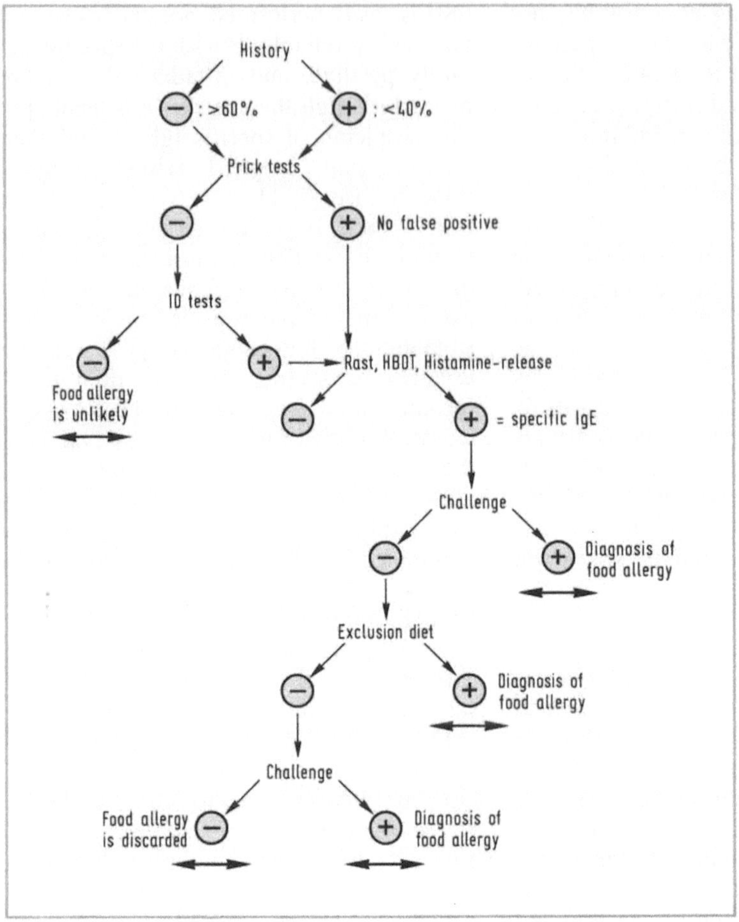

Fig. 38.1. The *decision tree* of IgE-dependent food allergy

duration (i.e., one month). Inhaled cromoglycate seems to be active in preventing asthma from additives and ingested cromoglycate has a better effect in IgE-dependent food allergy [24]. Rare cases of multiple food allergies present a difficult problem, for removal, even associated with disodium cromoglycate and antihistaminic drugs, fails to improve the breathing. Hyposensitization, which is only recommended in life-threatening anaphylaxis to foods, might be considered as a last resort.

References

1. Atkins FM, Steinberg SS, Metcalfe DD (1985) Evaluation of immediate adverse reactions to foods in adult patients. J Allergy Clin Immunol 75:356–363
2. Bjorksten F, Halnepuro L, Hannuksela M, Lahti A (1980) Extractions and properties of apple allergens. Allergy 350:671–677
3. Bock SA (1983) Food-related asthma and basic nutrition. J Asthma 20:377–381
4. Burr ML, Fehily AM, Stott NCH, Merrett TG (1985) Food-allergic asthma in general practice. Human Nutr Appl Nutr 39A:349–355
5. Cartier A, Malo JL, Forest F, Lafrance M, Pineau L (1984) Occupational asthma in snow-crab processing workers J Allergy Clin Immunol 74:261–269
6. Eriksson NE (1978) Food sensitivity reported by patients with asthma and hay fever. A relationship between food sensitivity and acetylsalicylic acid intolerance. Allergy 33:189–196
7. Freedman BJ (1977) Asthma induced by sulphur dioxide, benzoate and tartrazine contained in orange drinks. Clin Allergy 7:407–415

8. Ganderton MA (1978) Diet and asthma. Br Med J 1:1624
9. Girard JP, Gumowski P (1983) Contribution du test de provocation par inhalation au diagnostic de l'asthme bronchique d'origine alimentaire. Rev Fr Allergol 23:113–117
10. Hariparsad D, Wilson N, Dixon C, Silverman M (1984) Oral tartrazine challenge in childhood asthma: effect on bronchial reactivity. Clin Allergy 14:81–85
11. May CD (1976) Objectival clinic and laboratory studies of immediate hypersensibility reactions to food in asthmatic children. J Allergy Clin Immunol 58:500–515
12. Moneret-Vautrin DA, Andre CL (1983) Immunopathologie de l'allergie alimentaire et fausses allergies alimentaires. Masson, Paris
13. Moneret-Vautrin DA, Mohr N, Gérard H, Nicolas JP, Lacoste J, Grilliat JP (1986) Incidence de l'allergie alimentaire IgE-dépendante dans la maladie asthmatique. Méd Hyg 44:926–933
14. Nelson HS (1984) Gastroesophageal reflux and pulmonary disease. J Allergy Clin Immunol 73:547–556
15. Oehling A (1981) Importance of food allergy in childhood asthma. Respiration 42 [Suppl I]:44
16. Ortolani C, Pastorello E, Laraghi MT (1984) Diagnosis of intolerance to food additives. Ann Allergy 53:587–591
17. Palma-Carlos AG, Inacio F, Clode MH, Souza A (1985) Asthme par ingestion d'escargot. Allerg Immunol 17:5–6
18. Papageorgiou N, Lee TH, Nagakura T, Cromwell O, Wraith DG, Kay AB (1983) Neutrophil chemotactic activity in milk-induced asthma. J Allergy Clin Immunol 72:75–82
19. Pauli G, Peltre G, Bessot JC, Braun PF, David B (1984) Allergy to celery root coincident with mugwort pollen sensitivity. J Allergy Clin Immunol 73:114
20. Rowe AM (1972) Food allergy. Its manifestations and control, and the elimination diets: a compendium. Thomas, Springfield, p 687
21. Sheffer A, Austen KF (1980) Exercice induced anaphylaxis. J Allergy Clin Immunol 66:106–111
22. Stevenson DD, Simon RA (1981) Sensitivity to ingested metabisulfites in asthmatic subjects. J Allergy Clin Immunol 68:26–32
23. Wilson N, Silerman M (1985) Diagnosis of food sensitivity in childhood asthma. J R Soc Med 78:11–16
24. Wraigth DG (1987) Food-related asthma. In: Brostoff J, Challacombe SJ (eds) Food allergy and intolerance. Baillière Tindall, London, pp 486–497
25. Zanussi C (1982) Food allergy treatment. In: Brostoff J, Challacombe SJ (eds) Clinics in immunology and allergy. Food Allergy, vol. 2. Saunders, London, pp 221–240

39. Drug-induced Asthma

J. Bousquet, E. Fernandez, B. Guérin

Adverse reactions to drugs are increasing in number and represent a major cause of disease. About 30% of patients in hospitals present an adverse reaction to one or several drugs. Drug hypersensitivity or allergy is only observed in 5 to 30% of patients who suffer from iatrogenic disease, but the allergic reactions are the most severe and a fatal outcome is not exceptional. Drugs or drug additives have the potential to induce asthma by many mechanisms, among which allergy and idiosyncrasy are the most common and well-known, but other possible mechanisms have been observed. Some drugs generally produce one type of reaction, but others can trigger a number of effects [1, 21, 29, 32, 40].

39.1 Allergic Reactions

Mechanisms: IgE-mediated mechanisms are the most common and cause anaphylactic symptoms. Other types of immune reactions may be also observed but they are rarely seen in asthma. Few drugs are complete antigens [10, 27, 37, 38, 42] which can mount an immune response and trigger the activation of basophils and mast cells [33]. Often, drugs act as chemically reactive haptens [5, 30, 31] which link to human proteins (free or cell-bound) and become antigenic and allergenic and the complex may be either a metabolic derivative or the native molecule itself which is the antigenic determinant [43].

Symptoms: Inhaled drugs usually cause a bronchial obstruction which may be severe, whereas drugs administered by other routes can lead to an isolated asthma attack or systemic anaphylaxis in which asthma is only a part of the reaction. Bronchial obstruction usually may be a prominent feature of systemic anaphylaxis, but laryngeal edema seems to be more common and severe. In many instances, a minor asthmatic reaction is the first symptom that reveals drug allergy and is often undiagnosed, with a subsequent life-threatening reaction. It is therefore extremely important to recognize the early and minor symptoms of drug allergy as the bronchial obstruction induced by a drug allergy may be extremely severe and can be complete and irreversible within 1 to 3 min.

Diagnosis: Drug allergic reaction as a cause of asthma may be difficult to diagnose since all drugs are putative elicitors, patients usually take more than one drug, the allergic reaction is clinically undistinguishable from an idiosyncratic one and drug additives may also be involved. There are, however, some clinical criteria for drug allergy which may help in the diagnosis (Table 39.1).

When a drug is incriminated, as always in allergy, it is desirable to skin test the patient with the drug itself or with special extracts made for the purpose. Skin tests can be dangerous and fatal reactions have occurred while they are being made, so it is always necessary to start cautiously with a prick test and if it is negative to continue with intradermal tests. For a very few drugs, such as penicillin (penkit®), allergen extracts have been prepared to reduce the number of potential systemic reactions and to increase the efficiency of the diagnosis. For penicillin allergy, allergy to proteins and in some cases such as myorelaxants, skin tests are valuable. In penicillin allergy [2, 37, 39] it has been observed that patients who previously reacted with the drug but who had a negative skin test could, in the vast majority, tolerate the drug when it was readministered. For other drugs, except for nonspecific mast cell activators, a positive skin test is in favor of drug allergy, but a

Table 39.1. Clinical criteria for drug allergy. [According to 40, modified]

1. Allergic reactions occur in only a minority of patients receiving the drug.
2. The observed manifestations do not resemble the pharmacological action of the drug nor its toxic effects.
3. The reaction may conform to manifestations generally accepted as allergic, but may not be.
4. A required induction period, commonly 7 to 10 days, upon exposure to the drug. Some hidden drugs are present in foods and may sensitize the patient so that the reaction may appear on "first" exposure.
5. The reaction may be reproduced by other agents possessing similar and cross-reactive chemical structures.
6. The reaction may be reproduced even by minute amounts of the drug.
7. The reaction should resolve after the drug has been discontinued.
8. Blood and/or tissue eosinophilia may be present.
9. Raised serum total IgE levels may be present in nonatopic and atopic individuals.

negative skin test cannot eliminate its absence since the allergenic determinant may be a hapten or a non-cross-reactive metabolite.

Bronchial challenges can be performed if an inhaled drug is suspected, but should be done carefully since they are potentially harmful.

In vitro tests may help in the diagnosis of an IgE-mediated drug allergy but RAST discs are not easy to prepare by means of the cyanogen bromide method since the reactive determinants of the drugs are seldom suitable for the coupling procedure, as they do not contain the necessary amino groups. Human serum albumin may be used as a carrier protein in the coupling procedure and many drugs can be bound to RAST discs. However, this method is relatively difficult. Polystyrene is also available for coupling drugs and might be an alternative (chymo-FAST) but more studies are required for its final evaluation. At present, only penicillin and insulin-specific IgE [14] can be titrated easily. Another pitfall is represented by the isotype of the immunoglobulins specific to the drugs as IgG may be more important in some reactions than IgE. Other in vitro tests include basophil degranulation, histamine release, lymphocyte transformation tests and other tests of delayed-type hypersensitivity. None of these tests used routinely was shown to correlate significantly with drug-allergic reactions, whereas when used as a research tool they sometimes proved to be extremely valuable.

Drugs commonly involved in allergic reactions: Any drug that can cause IgE-mediated allergy can be responsible for a bronchial obstruction (Tab. 39.2).

Many drugs administered by the aerosol route or by the inhalation of a powder are potent sensitizers. These include enzymes and macromolecular components such as pituitary snuffs and antibiotics. In other cases, the true cause of an allergic reaction has to be demonstrated or may be lacking (quinine, quinidine). The most common effects of inhaled sodium cromoglycate are throat irritation, hoarseness, cough and transient bronchospasm, which are not allergic but potentially life-threatening reactions have been exceptionally reported and include anaphylaxis and bronchial obstruction [7, 26, 35].

39.2 Nonallergic Reactions

Many drugs acting through various mechanisms may elicit an anaphylactoid reaction which mimics anaphylaxis but that is not allergic in origin. Moreover, some drugs may induce a bronchial obstruction by acting directly on the bronchial cells.

Aspirin and related drugs: Aspirin and other cyclooxygenase inhibitors, such as nonsteroidal anti-inflammatory drugs, interfere in the metabolism of the arachidonic acid and in susceptible individuals cause a variety of untoward reactions including severe asthma.

Drugs activating basophils and mast cells nonspecifically: The activation of basophils and mast cells through nonimmunological mechanisms has been known for a long time. These drugs were usually classified as nonspecific histamine release compounds,

Table 39.2. Adverse effects of drugs on asthma (only drugs commonly involved are listed)

Drugs	Allergy		Mast cell activation	Autonomic nervous system	Pulmonary infiltrates	Other mechanisms
	IgE	Other				
Diabetes						
Insulin	++					
Chlorpropamide					+	
Dyes and additives						
Parabens	+					
Sulfites	?		?			Idiopathic
Azo dyes	+		?			arachidonic
Ethylene diamine	+	IV				acid?
Other dyes	+					
Enzymes						
Trypsin (inhaled)	+					
Chymopapain	+++					
Other enzymes	+					
Hemodialysis						
Ethylene oxide	++					
Formaldehyde	++		?			
Phthalates	++					
Hormones						
Pituitary stuff	+					
ACTH	++		+			
Other proteins	+					
Neurology						
Opiates			++			
Meprobamate	+					
Methyldopa				+		
Carbamazepine					+	
Imipramines					+	
Diazepam	+					
Parasympathomimetics						
Neostigmine				+		
Radiographic contrast media			+			Complement activation
Rheumatology						
Gold salts	?				+	
Colchicine	+					
Probenecid	+					
Vaccines						
Tetanus toxoid	+					
Egg-containing vaccines (viral)	+					
Vitamins						
Folic acid	+					
Thiamine	+					
B_{12}	+					
Others						
Deferoxamine						
Allergy-asthma						
Allergens	+++					
Cromolyn	+		?		+	
Antihistamine						?
Acetylcysteine						Irritation
Beclomethasone						

Table 39.2. (continued)

Drugs	Allergy		Mast cell activation	Autonomic nervous system	Pulmonary infiltrates	Other mechanisms
	IgE	Other				
Anesthetics						
Tubocurarin	+ +		+	?		
Succinylcholine	+ + +		+	+		
Althesin	+					
Halothane	+					
Ethyl ether	+					
Dextran	+					
Dantrolene	+					
Gallamine	+					
Thiopental	+					
Mephenesins					+	
Antimicrobials[a]						
β-lactams	+ + +	III			+	
Nitrofurantoin	+				+ + +	
Polymyxin	+			+ +		
Sulfonamides	+	III			+	
Aminosalicylic acid	+				+	
All others	+					
Anti-inflammatory						
Aspirin	?					Inhibition of cyclooxygenase
Indomethacin						
Glafenin	+				+	
Aminopyrine	+					
Antiparasitic[a]						
Bithionol	+					
Diethylcarbamazine	+					
Quinine	+					Idiopathic
Trivalent antimonial agents	+					
Pentamidine	?		+			
Stilbamidine			+			
Antiserum						
Antitoxins (animal)	+	III				
Antilymphocyte	+	III				
Cardiology						
Propanolol				β		
Timoptol[b]				blockade		
Reserpine				+		
Hydralazine			+			
Dipyramidole						Adenosine agonist
Heparin		+				+
Mecamylamine					+	
Mercurial diuretic	+					
Hydrochlorothiazide					+	
Cytostatics						
Cisplatin	+					
Cyclophosphamide	+					
Cytosine arabinoside	+					
Daunorubicin			+			
Methotrexate	?					Complement

[a] Common drugs involved, for review of all drugs involved in anaphylaxis see Sullivan [38]
[b] β-adrenoreceptor antagonist used in ophthalmology
I and IV: classification of Gell and Coombs

but recent data on mast cell activation has shown that histamine was only one of the released mediators in most instances. Several mechanisms may explain this reaction: Some compounds such as compound 48/80 produce histamine release by a primary pharmacological action, others may be cytotoxic, or directly activate complement leading to the generation of anaphylatoxin, others act on the displacement of histamine in the granule and others may directly activate the cell. In addition, basophils and mast cells may not respond identically to these agents. Finally, to increase the complexity still further, some of these drugs can also elicit an IgE-mediated allergic reaction (myorelaxants, ACTH) [3, 4, 9, 41].

Some patients such as those who have a systemic mastocytosis or an increased number of mast cells have a greater susceptibility to these agents, and are especially prone to experience anaphylactoid reactions or asthma. Asthmatics who have a nonspecific bronchial hyperreactivity may also develop symptoms when these drugs are inhaled.

Among the drugs able to trigger mast cells, polymyxin, colistin, the ACTH tetracosapeptide, iodinated radiocontrast media, morphine, codeine, myorelaxants, deferoxamine, pentamidine and stilbamidine or trimethaphan are the most widely recognized [6, 15].

Diagnosis of these reactions is often difficult as skin tests are of little value since many subjects can have a wheal and flare reaction with these drugs. Bronchial challenges are of interest when they are positive but this is not always the case. In vitro tests are of little or no value at all.

Adenosine agonists: Adenosine is a naturally occurring purine nucleotide involved in the synthesis of CAMP. In normal subjects adenosine seems to have no effect on airway caliber though in asthmatics this nucleoside was shown to be a bronchoconstrictor mediator [18]. Some drugs, such as dipyridamole, are adenosine agonists and they were shown to elicit a bronchial obstruction in some patients [personal observation].

β-adrenoreceptors blocking agents: β-blockers are widely used throughout the world. The first compounds that were synthesized did not have a cardiac selectivity (β_1- and β_2-antagonism). As a consequence, severe asthmatic reactions were observed with practolol and propanolol administered to asthmatic subjects [8, 19, 44, 45]. Eye drops of timoptol also induced severe asthmatic reactions in susceptible individuals [25]. Newly developed drugs are not totally safe in all asthmatics but they may be tested in subjects suffering from hypertension or coronary insufficiency. When they cannot be used they may be replaced by calcium antagonists.

Other drugs interfering with the autonomic nervous system: Asthma is a recognized side effect with anticholinesterase drugs, α-adrenergic agonists, cholinergic agonists or reserpine [17].

Antihistamines: The exact role of antihistamine in asthma is difficult to determine. It appears that some anti-H_1-antagonists such as astemisole or clemastine [28] are able to cause a bronchodilatation although in some children anti-H_1-antagonists were found to elicit a bronchoconstrictive response [34]. The effects of anti-H_2-antagonists are even more unclear.

39.3 Drug-induced Eosinophilic Lung Disease

Two different patterns of pulmonary eosinophilia occur in response to drug therapy: a Loeffler-like syndrome caused by a variety of drugs and a diffuse reticular syndrome elicited by nitrofurantoin [11].

Loeffler-like syndrome: Many drugs can cause the transient nonsegmental peripheral consolidation characteristic of the Loeffler's syndrome [12, 13]. An allergic mechanism may be postulated although it has been rarely documented. Asthma is a common symptom occurring during the pulmonary infiltrates. A list of the drugs involved is given in Table 39.2.

Nitrofurantoin-induced eosinophilic lung disease: Nitrofurantoin produces acute changes in the lung with fever, cough, diffuse pulmonary infiltration, asthma or other patterns. More sustained exposure leads to chronic pulmonary fibrosis. An allergic etiology is suggested by the frequent presence of eosinophils, rash and rapid recurrence of symptoms after challenge with the drug [24, 29]. From many immunological studies it appears that nitrofurantoin is immunogenic and that cellular or less likely humoral immunity is involved in acute clinical reactions to the drug [29].

39.4 Drug Additives

Additives are widely employed in the pharmaceutical industry. Some dyes and preservatives have been implicated in asthma or anaphylactoid reactions, but most of the agents used appear to be harmless [20].

Tartrazine, an azo dye, has been shown to elicit asthma by an idiosyncratic mechanism still poorly understood. IgE to tartrazine has been found but its exact relevance has to be demonstrated [16]. It was suggested without real proof that aspirin-intolerant patients may be prone to develop a reaction to this azo dye [20] but conflicting results have been produced. Reactions to azo dyes other than tartrazine and non-azo dyes are far less common [36].

Parabens are aliphatic esters of parahydrobenzoic acid cross-reacting with sodium benzoate. They are common sensitizers in contact allergic dermatitis but they can also mount an IgE immune response and there are three reports in the literature concerning anaphylaxis to parabens used with local anesthetics [36].

Metabisulfites are known to induce severe life-threatening asthmatic reactions when they are ingested as a food preservative [36]. It has also been shown that sulfites present in drugs can cause a bronchial obstruction. Among the drugs that contain sulfites are some bronchodilators such as isoetharine [22]. Asthma reactions occurred either with drugs administered by inhalation or by parenteral route. The mechanisms underlying these reactions seem to be nonallergic in nature.

Ethylene diamine is also able to induce asthma by an allergic mechanism [23].

39.5 Treatment

The treatment of the anaphylactic or anaphylactoid reaction often requires epinephrine and/or the adequate correction of the bronchial obstruction. If the drug is absolutely necessary to the patient a specific desensitization may be attempted with either an allergic drug such as penicillin or insulin, or with a drug that elicits an idiosyncratic reaction, such as aspirin or deferoxamine.

References

1. Adkinson NF Jr (1984) Risk factors for drug allergy. J Allergy Clin Immunol 74:567–572
2. Adkinson NF Jr, Thompson WL, Maddrey WC, Lichtenstein LM (1971) Routine use of penicillin skin testing on an impatient service. N Engl J Med 285:22–36
3. Assem ESK (1983) Neuromuscular blocking drugs. In: de Weck AL, Bundgaard H (eds) Allergic reactions to drugs. Springer, Berlin Heidelberg New York Tokyo, pp 299–312
4. Bataille A, Kienlen J, Vergnenègre A, Skassa-Brociek W, Bousquet J (1986) Allergie aux anesthésiques généraux. Rev Fr Allergol (in press)
5. Bousquet J, Rivory JP, Maurice F et al (in press) Double-blind intravenous challenges with formaldehyde in patients undergoing chronic hemodialysis. Clin Allergy
6. Bousquet J, Navarro M, Robert G, Aye P, Michel FB (1983) Rapid desensitization to deferoxamine. Lancet II:859–860
7. Brown LA, Kaplan RA, Benjamin PA, Hoffman LS, Shaerer WT (1981) Immunoglobulin E-mediated anaphylaxis with inhaled cromolyn sodium. J Allergy Clin Immunol 68:416–420
8. Carlson C, Järvinen KAJ (1978) Comparison of the effect of the beta 1-blocking drugs atenolol and metoprolol on bronchial asthma. Allergy 33:147–151
9. Charpin J, Aubert J, Boutin C (1967) The allergenic properties of the newer adrenocorticotrophic hormones. Acta Allergologica 22:297–298
10. Fireman P, Fineberg SE, Galloway JA (1982) Development of IgE antibodies to human (recombinant DNA), porcine and bovine insulins in diabetic subjects. Diabetes Care 5:119–125
11. Fraser RG, Paré JAP (1981) Eosinophilic lung disease of specific etiology. In: Fraser RG, Paré JAP (eds) Diagnosis of Diseases of the Chest. Saunders, Philadelphia, pp 906–911

12. Friedman H, Tworag FJ, Voss HE, Codeman M (1978) Eosinophilic pneumonia in association with the use of beclomethasone dipropionate aerosol. J Allergy Clin Immunol 61:150–159
13. Gheysens B, van Miedghen W (1984) Pulmonary infiltrates with eosinophilia due to glafenine. Eur J Respir Dis 65:456–459
14. Grammer LC, Patterson R (1984) Proteins: chymopapain and insulin. J Allergy Clin Immunol 74:635–640
15. Greenberger PA (1984) Contrast media reactions. J Allergy Clin Immunol 74:600–605
16. Guérin B, Brighton WD, Girard P (1985) Allergy to dyes. J Allergy Clin Immunol 75:107
17. Harries MG, Newman Taylor A, Wooden J, McAuslan A (1979) Bronchial asthma due to alpha-methyl dopa. Br Med J 1:1461
18. Holgate ST, Mann JS, Cushley MJ (1984) Adenosine as a bronchoconstrictor mediator in asthma and its antagonism by methylxanthines. J Allergy Clin Immunol 74:302–306
19. Jacobs RL, Rake GN, Fournier DC et al (1981) Potentiated anaphylaxis in patients with drug-induced beta-adrenergic blockade. J Allergy Clin Immunol 68:125–127
20. Juhlin L (1983) Intolerance to food and drug additives. In: de Weck AL, Bundgaard H (eds) Allergic reactions to drugs. Springer, Berlin Heidelberg New York Tokyo, pp 639–656
21. Kilburn K (1981) Pulmonary diseases induced by drugs. In: Fishman AP (ed) Pulmonary diseases and disorders. McGraw-Hill, New York, pp 707–724
22. Koepke JN, Selner JC, Dunhill AL (1983) SO_2 derived from bronchodilator solutions. J Allergy Clin Immunol 71:147
23. Lam S, Chan-Yeung M (1980) Ethylenediamine-induced asthma. Am Rev Respir Dis 121:151–155
24. Lebecque F, Mairesse M (1983) Pneumopathie à la nitrofurantoïne. Poumon Coeur 39:101–111
25. Lockey SD Sr (1981) Bronchospasm precipitated by ophthalmic instillations of timolol. Ann Allergy 46:267–270
26. Menon MPS, Das AK (1977) Asthma and urticaria during disodium cromoglycate treatment. Scand J Respir Dis 58:145–152
27. Newfield P, Roizen MF (1979) Hazards of rapid administration of vancomycin. Ann Intern Med 91:581
28. Nogrady SG, Hartley JPR, Handslip PDJ, Hurst NP (1978) Bronchodilatation after inhalation of the antihistamine clemastine. Thorax 33:479
29. Parker CW (1980) Drug allergy. In: Parker CW (ed) Clinical Immunology. Saunders, Philadelphia, pp 1219–1260
30. Pepys J (1984) Allergy of the respiratory tract to low molecular weight chemical agents. Clin Immunol Allergol: 163–186
31. Rivory JP, Maurice F, Larsson P, Johansson SGO, Bousquet J (1985) Anaphylactic shock with formaldehyde. J Allergy Clin Immunol 75:209
32. Rosenow EC III (1972) The spectrum of drug induced pulmonary disease. Ann Intern Med 77:977–991
33. Schneider CH (1983) Immunochemical basis of allergic reactions to drugs. In: de Weck AL, Bundgaard H (eds) Allergic reactions to drugs. Springer, Berlin Heidelberg New York Tokyo, pp 3–36
34. Schuller DE (1983) Adverse effects of bromptpheuniramine on pulmonary function in a subset of asthmatic children. J Allergy Clin Immunol 72:175–179
35. Sheffer AL, Rocklin RE, Goetzl EJ (1975) Immunologic components of hypersensitivity reactions to cromolyn sodium. N Engl J Med 293:1220–1225
36. Simon RA (1984) Adverse reactions to drug additives. J Allergy Clin Immunol 74:623–630
37. Sogn DD (1984) Penicillin allergy. J Allergy Clin Immunol 74:589–593
38. Sullivan TJ (1984) Allergic reactions to antimicrobial agents: A review of reactions to drugs not in the beta-lactam antibiotic class. J Allergy Clin Immunol 74:594–599
39. Sullivan TJ, Wedner HJ, Shatz GS, Jecies LD, Parker CN (1981) Skin testing to detect penicillin allergy. J Allergy Clin Immunol 68:171–180
40. de Swarte RD (1980) Drug Allergy. In: Patterson R (ed) Allergic Diseases – Diagnosis and Management, 2nd edn. Lippincott, Philadelphia, pp 452–583
41. Vervloet D, Nizanskowska E, Arnaud A, Senft M, Alazia M, Charpin J (1983) Adverse reactions to suxamethonium and other muscle relaxants under general anesthesia. J Allergy Clin Immunol 71:552–559
42. de Weck AL (1962) Studies on penicillin hypersensitivity. Int Arch Allergy 21:20–31
43. de Weck AL (1983) Immunopathological mechanisms and clinical aspects of allergic reactions to drugs. In: de Weck AL, Bundgaard H (eds) Allergic reactions to drugs. Springer, Berlin Heidelberg New York Tokyo, pp 75–135
44. de Weck AL (1983) Prevention and treatment of drug allergy. In: de Weck AL, Bundgaard H (eds) Allergic reactions to drugs. Springer, Berlin Heidelberg New York Tokyo, pp 227–242
45. Williams IP, Millard FJC (1980) Severe asthma after inadvertent ingestion of oxprenolol. Thorax 35:160

H. Clinical Features and Diagnosis in Children and Adults

40. Clinical Aspects of Asthma

P. S. Norman

Definitions of asthma are usually stated in terms that emphasize repeated short-term variations in resistance to airflow in the intrapulmonary airways. The clinical diagnosis of asthma is ordinarily not difficult from history and physical examination, as the history of recurrent attacks of wheezing and shortness of breath with relative freedom from respiratory difficulty between attacks and the finding of inspiratory and expiratory wheezes and relative hyperinflation of the chest during episodes are characteristic. It is, however, valuable to document changes in pulmonary function by objective measurement and, furthermore, occasional patients will present either with severely impaired function or conversely with completely normal function and it becomes necessary to resort to some maneuver to bring out the variability in airflow. Cockcroft (see Chapter 47) reviewed pulmonary function tests and pointed out that FEV_1 (forced expiratory volume in one second) and PFR (peak flow rate) are the most easily performed and sensitive tests. The ease of use allows repeated tests to be performed and thus to demonstrate the variability in airways resistance over time. At the same time the severity of the disease may be monitored.

When ventilatory function is impaired, the responsiveness to bronchodilator drugs may be tested and Cockcroft discussed the difficulty in measuring and defining a significant response. On the other hand, in the patient with normal pulmonary function but a history of attacks of dyspnea, it becomes useful to demonstrate hyperreactivity of airways to chemical or physical stimuli. Exposure to methacholine is most often used in this regard. Airways hyperresponsiveness, however, is subject to change (sometimes in seasonal allergic patients it disappears between seasons) and may be present in hay fever patients without asthma.

Lung function tests and several tests to demonstrate bronchial responsiveness are discussed by Wahn (see Chapter 42) who also recommends that a peak flowmeter be used at home and the PFR be recorded over several days or weeks. Scheinmann and Paupe (see Chapter 41) pointed out that the list of disorders which must be differentiated from asthma in childhood is long, but that bronchiolitis obliterans as a sequela of viral pneumonia is often confused with asthma. The dyspneic bouts in this disease differ from asthmatic attacks by their constant bacterial superinfection, the poor efficacy of bronchodilators and corticosteroids, and the presence of fixed peripheral atelectasis or obstructive emphysema. Bronchiectasis and cystic fibrosis lead to digital clubbing much more often than chronic asthma. All children with chronic respiratory disorders or nasal polyps should have a sweat test for cystic fibrosis. Ménardo and colleagues (see Chapter 45) also mentioned foreign bodies in the bronchi as a cause of wheezing dyspnea in attacks particularly when obstruction is not greatly improved by sufficient bronchodilator treatment. At times, symptoms do not arise immediately after aspiration and may have a latent period of months or years. Severe or fixed *asthma* calls for a bronchoscopy especially when there are radiographic abnormalities. Vascular rings constricting the trachea, hyperventilation syndrome and extrinsic allergic alveolitis are also mentioned as possibilities for *asthmatic attacks.* The point is made that two thirds of patients with α_1-antitrypsin deficiency are also atopic. This diagnosis is easy to make by laboratory test once it is suspected.

The laboratory tests necessary for evaluation of an asthmatic child is the topic of discussion by several authors. Although the point is made that an extensive laboratory evaluation is not ordinarily called for, certain tests are important to rule out other disease and to decide on the proper treatment. Wahn (see Chapter 42) indicated that complete blood counts should be done and a chest x-ray is essential to look for not only other conditions such as mentioned above, but also complications of asthma such as atelectasis, pneumothorax, and pneumomediastinum. X-rays of the paranasal sinuses are needed in patients with chronic or recurrent headache or nasal disease. A sweat chloride should be performed, as 20% of cystic fibrosis patients may have respiratory allergy. Lung function tests have also been mentioned. Finally, an evaluation for allergy is essential and requires not only a history and an examination for allergic stigmata such as allergic *shiners,* an allergic crease of the nose, acute or chronic otitis media, and atopic dermatitis, but also objective tests for allergic sensitivities.

Skin tests are most often chosen for this purpose and several techniques are described by Ménardo and colleagues (see Chapter 45). Intradermal tests are the most sensitive and should not be performed with solutions stronger that 1–1,000 wt/volume to avoid false positive reactions. Systemic reactions may occur in highly allergic children if concentrations less than 1–1,000 are not used for the first test with potent allergens. Prick tests are more frequently used in children and are quite safe. Recently introduced standardized devices for pricking the skin (Morrow-Brown needle, Stallerpointe, Allergy-Pricker, MULTI-TEST) improve reproducibility. Solutions preserved by 50% glycerol diminish the risk of false negative reactions due to loss of allergenic potency. When a prick test is negative with a strongly suspected allergen, an intradermal test with a 1–1,000 wt/volume may safely be performed. It is also useful to measure the response and several techniques are described. Negative controls with diluent alone are important and a positive control with histamine, 48/80, or codeine is also useful.

Adkinson (see Chapter 46) discussed the diagnostic value of serum determinations of IgE and IgE antibodies. Patients with allergic disease have higher levels of serum-IgE than nonatopic controls and levels can be especially high in individuals with eczema. Nevertheless, there is considerable overlap between atopic and nonatopic people in the range of 20–100 IU/ml so that total IgE is often not diagnostic. Furthermore, a number of nonallergic disorders are associated with increased IgE production. These include Wiskott-Aldrich syndrome, the hyper-IgE syndrome, Hodgkin's lymphoma, helminthic infections, drug-induced interstitial nephritis, idiopathic nephrotic syndrome, bullous pemphigoid, chronic nonatopic dermatoses, acute and chronic liver disease, cystic fibrosis and allergic bronchopulmonary aspergillosis.

Specific serum-IgE antibody assays by RAST and other methods are reliable and reproducible when properly performed and give semiquantitative or quantitative information depending on technique. Adkinson (see Chapter 46) compared them with skin tests and pointed out that skin tests give immediate answers and when done intradermally are more sensitive. Serum assays have a special use when skin testing cannot be interpreted because of dermatitis or the use of interfering drugs which cannot be withdrawn. When RAST and skin test are compared using identical allergens, the agreement between the *in vitro* and the *in vivo* tests is excellent. Choice between the methods depends more on convenience and price than any intrinsic advantage of one over the other.

A potential alternative is a basophil degranulation test performed with the patient's own cells. This test is described by Leynadier who has found good agreement with skin tests when *Dermatophagoides pteronyssinus* was the allergen. Concordance with RAST employing multiallergenic slides was about 65%. The technique appears less time consuming than in vitro histamine release studies.

Direct bronchial challenge might be considered the ultimate test as it should represent a laboratory reproduction of the disease. Spector (see Chapter 48) stated that it has been employed when there was insufficient information or discrepancies between history and skin tests or in vitro test results. He has found good agreement between skin tests and bronchial inhalation challenge with the same antigens. Only 4%

of his subjects tested had a positive bronchial inhalation challenge despite a negative skin test. Inhalation challenges can cause severe or prolonged asthmatic attacks, so that stepwise increases in antigen concentration, so as not to exceed clinically meaningful concentrations, are mandatory. Spector has never observed a permanent decrement in lung function. Ordinarily, bronchial challenges with allergens will not be necessary and need not be a routine office procedure. Challenges with methacholine, histamine, exercise or cold air, on the other hand, may be useful to demonstrate bronchial reactivity and can be adapted to office practice.

Bronchial challenge is useful as a research tool in the identification of new allergens, evaluation of blocking agents, and new treatments. In the patient with a negative response it may be useful in convincing him that a suspected allergen is not responsible for his symptoms.

Some complications of asthma occur with a sufficient frequency in children, so that every physician who deals with the condition should be aware of them. These complications are listed by Ménardo and colleagues (see Chapter 45). Pneumomediastinum occurred in 15% of children older than 10 in one survey. On the other hand, this complication was very rare in children under 2 presumably because infants are unable to generate high intrathoracic pressures. Pneumothorax is rarer than pneumomediastinum (1.1 to 2.6% of children hospitalized for asthma) but should be suspected when there is a rapid deterioration of the patient's condition accompanied by increasing dyspnea. Chest pain is often present. Atelectasis is quite common in children (10.6–16.6% of hospitalized asthmatics) and perhaps can be explained by the small number of alveolar pores before the age of seven. Allergic bronchopulmonary aspergillosis is rare in childhood, but must be considered when progressive fatigue and weight loss develops, particularly in the presence of high total IgE titers or large numbers of eosinophils or pulmonary infiltrates. Arterial oxygen desaturation during sleep may be experienced by children when their asthma is unstable. The mean decrease is usually modest but sometimes may be ominous and require supplemental oxygen during sleep. The problem improves as daytime pulmonary function improves.

Inappropriate secretion of antidiuretic hormone can occur in children with acute bronchial asthma and complicate fluid therapy to promote fluid secretions which can be raised more easily. Postasthmatic pseudo polio (Hopkins syndrome) is an uncommon entity characterized by paralysis of an arm or a leg about 5 days after an attack and is preceded by pain in the affected limb. Residual weakness and muscle wasting are usual. In addition to cough syncope, seizures occur rarely in children during asthma attacks. Hypoxia, electrolyte disturbances and theophylline toxicity are possible causes of this problem.

Status asthmaticus and respiratory failure are the most familiar and feared of the complications. Its treatment is better regarded as prevention. In children who seem prone to recurrent status asthmaticus prompt and vigorous treatment of the attack early in its generation should prevent dangerous deterioration of the situation. This emphasizes that training programs for asthmatic children and their parents are a necessity.

41. Asthma in Childhood

P. Scheinmann, J. Paupe

Asthma is the most common of all chronic childhood diseases. It is frequently underdiagnosed and undertreated [1]. Early diagnosis and accurate assessment of the severity of asthma are necessary to minimize its physical, psychological and socioeconomic consequences both in childhood and in adulthood.

This chapter will emphasize some aspects of childhood asthma which daily experience shows to be essential for its management, yet which are frequently misunderstood and/or neglected (Table 41.1).

Table 41.1. Asthma history

Asthmatic attacks	
Rhythm (seasonal or perennial asthma)	
Frequency and duration	
Previous treatments (nature and efficacy)	
Number of emergency hospitalizations	
Prodromal phase	
Precipitating factors	
Inhalant allergens (house dust, pollens, animal danders, molds)	
Exercise (free running)	
Viral infections	
Changes in weather, climate and residence	
Emotional stress	
Irritant (cigarette smoking)	
Foods (and additives), drugs (aspirin and non-steroidal anti-inflammatory agents)	
Individual factors	
Symptoms having heralded overt asthma	
Recurrent rhinitis, otitis media, croup, bronchiolitis	
Atopic dermatitis	
Family history of atopic disease	
Impact of asthma	
On child:	Restriction of physical activities and school attendance, physical and emotional disturbances
On family:	Disturbed family relationships
Cooperation with the patient and family	

41.1 Clinical Patterns

Asthmatic attacks: Acute asthmatic attacks are the main reason for seeking medical advice. Some attacks have an abrupt onset. Generally, frank nocturnal dyspnea, with tachypnea and sometimes low-grade fever in younger children, develops more gradually. Cough is frequent and may induce vomiting. Wheezing, like dyspnea, predominates during expiration.

Little information is essential before initiating treatment at the time of an acute attack: the apparent precipitating factor, the duration of dyspnea, the amount and effect of drugs already administered and the outcome of previous episodes.

With immediate therapy mild asthmatic attacks show definite improvement within two hours. Yet all attacks must be closely watched. Patients at higher risk of acute respiratory failure are children under 5 years and those with severe asthma and/or a history of status asthmaticus. Ominous symptoms include a poor response to treatment, cyanosis, diminished breath sounds in spite of marked respiratory effort with use of accessory respiratory muscles, pulsus paradoxus $\geqq 20$ mmHg, appearance of weariness and altered state of consciousness. Hospitalization is required for immediate laboratory investigations (particularly blood gases determination) and intensive treatment.

Assessment of the asthmatic child: After reversal of acute bronchial obstruction, particularly if there is a history of previous episodes, a confident and prolonged physician-patient family relationship must be developed. The keystone of successful management of asthma is its clinical history [2].

History: The main factors involved in proper management of asthma are summarized in Table 41.1. Some of them deserve further comment.

As asthmatic attacks constitute the most troublesome event in the child's life, great attention should be paid to triggering factors. They can vary with age (for example virus-induced attacks are more frequent in early than in later childhood). They vary from one child to another. Some triggering factors are overlooked although they regularly precipitate attacks in many asthmatic children. These include long trips, or returning home after hospitalization or residential schooling and reopening of school. With preventive intensification of treatment numerous attacks would not occur.

A key element of the history is the recognition of the prodromal phase (most often rhinitis or cough) which precedes the overt attack by a few hours or days and is the optimal moment for adjusting treatment. Teaching a family to detect and to cope with early worsening of respiratory status decreases the number and severity of asthmatic attacks and is essential in building self-confidence in the child and family [3].

Classification of asthma: Defining the grade of asthma is often easy and is essential for tailoring treatment to the needs of each individual child.

Most children, at least 75%, have a mild or moderate form of asthma with infrequent attacks and normal interim pulmonary function. In contrast, severe asthma is generally characterized, from its onset, by frequent and distressing attacks with a varying degree of corticosteroid dependence.

However the diagnosis of severe asthma may be questioned in a family with a history of mild or quiescent asthma. It should be remembered that wheezing may represent only the tip of an iceberg and that significant airway obstruction and hyperinflation may persist after obvious signs of asthma have cleared. The failure of self-assessment of asthma emphasizes the value of objective signs: barrel-chest deformity correlated with roentgenologic hyperinflation, air trapping with diminished diaphragmatic excursion and persistent hyperinflation at repeated pulmonary function studies during symptom-free intervals [4].

Much time and skill will be required of the medical team for maximum prevention of the major complications of severe asthma. In practice, only severe asthma can lead to status asthmaticus or even death. These accidents can frequently be prevented by early recognition and treatment. Regular home measurements of PEFR may prove very helpful.

When the child reaches adulthood, height can be expected to be normal [5] except in those who received continual and excessive corticosteroid treatment.

Previous school absenteeism can have disastrous consequences when the individual enters the labor market.

Finally, numerous factors (especially associated persistent atopic dermatitis) seem to predispose to chronic asthma in adulthood, the most important of which is the severity of asthma at its onset [6].

Equivalents of asthma: Chronic cough may be the main manifestation of asthma. It is poorly responsive to antitussive and anti-infectious drugs as well as to adenoidectomy and tonsillectomy (which sometimes seem to precipitate overt asthma). Chronic nocturnal cough thus remains distressing for most parents. Diagnosis is facilitated by the presence of an atopic background, an increased airway reactivity and the efficacy of bronchodilators and/or immunotherapy.

The same comments apply to persistent or recurrent pneumonia [7] which may occur as the initial symptom of asthma. The right middle lobe is the one most commonly involved.

41.2 Differential Diagnosis

The diagnosis of asthma is generally evident especially in older children. A comprehensive list of the conditions to be differentiated from asthma is found elsewhere [8]. Only the most common will be discussed. Many of them may coexist with asthma or be accompanied by bronchial hyperreactivity.

A foreign body must be suspected at any age, even in the absence of suggestive initial symptoms. Sometimes only the systematic chest radiograph in full expiration leads to the discovery of localized air trapping and then to bronchoscopy.

Digital clubbing may be seen in chronic asthma, but rather suggests the presence of bronchiectasis (due or not to primary ciliary dyskinesia) and above all cystic fibrosis. A sweat test should be performed in all children with chronic respiratory disorders and/or nasal polyps.

Gastroesophageal reflux (GER) has been claimed to induce night cough, acute laryngitis and wheezing. In our experience this appears to be true only in nonallergic children. Medical treatment of GER is then effective. In contrast, although a high incidence of GER has been documented in severe atopic asthma its role in the pathogenesis of nocturnal symptoms awaits more definitive confirmation.

Bronchiolitis obliterans as sequelae to severe viral pneumonias (especially measles and adenovirus) are often confused with asthma. Dyspneic bouts differ from asthmatic attacks by their constant bacterial superinfection, the poor efficacy of bronchodilators and corticosteroids and the presence of fixed peripheral atelectasis and/or obstructive emphysema (source of definitive perfusion defects) [9].

41.3 Positive Diagnosis

The diagnosis of asthma is based on personal and familial history and physical findings. Attention should be focused not only on the chest but also on the upper respiratory tract, the eyes and the skin which often are a source of great disability.

Moreover the finding of allergic conjunctivitis and/or pale or purplish nasal mucosa and/or atopic dermatitis is of high diagnostic value. There is virtually no other possible diagnosis than asthma in a wheezing child with xerosis and/or retroauricular folds.

In current practice few laboratory procedures are necessary. Chest radiographs exposed in full inspiration and maximal expiration are indicated as a baseline to which later films can be compared and are indispensable in the differential diagnosis of asthma. Eosinophilia in peripheral blood, in nasal secretions and above all in sputum should be sought. Even very young symptomatic children produce sufficient sputum to be collected by pulmonary physiotherapy [10].

The prominent role of allergy in asthmatic children makes skin testing necessary. Allergens are selected and positive responses are interpreted on the basis of history.

Serum-IgE are frequently but not always increased. RAST should be reserved for children who cannot be adequately skin tested (i.e., atopic dermatitis, dermographism, poor respiratory condition).

Respiratory function studies cannot be overemphasized as a diagnostic tool (increased bronchial reactivity to histamine or cholinergic agents, reversibility of bronchospasm with bronchodilators or exercise-induced asthma) and as an objective means of assessing the severity of asthma and the effectiveness of treatment. Nasal and bronchial provocation tests are usually performed only when the identification of a specific allergen is impossible with conventional investigations and is the prerequisite of immunotherapy.

References

1. Speight ANP, Lee DA, Hey EN (1983) Underdiagnosis and undertreatment of asthma in childhood. Br Med J 286:1253–1256
2. Leffert F (1980) The management of chronic asthma. J Pediatr 97:875–885
3. Leffert F (1980) The management of acute severe asthma. J Pediatr 96:1–12
4. Kraemer R, Meister B, Schaad UB, Rossi E (1983) Reversibility of lung function abnormalities in children with perennial asthma. J Pediatr 102:347–350
5. Martin AJ, Landau LI, Phelan PD (1981) The effect on growth of childhood asthma. Acta Paediatr Scand 70:683–688
6. Blair H (1977) Natural history of asthma, 20-year follow-up. Arch Dis Child 52:613–619
7. Eigen H, Laughlin JJ, Homrighausen J (1982) Recurrent pneumonia in children and its relationship to bronchial hyperreactivity. Pediatrics 70:698–704

8. Spiegel SC, Katz RM, Rachelefsky GS (1983) Asthma in infancy and childhood. In: Middleton E Jr, Reed CE, Elliot EF (eds) Allergy, principles and practice, 2nd edn. Mosby, St. Louis Toronto, pp 863–900
9. Meyer B, de Blic J, Pariente D, Lamour C, Benoist MR, Nezelof C, Scheinmann P (1983) La bronchiolite oblitérante: moyens d'exploration et de diagnostic. Ann Pediatr 30:351–355
10. de Blic J, Scheinmann P, Dhont P, Pfister A, Paupe J, da Lage C (1982) Deciding in need for antibiotics in children with acute asthma. Lancet 1:629–630

42. Diagnosis of Asthma in Childhood

U. Wahn

Although the pathophysiological mechanisms involved in childhood asthma are similar as in adults, several factors account for specific problems in different age groups. They include variations of different age levels in anatomic, physiological, pathological, immunologic and psychological patterns. Differences between adult and childhood asthma are obvious, especially in younger children. Therefore, diagnosis and management of bronchial asthma during infancy and childhood include features that may be different and distinct from those during adulthood.

In some children it is possible to induce an asthmatic reaction to substances, to which serum-IgE antibodies can be demonstrated. In others, allergens may play only a negligible role. Allergic reactions may induce bronchoconstriction directly. It may be more important for the understanding of perennial allergic asthma, that unspecific tracheobronchial reactivity is increased by allergen-induced late asthmatic response [1, 2]

Allergy can only partly explain the pathogenesis of asthmatic symptoms. Even in atopic children mechanisms other than the IgE mast cell system are probably relevant in generating asthmatic attacks. Upper and lower respiratory tract irritants have been demonstrated to induce asthma. These include cigarette smoke, cold air, odors from spray of perfumes and chemicals. Atmospheric changes may be associated with an increase in asthmatic activity, too.

The most common infectious agents which are responsible for triggering asthma are viruses [3]. While in preschool children RSV are by far the most relevant pathogens (Table 42.1), in school children and adolescents, infections with mycoplasma pneumoniae become more common [4]. An increase in bronchial reactivity after lower respiratory tract infections has been shown in children [5, 6].

Exercise, especially running or bicycle riding may be a major asthmatogenic factor. It occurs in up to 90% of asthmatic children [7]. Sometimes it may be the first manifestation of childhood asthma. Characteristically it starts after 5 min of heavy exercise and may last for more than an hour. It is generally accepted, that the major triggering factor in exercise-induced asthma is airway cooling caused by hyperventilation [8]. The heat loss of the bronchial mucosa may cause the release of mediator and act locally via neuroreflexes to produce bronchoconstriction.

Emotional factors in a minority of children may aggravate asthma. However, there is no evidence indicating psychological factors to be the basis for asthma.

Acute or chronic sinusitis is frequently associated with asthma; asthmatic attacks may be induced through irritant or *reflex mechanisms.*

The pathogenic role of gastroesophageal reflux for chronic nocturnal asthma in children is still under controversy [17–19].

In contrast to adults, aspirin intolerance, which may induce asthma is rarely seen in children. In the majority of asthmatic children several factors, which have been mentioned above, may have an additive effect in precipitating asthmatic attacks (Table 42.2).

42.1 History

An accurate chronological history provides helpful information for diagnosis and generally gives the clues, which are necessary for further diagnostic tests.

A positive family history of atopic disease may indicate a pathogenic role of atopic allergens for the disease of the child.

Table 42.1. Infectious agents triggering childhood asthma

Preschool age	School age	Adolescents
RSV Parainfluenza virus Adenovirus	Rhinovirus Mycoplasma pneumoniae Parainfluenza virus RSV	Mycoplasma pneumoniae Rhinovirus Parainfluenza virus

Table 42.2. Precipitants of asthmatic symptoms in infancy and childhood. [Modified from 8]

	Infancy	Early childhood	Late childhood
Viral infection	+ + + +[a]	+ + +	+(+)
Exercise	+	+ +	+ + +
Irritants	+	+ +	+ + +
Foods	+ +	+	(+)
Indoor inhalants	+(+)	+ + +	+ + +
Pollens		+ +	+ + +
Emotions	(+)	(+)	(+)

[a] Denotes relative importance

In most cases the child's history has to be taken from the mother, who may be unaware of important details or may interpret her observations in her own version. Older children frequently tend to deny their illness. Symptoms may begin in infancy. Since younger children are more susceptible to viral infections leading to frequent upper respiratory symptoms, persistant nasal and chest symptoms are readily attributed to this, and allergy may be overlooked. When allergy is recognized, a number of children will already have had tonsillectomy or adenoidectomy or may have tympanotomy tubes.

Many asthmatics are called *bronchitics* for a number of years, because cough is an obvious symptom in the younger child. When trying to decide if the child has asthma, attention should be given to the episodic nature of symptoms and to the fact, that attacks may be provoked either by upper respiratory infections (fever?), by exercise or allergens [9].

It is most important to get detailed information of the symptoms related to time of day or week (many children are worse during the night and improved during the day), to meals, to being indoors or outdoors or to contact with specific animals, substances, or places.

Sometimes it may be helpful to get information about prior response to previous treatment that the child had received.

42.2 Physical Examination

For the evaluation of an asthmatic child a complete physical examination may give important information. Special attention has to be given to height and weight, which may indicate the degree of severity of asthma, since children with chronic symptoms may demonstrate a failure of growth. The eyes may show the classic dark circles (allergic shiners), the nose an allergic crease at the edge or nasal obstruction and in the ears acute or chronic otitis media is frequently found. The skin has to be investigated for atopic lesions. Examination of the chest should focus on sounds of airways obstruction, to a barrel-chest deformity and to symptoms of hyperinflation like increased resonance, subcostal recession, tracheal tug and excessive muscle activity. Clubbing of the nails mostly suggests an alternative diagnosis.

42.3 Laboratory Procedures

A number of laboratory examinations are necessary for the evaluation of an asthmatic child at the first visit. Complete blood counts (eosinophilia) should be routinely done, as well as tuberculine testing by multiple puncture test. An x-ray film of the chest should be obtained in every patient in order to exclude complications of asthma (atelectasis, pneumothorax, pneumomediastinum) or other diseases (foreign body). In many cases x-ray films of paranasal sinuses are also indicated. A sweat test for chloride determination should be performed, since 20% of cystic fibrosis patients may have respiratory allergy.

Skin tests can be performed in children as in adults. The prick technique, which is most appropriate for children, has been shown to give well-reproducible results [10]. In general, skin tests can be performed in children older than 3 years. In younger children and even in infants they may be performed on special indications, but they are rarely necessary. Interpreting skin tests in infancy hyporeactivity to both histamine and allergens has to be taken into consideration [11]. For this age group the RAST for allergen-specific serum-IgE is the appropriate test identifying offending allergens from the environment or foods. It is also the diagnostic procedure of choice in children with severe eczema, who cannot be skin tested. It should be performed and interpreted by an allergist. In contrast, the determination of total serum-IgE has been shown not to be a very useful screening technique for allergic asthma. It has a predictive value for atopic disease only in cord blood or in early infancy [12].

The laboratory tests should be completed by quantitative determination of serum-immunoglobulins (IgG, IgA, IgM) and α_1-antitrypsin (Table 42.3).

Lung Function Tests

Simple lung function tests should be carried out on asthmatic children at the time of initial visit and during therapy. Normal values for pulmonary function tests in children are available [13].

While for preschool children the use of a peak flowmeter is most appropriate, spirometry, which is more complicated for children, as a more reliable method should be applied in children older than 6 years. Generally, a child which is investigated by forced expiratory maneuvers, has several attempts, out of them the best values for FVC, FEV_1, or peak flow are recorded and compared to the predicted values, which are related to the child's height. Flow-dependent measurements by spirometry or peak expiratory flowmeters reflect primarily large airway obstruction.

Since bronchial obstruction occasionally may be induced by forced expiration, more complex and not effort-dependent lung function tests, including the more sensitive whole body plethysmography, have been recommended for children. Recently techniques have become available, which allow the measurements of resistances by an oscillatory method, which appears to be a

Table 42.3. Diagnostic procedures in childhood asthma

Routine:	Complete blood count, sedimentation rate Serum-IgG, IgA, IgM, α_1-antitrypsin Total IgE, specific serum-IgE (RAST) Chest x-ray, paranasal sinus x-ray Skin test, tuberculine test, lung function test with response to bronchodilators
Provocation tests:	Histamine Exercise Antigen inhalation
At special indications:	– Sweat test – Precipitating antibodies – Bronchoscopy – Bronchography

promising alternative, especially in children [14].

For the interpretations of all lung function tests it has to be taken into account, that the findings in asthmatic children vary markedly from day to day and even from hour to hour. Lung function tests at an initial evaluation should be completed by a measurement of the response to bronchodilators.

Provocation Test

Bronchial responsiveness is measured by testing the bronchial reaction to pharmacological agents, which can be inhaled in increasing doses. Beside histamine, methacholine and carbachol are often applied [20]. Most often the dose of the agonist is increased by increasing concentrations, while the inhaled volume remains constant. After establishing a baseline lung function, saline is inhaled in order to detect nonspecific responses. Thereafter, the agonist is given, starting for example with a histamine dose of 0.125 g/l and increasing it up to 8 g/l. For assessing the bronchial response either peak flow rates (PEFR), forced expiratory volumes in one second (FEV_1) or airway resistance (Raw) can be measured [21, 22].

Exercise Tests

Standardized exercise in asthmatic children can provoke bronchial obstruction, the degree of which is related to the degree of bronchial responsiveness to inhaled histamine [20]. Therefore exercise tests are used as alternative tests to assess bronchial responsiveness. As has been shown by Godfrey [23], standard steady-state running tests give more reproducible responses than stepping or running up- and downstairs or cycling. For clinical purposes it is sufficient to have a child run for 6 min and measure lung function before exercise and 3 to 5 min after exercise. A postexercise fall of 20% of the peak flow rates or the FEV_1 is abnormal. There is a correlation between the severity of the fall and the severity of asthma in a child [20].

Inhalation of Cold Air

As it has been shown by several investigators, the heat loss due to isocapnic voluntary hyperventilation is the same as the heat loss of the bronchi during exercise [15], leading to a similar degree of bronchial obstruction. Therefore tests have been proposed using isocapnic hyperventilation of cold air (−18 °C and 0% humidity) as a stimulus [16].

PEFR Recording at Home

Characteristically lung function values, particularly in children, vary during the day. Therefore random measurement of lung function for the clinical evaluation is sometimes of little use. In order to evaluate a child's asthma more thoroughly, peak flowmeters should be used at home for several days or weeks. The best PEFR of 3 attempts, recorded in the morning and in the evening before the medication is taken, can be used for evaluation and response to treatment.

Allergen Inhalation Tests

Provocation studies with allergens together with pulmonary function tests can be used to determine the significance of environmental allergens for asthma in children. Airway reactions to allergens at increasing concentrations are dependent on both the degree of unspecific bronchial reactivity and the degree of sensitivity to the allergen involved [20]. Provocation tests are indicated before the consideration of immunotherapy with perennial allergens.

Bronchological Examinations

Since asthmatic symptoms can be caused by a number of malformations or acquired anatomical disorders, in selected cases, bronchoscopy and bronchography may be indicated [17].

References

1. Cartier A, Thomson NC, Frith PA, Roberts BS, Tech M, Hargreave FE (1982) Allergen-induced increase in bronchial responsiveness

to histamine: relationship to the late asthmatic response and change in airway caliber. J Allergy Clin Immunol 70: 170
2. Cockcroft DW (1983) Mechanism of Perennial Allergic Asthma. Lancet II: 253–255
3. Frick OL (1983) Role of Viral Infections in Asthma and Allergy. Clin Rev Allergy 1:5–17
4. Carlsen KH, Ørstavik I, Leegaard J, Høeg H (1984) Respiratory virus infections and aeroallergens in acute bronchial asthma. Arch Dis Child 59: 310–315
5. Mok JYO, Simpson H (1984) Symptoms, atopy, and bronchial reactivity after lower respiratory infection in infancy. Arch Dis Child 59: 299–305
6. Eigen H, Laughlin JJ, Homrighausen J (1982) Recurrent Pneumonia in Children and Its Relationship to Bronchial Hyperreactivity. Pediatrics 70: 698–704
7. Godfrey S (1977) Childhood Asthma. In: Clark TJH, Godfrey S (eds) Asthma. Chapman and Hall, London, pp 324–366
8. Pearlman DS, Bierman CW (1980) Asthma (Bronchial Asthma, Reactive Airways Disorder). In: Bierman CW, Pearlman DS (eds) Allergic Diseases of Infancy, Childhood and Adolescence. Saunders, Philadelphia, pp 581–604
9. König P (1981) Hidden Asthma in Childhood. Am J Dis Child 135: 1053–1055
10. Malling H-J, Andersen CE, Boas M-B, Holgersen F, Munch EP, Weeke B (1982) The Allergy Pricker. Qualitative Aspects of Skin Prick Testing Using a Precision Needle. Allergy 37: 563–567
11. Ménardo JL, Bousquet J, Rodière M, Astruc J, Michel FB (1985) Skin Test Reactivity In Infancy. J Allergy Clin Immunol 75: 646–651
12. Bousquet J, Ménardo JL, Robinet-Levy M, Michel FB (1983) Möglichkeiten der Vorhersage allergischer Erkrankungen im Säuglingsalter. In: Wahn U (Hrsg.) Aktuelle Probleme der Pädiatrischen Allergologie. Gustav Fischer, Stuttgart, pp 43–54
13. Polgar G, Promadhat V (1971) Pulmonary function testing in children. Saunders, Philadelphia
14. Berdel D, Holle JP, Hartmann V, Magnussen H (1981) Die Bedeutung der oszillatorischen Atemwiderstandsmessung im Kindesalter. Klin Pädiatr 193: 73–76
15. Tal A, Pasterkamp H, Serrette C, Leahy F, Chernick V (1984) Response to cold air hyperventilation in normal and in asthmatic children. J Pediatr 104: 516–521
16. McLaughlin FJ, Dozor AJ (1983) Cold Air Inhalation Challenge in the Diagnosis of Asthma in Children. Pediatrics 72: 503–509
17. Szekely E, Farkas E (1978) Pediatric bronchology. Akademiai Kiadó, Budapest, University Park Press, Baltimore, pp 300, 401
18. Martin ME, Grunstein MM, Larsen GL (1982) The Relationship Of Gastroesophageal Reflux To Nocturnal Wheezing In Children With Asthma. Ann Allergy 49: 318–322
19. Hughes DM, Sper S, Rivlin J, Levison H (1983) Gastroesophageal reflux during sleep in asthmatic patients. J Pediatr 102: 666–672
20. Neijens HJ, Duiverman EJ, Kerrebijn KF (1983) Bronchial Responsiveness in Children. Pediatr Clin North Am 30: 829–846
21. Townley RG, Bewtra AK, Nair NM, Brodkey FD, Watt GD, Burkem KM (1979) Methacholine Inhalation Challenge Studies. J Allergy Clin Immunol 64: 569–574
22. Woolcock AJ, Yan K, Salome C (1983) Methods for assessing bronchial reactivity. Eur J Respir Dis 64: 181–194
23. Godfrey S (1974) Exercise testing in children. Saunders, London

43. Treatment of Childhood Asthma

J. O. Warner

"I have no magic cure to report... Asthma has many aetiological aspects and should be treated according to the various causes that bring it about", Maimonides, 12th century [1].

There have been considerable advances in the development of palliative therapies for asthma over the last quarter of a century, but we have advanced no further than Maimonides in terms of finding a cure. Thus we must follow his dictum of a multidisciplinary approach to this multifactorial condition. Treatment will involve the employment of allergy therapy, pharmacology and psychiatry.

As there is a wide spectrum of severity of disease, the management must be tailored to the individual. To a considerable extent, the ideal recipe will be achieved by a process of trial and error, utilizing a rational sequence of therapeutic approaches from the simplest and safest to the more complex schedules. At each stage in the trial of therapy, a careful assessment of response, which should include at least twice daily measurements of peak expiratory flow rates, which is possible in any child above five years of age, and a daily diary card record of symptoms is needed [2]. The goal of treatment should be to return the child to an absolutely normal existence, allowing participation in all usual childhood activities. This is achievable in all but a very small minority of cases.

43.1 General Measures

Allergen avoidance: The vast majority of asthmatic children are clearly atopic, with family histories of allergy and positive prick skin tests to one or more common allergens [3]. The dramatic benefit following removal from occupational allergen exposure provides the example which pediatricians would like to emulate in common allergen avoidance [4]. However, the relationship between positive prick skin tests and clinical history of the provoking factors is often unclear. Furthermore, the correlation between positive skin tests and reaction to the same allergen on bronchial challenge is not at all good [5]. Thus, drastic allergen avoidance measures must be preceded by accurate allergy diagnosis. Even in ideal circumstances most avoidance techniques have, to date, been disappointing.

House dust mite: The most common allergen which is likely to be important in childhood asthma is the house dust mite, Dermatophagoides pteronyssinus [6]. Avoidance of the house dust mite was first recommended 50 years ago before confirmation that mites were the principal allergen in dust [7]. As children spend a considerable proportion of their day in the bedroom, in close proximity to house dust mites, and asthmatics frequently have nocturnal symptoms, it is attractive to hypothesize that mites and nocturnal asthma are causally related. Trials of house dust mite avoidance, however, have been rather disappointing. Techniques involving the use of plastic mattress covers, removal of soft toys and feather bedding, and regular vacuuming, have been described [8], but found wanting in several recent controlled trials [9, 10]. It remains to be seen whether acaricides [11] or alternative mite elimination techniques [12] are clinically valuable.

Pets: Recommendation to banish the much loved family pet is difficult without convincing evidence that it is a major cause of problems. Parents frequently dispute the relevance of animal dander allergy when they do not observe acute reactions in their child, because there is a continuous exposure in the house. It may take up to three months for the dander to be totally removed after banishment of the pet. Once home exposure ceases, it often becomes more obvious that the allergy is relevant, with subsequent encounters producing acute reactions. It is preferable for asthmatic children to have no pets at all, or at least none should be allowed in their bedrooms.

Pollens and molds: Avoidance of aeroallergens, such as pollen grains and mold spores, is impossible, unless children are restricted to an air-filtered, closed building. Pollens in the house may be minimized by keeping windows shut during the day and installing window air conditioners [13]. The use of air filters or electrostatic precipitators inside the house has not been validated by controlled study [14] and there has been conflicting information from trials on the use of ionisers [15, 16]. The wearing of helmets with visors and air compressors may be effective in special circumstances, but this is hardly practicable for children.

Foods: Some children have a clear history of asthma precipitated by a variety of foods, drinks, and artificial additives [17]. Under such circumstances dietary manipulation is obviously indicated. However, there is no evidence that foods, drinks, food residues or additives are particularly involved in exacerbation of the majority of asthma. Thus, trial diets are very rarely indicated as primary treatment for asthma, though they may be of value for the control of other atopic problems, such as ezcema [18].

Psychotherapy: Emotional disturbance can clearly trigger asthmatic attacks and psychogenic factors commonly compromise asthma control [19]. It is imperative that the child and family should be helped to gain a realistic understanding and acceptance of the condition, and that specific psychological problems should be treated. This requires sensitivity and patience from the pediatrician and extra time devoted to consultation. Parents and children should be allowed to air their anxieties and misconceptions about the disease. Careful and clear explanations, which can be aided by diagrams and written instructions, are essential. Most emotional problems relating to asthma can be effectively managed by the pediatrician, but occasionally psychiatric intervention from a specialist may be required. However, psychopathology in the family may not be obvious to the clinician without a careful assessment [20]. Where there is severe psychopathology in the parent or family or where appropriate treatment has failed, referral is indicated. Several psychotherapeutic approaches have been assessed and shown to be of value in asthma and can be a useful adjunct to standard treatment [21].

Physiotherapy: Physiotherapists can most usefully train children to use their inhalers correctly and supervise the issuing and maintainance of their air compressor and nebulizer units. Controlled breathing can encourage relaxation and may be of value during acute attacks, but no trial has been conducted to support this contention. Postural drainage is only necessary when there is lobar collapse or during the recovery stage after an acute, severe attack when expectoration of secretions and plugs can be aided. Routine chest physiotherapy may adversely affect asthmatic children as coughing can initiate bronchoconstriction.

Exercise: Encouragement to participate in all physical activities is important, as asthmatic children tend to lead a sedentary life. There are a disproportionate number of goalkeepers among the football playing asthmatic children. Improved physical fitness is of value to all and participation in sporting activity encourages assimilation of the asthmatic child into a normal environment. However, physical fitness *per se* has no specific effect on asthma. Swimming is the least likely to induce bronchospasm, but properly designed activities outside the swimming pool can be equally safe [22]. Emphasis should be placed on the use of prophylactic medications taken immediately before any exercise, which will protect the majority of children from exercise-induced bronchospasm.

Social management: Asthma is a common cause of school absenteeism, but appropriate prophylactic therapy can reduce this very considerably [23]. The demand for special schooling or institutional care has fallen considerably. Where a child's education has been compromised despite optimal therapy, residential schooling may be of value and this usually arises where there are additional psychosocial problems in the family. As children often improve during holidays away from home, parents often ask whether a move to a different climate would be of value. While a change of environment may lead to an improvement, this is usually temporary, and asthma has been found in all countries and climates around the world. The aim of treatment is to allow children to live in good health in their home environment and this is predominantly achieved by appropriate pharmacological therapy.

43.2 Drug Treatment

Asthma Under Two Years of Age

As responses to treatment differ somewhat in infants below 18–24 months of age, they are considered separately. Most wheezing in infancy is associated with upper respiratory tract infection, but as this is virtually always viral in origin, antibiotics are not required. The wheeze is often loud and persistent, but in most cases causes no distress to the infant, though considerable upset to parents. It may well be unnecessary to use any treatment, though this approach is often difficult to sell to parents. The respiration rate and degree of recession will be more reliable indicators of severity of disease rather than the wheeze itself.

Infant wheezers are often rather poorly responsive to β-agonists, even when administered by nebulizer [24]. However, these drugs are still worthy of trial as occasionally they are effective even in very young infants. Nebulized ipratropium bromide does, in 40% of salbutamol-resistant wheezers, temporarily relieve airflow limitation and may be of value [25]. Oral theophyllines are sometimes helpful and are available in elixir form, which is suitable for small infants. However, the unpleasant taste often hampers adequate administration. Doses must be carefully estimated with blood or salivary theophylline level measurements if high doses are utilized [26]. Rectal administration is unsatisfactory as absorption is eratic. Frequent episodes may be controlled by either regular theophyllines [27] or three to four times daily sodium cromoglycate, administered by a nebulizer [28]. Only the very severe acute cases may require short courses of steroids and such children certainly require hospital admission for assessment. There are no published trials of steroid therapy in this situation which give any guidance on their value, but in the absence of further information, they remain mandatory for severe, acute asthma unresponsive to bronchodilators. In the occasional infant with frequent, severe wheezing, long-term steroids may be required. They are more safely administered on alternate days with little or no adrenal or growth suppression resulting [29].

Asthma Over Two Years of Age

Mild, episodic asthma: Children with mild, episodic asthma, grow normally, miss little school and have minimal or no lung function abnormality between attacks. Most will be satisfactorily treated with sympathomimetic drugs administered orally for individual attacks. The β_2-specific agonists are preferred and are most rapidly effective when administered by an inhaler. Using some of the newer inhalation devices it is possible to train children even younger than three years of age to use the inhaled therapy efficiently [30]. Where children develop exercise-induced asthma a dose of inhaled bronchodilator immediately prior to the activity will be protective in most children [31]. It is probably easier to control episodes of bronchospasm if the bronchodilators are commenced early in the course of the illness.

Frequent, episodic asthma: When attacks become relatively frequent, more than once every two weeks, it will be necessary to consider the use of regular prophylactic therapy. Here the choice lies between regular theophylline preparations, preferably in a slow release form [32], or sodium cromoglycate, either by a nebulizer in the young and poorly coordinated child, or spinhaler [28, 33]. Recent trials suggest that the pressurized aerosol form of sodium cromoglycate is not as effective as the spinhaler in children [34]. The sodium cromoglycate must be taken at least three, and preferably four, times daily, because of its relatively short duration of action. Because of its exclusive prophylactic effect it must be administered continuously to prevent attacks, and is, in fact, of little or no value during acute episodes. Most failures of this treatment are due to failure to use the inhaler correctly. Thus, time spent on education on inhaler usage is invaluable. Like β_2-agonists, it also has a prophylactic role taken prior to exercise. When using theophylline preparations, the dose must be tailored to the individual patient. While an optimal dose in mg per kg can be evolved for individual slow release preparations [35], it is always necessary to monitor the therapy with theophylline level measurements, particularly with the wide range of preparations available [26]. The decision on whether to use either sodium cromoglycate or high dose, slow release theophylline will be primarily based on the child's preferences. There is little to choose between the two treatments and in fact one study has suggested that using both has no additional effect [36].

Any breakthrough wheezing on prophylactic therapy can usually be controlled by β-agonists, again preferably by inhalation, as necessary, up to a maximum of once every four hours. Failure to control an acute exacerbation on this schedule indicates that the attack is severe and requires medical attention.

Chronic, perennial or severe episodic asthma: Children with severe asthma will often fail to respond to regular sodium cromoglycate or high dose, slow release theophyllines, and in these cases steroid therapy will be required. There is little to be gained from continuing with sodium cromoglycate once this has become ineffective [37]. There is no doubt that corticosteroid treatment has had a dramatic effect on the management of asthma. However, in the past caution was required because of the effects of systemic corticosteroid treatment. Nevertheless, its use in very severe cases showed that the ill effects were greatly outweighed by the benefits of such therapy [38]. Attempts to use corticotropin as an alternative to oral prednisolone was suggested as having less growth inhibition [39] but this has not been proven through subsequent clinical experience. The development of potent, topically active steroid preparations, such as beclomethasone dipropionate [40], betamethasone valerate [41] and budesonide [42] by inhalation has dramatically improved the management of moderate to severe asthma. These inhaled preparations are extremely potent in controlling asthma but, unless high doses are used, have no detectable effect on the hypothalamic pituitary adrenal axis. This has been shown by numerous studies [40, 42]. Provided the daily dose of beclomethasone dipropionate is less than 800 µg, adrenal suppression is very rare. A dose between 800 and 1,600 µg per day, results in infrequent side effects. Oral candidiasis occurs relatively rarely in childhood, though it does appear to be more common in adults [43].

There are now several modes of delivery of corticosteroids for inhalation. All are available as a pressurized aerosol with or without a spacer device. The latter may improve distribution of the drug through the lungs [42]. However, many small children find the pressurized aerosol rather difficult to use. Such children may manage the dry powder form via the rotahaler [44]. We are currently investigating the value of the 750 ml pear-shaped spacer inhaler (Nebuhaler) for the administration of budesonide to small children. This may have some advantages, particularly for infants [45].

While the original trials of beclomethasone dipropionate suggested that a four times daily schedule of treatment was optimal, there is some evidence that it can be used optimally on a twice daily schedule [46]. The same is true of budesonide [42]. Sometimes as children become wheezy, they are no longer able to take the inhaled steroid therapy effectively and the condition rapidly declines. It may be of benefit to administer a dose of inhaled bronchodilator, five minutes before the inhaled steroids in such situations, though this has never really been established by a controlled study [47]. If children develop a severe attack while on inhaled corticosteroid therapy, it may be necessary to resort to a course of oral prednisolone. Should this occur repeatedly, then it may be necessary to use long-term alternate day steroid orally, in addition to the inhaled preparation. Patients on steroids should always be given regular bronchodilator therapy as well. This may either be with oral, slow release theophylline or β-agonist, whilst inhaled β-agonists can be kept in reserve for any exacerbations. One of the important effects of steroids is to facilitate the bronchodilator response and this should be capitalized upon in chronic asthma [48, 49]. Ipratropium bromide inhalations may also have a role in chronic asthma, but this has yet to be defined [50]. There are a very small percentage of severe, chronic asthmatics in childhood who do not respond to steroids. These patients, as in adults, have very considerable fluctuations in their degree of air flow limitation. Management can be extremely difficult but best achieved with optimal doses of slow release theophyllines, inhaled β-agonists and ipratropium bromide [51].

43.3 Acute Exacerbations of Asthma

Acute exacerbations of asthma have been termed *status asthmaticus,* but this is an ill-defined term and is probably best avoided. Acute attacks are potentially lethal and therefore great care is required in assessment and if the attack is considered severe the patient will require treatment with full intensive care facilities. In adults it is clear that many asthma deaths are probably avoidable [52]. However, in childhood, while some deaths may well be avoidable, occasionally totally unexpected deaths occur [53]. There has been much dispute as to the cause of death in many asthmatics, particularly during the epidemic of deaths during the 1960s. This dispute has been renewed because of a further increase in deaths in New Zealand in the last few years [54]. There are disturbing indications that a similar increase in deaths is beginning to be apparent in the United Kingdom over the last few years.

A dose of β-agonist administered by a nebulizer is both diagnostic and therapeutic in this situation. The clinical state should be assessed before and 10 min after such treatment. A response, which must be documented objectively, preferably with the use of a peak flowmeter, will allow admission to an open ward and continuation of nebulized therapy. However, failure to respond to this treatment or a relapse within two hours of a single dose, denotes severe acute asthma and requires treatment with full intensive care.

Oxygen should be administered to all cases. As there is no concern about chronic CO_2 retention, concentrations of up to 100% may be used as required. An intravenous infusion should be established immediately after there has been a failure to respond to inhaled β-agonists. Fluid replacement should be based on an assessment of the degree of dehydration. This may occur because of poor fluid intake and evaporative loss from the airways during a prolonged attack. However, overhydration can hinder recovery because pulmonary edema is easily precipitated. Therefore intravenous fluid should be calculated between 100 and 125% of normal daily requirements as 4.3% dextrose and one fifth normal saline. Children on steroids may require additional potassium based on electrolyte estimations. The role of bicarbonate therapy is slightly controversial. It has been suggested that a low pH may cause a loss of adrenergic responsiveness. In practice, bicarbonate is rarely required unless there is a persistent metabolic acidosis, in which case a calculated half correction can be made using the formula

$$\text{base deficit} \times \text{weight in kilos} \times 0.15$$

as millimoles of sodium bicarbonate administered by slow infusion.

The mainstay of treatment will be bronchodilators and steroids. Provided the patient has not received theophylline preparations in the previous 12 hours, aminophylline should be administered at a dose of 5.6 mg per kg given slowly over 20 min. Thereafter a continuous infusion of 0.9 mg per kg per hour should be maintained [55]. If theophyllines have been used within the previous 12 hours it should be possible to get a blood level measurement within half an hour, so that doses for intravenous therapy can be judged accordingly. Where there is doubt about the blood level of theophylline, intravenous salbutamol 10 µg per kg, can be administered and followed with a continuous infusion of up to 0.25 µg per kg per min. Failure to respond immediately to the initial dose of intravenous bronchodilator is an indication for intravenous hydrocortisone in a dose of 4 mg per kg every four hours. The vast majority of patients will respond to this treatment within four to six hours, though intravenous treatment should be maintained for at least 24 to 48 hours before slowly converting to an oral and inhaled regime. It is appropriate to combine intravenous aminophylline with salbutamol, either by a nebulizer or intravenously [56].

There has been some dispute concerning the role of corticosteroids in acute asthma and very few controlled studies have been conducted [57]. However, at present there should be no hesitation in the use of this treatment, with one recent controlled study demonstrating a favorable response [58]. Indeed, strong indications from studies of asthma deaths showed that failure to use steroids is a major cause of death [59].

It is very rare for a patient to progress to respiratory failure and require ventilation, but this is more likely in infants. The decision to institute ventilation is clinical, but will be strongly influenced by the serial arterial blood gas records. A $paCO_2$ of greater than 8.5 kPa and rising, particularly if associated with decreased air entry, cyanosis despite 40% oxygen, depressed level of consciousness, poor muscle tone and exhaustion, will indicate that intervention is necessary. Intubation should be done under an anesthetic and muscle relaxation is best achieved with pancuronium bromide, which will not produce histamine release as with the other muscle relaxants. Ventilation usually requires high pressures initially and this may lead to complications with reduced cardiac output and gas leaks from the lung. Heavy sedation and paralysis is usually required to achieve adequate ventilation, which should be maintained until arterial pCO_2 is near normal with low pressure ventilation [60]. Antibiotics are not indicated for the management of acute asthma alone [61]. It is imperative that treatment is maintained for a considerable length of time after recovery from the acute attack. Furthermore it will usually be necessary to adjust the prophylactic therapy in order to maintain good control of the condition [62].

43.4 Immunotherapy

Allergy is common among asthmatic children and this has led to a considerable amount of immunotherapy being prescribed primarily for this condition. The impression from many trials is that children have a greater clinical response than adults [63]. However, it is clear that therapy must be used for longer periods, of at least two years, in order to maintain the benefit [64]. The only allergens which should be considered for immunotherapy in asthmatic subjects are house dust mite and perhaps grass pollens. Currently the evidence to support the use of other preparations is lacking [65].

43.5 Inhalers

There is now a bewildering array of delivery devices to administer inhaled medications. Simple pressurized aerosols require good coordination to be used optimally. Ideally the child should relax to the end tidal position and then take a long, slow inhalation starting just before actuation of the aerosol. At full inspiration the child should maintain a 10 s breath hold. This procedure is often impossible for small children. They usually find the rotahaler easier. However, it is still necessary for the child to generate a reasonable inspiratory flow. It has recently been shown that placing a spacer device between pressurized aerosol and the patient improves the delivery and distribution of medication. The latest development, known as a Nebuhaler, has a valve incorporated into a 750 ml conical reservoir, which allows its use in very small children [66]. Nebulizers with appropriate air compressors may be necessary in very small children who are unable to use any form of simple inhaler. They are only very rarely required in older children on a domiciliary basis, unless it can be proven that this form of delivery produces greater degrees of bronchodilatation than a simple device.

References

1. Maimonides M (1963) Treatise on Asthma. Translator: Muntner S. Lippincott, Philadelphia Montreal
2. Connolly N, Godfrey S (1970) Assessment of the child with asthma. J Asthma Res 8:31–36
3. Russell G, Jones SP (1976) Selection of skin tests in childhood asthma. Br J Dis Chest 70:104–106
4. Chan-Yeung M, Lam S, Koerner S (1982) Clinical features and natural history of occupational asthma due to western red cedar (*Thuja plicata*). Am J Med 72:411–415
5. Warner JO (1977) Bronchial provocation tests. Arch Dis Child 52:750–751
6. Warner JO, Price JF (1978) House dust mite sensitivity in childhood asthma. Arch Dis Child 53:710–713
7. Dekker H (1928) Asthma and mites. MMW 75:515
8. Sarsfield JK, Gowland G, Toy R, Norman ALE (1974) Mite-sensitive asthma in childhood. Arch Dis Child 49:716–721
9. Burr ML, Dean BU, Merrett TG, Neale E, St. Leger AS, Verrier-Jones ER (1980) Effects of anti-mite measures on children with mite sensitive asthma: a controlled trial. Thorax 35:506–512
10. Kosgaard J (1982) Preventive measures in house dust allergy. Am Rev Respir Dis 125:80–84
11. Penaud A, Nourrit J, Timon-David P, Charpin J (1977) Results of a controlled trial of the acaricide Paragerm on Dermatophagoides spp. in dwelling houses. Clin Allergy 7:49–53
12. van de Maele B (1983) A new strategy in the control of house dust mite allergy. Pharmatherapeutica 3:441–444
13. Solomon WR, Barge HA, Boise JR (1980) Exclusion of particulate allergens by window air conditioners. J Allergy Clin Immunol 65:305–308
14. Mitchell EA, Elliott RB (1980) Controlled trial of an electrostatic precipitator in childhood asthma. Lancet II:559–561
15. Nogrady SG, Furnass SB (1983) Ionisers in the management of bronchial asthma. Thorax 38:919–922
16. Ben-Dov I, Amirav I, Schochina M, Amitai I, Bar-Yishay E, Godfrey S (1983) The effect of negative ionisation of inspired air on the response of asthmatic children to exercise and inhaled histamine. Thorax 38:584–588
17. Wilson N, Vickers H, Taylor G, Silverman M (1982) Objective test for food sensitivity in asthmatic children: increased bronchial activity after cola drinks. Br Med J 284:1226–1228
18. Minford AMB, Macdonald A, Littlewood JM (1982) Food intolerance and food allergy in children: a review of 68 cases. Arch Dis Child 57:742–747
19. Lask B (1979) Emotional factors in wheezing children. J R Soc Med 72:56–59
20. Goldsworthy S, Ancill RJ, Carr AC, Warner JO (1981) Computer-aided assessment of depression and anxiety. Prog Respir Res 17:277–281
21. Coher SI, Lask B (1983) Psychological factors. In: Clarke T, Godfrey S (eds) Asthma, 2nd edn. Chapman and Hall, London, pp 184–201
22. Oseid S, Edwards AM (1983) The asthmatic child in play and sport. Pitman, London
23. Speight ANP, Lee DA, Hey EN (1983) The underdiagnosis and undertreatment of asthma in childhood. Br Med J 286:1253–1256
24. Lenney W, Milner AD (1978) At what age do bronchodilator drugs work? Arch Dis Child 53:532–535
25. Hodges IGC, Groggins RC, Milner AD, Stokes GM (1981) Bronchodilator effect of inhaled ipratropium bromide in wheezy toddlers. Arch Dis Child 56:729–732
26. Goldsworthy SJ, Kemp M, Warner JO (1981) Salivary and urine theophylline levels in the management of childhood asthma. J R Soc Med 74:415–418
27. Stratton D, Carswell F, Hughes AO, Fysh WJ, Robinson P (1984) Double-blind comparisons of slow-release theophylline, ketotifen and placebo for prophylaxis of asthma in young children. Br J Dis Chest 78:163–167
28. Lenney W, Milner AD (1978) Nebulised sodium cromoglycate in the pre-school wheezy child. Arch Dis Child 53:474–476
29. Fallier CJ, Chai H, Molk L, Bane H, Cardoso RR de A (1972) Pulmonary and adrenal effects of alternate day corticosteroid therapy. J Allergy Clin Immunol 49:156–166
30. Lenney W, Milner AD, Hiller EJ (1978) Use of salbutamol powder in childhood asthma. Arch Dis Child 53:958–961
31. Anderson SD, Seale JP, Rosea P, Bandler L, Thesbald G, Lindsay DA (1976) Inhaled and oral salbutamol in exercise induced asthma. Am Rev Respir Dis 114:493–500

32. McKenzie SA (1982) Sympathomimetics and theophylline derivatives in the management of childhood asthma. Topics in paediatrics 3, Royal College of Physicians. Pitman, London, pp 62–71
33. Morrison Smith J, Devey GF (1968) Clinical trial of disodium cromoglycate in treatment of asthma in children. Br Med J II: 340–344
34. Robson RA, Taylor BJ, Taylor B (1981) Sodium cromoglycate spincaps or metered dose aerosol. Br J Clin Pharmacol 11: 383–384
35. McKenzie SA, Baillie E (1978) Serum theophylline levels in asthmatic children after oral administration of two slow-release theophylline preparations. Arch Dis Child 53: 943–946
36. Hambleton G, Weinberger M, Taylor J, Cavanaugh M, Ginchansky E, Godfrey S, Tosley M, Bell T, Greenberg S (1977) Comparison of cromoglycate (cromolyn) and theophylline in controlling symptoms of chronic asthma – a collaborative study. Lancet I: 381–385
37. Mitchell I, Paterson IC, Cameron SJ, Grant IWB (1976) Treatment of childhood asthma with sodium cromoglycate and beclomethasone dipropionate aerosol simply and in combination. Br Med J 2: 457–458
38. Smith JM, Pizarro YA (1973) Evaluation of systemic steroid treatment in children with asthma. Practitioner 211: 664–668
39. Friedman M, Strang LB (1966) Effect of long-term corticosteroids and corticotrophism on the growth of children. Lancet 2: 568–572
40. Godfrey S, Balfour-Lynn L, Tosley M (1978) A three-to-five year follow up of the use of the aerosol steroid beclomethasone dipropionate in childhood asthma. J Allergy Clin Immunol 62: 335–339
41. Taylor B, Norman AP (1975) Betamethasone 17-valerate in childhood asthma. Acta Paediatr Scand 64: 234–240
42. Field HV, Jenkinson PMA, Frame MH, Warner JO (1982) Asthma treatment with a new corticosteroid aerosol, Budesonide, administered twice daily by spacer inhaler. Arch Dis Child 57: 864–866
43. Kerrebijn KF (1976) Beclomethasone dipropionate in long-term treatment of asthma in children. J Pediatr 89: 821–826
44. Edmunds AT, McKenzie S, Tosley M, Godfrey S (1979) A clinical comparison of beclomethasone dipropionate delivered by pressurised aerosol and as a powder from a rotahaler. Arch Dis Child 54: 233–235
45. Reiser J, Frame MH, Warner JO (1986) The potential value of a 750 ml spacer for the administration of inhaled corticosteroids to children. Pediatr Pulmonol 2: 237–243
46. Mecoy RJ, Laby B (1982) Beclomethasone dipropionate in a twice daily treatment of asthma. Aust Fam Physician 9: 721–727
47. Muers M, Dawkins K (1983) Effect of a timed interval between inhalations of beta agonist and corticosteroid aerosols on the control of chronic asthma. Thorax 38: 378–382
48. Clarke RA, Anderson PB (1978) Combined therapy with salbutamol and beclomethasone inhalers in chronic asthma. Lancet II: 70–73
49. Nassif EG, Weinberger M, Thompson R, Huntley W (1981) The value of maintenance theophylline in steroid dependant asthma. N Engl J Med 304: 71–75
50. Mann NP, Hiller EJ (1982) Ipratropium bromide in children with asthma. Thorax 37: 72–74
51. Carmichael J, Paterson IC, Diaz P, Crompton GK, Kay AB, Grant IWB (1981) Corticosteroid resistance in chronic asthma. Br Med J 282: 1419–1422
52. British Thoracic Association (1982) Death from asthma in two regions of England. Br Med J 285: 1251–1255
53. Mellis CM, Phelan PD (1978) Asthma deaths in childhood – a continuing problem. Thorax 32: 29–34
54. Wilson JD, Sutherland DC, Thomas AC (1981) Has the change in tetra-agonists combined with oral theophylline increased cases of fatal asthma? Lancet I: 1235–1237
55. Mikenko PA, Ogilvie RI (1973) Rational intravenous doses of theophylline. N Engl J Med 289: 600–603
56. Edmunds AT, Godfrey S (1981) Cardiovascular response during acute severe asthma and its treatment in children. Thorax 35: 745–750
57. Luksza AR (1982) Acute severe asthma treated without steroids. Br J Dis Chest 76: 15–19
58. Shapiro GG, Furukawa CT, Pierson WE, Gardinier R, Bierman CW (1983) Double-blind evaluation of methylprednisolone versus placebo for acute asthma episodes. Pediatrics 71: 510–514
59. Grant IWB (1982) Are corticosteroids necessary in the treatment of severe acute asthma? Br J Dis Chest 76: 125–129
60. Branthwaite MA (1978) The management of severe asthma. In: Baderman H (ed) Management of medical emergencies. Pitman, Tunbridge Wells, pp 48–56
61. Shapiro GG, Eggleston PA, Pierson WE, Ray CG, Bierman CW (1974) Double-blind study of the effectiveness of a broad spectrum antibiotic in status asthmaticus. Pediatrics 53: 867–872

62. McKenzie SA, Edmunds AT, Godfrey S (1979) Status asthmaticus in children. Arch Dis Child 54:581–586
63. Warner JO (1981) Hyposensitisation in asthma: a review. J R Soc Med 74:60–65
64. Price JF, Warner JO, Hey EN, Turner MW, Soothill JF (1984) A controlled trial of hyposensitisation with adsorbed tyrosine Dermatophagoides pteronyssinus antigen in childhood asthma: in vivo aspects. Clin Allergy 14:209–220
65. Warner JO (1984) Immunotherapy. In: Lessof MH (ed) Allergy. John Wiley, Chichester, pp 447–464
66. Newman SP, Clarke SW (1983) Therapeutic aerosols: 1 – Physical and practical considerations. Thorax 38:881–886

44. Asthma in Adults

J. Bousquet, Ph. Godard, F. B. Michel

Asthma is not a disease restricted to childhood. Many adults and even old age patients suffer from asthma. Allergy is less important than in children and the so-called *intrinsic* asthma increases in frequency with age. Owing to a sustained bronchial inflammation, there is an accelerated decline of the pulmonary function of adult asthmatics leading to pulmonary impairment.

44.1 Natural History

Asthma is a common disease and the first attack may appear at any age, although the onset of allergic asthma is almost invariably before the age of 25 years, whereas the nonallergic variety occurs more commonly in middle age. In children, males have asthma more often than females, while in adults this male sex predominance is not seen.

Although progress has been made in treating asthmatic patients, it still remains exceedingly difficult to forecast the course of any individual's disease. Some children outgrow bronchial asthma, but the exact percentage is still a matter of debate ranging from 28 to 78% according to the investigator and definition of the disease. Moreover, if pulmonary function tests are performed in adults who had presented asthma in childhood, it appears that many so-called symptom-free patients have a reversible airway obstruction. Although individual variations do exist, it seems that if an individual develops asthma as an adult, the disease is often more severe and persistent. An earlier onset usually means a better prognosis, except when asthma begins in infancy. Patients suffering from nonallergic asthma may have remissions occurring at the beginning of the disease, but they tend to be less frequent and of shorter duration than in allergic asthma [1].

Asthma is a major factor contributing to an accelerated decline of the pulmonary function. It has been recently shown in a prospective study performed in a community that the rate of decline of FEV_1 was more rapid in asthmatic patients (50 ml/year) than in smokers (45 ml/year) and in normal nonsmoking subjects (32 ml/year) [2]. These findings were confirmed in a study of the pulmonary function of house dust mite allergic asthmatics (Fig. 44.1).

44.2 Provoking Factors

Allergy: Aeroallergens represent a very common provoking factor of asthma in children but their role in adults is less important, although it must not be forgotten. Foods are less likely to cause asthma in adults by an allergic mechanism (Fig. 44.2) [3]. Allergic asthmatics frequently present other manifestations of atopy such as rhinitis, conjunctivitis or atopic dermatitis. These patients usually developed asthma during childhood.

Many patients who suffer from allergic rhinitis and asthma tend to improve spontaneously after the fifth decade maybe since the number of mucosal mast cells decays or because the IgE responses are less intense. However, this is not the case in every subject.

Occupational asthma: Occupational asthma is, of course, mostly observed in adults. It can be due to allergic, irritative or pharmacological factors. Both atopic and nonatopic individuals can have occupational asthma (see corresponding chapters).

Aspirin sensitivity: In contradistinction with allergy, aspirin sensitivity is less common in children than in adults. Patients who present an intolerance to aspirin have asthma

Fig. 44.1. Evolution of FEV_1 and $FEV_{25-75\%}$ in asthmatic patients allergic to house dust mites according to their age. 315 asthmatic subjects were tested. ($p < 0.001$, F test)

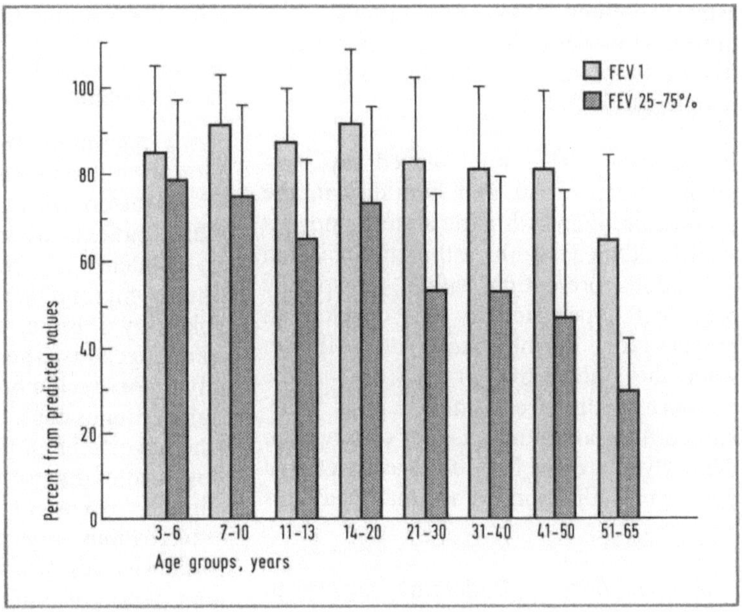

with many other analgesics that elicit an inhibition of the cyclooxygenase pathway of arachidonic acid, but it appears, from many studies, that most of them are not intolerant to tartrazine [4].

Preservatives and metabisulfites: Many preservatives present in foods and drugs have been associated with asthma exacerbations. However, in most cases observations are anecdotal. On the other hand ingested metabisulfites and inhaled SO_2 are common provoking agents. There are widely used as antioxidants in foods and even in some drugs such as β_2-agonists. Like analgesics, these preservatives are not often involved in childhood asthma [5].

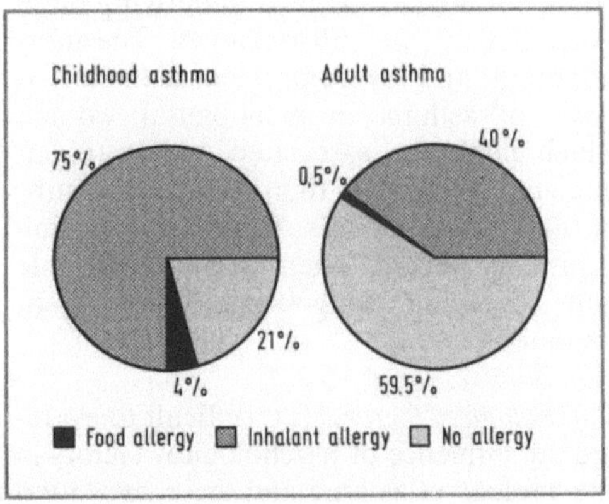

Fig. 44.2. Etiologies of asthma in children and adults. 300 asthmatic patients were studied

Infections: Upper respiratory infections of viral origin are common triggers of asthma in infancy and early childhood, but their role is still important in adults. Sinusitis may also cause asthma in adults. On the other hand, respiratory infections of bacterial origin seldom appear to precipitate asthma (see corresponding chapter).

Gastroesophageal reflux: Many asthmatic patients have a spontaneous or iatrogenic gastroesophageal reflux since drugs like theophylline can cause or aggravate it. However, it is often difficult to prove that this etiology is directly involved in the precipitation of asthma. Often, it is only one of the causes of asthma or it does not trigger it. The treatment of the reflux only improves a rather small subset of patients.

Exercise: Most asthmatics, whatever their age, become increasingly dyspneic following exertion, but true exercise-induced asthma, defined by an asthma attack in the minutes following the exercise in patients free of symptoms at rest, seems to be rarer than in childhood.

Environment: The role played by pollutants, temperature and humidity in the production of an asthmatic attack is not yet totally defined. Both asthmatic children and adults presenting with a nonspecific bronchial hyperreactivity can develop an exacerbation during peaks of pollution when they inhale SO_2 or NO_2 and in the presence of tobacco smoke. It is well-known that pollution episodes observed in Pennsylvania or in London directly caused many hospitalizations of asthmatic patients [6].

Hormonal factors: Endocrine factors in asthmatic women exert unusual contributory effects, none of which is completely understood. Some women report cyclic exacerbations of wheezing during menstruation, but the mechanisms underlying these exacerbations are still unknown. The most important and severe problem is the initial onset of asthma in menopausal women which might be associated with estrogen depletion, although there is no data supporting this hypothesis. This type of asthma is usually severe, often being intractable and requiring long-term corticosteroid treatment.

Psychological factors: It is difficult to evaluate the influence of psychological factors in the etiology of asthma and the provocation of individual attacks. However, in patients with unstable asthma they are likely to be of importance. Considerable difference of opinion exists as to whether emotional disturbances are an etiological factor or a consequence of asthma.

Drugs: Many drugs are shown to cause asthma by allergic, pharmacological mechanisms or mast cell activation. Iatrogenic asthma appears to increase in frequency (see corresponding chapter).

44.3 Presentation of Asthma in Adults

Asthma is a heterogeneous disease and can be observed in various situations.

Acute intermittent asthma: This is a common form of asthma in young subjects and is characterized by long periods during which patients are symptom-free and show no evidence of respiratory impairment. Their symptomatic periods are usually provoked by seasonal allergens or respiratory tract infections. These patients present usually a nonspecific bronchial hyperreactivity during remissions. However, in patients who have perennial intermittent symptoms, this form of disease tends to be replaced by chronic persistent asthma with acute exacerbations, especially if they smoke. Oral corticosteroids are rarely required for a long period of time, but may help in some situations.

Chronic persistant asthma: Individuals with chronic persistant asthma are usually easily recognized. The bronchial obstruction is constantly present and therefore they need constant medication. This group includes patients who have the intrinsic form of asthma, those who are sensitized to perennial allergens such as house dust mites, or patients intolerant to aspirin. Inhaled or eventually oral corticosteroids represent the drugs of choice to decrease the sustained inflammation of the airways. These patients are susceptible to developing chronic progressive respiratory impairment and cor pulmonale.

Many patients with chronic asthma present morning and nocturnal exacerbations that represent a troublesome, sometimes serious and even fatal feature of asthma [7]. Nocturnal asthma can be attributed to many factors among which an exaggeration of a normal circadian rhythm in airway caliber or in the secretion of catecholamines and adrenaline has been implicated. The treatment of this form of asthma can be very difficult. Mild cases may respond to simple bronchodilator treatment but this should be given regularly throughout the day to stabilize the airways, even though patients do not have symptoms at this time. In severe cases, all treatments may fail.

Chronic intractable asthma: In some adult asthmatics bronchoconstriction never remits and such patients are considered to have chronic intractable asthma [8]. Occasionally this may represent a combination of asthma and chronic bronchitis induced by heavy cigarette smoking. Sometimes there is little variation in obstruction from day to day and the persistent wheezing is more suggestive of asthma than bronchitis. A personal or familial history of atopy and the finding of eosinophils point to a diagnosis of asthma, but frequently the clinical presentation suggests the combination of both asthma and chronic bronchitis with intermittent exacerbations of bronchospasm. These patients usually respond poorly to β_2-agonists and it is advisable to treat them with high doses of oral or parenteral corticosteroids of up to 2 mg/kg of body weight for several days to assess the reversibility of the bronchial obstruction.

Hidden asthma: Many patients presenting with chronic cough are in fact misdiagnosed asthmatics since they may not have evidence of airways obstruction [9]. However, when nonspecific provocative challenges with histamine or methacholine are performed these patients behave like asthmatics.

Acute complications: Complications such as pneumonia, atelectasis, mucoid impactions and mucous plugging, or pneumomediastinum are more often seen in children than in adults [10].

Deaths caused by asthma occur predominantly in adults aged 40 to 60 years. Deaths resulting from asthma outside the hospital may occur suddenly and are often caused by a delayed efficient treatment, especially systemic corticosteroids [10].

Chronic complications: Sleep apnea may rarely coexist with asthma and such patients may only have mild hypoxemia while awake but have severe alarming hypoxemia at night because of obstructive apnea. Moreover there are many adults with chronic stable asthma who present irregular breathing and hypoxemia during sleep [11].

The accelerated decline of the pulmonary function of asthmatics occasionally leads, in patients chronically affected, to a chronic respiratory insufficieny and a cor pulmonale.

Oral corticotherapy is sometimes essential to the management of some cases of severe intractable asthma and the benefits to be obtained from these drugs far outweigh their potential hazards. However, they can lead to severe complications among which diabetes, mental disturbances, osteoporosis and vertebral compression fractures are the most common.

Asthma in pregnancy: Asthma in the pregnant patient affects the health of both the mother and the fetus. The most common threat to both is uncontrolled asthma leading to hypoxemia that present potential sources of mortality for the fetus and the initiation of premature labor. It appears that patients with mild asthma usually have either no change in their symptoms or they may even observe some improvement. On the other hand, patients with severe asthma may get worse. The treatment of the pregnant asthmatic is analogous to that of the nonpregnant patient although some drugs such as oral corticosteroids may have some unfavorable effects on the fetus [12].

Asthma in the elderly: The diagnosis of asthma in the elderly remains uncommon because in the mind of many doctors asthma is a disease of the young and the composite definition of asthma that would include etiological, clinical and even therapeutic characteristics is lacking. Asthma should be differentiated from the bronchial edema often seen during cardiac failure, pulmonary embolism or chronic bronchitis. In many patients asthma started early in life and although the allergic etiology does not represent a major provoking factor it cannot be excluded. When the onset of asthma was late, it is often intrinsic [13].

The treatment of asthma in the elderly is slightly different to that in adulthood since the clearance of theophylline is decreased and it appears that β_2-agonists may be less active. Moreover, some patients with cardiac arrhythmias may be worsened if theophylline and β_2-agonists are associated [14].

44.4 Treatment Particularities of Asthma in Adults

The treatment of asthma in adults is basically the same as that of children, but some drugs have slightly different effects. The clearance of theophylline is decreased in adults and dosages should be reduced; β_2-agonists may be less effective and anticholinergics may be more active in adults. Finally, specific immunotherapy should not be started in patients with an impaired pulmonary function ($FEV_1 < 70\%$ from predicted values), when there is a concomitant sinusitis or other etiologic factors, such as aspirin sensitivity. It was shown that this form of treatment is less effective in adults than in children [15].

References

1. Smith MJ (1983) Epidemiology and natural history of asthma, allergic rhinitis and atopic dermatitis. In: Middleton E Jr, Reed CE, Elliot EF (eds) Allergy, Principles and Practice, 2nd edn. Mosby, St. Louis, pp 771–804
2. Woolcock AJ, Peat JK, Cullen K (1986) The effect of asthma on rate of decline of lung function. Am Rev Respir Dis 133: A156
3. Onorato J, Merland N, Terral C, Michel FB, Bousquet J (1986) Double-blind food challenge in asthma. J Allergy Clin Immunol 78 (in press)
4. Stevenson T (1986) Adverse reactions to aspirin and nonsteroidal anti-inflammatory drugs. In: Reed CE (ed) Proceedings of the XIIth Congress of Allergology and Clinical Immunology. Mosby, St. Louis, pp 79–82
5. Simon RA (1986) Sulfite sensitivity. Ann Allergy 56:281–288
6. Bousquet J, Michel FB (1986) Environmental control in asthma. In: Reed CE (ed) Proceedings of the XIIth Congress of Allergology and Clinical Immunology, Mosby, St. Louis, pp 390–393
7. Hetzel MR, Clark TJH (1983) Adult asthma. In: Clark TJH, Godfrey S (eds) Asthma. Chapman and Hall, London, pp 457–486
8. Scoggin CH, Petty TH (1980) Clinical strategies in adult asthma. Lea and Febiger, Philadelphia
9. Corrao WM, Braman SS, Irwin RS (1979) Chronic cough as the sole presenting manifestation of asthma. N Engl J Med 12: 633–637
10. Bernstein IL (1983) Asthma in adults. In: Middleton E Jr, Reed CE, Elliot EF (eds) Allergy, Principles and Practice, 2nd edn. Mosby, St. Louis, pp 841–856
11. Caterall JR, Calverley PMA, Brezinova V et al (1982) Irregular breathing and hypoxaemia during sleep in chronic stable asthma. Lancet I:301–304
12. Weinstein AM, Dubin BD, Podleski WK, Spector SL, Farr RS (1979) Asthma and pregnancy. JAMA 241: 1161–1165
13. Burr ML, Charles TJ, Roy K, Seaton A (1979) Asthma in the elderly: an epidemiological survey. Br Med J 1: 1041–1044
14. Bousquet J, Clauzel AM, Michel FB (1987) Beta-adrenergic agonists in asthma. In: Barnes P, Kaliner M (eds) Neural regulation of the airways. Lung Biology in Health and Disease. Marcel Dekker, New York (in press)
15. Bousquet J, Michel FB (1986) Immunotherapy in asthma. In: Reed CE (ed) Proceedings of the XIIth Congress of Allergology and Clinical Immunology. Mosby, St. Louis, pp 394–396

45. Skin Tests

J. L. Ménardo, W. Skassa-Brociek, J. Bousquet

Skin tests represent, since Blackley introduced them in 1870, the primary diagnostic tool in allergology. They make it possible to demonstrate specific IgE bound on the cutaneous mast cell. Their characteristics, simplicity and rapidity of performance, interpretation, low cost and high sensitivity explain why the recent sophisticated method of RAST, commercialized some 100 years later, has not been able to oust the rank of key position that cutaneous testing occupies in allergology [1].

Cutaneous testing is a necessary investigation for asthmatic patients, and only immediate-type tests are performed since epicutaneous test and delayed hypersensitivity tests provide little information. A positive skin test does not necessarily mean that this allergen is a total explanation for the patient's asthma. A positive provocative challenge would be a better indication of undoubted allergic sensitization. However, a precise and concordant clinical story can be considered as satisfactory, in so far as the quality of skin testing has been largely improved with the recent efforts of standardization.

45.1 Methods

Intradermal reaction (IDR): The allergen extract is injected intracutaneously from a 1 ml tuberculin syringe filled with approximatively 0.1 ml of the solution through a 26 gauge by ⅜ inch needle.

Before injection, all bubbles must be carefully eliminated in order to avoid *splash* reactions which could be mistakenly interpreted. The test is performed on the volar surface of the arm or the forearm, the syringe placed at an angle of 45 ° to the arm, the level of the needle downwards, facing the skin, and penetrating entirely, but not going any deeper. A volume of approximatively 0.02 ml is gently injected in order to produce a 3 mm bleb.

Solution concentrations must never be stronger than $1/1000$ weight by volume (wt/v) in order to avoid false positive reactions related to nonspecific irritant factors [2]. If the patient is clinically suspected to be allergic, lower concentrations for this allergen extract must be chosen as systemic reactions could occur.

IDR is the most sensitive method for skin testing and its use is recommended for extract of low allergenic concentrations such as venoms or drugs as other methods usually give negative reactions.

Prick test (PT) (Fig. 45.1): This method was first described in the twenties, and used later again by Squire [3], but it became a widespread tool in the seventies [2, 4] and currently, it tends to supplant the other methods. It is performed by directing a needle ($32 \times 7/10$ mm) through a drop of the allergen solution at an angle of 60 to 70° at the same time lifting the skin, thus making a canal through which the extract penetrates. No bleeding must occur. Such a method results in an injection of an amount of about 3 millionths of a ml into the skin [3]. The drop can be removed immediately after the skin has been pricked [5].

PTs appear to have several advantages over IDR: (i) They are simply and quickly performed; (ii) they do not provoke any harm and are thus easily performed on infants; (iii) if negative, they do not elicit any change in the aspect of the skin making the interpretation easier; (iv) if positive, the wheal and flare reaction size is small (rarely exceeding 10 mm) making it possible to perform as many as 20 tests on a forearm; (v) we noticed only one systemic reaction in more than 4,000 patients undergoing prick testing; (vi) their reproducibility can be improved by using the recent standardized

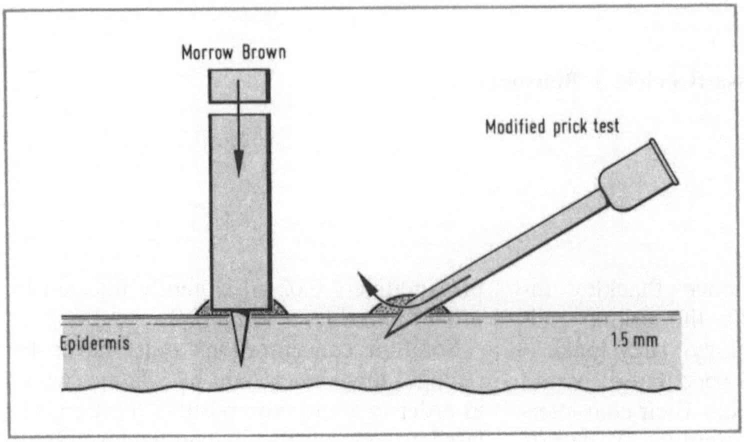

Fig. 45.1. Two methods of prick testing. The Morrow-Brown needle makes it possible to standardize the depth of the penetration

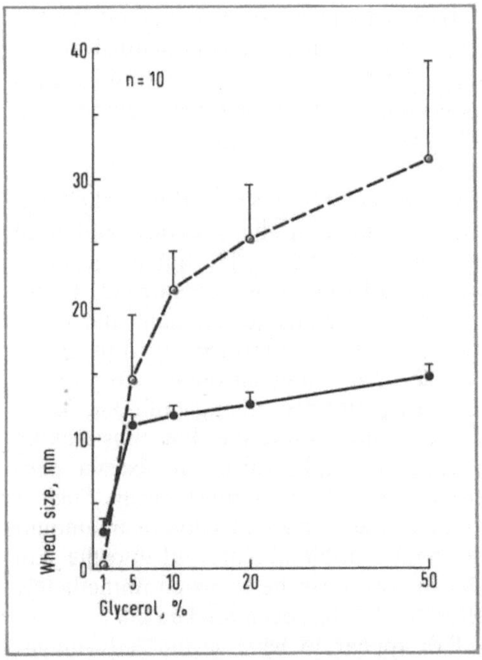

Fig. 45.2. Intradermal injection of glycerol solution at different concentrations. —— wheal size; ---- erythema

devices like the Morrow-Brown Needle or Stallerpointe [6], the Allergy-Pricker [7], or the MULTI-TEST [8]; (vii) allergen extract solutions used for PT are more concentrated than for ID route (usually 5×10^{-2} wt/v) and are diluted in 50% glycerol. These conditions prolong the storage life of the allergen solutions and thus diminish the risk of false negative reactions due to the loss of allergenic potency of the extract solution [9]; and (viii) IDR results in a less precise separation of allergic and nonallergic subjects than PT evaluation owing to a great number of false positive reactions [10].

Finally, like IDR, PT makes it possible to determine the end point titration by injecting three fold lower concentrations and searching for the lowest one which gives a reaction.

Scratch test: The superficial layers of skin are abraded by a needle or a scarifier without causing any bleeding and a drop of allergenic extract is applied over the scratch.

Prick and scratch tests are, thus, closely related. However, (i) the scratch test introduces a variable amount of antigen into the epidermis and is therefore difficult to standardize; and (ii) false positive reactions do occur if the patient exhibits dermographism. Owing to these flaws the scratch test should not be used anymore.

Diluents: Glycerol must not be used for intradermal tests [11] at a concentration over 2% (Fig. 45.2) as it provokes nonspecific irritant reactions which do not appear to be related to histamine release [12]. It is, however, possible to dilute extracts for IDR from concentrated allergens preserved in 50% glycerol. On the other hand, human serum albumin (HSA) induces very few reactions [12].

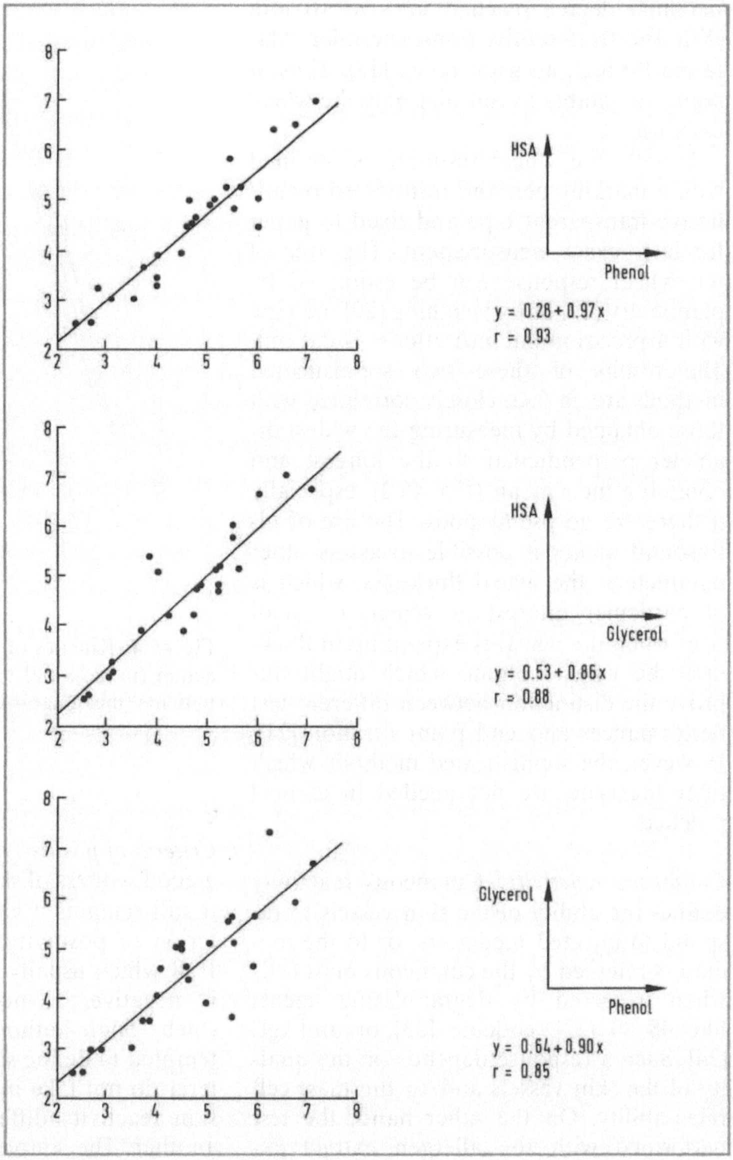

Fig. 45.3. Comparison of the size of the wheals induced by a Dermatophagoides pteronyssinus extract diluted in human serum albumin (HSA), 50% glycerol or phenol and tested by prick

HSA, phenol or glycerol may be equally successfully employed for prick testing although they have slightly different behavior related to different viscosity [12] (Fig. 45.3).

45.2 Interpretation

Measurement: Whatever the method, the immediate skin test induces a response which reaches a peak in 10 to 17 min [13]. Delayed reactions can be observed and generally reflect the late phase reaction [14, 15] and its occurrence seems to be related to the size of the immediate reaction [16], but sometimes reveal (when IDR is chosen) a precipitin-induced reaction. The wheal results from the direct action on capillaries of mediators released by the cutaneous mast cell; the mast cell shows alterations within 15 s after allergen injection with a maximal degree reached in 5 to 10 min [17]. The flare results from arteriolar dilatation through an axon reflex [18]. Thus, it seems preferable to consider only the wheal response.

Usually the wheal response is outlined with a marking pen and transferred by adhesive transparent tape and fixed to paper for later exact measurement. The area of the wheal response can be estimated by planimetry [19] or by weighing [20] the tape with a precision balance after it is cut out. The results of these two sophisticated methods are, in fact, closely correlated with those obtained by measuring the widest diameter perpendicular to the longest and obtaining their mean (Fig. 45.2), especially if there are no pseudopods. The use of ultrasound makes it possible to assess other parameters: the wheal thickness, which is of particular interest in wheals of small size; when the wheal is expanding in thickness the wheal volume which might improve the distinction between different test performances and end point titration [21]. However, the sophisticated methods which offer precision are not needed in clinical practice.

Cutaneous reactivity: Cutaneous reactivity defines the ability of the skin vessels to respond to injected mediators, or to the mediators released by the cutaneous mast cells when triggered by degranulating agents like 48/80 [22], codeine [23] or anti-IgE [24]. Such a response depends on the quality of the skin vessels and/or the mast cell releasability. On the other hand, the test performed with the allergen extract explores not only the cutaneous reactivity, but also the *cutaneous sensitivity* determined by specific IgE sensitizing the cutaneous mast cell.

Timing: The kinetics of the whealing response is different for the different agents. The peak is obtained at 5 min for histamine with a rapid decrease in the size, whereas the peak is obtained after the 7th min for codeine and 48/80 and lasts longer than histamine (Fig. 45.4). The kinetics of the allergen-induced wheal is very similar to those of the degranulating agents [Ménardo, unpublished data].

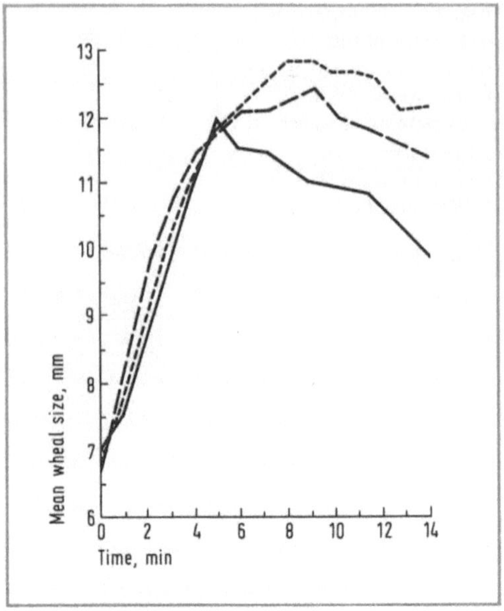

Fig. 45.4. Kinetics of the wheal size-induced reaction (intradermal test) in 15 adult nonallergic patients (mean age = 29 ± 6) using —— histamine, - - - - codeine, — — — 48/80

Criteria of positivity: If the size of the test is a good witness of skin-fixed IgE antibodies, it still remains a vague and subjective criterion of positivity, especially when using IDR which usually induces, even if the test is negative, a modification of the skin (bleb). Some authors using PT [25] have attempted to define size criteria, but such criteria do not take into account the fact that skin reactivity differs from one subject to another. The simplest criterion is a ratio of the size of the test induced by the allergen to the size of that induced by a degranulating agent like 48/80 or codeine [8]. Histamine can be used as a positive control for this ratio, but it does not explore the mast cell releasability. Others use a close ratio including the possible reaction induced by the negative control solution (diluent) [26], but the ratio (size of allergen test/size of positive control test) is very easy to appreciate and appears to be satisfactory. With a codeine phosphate 5% solution, we used a threshold of 80%, since most of the subjects who reach this threshold also have a positive RAST to the allergen (Fig. 45.5). Such

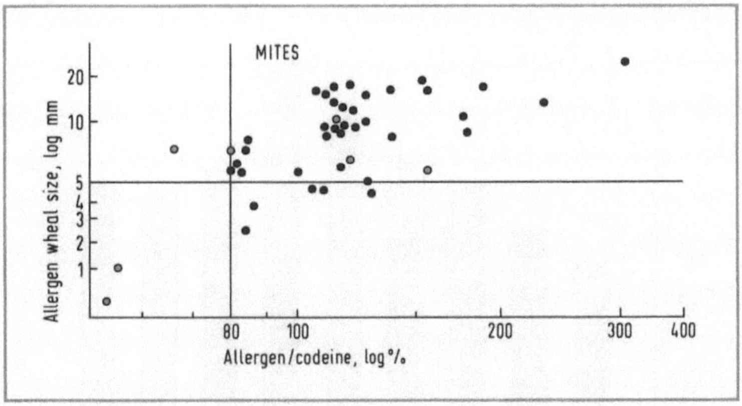

Fig. 45.5. Index of positivity: Most of the patients who have a positive RAST to Dermatophagoides pteronyssinus have an index

$$\frac{\textit{size of allergen test}}{\textit{size of 5\% codeine test}}$$

over 80% even if the wheal size is under 5 mm (green circles = patients with a negative RAST; black circles = patients with a positive RAST)

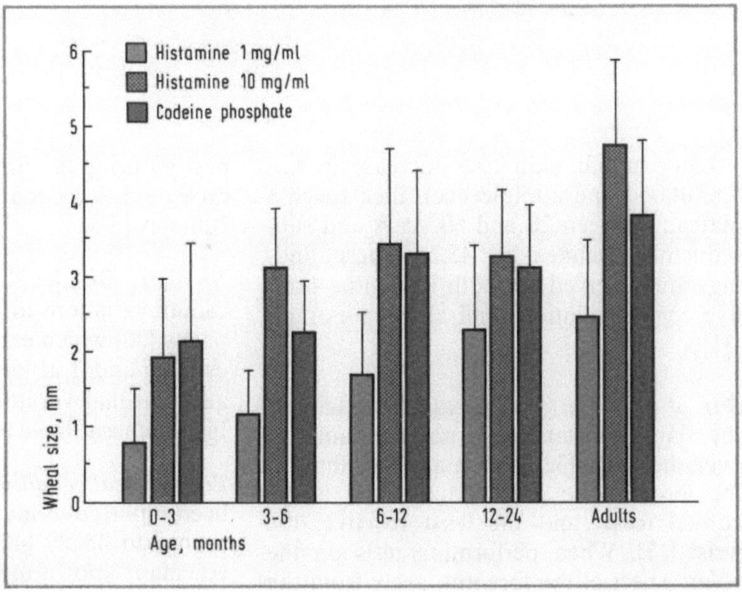

Fig. 45.6. Mean wheal size of different control solutions in 78 infants and 30 adults

a criterion makes it possible to decrease the number of RAST performed on a patient and consequently reduces the cost of the investigation.

45.3 Factors Affecting the Cutaneous Response

Many factors can affect the quality of skin testing and their occurrence in a patient can be easily demonstrated by the use of a positive control test (histamine, codeine) which must always be injected prior to testing.

Age: It is important to reject the tenet according to which children under 3 years cannot be tested [27, 28] because there are no precise grounds for it. Skin test size is smaller in infants [3, 29], but PT permits skin testing in infants without any difficulty. The texture of their skin makes it very easy for the wheal to grow and become obvious although, in the first year of life there is a histamine hyporeactivity and a less important but undeniable codeine hyporeactivity (Fig. 45.6) [30]. These characteristics tend to fade as the child enters his second year, but the size of the wheal (PT) remains generally under 2 mm.

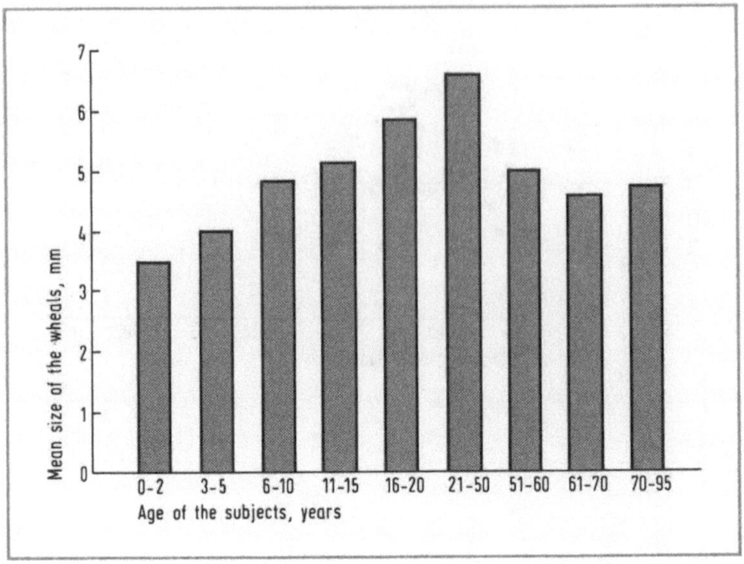

Fig. 45.7. Mean wheal size of histamine (1 mg/ml) according to the age of the subjects

Later in life, skin tests increase in size (childhood and adolescence), then reach a plateau between 20 and 50 years and subsequently decline (Fig. 45.7). These findings are observed for both histamine positive control solutions and allergen extracts [31].

Site of injection: The whealing capacity of the skin to histamine is not the same all over the body [32] and it appears that on the forearm the most reactive site is the cubital fossa, and the least reactive, the wrist [13]. When performing tests on the volar aspect of the forearm, away from the wrist and the antecubital fossa, the wheal size is not altered by varying the position of testing within this area [33]. The back can also be chosen for PT because it appears to be one of the most reactive sites. It must be noted that studies on mast cell content in normal human skin have reported conflicting results upon variations in relation to body regions [34].

Sex: Skin reactivity differences in male and female patients appear essentially related to the difference in the sensitization to allergens [35, 36], as no difference can be observed when using 48/80 [21]. However, it has been demonstrated that women exhibit the weakest histamine whealing capacity during the first day of the menstrual cycle and a second minimum around the 20th day [37].

Rhythms: Besides the menstrual cycle, circadian variations in histamine whealing capacity [38] which exhibits a peak in the late evening and is at its lowest in the morning, and seasonal variations, related to specific IgE synthesis, have been demonstrated [39].

Pathological conditions: Acute urticaria has been reported to increase the cutaneous response to 48/80 [40]. On the other hand, eczema is known to diminish the skin reactivity [41]. It also seems reasonable not to perform skin tests in areas where there is any skin lesion which might interfere with skin reactivity. Finally, in cases of previous systemic anaphylactic reaction, a delay of one week is preferable before skin testing.

Drugs

Some drugs can interfere with the whealing capacity of the skin thus making the interpretation of skin tests unclear. On the other hand, others largely used in asthmatic patients do not modify the cutaneous responsiveness:

Antihistamines: The H_1-antagonists which antagonize the capillary effects of histamine inhibit the wheal and flare reaction [42, 43] to histamine, and this effect can be used to demonstrate the antihistaminic activity of a drug and the duration of its effect [44]. Moreover, the H_1-antagonists reduce also the wheal reaction induced by degranulating agents or allergens in sensitized patients [45].

H_2-antagonists (cimetidine) alone have no significant effect on the whealing response to histamine, 48/80, or allergen [46, 47] though it is suggested that they can increase the allergic reaction by blocking the negative feedback control of histamine on mediator release [47].

Different studies on the combination of H_1- and H_2-antagonists have reported conflicting results; some mentioned an enhancement of the inhibitory effect [46, 48, 49], others did not [45, 50].

β_2-adrenergic agents: These drugs in the therapeutic range and routes used in the treatment of asthma do not inhibit allergen skin tests [51, 52], but when they are injected directly in the skin, at the site of the test the whealing capacity of the skin is diminished [53–55]. Such an effect seems to be due to an antianaphylactic property of β_2-adrenergic drugs rather than to a direct action on the dermal vasculature [54].

Theophylline: Results of these studies are in disagreement. Some studies have found that aminophylline and theophylline reduce the wheal size of skin tests either to histamine or allergen, and that this effect could be related to the blood level of this drug [42, 56]. However, other studies were unable to find any significant difference in the wheal size of the allergen or histamine-induced skin tests, before and after an acute or chronic administration of theophylline therapeutic range [57, 58].

Corticosteroids: Short-term (less than one week) administration of corticosteroids at therapeutic ranges used in asthmatic patients does not modify cutaneous testing with histamine, 48/80 or allergen [58, 59], even though the blood eosinophilia has lowered. Long-term corticotherapy modifies the skin texture and makes the interpretation of immediate skin tests more difficult.

Cromolyn: Disodium cromoglycate injected with, or prior to, allergens or degranulating agents, does not modulate skin whealing response [60, 61].

Ketotifen: This protective drug is a potent antihistamine (H_1) but possesses anti-anaphylactic and antiasthmatic properties. Its administration during three days at half the dosage usually used in the prophylactic treatment of asthma, induces a dramatic decrease in the size of the allergen-induced wheal reaction. Such an inhibitory effect does not seem to last longer than 5 to 7 days [62].

Imipramines and phenothiazines: Tricyclic antidepressants and neuroleptics have potent antihistamine effects which largely inhibit the whealing cutaneous response to histamine [63], and also to degranulating agents [Ménardo, unpublished data].

Specific immunotherapy: The diminution in skin test reactivity has been noticed by many authors in the patients undergoing immunotherapy with pollen extracts [64–66]. Rush immunotherapy protocols make it possible to notice a rapid decrease (1 week) in size and end-point titration for pollen extracts [67, 68], and also for mite extracts [69]. Such a rapid effect does not seem to be related to a specific IgG increase and concerns only the allergen used for the immunotherapy (the cutaneous reactivity assessed by codeine and histamine remains totally unchanged) [67].

References

1. Skin testing and radio-allergo sorbent testing (RAST) for diagnosis of specific allergens responsible for IgE-mediated diseases – Position statement. J Allergy Clin Immunol (1983) 72:515–517
2. Stenius B (1973) Skin and provocation tests with Dermatophagoides pteronyssinus in allergic rhinitis. Comparison of prick and intracutaneous skin test methods and correlation with specific IgE. Acta Allergologica 28:81–100
3. Squire RJ (1950) The relationship between horse-dandruff and horse serum antigens in asthma. Clin Sci 9:127–150

4. Pepys J (1975) Skin testing. Br J Hosp Med 14:412–417
5. Ownby DR, Anderson JA (1982) An improved prick skin test procedure for young children. J Allergy Clin Immunol 69:533–535
6. Brown HM, Thantrey N, Jackson FA (1979) Species specific grass pollen sensitivity. Clin Allergy 9:465–472
7. Østerballe O, Weeke B (1979) A new lancet for skin prick testing. Allergy 34:209–212
8. Ménardo JL, Bousquet J, Michel FB (1982) Comparison of three prick test methods with the intradermal test and with the RAST in the diagnosis of mite allergy. Ann Allergy 48:235–239
9. Norman PS, Marsh DG (1978) Human serum albumin and tween 80 as stabilizers of allergen solutions. J Allergy Clin Immunol 62:314–319
10. Brown WG, Halonen MJ, Kalteborn WT, Barbee RA (1979) The relationship of respiratory allergy, skin test reactivity and serum IgE in a community population sample. J Allergy Clin Immunol 63:328–335
11. Slavin RG (1974) Skin tests in the diagnosis of the immediate type. Med Clin North Am 58:65–69
12. Ménardo JL, Bousquet J, Bataille A, Réstagny G, Michel FB (1983) Effects of diluents on skin tests. Ann Allergy 51:535–538
13. Voorhorst R, van Krieken H (1973) Atopic skin test reevaluated. I. Perfection of skin testing technique. Ann Allergy 31:137–142
14. Kaliner M (1984) Hypotheses on the contribution of late phase allergic responses to the understanding and treatment of allergic diseases. J Allergy Clin Immunol 73:311–315
15. Dor PJ, Vervloet D, Sapene M, Andrac C, Bonerandi JJ, Charpin J (1983) Induction of late cutaneous reaction by kallikrein injection: comparison with allergic-like late response to compound 48/80. J Allergy Clin Immunol 71:363–370
16. Argawal K, Zetterström R (1982) Diagnostic significance of late cutaneous allergic responses and their correlation with radio allergo sorbent test. Clin Allergy 12:489–497
17. Ting S, Dunsky EH, Lavker RM, Zweiman B (1980) Patterns of mast cell alterations and in vivo mediator release in human allergic skin reactions. J Allergy Clin Immunol 66:417–423
18. Rebhun J, Botvin J (1980) Histamine flare, a neurovascular response. Ann Allergy 45:59–61
19. Sussman GL, Schocket AL (1981) Evaluation of skin test response using two techniques of measurement. American Academy of Allergy Meeting (abstract 246)
20. Ownby DR (1982) Computerized measurement of allergen-induced reactions. J Allergy Clin Immunol 69:536–538
21. Serup J (1984) Diameter, thickness, area and volume of skin-prick histamine wheals: measurement of skin thickness by 15 MH2 A mode ultrasound. Allergy 39:359–365
22. Voohorst R, Nikkels AH (1977) Atopic skin test reevaluated. IV. The use of 48/80 in routine skin testing. Ann Allergy 38:255–262
23. Sulzberger MB, Baer RL (1940) Whealing capacity of the skin of newborn or young infant. Arch Dermatol Syph 41:1029–1035
24. Stevenson D, Orgel HA, Hamburger RN, Reid RT (1971) Development of IgE in newborn human infants. J Allergy 48:61–72
25. Lessof MH, Buisseret PD, Merrett J, Merrett TG (1980) Assessing the value of skin prick tests. Clin Allergy 10:115–120
26. Schultze-Werninghaus G (1980) Comparison of standardized skin and provocation tests with RAST and histamine release from leucocytes in bronchial asthma. Allergy 35:259–261
27. Boutin C, Viallat JR (1980) Tests cutanés d'allergie. In: Charpin J (ed) Allergologie. Flammarion, Paris, pp 288–295
28. Aas K (1975) Diagnosis of immediate type respiratory allergy. Pediatr Clin North Am 22:33–42
29. van Asperen PP, Kemp AS, Mellis CM (1984) Skin test reactivity and clinical allergen sensitivity in infancy. J Allergy Clin Immunol 73:381–386
30. Ménardo JL, Bousquet J, Rodière M, Astruc J, Michel FB (1985) J Allergy Clin Immunol 75:646–651
31. Skassa W, Bousquet J, Ménardo JL, Michel FB (1985) Skin test reactivity from infancy to elderly. J Allergy Clin Immunol 75, 1 (part 2):362 (abstract)
32. Swain HH, Becker EL (1952) Quantitative studies in skin testing. V. The whealing reactions of histamine and ragweed pollen extract. J Allergy 23:441
33. Clarke CW, Mitchell J, Nunn AJ, Pepys J (1982) Reproducibility of prick skin tests to five common allergens. Clin Allergy 12:1–8
34. Eady RAJ (1979) The mast cell in diseases of the skin. In: Pepys J, Edwards AM (eds) The mast cell, its role in health and disease. Pitman, Bath, pp 544–549
35. Hendrick DJ, Davies RJ, d'Souza MF, Pepys J (1975) An analysis of skin prick test reactions in 656 asthmatic patients. Thorax 50:2–8
36. Haahtela T, Björksten F, Heiskala M, Suoneimi I (1980) Skin prick test reactivity to common allergens in Finnish adolescents. Allergy 35:425–431

37. Bosse K, Ladebeck HE (1972) Die kutane histamine Reaktion in Korrelation zum Cyclus der Frau. Z Haut Geschlechtskr 47:365–369
38. Lee RE, Smolensky MH, Leach CS, Mc Govern JP (1977) Circadian rhythms in the cutaneous reactivity to histamine and selected antigens, including phase relationships to urinary cortisol excretion. Ann Allergy 38: 231–236
39. Haahtela T, Jokela H (1980) Influence of the pollen season on immediate skin test reactivity to common allergens. Allergy 35:15–23
40. Juhlin L, Rune C (1962) Skin reactions to 48/80 in normal subjects and patients with urticaria and eczema. Acta Dermatol Venereol 42:11–16
41. Uehara M (1982) Reduced histamine reaction in atopic dermatitis. Arch Dermatol 118:244–250
42. Mosko M, Marshall RB Jr (1950) A study of the effect of various drugs on the whealing reaction. J Allergy 21:242–249
43. Galant SP, Zippin C, Bullock J, Crisp J (1972) Allergy skin tests. I. Antihistamine inhibition. Ann Allergy 30:53–63
44. Burns RBP, Shelanski MV (1977) Histamine wheal and flare inhibition by clemastine fumarate. Ann Allergy 38:339–344
45. Summers R, Sigler R, Shelhamer JH, Kaliner M (1981) Effects of infused histamine on asthmatic and normal subjects: comparison of skin test responses. J Allergy Clin Immunol 67:456–464
46. Harvey RP, Schoket AL (1980) The effect of H1 and H2 blockade on cutaneous response in man. J Allergy Clin Immunol 65:136–139
47. Smith JA, Mansfield LE, Nelson HS, Colonel MC (1979) The effect of Cimetidine on the immediate cutaneous response to allergens. Ann Allergy 42:353–354
48. Lichtenstein LM, Gillespie E (1975) The effects of the H1 and H2 anti-histamines on "allergic" histamine release and its inhibition by histamine. J Pharmacol Exp Ther 192:441–450
49. Smith JA, Mansfield LE, de Shazo RS, Nelson HS (1980) An evaluation of the pharmacological inhibition of the immediate and late cutaneous response to allergen. J Allergy Clin Immunol 65:118–121
50. Hutchcroft BJ, Moore EG, Orange RP (1979) The effect of H1 and H2 receptor antagonism on the response of monkey skin to intradermal histamine, reverse-type anaphylaxis and passive cutaneous anaphylaxis. J Allergy Clin Immunol 63:376–382
51. Imbeau SA, Harruf R, Hirscher M, Reed CE (1978) Terbutaline's effect on the allergy skin test. J Allergy Clin Immunol 62:193–196
52. Spector SL (1979) Effect of a selective beta 2 adrenergic agonist and theophylline on skin test reactivity and cardiovascular parameters. J Allergy Clin Immunol 64:23–28
53. Ting S, Zweiman B, Lavker R (1983) Terbutaline modulation of human allergic reactions. J Allergy Clin Immunol 71:437–441
54. Gronneberg R, Standberg K, Hagermark O (1980) Cutaneous responses to allergen after local pretreatment with beta-adrenoceptor stimulating and blacking agents. Allergy 34:409–412
55. Ohmi T, Mue S, Takahashi M, Ishihara M, Tamura G, Takashima T (1982) The inhibitory effect of isoproterenol and dibutyryl cyclic-AMP on the immediate skin reaction. Ann Allergy 48:40–43
56. Fine SR, Fogarty M, Goel Z, Grieco MH (1977) Correlation of serum theophylline levels with inhibition of allergen and histamine induced skin-tests. Ann Allergy 38:440 (abstract)
57. Chipps BE, Sobotka AK, Saunders JP, Teets KC, Norman PS, Lichtenstein LM (1980) Effect of theophylline and terbutaline on immediate skin tests. J Allergy Clin Immunol 65:61–64
58. Galant SP, Bullock J, Wong D, Maibach HI (1973) The inhibitory effect of anti-allergy drugs on allergen and histamine induced wheal and flare response. J Allergy Clin Immunol 51:11–21
59. Slott RI, Zweiman B (1974) A controlled study of the effect of corticosteroids on immediate skin test reactivity. J Allergy Clin Immunol 54:229–234
60. Ting S, Zweiman B, Lavker RM (1983) Cromolyn does not modulate human allergic skin reactions in vivo. J Allergy Clin Immunol 71:12–17
61. Ting S, Reimann F, Zweiman B (1984) Effects of cromolyn on codeine-induced histamine release in vivo. Allergy 39:493–497
62. Debelic M, Schiess W (1981) Beeinflussung der IgE-vermittelten Hauttestreaktionen durch Ketotifen. Dtsch Med Wochenschr 106:1704–1707
63. Sullivan TJ (1982) Pharmacologic modulation of the whealing response to histamine in human skin: identification of doxepin as a potent in vivo inhibitor. J Allergy Clin Immunol 69:260–267
64. Berg T, Nordvall SL, Lanner A (1980) Clinical studies of a purified timothy pollen extract. Desensitization therapy with a purified timothy pollen preparation compared to a crude timothy pollen extract. I. Results of test in vivo. Int Arch Allergy Appl Immunol 63:266–274

65. Colmes A (1932) Serial skin tests as a guide in the treatment of hay fever. J Allergy 3:449–454
66. Frostad AB, Grimer Ø, Sandvik L, Moxnes A, Aas K (1983) Clinical effects of hyposensitization using a purified allergen preparation from timothy pollen as compared to crude aqueous extracts from timothy pollen and a four grass-pollen mixture respectively. Clin Allergy 13:337–357
67. Bousquet J, Guérin B, Dotte A, Dhivert H, Djoukhadar F, Hewitt B, Michel FB (1985) Comparison between rush immunotherapy with a standardized allergen and an alun adjuved pyridine extracted material in grass pollen allergy. Clin Allergy 15:179–194
68. Freeman J (1930) Rush inoculation with special reference to hay fever treatment. Lancet I:744–747
69. Bousquet J, Calvayrac P, Dhivert H, Hejjaoui M, Guérin B, Michel FB (1985) Early benefits of rush immunotherapy with a standardized mite extract. J Allergy Clin Immunol 75, 1 (part 2):238 (abstract)

46. Diagnostic Value of IgE in Bronchial Asthma

N. F. Adkinson Jr

Since IgE-dependent mechanisms are commonly active in the vast majority of cases of childhood asthma, and in many cases of adult-onset asthma as well, the assessment of IgE can be an important adjunct to the evaluation of the asthmatic patient. The clinical usefulness of total serum-IgE assays and tests for IgE antibody depends, to some extent, upon the contribution of IgE-dependent mechanisms to a given patient's asthma. Even when reaginic mechanisms are unlikely, IgE assays can be useful in establishing this fact and validating the diagnosis of a cryptogenic or *intrinsic* form of asthma.

46.1 Serum-IgE Protein

Compared with other immunoglobulin classes (IgG, IgA and IgM), the concentrations of circulating IgE in serum are quite low, usually in ng/ml. Such low levels of IgE protein require sensitive immunoassays for quantitation. A number of suitable assays are available, both double antibody and solid phase in nature [1]. Competitive binding solid phase assays, in which an insolubilized anti-IgE antibody competes for radiolabeled or defined amounts of IgE protein, are to be avoided as this method tends to systematically overestimate IgE protein concentrations below 50 IU/ml [2].

Numerous studies have indicated that the basal levels of serum-IgE are under genetic control [3]. About 60 to 80% of the variance of serum-IgE levels can be accounted for by heredity. Although not firmly established, much of the data is compatible with a recessive mode of inheritance for low IgE serum levels.

In order to interpret measured values, it is imperative to have age-specific normative values taken from populations carefully screened to exclude subjects with atopic disorders, and other confounding influences such as parasitic infections. While IgG and IgM antibodies reach half-normal adult levels by one year of age, IgA and even more dramatically IgE are significantly delayed such that half-adult levels are commonly not achieved until age 6–8 [4]. Thus, age-adjusted normative values are necessary to interpret total serum-IgE levels in children younger than 12.

Several studies have now suggested that a distinctively elevated serum-IgE in the first year of life is associated with the early development of signs and symptoms compatible with IgE-dependent disease [5, 6]. These studies have not clearly shown whether the onset of childhood asthma is more likely in children with elevated total serum-IgE levels early in life, but this remains a reasonable presumption.

In adults, those patients with atopic disorders have, as a group, much higher levels of total serum-IgE than nonatopic controls. The study by Wittig et al summarized in Table 46.1 is typical, and illustrates that patients with eczema have higher IgE levels than those with allergic rhinitis alone [7]. Allergic asthma produces even higher IgE levels, and the combination of asthma and eczema is associated with the highest IgE levels. These levels are to be contrasted with geometric mean values of 25 IU/ml or less in non-atopic adult populations [4].

Table 46.1. Mean serum-IgE among atopic populations. [Data from 7]

Diagnosis	No.	IgE (IU/ml)
Asthma and eczema	48	985
Asthma	578	305
Eczema	49	273
Allergic rhinitis	244	171

(One international unit (IU) of IgE is equivalent to 2.4 ng.) Other studies have similarly confirmed elevation in total serum-IgE protein in allergic asthmatic patients throughout the world [4].

Although allergic individuals have higher serum-IgE values than nonallergics, there is much overlap between atopic and nonatopic populations [8, 9]. The overlap between atopic and nonatopic populations is greatest between 20–100 IU/ml. However, below 20 IU are only 5% of allergic patients, but 65% of nonallergic subjects. Similarly above 100 IU/ml there are only 5% of nonallergic adults, compared with 40% of allergic subjects. Thus, serum-IgE values < 20 IU/ml or > 100 IU/ml have the greatest utility for differential diagnosis.

It is important to recognize that there are a number of nonatopic disorders which are associated with increased IgE production [reviewed in 4]. Some immunodeficiency and neoplastic diseases fall into this category. Among these are the Wiskott-Aldrich syndrome, the hyperimmunoglobulin E syndrome (characterized by very high IgE levels, recurrent infections, and a cellular immune deficit), Hodgkin's lymphoma, and cytotoxic therapy given as preparation for bone marrow transplantation. Helminthic infections of all types produce marked elevations in IgE, probably through an effect of the parasite on the normal immunoregulation of IgE by host T-lymphocytes. Other diseases with associated increased IgE include drug-induced interstitial nephritis, idiopathic nephrotic syndrome, bullous pemphigoid, chronic nonatopic dermatoses, acute and chronic liver disease, cystic fibrosis, and allergic bronchopulmonary aspergillosis.

As with any laboratory test, the results of total serum-IgE evaluations must be interpreted by the context of the patient's symptoms, historical background, and other known medical problems. In general, low IgE levels (< 20 IU/ml in adults) suggest that IgE-dependent disease is not likely to be a major etiologic factor for the patient's asthmatic symptoms. Moderate levels are compatible with IgE-dependent mechanisms in asthmatic patients, while very high levels (> 1000 IU/ml) require consideration of other possible causes for elevated serum-IgE (especially, allergic bronchopulmonary aspergillosis, parasitic infections, and clinical states in which immune regulation may be abnormal).

46.2 IgE Antibody Determination

IgE antibody tests provide an opportunity to identify environmental allergens of clinical significance to a given patient with allergic asthma. Negative tests with extracts of aeroallergens common to the patient's environment are also useful in identifying cases where IgE mechanisms are not likely to be important. Traditional testing for classic reaginic, or IgE-dependent allergy has been by use of skin testing of the immediate-type. After the identification of reaginic antibody as IgE in 1966, it was possible to develop highly sensitive and specific immunoassays for IgE antibody circulating in serum, as distinct from the IgE fixed to tissue mast cells which is detected by skin testing. In 1967 Wide et al described the first such serological assay for IgE called the radioallergosorbent test [RAST] [10]. Inhalation challenge may also be used to assess IgE antibody using pulmonary resistance as the response variable. The principles of these tests and their practical application are discussed elsewhere in this volume.

For routine clinical use, the practical choice is usually between skin testing and RAST. In general, when compared using identical materials, the agreement between measurement of IgE antibody by RAST and by intradermal skin testing titrations is excellent [4]. This being the case, it is useful to review the advantages and disadvantages of each method.

Skin testing provides an immediate answer; an entire battery can usually be completed within 60–90 min. Since skin testing is a biological assay for IgE antibody, it assesses mast cell function as well as the presence of triggering IgE antibody. It can be argued that this test property is usefully related to the risk of allergic disease. Skin testing maximizes sensitivity; properly performed intradermal skin tests are almost always slightly more sensitive than RAST testing. Maximum sensitivity is important for anaphylactic states such as those involved in drug allergy and stinging insect allergy. However, it is not clear that the extra sensitivity afforded by skin testing is clinically significant for aeroallergy diseases such as allergic rhinitis and asthma. Finally, skin testing is more economical in most cases than currently available RAST testing.

There are certain inherent advantages of RAST testing which should be kept in mind. First, RAST provides quantitative estimates of IgE antibody which can be reproduced by other laboratories which use the same materials. Second, internal quality control of reagents can be maintained using known positive serum pools. Third, provided a reasonable threshold value for positivity is chosen, a positive RAST result usually indicates specific IgE antibody since biological variables, such as skin texture and quality, do not come into play. RAST can provide a means for assessing IgE antibody when skin testing cannot be properly interpreted because of extensive dermatitis or interfering drugs which cannot be withdrawn. Finally, as a laboratory test requiring only venipuncture for a small serum sample, both patient and physician time are conserved.

Tests for IgE antibody, whether skin tests or *in vitro* immunoassays, should be chosen on the basis of the patient's history and physical findings in order for the results to be clinically relevant. When concordant with history and physical findings, a positive test identifies an environmental allergen of potential clinical significance. When an IgE antibody test is negative the likelihood of clinical significance for that allergen is markedly reduced.

References

1. Adkinson NF Jr (1986) Measurement of total serum immunoglobulin E and allergen-specific immunoglobulin E antibody. In: Rose NR, Friedman H (eds) Manual of clinical immunology, 3rd edn. American Society for Microbiology, Washington, pp 664–674
2. Johansson SGO, Berglund A, Kjellman N-IM (1976) Comparison of IgE values as determined with different solid phase radioimmunoassay methods. Clin Allergy 6:91
3. Marsh DG, Meyers DA, Bias WB (1981) The epidemiology and genetics of atopic allergy. N Engl J Med 305:1551–1559
4. Knauer KA, Adkinson NF Jr (1983) Clinical significance of IgE. In: Middleton E Jr, Reed CE, Ellis EF (eds) Allergy – Principles and Practice, 2nd edn. Mosby, St. Louis, pp 673–688
5. Orgel HA, Hamburger RN, Bazaral M et al (1975) Development of IgE and allergy in infancy. J Allergy Clin Immunol 56:296–307
6. Frick OL, German DF, Mills J (1979) Development of allergy in children. I. Association with virus infections. J Allergy Clin Immunol 63:228
7. Wittig HJ, McLaughlin ET, Leifer KL, Beloit JD (1978) Risk factors in the development of allergic disease. Analysis of 2190 patient records. Ann Allergy 41:84–88
8. Barbee RA, Halonen M, Lebowitz M, Burrows B (1981) Distribution of IgE in a community population sample: correlations with age, sex, and allergen skin test reactivity. J Allergy Clin Immunol 68:106
9. Zetterstrom I, Johansson SGO (1981) IgE concentrations measured by PRIST in serum of healthy adults and in patients with respiratory allergy: a diagnostic approach. Allergy 36:537
10. Wide L, Bennich H, Johansson SGO (1967) Diagnosis of allergy by an *in vitro* test for allergenic antibodies. Lancet 2:1105

47. Pulmonary Function Tests in Asthma

D. W. Cockcroft

"A disease characterized by wide variations over short periods of time in resistance to flow in intrapulmonary airways" is the primary definition of asthma suggested by Scadding [1]. Asthma (currently symptomatic) is characterized by hyperresponsiveness of the tracheobronchial smooth muscle to numerous nonallergic (nonspecific) physical or chemical stimuli such as exercise, cold air, histamine, methacholine, etc. [2]. Thus, asthma may be diagnosed by demonstrating significant variability in pulmonary flow rates, resistance to airflow, or sequelae thereof, (e.g., changes in lung volume) either spontaneously or as a result of intervention. Thus, the pulmonary function laboratory plays a valuable role in the objective assessment of patients with asthma.

There is much scientific literature relating to pulmonary functions in asthma. This chapter will concentrate primarily on the clinical value of pulmonary functions in assessment of asthma rather than more detailed pathophysiological research. *Routine* pulmonary function studies as well as specialized, more sensitive tests will be reviewed; assessment of bronchial responsiveness by bronchoprovocation will be discussed in a subsequent chapter.

47.1 "Routine" Pulmonary Function

The four aspects of pulmonary function which are routinely measured in most laboratories include lung volumes, diffusion capacity, expiratory flow rates and bronchodilator response.

Lung volumes: The lung volumes, within the maximal breath or vital capacity (VC), are measured directly from a spirometer. The residual volume (RV), which is the volume of air remaining in the lung after maximal expiration must be measured indirectly either with an inert gas (usually helium) dilution technique, or with a plethysmograph [3]. From this, the functional residual capacity (FRC), the volume in the lung at the end of a quiet expiration, and total lung capacity (TLC = RV + VC) can be calculated.

Abnormalities in lung volumes generally relate to the degree of airflow obstruction and may vary from normal, to reduced VC with increases in FRC, RV, and sometimes TLC [3, 4]. Acute changes in TLC after intervention are usually small [5, 6], but occasionally may be large [7]. TLC, FRC, and RV decrease as asthma is treated [4] and on rare occasions improvement in asthma may be reflected mainly by improvement in lung volumes with little change in flow rates [3, 8]. Generally, however, lung volume measurements are most useful in quantitating the degree of physiological abnormality in asthma and of limited value diagnostically, i.e., in differentiating asthma from the other obstructive airways diseases.

Pulmonary diffusion: The integrity of the alveolar capillary membrane is estimated by measurement of the pulmonary diffusing capacity for carbon monoxide D_LCO [9]. In this test, the rate at which CO leaves the alveolar (inspired) gas to attach to the intracapillary hemoglobin is measured. Results depend on both the surface area (reduced in emphysema) and the thickness (increased in interstitial lung disease) of the alveolar capillary membrane, as well as the volume of blood in the pulmonary capillaries (reduced in severe anemia, pulmonary embolus, etc.) [9].

In asthmatics D_LCO is usually normal, but has been reported as being sometimes increased [3]. This latter feature, however, is likely due to a systematic overestimation of D_LCO by usual methods in the presence of airflow obstruction [10]. When appropriate methods are used, the D_LCO in bronchial asthmatics is not altered. The limited clinical value of measurement of D_LCO relates chiefly to differential diagnosis from chronic obstructive airways disease in which D_LCO is often reduced.

Expiratory flow rates: Expiratory flow rates may be assessed by spirogram or maximum expiratory flow-volume curve. The spirogram is a tracing of forced expiration from TLC to RV in which lung volume is plotted against time. Measurements include the forced expiratory volume in one second (FEV_1) the forced VC (FVC), the ratio of FEV_1 to VC or FVC, and flow over the middle 50% of FVC referred to as maximum midexpiratory flow rate (MMFR) or forced expired flow between 25 and 75% of VC (FEF_{25-75}) [3, 6]. From the flow-volume curve, where maximal expired flow is plotted against lung volume, flow at various lung volumes, e.g., 50 and 25% of VC ($\dot{V}_{max\,50}$, $\dot{V}_{max\,25}$) and peak flow ($\dot{V}_{max}$, or PFR) can be calculated [11]. Flow volume curves require an expensive apparatus for calculation, whereas spirograms may be obtained with large expensive laboratory spirometers, or with small portable "office" spirometers. Portable peak flowmeters are also available for office or home determination of PFR.

Expiratory flow rates are valuable to assess the presence and degree of airflow obstruction in asthma. It is said that flows occurring at high lung volumes (early in expiration) e.g., PFR, FEV_1 reflect large airway function, while those occurring at lower lung volumes (MMFR, $\dot{V}_{max\,25}$) reflect small airway function. Airflow obstruction is characteristic of symptomatic asthma, however it is also seen in other obstructive airways diseases. Inspiratory airflow obstruction may be useful to diagnose extrathoracic airway (e.g., laryngeal) obstruction which may mimic asthma [12].

Bronchodilator response: Bronchodilator responsiveness is the most valuable of the *routine* pulmonary functions in bronchial asthma. Expiratory flow rates are repeated at the appropriate time after an inhaled bronchodilator e.g., 20 min after 200 μg inhaled salbutamol (Fig. 47.1). If the flow rates are technically accurate a *significant* improvement indicates the diagnosis of asthma or an asthmatic component to an underlying disease.

Since bronchodilator response is widely used diagnostically, a number of precautions must be discussed. Firstly, a *significant* increase depends on the variability

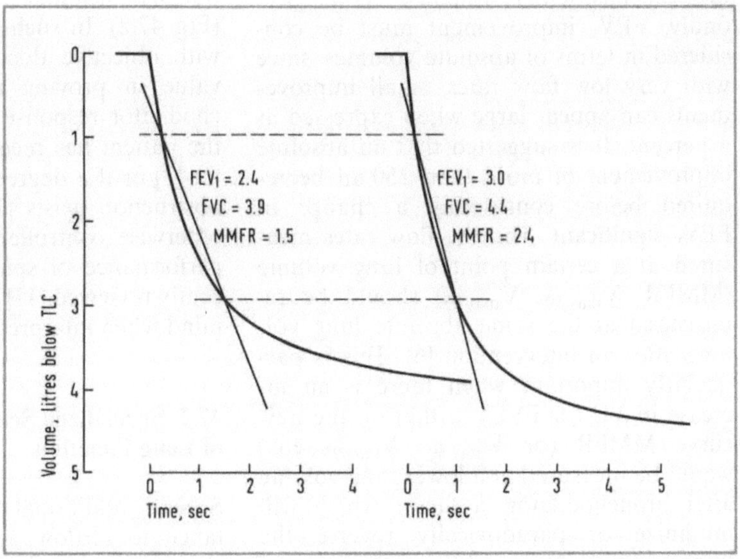

Fig. 47.1. Spirogram before and after 200 μg salbutamol in a subject with bronchial asthma. Lung volume in liters below TLC is on the vertical axis and time in seconds on the horizontal axis. The two spirograms also show the volume adjustment method of measuring MMFR, so that the post-bronchodilator MMFR is measured at the same lung volume as the prebronchodilator MMFR (horizontal dashed lines)

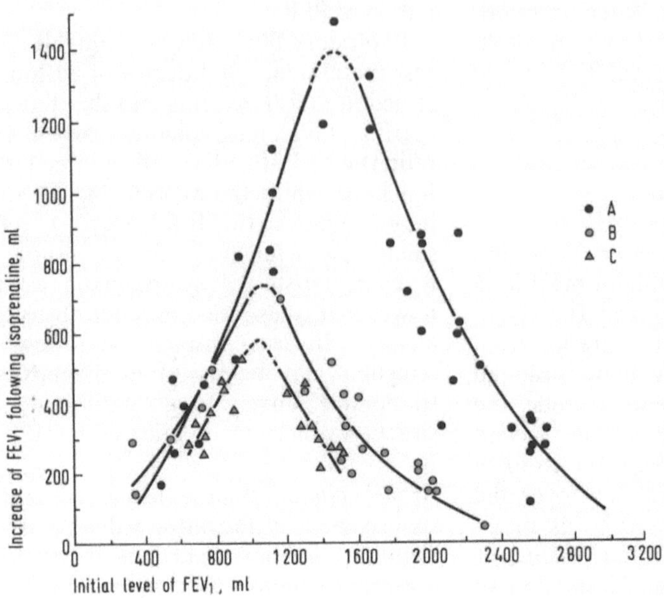

Fig. 47.2. Bronchodilator response (FEV_1 improvement on the vertical axis) relate to initial level of FEV_1 (ml, horizontal axis) in three subjects with asthma. Decreased responsiveness is seen when the FEV_1 is high as well as when the FEV_1 is markedly reduced. (From KM Hume and B Gandevia, Thorax 1957, 12:276, reproduced here with permission of the authors and Thorax)

of the test and bronchodilator-induced improvement in normals [3, 13]. Therefore the FEV_1 must improve only 15% to be significant [3], whereas the more sensitive and more variable MMFR must improve ≧50% to be significant [13]. When this is taken into account the less sensitive, but more reproducible FEV_1 appears to be the *best test* for evaluating bronchodilator (and possibly bronchoconstrictor) response [14]. Secondly, FEV_1 improvement must be considered in terms of absolute volumes, since with very low flow rates, small improvements can appear large when expressed as a percent. It is suggested that an absolute improvement of more than 250 ml be required before considering a change in FEV_1 significant. Thirdly, flow rates measured at a certain point of lung volume (MMFR, $\dot{V}_{max\,50}$, $\dot{V}_{max\,25}$) should be remeasured at the same absolute lung volume after an intervention [6]. This is particularly important when there is an increase in VC (or FVC) so that on the new curve MMFR (or $\dot{V}_{max\,50}$, $\dot{V}_{max\,25}$ etc.) would be measured at a lower lung volume after bronchodilator, a factor which will minimize or paradoxically reverse the improvement. Thus *volume adjustment* of MMFR (or $\dot{V}_{max\,50}$, $\dot{V}_{max\,25}$) is important when considering bronchodilator response [6] (Fig. 47.1). Finally, it must be noted that absence of a bronchodilator response does not rule out bronchial asthma. Bronchodilator response may be absent when asthma is well-controlled and thus flows near normal, and alternatively, the response may be absent when severe *refractory* asthma has developed [15] (Fig. 47.2). In such cases a trial of steroids with objective documentation may be of value in proving reversibility [3]. Bronchodilator response may also be absent if the patient has recently used bronchodilator [3] or if a degree of irreversible airflow obstruction exists [16], but symptoms are otherwise controlled. Technical pitfalls in performance of spirometry have been recently reviewed [17] and should be borne in mind when interpreting spirometric data.

47.2 Specialized Sensitive Tests of Lung Function

Several additional tests of airflow/resistance to airflow and/or pulmonary mechanics are available. Since resistance to airflow is maximal in the large central airways, the small (< 2 mm diameter) airways represent a *silent* zone of the lung in which significant pathology can be present with little or no alteration in most *routine* lung functions [18]. The tests outlined below are reported to be more sensitive or to more clearly demonstrate small airways dysfunction or both. Most require an expensive sophisticated apparatus and therefore are more suited to research studies; there is little evidence that routine clinical use of these tests in asthma is of value. Therefore, the tests will be only briefly described.

Airways resistance: A number of methods are available for the indirect measurement of airways resistance (Raw) and its reciprocals, conductance (Gaw) and specific Gaw (SGaw = Raw/FRC). The most common method applies Boyle's law to measurements of pressure and flow using a constant volume variable pressure plethysmography [19]. Raw is dependent on central large airway diameter and may be influenced by laryngeal caliber [20]. Much like the MMFR, large changes (> 50% in SGaw, ~ 40% for Raw) are required for significance in bronchodilator studies [13].

Compliance: Pulmonary compliance is determined as the slope of the pressure-volume curve ($\Delta V/\Delta P$) and requires an esophageal balloon and plethysmograph for measurement [21]. Although compliance may be significantly reduced in asthmatic airways obstruction, compared with normals and emphysema patients (increased compliance) [22], the measurement of compliance has little clinical value in asthma.

Frequency dependence of compliance: A fall in pulmonary compliance with increasing respiratory rate is termed *frequency dependence* [18] and is regarded as the *gold standard* measurement of small airways dysfunction [23]. Although frequency dependence may be present in asthmatics with normal lung function [18], its clinical relevance has not been established and the test is too tedious for routine use.

Helium flow volume curves: Turbulent airflow (large airways) is density-dependent and will increase if gas density is reduced, whereas laminar airflow (small airways) shows no density-dependent change. Comparison of flow volume curves breathing 80% helium (low density) vs air has been suggested as a test of small airways disease [24]. The increase in $\dot{V}_{max\,50}$ breathing helium ($\dot{V}_{max\,50}$) falls as resistance to airflow becomes more laminar (i.e., small airways) and thus less density-dependent. The *volume of isoflow,* where the two curves cross, also increases with small airways obstruction [24]. This approach has been suggested as a test of early lung disease in smokers [24] and has been used to determine the site of various airways responses in asthma [25]. However, questions raised regarding the high, within and between individual variability and its ability to pinpoint small airways disease has been recently summarized [23]. Although valuable in research, clinical application is limited.

Single breath nitrogen washout: The single breath nitrogen (washout) test or closing volume curve [26] is perhaps the most valuable test for determining early and/or small airways dysfunction [23, 27]. A single breath of 100% oxygen is inspired to TLC, and the exhaled N_2 concentration is measured continuously during a slow VC exhalation. The N_2 vs volume curve has four phases: phase I = dead space washout ($N_2 = 0$); phase II = rapid equilibration; phase III = alveolar plateau (slow N_2 rise); and phase IV = rapid N_2 rise as airways start closing [26]. Increase in the slope of phase II (N_2/l) or in the closing volume (%CV/VC) where phase III meets phase IV, are thought to be early indicators of small airways dysfunction [27]. This test shows promise in the early detection of lung disease and is frequently abnormal in even well-controlled asthmatics, however the test currently remains largely used as a research tool [23].

Site of airway response: The predominant site of airways responses in asthma has been studied extensively [25, 28]. Bronchoconstriction in asthma may occur predominantly in either large or small airways or both. The major clinical correlation is that severity of asthma and/or of preexisting airways obstruction appears to be more severe in *small airways responders* [28]. Although, perhaps of some therapeutic value, as atropine may preferentially inhibit large airways responses [28], the clinical value of differentiating between large airway and small airways responders appears limited.

47.3 Clinical Role of Pulmonary Function in Asthma

Pulmonary functions may prove useful clinically in three areas: diagnosis; assessment of severity; and follow-up of asthmatics. The clinical value of pulmonary function testing will be discussed under these three headings.

Diagnosis: It has been stated that "in general, lung-function tests do not make diagnoses but uncover functional disturbances..." [29]. Asthma is, however, probably the only disease which may be diagnosed by pulmonary function (bronchodilator response) alone. Nevertheless, in the 5–10% of the population with a cumulative prevalence of asthma (of widely varying severity), the majority of asthmatics will have normal pulmonary functions, the majority of the time. Thus, applying diagnostic test evaluation [30], the bronchodilator response is a test with high specificity (few false positives) but with very low overall sensitivity. Such analysis, however, is hindered by a lack of *gold standard* for the diagnosis of asthma. The relative roles of asthma-diagnostic techniques are outlined below; as this is a controversial area, the views expressed are the author's personal approach.

Asthma, as currently defined, is a disease characterized by symptoms due to increased responsiveness of the tracheobronchial smooth muscle and associated with wide variations in resistance to airflow [1]. Since pulmonary function (and even airways responsiveness, see below) are often normal in asthmatics the **clinical evaluation,** although less than perfect [31], remains the best *gold standard* for the diagnosis of asthma. The presence of *variable* and frequently nocturnal chest symptoms (wheeze, dyspnea, chest tightness, cough) particularly when associated with specific exposures (seasonal, allergen, occupational, ASA, etc.) and the historical response to asthma treatment should strongly alert the clinician to the diagnosis of asthma. Clinical evaluation will have reduced specificity but much improved sensitivity, compared to pulmonary function.

Bronchial responsiveness to physical and chemical stimuli (exercise, cold air, histamine, methacholine) is increased in virtually all symptomatic asthmatics [2]. Recently, one group has suggested that the methacholine inhalation test be used as a *gold standard* for the diagnosis of asthma [31]. There is little doubt that measurement of airway responsiveness to histamine or methacholine is the best gold standard test available, however some important points should be made when interpreting results of airway responsiveness. Just as with pulmonary functions, airway responsiveness may vary with fluctuations in the clinical picture. Seasonal asthmatics tested out of season may have normal responsiveness [32]. Occupational asthmatics may have normal tests when away from work for as little as 3 days, early in their illness [33] or for several months in established disease [34]. Positive tests also occur in normals and rhinitis subjects with no chest symptoms [32]. In a random population of 500, positive tests in subjects lacking chest symptoms ($n=33$) exceeded the number of positive tests in asthmatics ($n=25$) [35, Cockcroft, unpublished data]. Definitions may eventually change so that these subjects are recognized as asymptomatic or latent asthmatics. With these caveats in mind, measurement of airways responsiveness rank a clear second to clinical evaluation in the diagnosis of asthma.

Pulmonary function tests rank third in diagnostic efficacy. In a random population study of 500 subjects, 52 subjects with past or present asthma were identified; all had a normal FEV_1 and 27, or over 50%, (all past or seasonal asthmatics) had normal airway responsiveness to histamine [Cockcroft, unpublished data]. In a more selected group of asthmatics the FEV_1/FVC ratio was normal in most [31]. However, the sick "tip of the iceberg" asthmatics who present more commonly for treatment include a larger percent with baseline airway obstruction, and with *positive* bronchodilator or steroid response on lung function tests. Such tests provide a useful adjunct to clinical evaluation and measurements of airways responsiveness in the diagnosis of asthma. In our chest clinic, we see a large number of asthmatics with normal pulmonary functions in whom history and airways responsiveness are used to make the diagnosis; this number is estimated to represent close to, but less than 50%, of our asthma diagnoses. In an allergy clinic, the proportion of asthmatics with normal lung function would likely be greater, and as noted above in a random population, this is the rule rather than the exception. Pulmonary functions define the extent of the physiological abnormality [29] and are useful in differential diagnosis between asthma and diseases producing similar symptoms [3].

Assessment of severity: The degree of lung function abnormality is a reliable guide to assessment of severity of airflow obstruction of an individual *attack* at a given point in time, and the degree of *irreversible* change may reflect overall asthma severity [16]. However, in a variable, and controllable disease, such as asthma (and e.g., hypertension) the overall severity of disease may be poorly reflected by isolated measurements of physiological abnormality. Many *severe* asthmatics may (? should) maintain normal or near normal lung function at the expense of much medication, whereas otherwise *mild* asthmatics may develop an episode of severe obstruction after exposure to a relevant triggering factor. Once again the clinical picture, particularly the minimum medication requirement needed to achieve acceptable control [32, 36], is most valuable in assessing overall severity of chronic asthma.

Follow-up and patient monitoring: Probably the most valuable role of pulmonary functions clinically, is in the area of acute and chronic patient monitoring. Clinical evaluation (e.g., nocturnal symptoms, exercise limitation, days missed from school/work, emergency/hospital visits etc.) is once again acceptable and preferred for most asthmatics. However it is noted that there is a less than ideal correlation between symptoms and degree of airflow obstruction in asthmatics [37]. Increases in airflow obstruction are perceived less often in subjects with greater airway hyperresponsiveness and greater preexisting airflow obstruction [37]. These, of course, are the subjects most likely to develop severe asthmatic episodes requiring chronic treatment. There are a number of patients whose perception of increasing airflow obstruction appears to be almost absent. In the acute hospitalized asthmatic, symptoms resolve well before pulmonary function [38]. Thus monitoring of pulmonary functions has an important role to play in assessing recovery from acute asthma and in assessing treatment in long-term chronic asthma particularly in *brittle* asthmatics and poor perceivers of symptoms [39]. Although chronic treatment for asthma is usually based on symptoms, in these latter groups of asthmatics, therapeutic changes may be dictated by falling pulmonary flow rates.

The best test and clinical application: The ideal test of lung function as applied to asthma, is a direct measure of airflow/resistance to airflow which is reproducible, and reflects significant changes in bronchomotor tone occurring either spontaneously or due to bronchodilator or bronchoconstrictor exposure. Additionally, ease of patient performance, availability, cost and portability of equipment are also important. Of the many tests of airflow/resistance to airflow available, the FEV_1 is widely used particularly in North America, while PFR is also widely used, especially in the U.K. The FEV_1 has been shown to be superior to more *sensitive* tests [14], is reproducible, easy to perform and may be carried out on inexpensive portable equipment. The PFR, although perhaps more effort-dependent, is also reproducible, easy to perform, and very portable inexpensive equipment is available. Home or work measurement of PFR is reliable [40] and valuable in the home monitoring of high risk asthmatics [39, 40] and

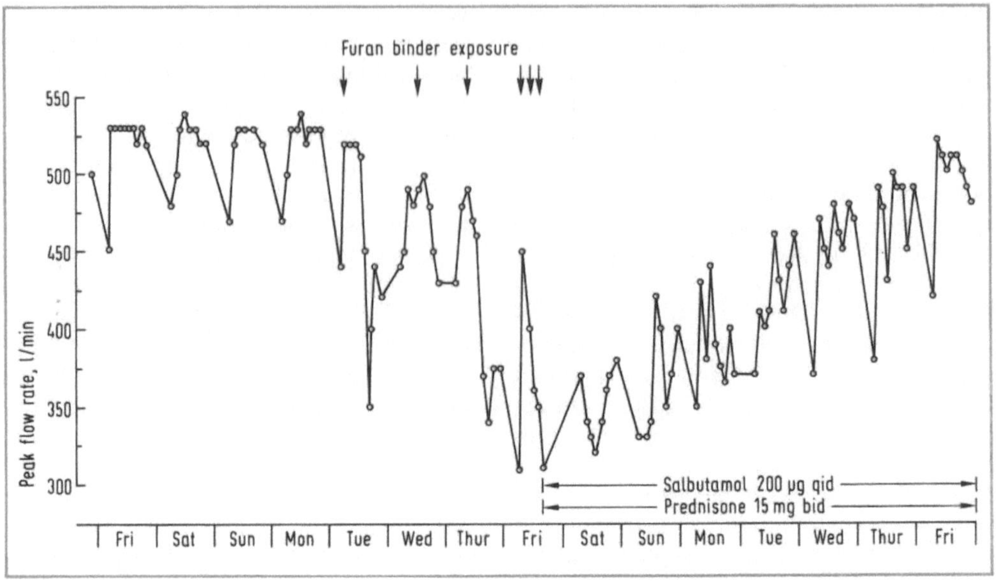

Fig. 47.3. Value of outpatient measurement of PFR in the assessment of occupational asthma. PFR in l/min measured several times per day is graphed on the vertical axis against days of the week on the horizontal axis. A fall in PFR related to occupational exposure to a furan-based binder system can be seen; this was followed by recovery with salbutamol and prednisone treatment. (From Cockcroft et al, J Allergy Clin Immunol 1980, 66:458, reproduced here with permission of the authors and the Journal of Allergy and Clinical Immunology)

in the diagnosis and monitoring of occupational asthma [41, 42] (Fig. 47.3). Monitoring PFR or FEV_1 in the outpatient clinic is a valuable adjunct to clinical evaluation of asthmatics, particularly when flow rates suggest severe airflow obstruction not reflected by symptoms. An added benefit to measuring flow rates before and after inhaled bronchodilator is the chance to observe technique of inhaler use. The poor performance with metered dose inhalers in many asthmatics suggests the need for repeated observation and reinstruction [43]. Measurements of flow rates are not particularly valuable in the acute hospitalized asthmatic and may be difficult and unreliable in performance. Nevertheless, there appears to be a reasonable role for assessment of lung function in the recovery phase [38].

47.4 Conclusions

Pulmonary function studies in asthma have been reviewed with particular emphasis on their clinical value. For clinical purposes, simple reproducible tests such as FEV_1 and PFR are most valuable. Although useful in assessing diagnosis, severity, and follow-up of asthma, for most patients these tests are less important than the clinical evaluation and/or bronchial responsiveness measurement. Pulmonary functions are particularly valuable, occasionally, in differential diagnosis, assessment of severity of physiological abnormality at a point in time, and monitoring certain asthmatic patients. This latter point is useful in occupational asthmatics and is particularly valuable in certain high risk patients who do not perceive increasing airflow obstruction well.

Acknowledgement: The author wishes to thank J. Conan for preparing the manuscript.

References

1. Scadding JG (1983) Definition and clinical categories of asthma. In: Clark TJH, Godfrey S (eds) Asthma, 2nd edn. Chapman and Hall, London, p 5
2. Hargreave FE, Ryan G, Thomson NC, O'Byrne PM, Latimer K, Juniper EF, Dolovich J (1981) Bronchial responsiveness to histamine or methacholine in asthma: measurement and clinical significance. J Allergy Clin Immunol 68:347–355
3. Kanner RE, Watanabe S (1981) The role of the pulmonary function laboratory in patients with bronchial asthma. In: Gershwin ME (ed) Bronchial Asthma: Principles of Diagnosis and Treatment. Grune and Stratton, New York, pp 101–115
4. Woolcock AJ, Read J (1966) Lung volumes in exacerbations of asthma. Am J Med 41:259–273
5. Holmes PW, Campbell AH, Barter CE (1978) Acute changes of lung volumes and lung mechanics in asthma and in normal subjects. Thorax 33:394–400
6. Cockcroft DW, Berscheid BA (1980) Volume adjustment of maximal midexpiratory flow: importance of changes in total lung capacity. Chest 78:595–600
7. Peress L, Sybrecht G, Macklem PT (1976) The mechanism of increase in total lung capacity during acute asthma. Am J Med 61:165–169
8. Woolcock AJ, Read J (1965) Improvement in bronchial asthma not reflected in forced expiratory volume. Lancet 2:1323–1325
9. West JB (1979) Respiratory Physiology – the essentials, 2nd edn. Williams and Wilkins, Baltimore, pp 22–31
10. Graham BL, Mink JT, Cotton DJ (1984) Overestimation of the single-breath carbon monoxide diffusing capacity in patients with air-flow obstruction. Am Rev Respir Dis 129:403–408
11. Knudson RL, Slatin RC, Lebowitz MD, Burrows B (1976) The maximal expiratory flow-volume curve. Am Rev Respir Dis 113:587–600
12. Christopher KL, Wood RP, Eckert RC, Blager FB, Raney RA, Souhrada JF (1983) Vocal-cord dysfunction presenting as asthma. N Engl J Med 308:1566–1570
13. Watanabe S, Renzetti AD Jr, Begin R, Bigler AH (1974) Airway responsiveness to bronchodilator aerosol. 1. Normal human subjects. Am Rev Respir Dis 109:530–537
14. Light RW, Conrad SA, George RB (1977) The one best test for evaluating the effects of bronchodilator therapy. Chest 72:512–516
15. Hume KM, Rhys Jones E (1961) The response to bronchodilators in intrinsic asthma. Q J Med 30:189–199
16. Brown PJ, Greville HW, Finacune KE (1984) Asthma and irreversible airflow obstruction. Thorax 39:131–136
17. Lewis BM (1981) Pitfalls of spirometry. J Occup Med 23:35–38
18. Woolcock AJ, Vincent NJ, Macklem PT (1969) Frequency dependence of compliance as a test for obstruction in the small airways. J Clin Invest 48:1097–1106
19. West JB (1979) Respiratory Physiology – the essentials, 2nd edn. Williams and Wilkins, Baltimore, pp 155–156
20. Nadel JA (1979) In Discussion. In: Sadoul P, Milic-Emili J, Simonsson BG, Clark TJH (eds) Small Airways in Health and Disease. Excerpta Medica, Amsterdam, p 30
21. West JB (1979) Respiratory Physiology – the essentials, 2nd edn. Williams and Wilkins, Baltimore, pp 153–155
22. Colebatch HJH, Finacune KE, Smith MM (1973) Pulmonary conductance and elastic recoil relationships in asthma and emphysema. J Appl Physiol 34:143–153
23. Buist SA (1984) Current status of small airways disease. Chest 86:100–105
24. Dosman J, Bode F, Urbanetti J, Martin R, Macklem PT (1975) The use of a helium-oxygen mixture during maximum expiratory flow to demonstrate obstruction in small airways in smokers. J Clin Invest 55:1090–1099
25. Ingram RH Jr, McFadden ER Jr (1977) Localization and mechanisms of airway responses. N Engl J Med 297:596–600
26. Buist AS, Ross BB (1973) Predicted values for closing volumes using a modified single breath nitrogen test. Am Rev Respir Dis 107:744–752
27. Dosman JA, Cotton DJ, Graham BL, Hall DL, Li R, Froh F, Barnett GD (1981) Sensitivity and specificity of early diagnostic tests of lung function in smokers. Chest 79:6–11
28. McFadden ER Jr, Ingram RH Jr (1979) Site of airway responses in asthma. In: Sadoul P, Milic-Emili J, Simonsson BG, Clark TJH (eds) Small Airways in Health and Disease. Excerpta Medica, Amsterdam, pp 156–160
29. Macklem PT (1975) New tests to assess lung function. N Engl J Med 293:339–342
30. Department of Clinical Epidemiology and Biostatistics, McMaster University Health Sciences Centre (1981) How to read clinical journals. II. To learn about a diagnostic test. Can Med Assoc J 124:703–710
31. Pratter MR, Hingston DM, Irwin RS (1983) Diagnosis of bronchial asthma by clinical evaluation: an unreliable method. Chest 84:42–47

32. Cockcroft DW, Killian DN, Mellon JJA, Hargreave FE (1977) Bronchial reactivity to histamine: A method and clinical survey. Clin Allergy 7:235–243
33. Cockcroft DW (1982) Acquired persistant increase in nonspecific bronchial reactivity associated with isocyanate exposure. Ann Allergy 48:93–95
34. Lam S, Wong R, Yeung M (1979) Nonspecific bronchial reactivity in occupational asthma. J Allergy Clin Immunol 63:28–34
35. Cockcroft DW, Murdock KY, Berscheid BA (1984) Relationship between atopy and bronchial responsiveness to histamine in a random population. Ann Allergy 53:26–29
36. Juniper EF, Frith PA, Hargreave FE (1981) Airway responsiveness to histamine and methacholine: relationship to minimum treatment to control symptoms of asthma. Thorax 36:575–579
37. Burdon JGW, Juniper EF, Killian KJ, Hargreave FE, Campbell EJM (1982) The perception of breathlessness in asthma. Am Rev Respir Dis 126:825–828
38. McFadden ER Jr, Kiser R, de Groot WJ (1973) Acute bronchial asthma: Relations between clinical and physiologic manifestations. N Engl Med J 288:221–225
39. Hetzel MR, Clark TJH (1983) Adult asthma. In: Clark TJH, Godfrey S (eds) Asthma, 2nd edn. Chapman and Hall, London, pp 457–489
40. Hetzel MR, Williams IP, Shakespeare RM (1979) Can patients keep their own peak-flow records reliably? Lancet 1:597–599
41. Burge PS, O'Brien IM, Harries MG (1979) Peak flow rate records in the diagnosis of occupational asthma due to colophony. Thorax 34:308–316
42. Cartier A, Pineau L, Malo J-L (1984) Monitoring of maximum expiratory peak flow rates and histamine inhalation tests in the investigation of occupational asthma. Clin Allergy 14:193–196
43. Epstein SW (1983) Aerosol devices and techniques. In: Anticholinergic Therapy with Atrovent: an important new advance in asthma and bronchitis therapy. MedMark, Pointe Claire, pp 25–30

48. Bronchial Provocation Tests

S. L. Spector

Supported in part by the Allergy Research Foundation.

More and more investigators are performing bronchial inhalation challenge procedures to provide answers regarding experimental and clinical considerations in normals and in asthmatic subjects. Inhalation challenges have been compared to other provocative challenges such as exercise or the inhalation of cold air. The mediators released from these challenges have provided insight into mechanisms yet to be understood. Provocation challenges are here to stay. Current concepts regarding their use are herein reviewed, but other sources should be consulted for more details [1–3].

48.1 Preparatory Considerations Prior to Bronchoconstrictive Challenges

Certain baseline considerations are essential before a proper study can be completed. These are summarized in Table 48.1. Before a bronchial challenge patients should be instructed that the inhaled substance may result in an increase, a decrease, or no change in their pulmonary function. Subjects are best tested in an asymptomatic state. Smoking, cola drinks, and chocolate should be discontinued at least 6 hours before testing. Air pollution exposure and exercise should be avoided 2 hours before bronchial challenge. If possible, medications should be stopped. Realizing this is not always possible for patients requiring chronic medications, I recommend withholding medications for 8 hours with β-adrenergic stimulating agents, short acting theophylline derivatives, α-adrenergic blocking and anticholinergic agents. Other medications should be withheld longer: 12 hours for sustained release β-agonists; 24 hours for cromolyn sodium or sustained release theophylline agents, 48 hours for the usual antihistamines, and 96 hours for hydroxyzines or similar long acting medications. The metabolism of the medications is often such that a person may remain under the influence of the substance for a longer time than is presumed from the listed recommendations. This effect can be minimized if challenges are done at consistent times in relation to a given medication.

Characteristically two different methods are used to measure airway response: maximal expiratory flow maneuvers and submaximal flow maneuver such as airway resistance. A deep inspiration or expiration may cause bronchoconstriction in asthmatic patients, which is prevented by anticholinergics such as atropine.

The ability to abolish changes in bronchomotor tone with a deep inspiration may render the forced expiratory volume in one second (FEV_1) relatively insensitive in those showing this response. Although the FEV_1 maneuver can be criticized for being an effort-dependent test, it has survived the test of time as a useful, convenient, and

Table 48.1. Considerations prior to performing a presumed bronchoconstrictive challenge

1. Avoid the suggestion that the inhaled substance might produce a given effect.
2. Prepare patient so that pulmonary function is stable and the patient is asymptomatic.
3. Avoid possible triggers prior to challenge such as air pollution, smoking, viral infections or exercise.
4. Avoid possible dilators or blockers of a constrictor response, such as bronchodilator medications, coffee, chocolate, or cola drinks.
5. Assess bronchial lability produced by the pulmonary function maneuver itself.
6. Assess the effect of the diluent itself at a given temperature, pH and osmolarity.

minimally variable test of pulmonary function. Unfortunately, the body plethysmograph is expensive to make or purchase and not widely available, and the panting maneuver itself might be affected by laryngeal narrowing induced by a particular drug administered during bronchial provocation.

The diluent in which the bronchoconstrictive substance is dissolved should not cause bronchial obstruction. If it does, the subject must be tested on another day, or he may prove unsuitable for challenge with this substance. The method of delivery, pH, osmolarity and preservatives may be important.

48.2 Inhalation Challenges with Agents Other than Antigens

Asthmatic patients are often said to be hyperreactive to almost any so-called *nonspecific stimulus* to a comparable degree; however, this is not really the case [4–6]. Some of the differences between these agents will be discussed. Most of the commonly employed agents are listed in Table 48.2. Ultrasonically nebulized distilled water has been suggested as a test for bronchial reactivity since asthmatic subjects, unlike patients with chronic bronchitis or normal nonsmokers, are reported to undergo bronchoconstriction in response to ultrasonically nebulized distilled water but not to nebulized saline [7, 8]. We have observed some asthmatics who do have a fall in FEV_1 after isotonic saline. Thus the universality of the above observation is questionable. Although the close correlation between responsiveness to methacholine and histamine has been emphasized, these challenges are not exactly comparable. There is a small subgroup of asthmatic subjects who tolerated increasing doses of histamine without a corresponding fall in FEV_1, becoming unresponsive to the highest test dose [9]. Similar findings were reported by others [10, 11]. We [7] reported one patient highly reactive to histamine inhalation who responded to the lowest concentration and who subsequently showed marked improvement after oral antihistamine.

Histamine and methacholine reactivity can also be distinguished by the ability of hexamethonium (a ganglionic blocking

Table 48.2. Agents employed to assess "nonspecific" reactivity by inhalation challenge procedures

Agent	Popularity in the United States	Advantages or disadvantages
Distilled water	Growing	Experience still inadequate Solution readily available No unpleasant taste
Acetylcholine (ACh)	Minimal	Effect is short-lived
Carbachol	Greater than ACh	Very stable in solution ? Adverse vagal-like reactions
Histamine phosphate	Great	Stable in solution Direct and reflex smooth muscle constrictor Results similar to those of methacholine
Prostaglandin $F_{2\alpha}$	Minimal	Asthmatics 8000× more sensitive than healthy controls Wide dose range, reactive bronchodilation Unpleasant side effects ASA-sensitive asthmatics less reactive
Serotonin	Negligible	Importance in humans speculative Released from platelets in humans May potentiate vagal effects Many salts unstable in solution

ASA = acetylsalicylic acid

agent) to block histamine but not methacholine aerosol [12]. Since SCH 1000, an atropine analog, prevented methacholine-induced but not histamine-induced bronchoconstriction, and chlorpheniramine prevented histamine-induced but not methacholine-induced bronchoconstriction, Woenne and co-workers [13] reasoned that the mechanism and receptor sites involved in bronchial provocation by histamine and methacholine were distinctly different. From a technical viewpoint, there is a small but significant cumulative dose effect with methacholine ($p<.01$) but not with histamine.

Histamine response also has been compared with acetylcholine by inhalation, with similar reactivity shown [14, 15]. When inhaled histamine and methacholine have been compared to inhaled prostaglandin F_{2alpha} ($PGF_{2\alpha}$) it has been found that aspirin-sensitive asthmatic patients are less sensitive to $PGF_{2\alpha}$ than are non-aspirin-sensitive asthmatic patients [16, 17]. Hajos [18] studied 158 asthmatic subjects, 18% of whom reacted only to 0.2% serotonin and not to histamine or acetylcholine.

Histamine and methacholine challenges have been compared to exercise airway reactivity in normal and asthmatic subjects [19]. Although histamine and methacholine sensitivity were correlated, methacholine was better than histamine in differentiating asthmatics from normal subjects. Methacholine and histamine sensitivity correlated better with FEV_1 than with SGaw, presumably because of greater variation in SGaw measurements. No significant correlation was found between exercise response and histamine sensitivity ($r=0.44$, $p<1.1$). However, there was a significant correlation with exercise response and methacholine reactivity ($r=0.54$, $p<0.05$). Development of postexercise bronchospasm in asthmatic subjects correlated poorly with minute ventilation ($r=-0.20$) and with respiratory heat loss ($r=0.17$). There were more side effects with histamine than methacholine. Others have commented on the positive correlation between exercise-induced asthma and sensitivity to methacholine [5, 6]. Exercise appears to be a less sensitive test than histamine or methacholine bronchial inhalation tests as a measure of nonspecific bronchial responsiveness [5, 6, 19–21].

Bronchial responsiveness to methacholine has been compared to responsiveness to respiratory heat loss. Although there was good correlation in general, some individuals were relatively more responsive to methacholine than heat loss and vice versa [22]. Kivity and Souhrada [23] concluded that there was no correlation between eucapnic hyperventilation and methacholine responsiveness, yet O'Byrne and associates [24] found a good correlation between the two. The equipment required for the former is expensive, necessitating complex calculations and several measurements that are technically difficult. It is clear that further research is required in this subject.

48.3 Purposes of Performing Bronchial Inhalation Challenge to Presumed Bronchoconstrictive Substances Other than Antigens

Define atypical or variant asthma: An increased reactivity, compared with normal persons, to a variety of bronchoconstrictive substances is characteristic of individuals with asthma [1, 2, 11, 25–27] including those with cough or chest tightness as their primary manifestation [28].

Relate reactivity to other descriptive or predictive factors: Various investigators have linked reactivity of the airways as measured by histamine or acetylcholine challenge to the severity of asthmatic symptoms and duration of asthma [14, 29, 30]. Townley and co-workers [27], however, did not find such a relationship with duration of symptoms but did note that reactivity was less in patients who were free of symptoms for more than 2 years. On the other hand, subjects with the greatest reactivity to histamine and methacholine were admitted for intensive in-patient care at a younger age and had an earlier age of onset and asthma longer than patients with less airway reactivity [31]. In another study, those patients who could tolerate a high concentration of methacholine had the least severe asthma, as measured by discharge dose of corticosteroids [9]. Cockcroft and associates

[32] expressed a similar idea by demonstrating the correlation between mean degree of airway reactivity and severity of asthma, as assessed by medication requirements for symptom control. Other workers noted that asthmatic subjects with airways highly reactive to histamine and low panic-fear psychological profiles were hospitalized at exceptionally high rates relative to others [33]. Muranaka and colleagues [34] reported that asthmatics with long-term remissions had lower thresholds of bronchial reactivity than did those who were currently symptomatic.

A reciprocal relationship between the so-called *nonspecific* bronchial reactivity and reactivity to an allergen mixture has been commented on by various groups [35–37]. However, the design of studies dealing with these relationships should be scrutinized, especially with regard to the concentration of antigens administered and pulmonary function test utilized to assess response [1, 38–40]. The greater the hyperreactivity and diurnal fluctuations, the lower the peak expiratory flow rate (PEFR) on awakening and the greater the response to albuterol, according to Ryan and co-workers [41]. There also is a relationship between bronchial responsiveness and the level of treatment required for control of symptoms [22].

Relate blocking effects to usefulness in treatment of hyperreactive airways: Pharmaceutical companies have assumed that if an increase in nonspecific bronchial reactivity is the hallmark of asthma, agents that block or normalize this reactivity may be useful in the treatment of asthma [42].

Define and understand occupational asthma: During investigations of occupation-related asthma, an increased reactivity to methacholine or histamine after exposure to an offending substance is accepted as confirmatory evidence of the relevance of that substance [43, 44]. With most of these agents it would appear that augmented bronchial reactivity is the result of chronic exposure rather than a necessary predisposing condition for the development of occupational asthma [4, 44].

Factors affecting response to bronchoconstriction substances other than antigens: Table 48.3 summarizes the factors or circumstances that will alter the response to a bronchoconstrictor other than antigens.

48.4 Bronchial Provocation with Antigens

Most patients with allergic asthma appear to have symptoms caused by the common allergens for which there are skin test reagents and extracts available. The type of antigen used is only one factor that determines whether the bronchial response to the allergen is immediate, late, or a combination of these.

Immediate response: An immediate response is the most common reaction observed during bronchoprovocation tests. Acute bronchospasm sufficient to change lung function values develops within minutes after the antigen inhalation. Frequently hyperinflation and sometimes clinical symptoms of airways obstruction, including cough, become apparent. Antigen inhalation probably produces an IgE-linked release of chemical mediators [1], although theoretically IgG_4 skin sensitizing antibody may be implicated. The immediate reaction usually peaks at 20 or 30 min and clears by 2 or 3 hours. It is not only influenced by the IgE titer but by the concentration of antigen as well. It is characteristically inhibited by cromolyn sodium. Although corticosteroids are not thought to inhibit the immediate reaction, this concept recently has been challenged [45].

Late response: Late responses develop usually 4–6 to 16 hours after exposure to inhaled antigenic material and can last 36 hours or longer after antigen and occupational exposure [46–51]. Late responses probably result from inflammation, intraluminal mucous accumulation, and smooth muscle contraction. The mechanisms responsible for the late reactions are not entirely clear, but both IgE and IgG seem necessary. They are occasionally associated with fever and leukocytosis, and may induce recurrent nocturnal exacerbations.

Perhaps the more important factors responsible for late reactions are the concen-

Table 48.3. Factors affecting response to bronchoconstrictors

Agent	Direction of response
Viruses, viral vaccines, or bacterial vaccines	Usually lowering of threshold Occasionally no change
Air pollutants (including cigarette smoke)	Usually lowering of threshold Occasionally no change
Recent antigenic challenge	Usually lowering of threshold Occasionally no change
Occupational exposure	Usually lowering of threshold
Baseline degree of response	Probably no effect
Medications:	
β-agonists	Raising threshold
β-antagonists	No effect Lowering of threshold
Cromolyn sodium	Usually raising threshold Occasionally no effect
Ascorbic acid	Raising threshold or no effect
Anticholinergic agents	Usually some raising of threshold
α-blocking agents	Usually raising of threshold
Corticosteroids	Usually no effect Occasionally raising of threshold
Antihistamines (H_1)	Raising of threshold
Antihistamines (H_2)	Lowering of threshold No effect
Nifedipine	Raising of threshold
Lidocaine	Raising of threshold
Emotions	Lowering of threshold
Circadian or other body rhythms	Variable threshold
Allergic skin test reactivity or total IgE	Lowering of threshold or no effect

tration of antigen used and the nature of the antigen itself, since more late reactions occur after exposure to house dust and mold than after exposure to certain pollens [27]. High levels of specific IgE have an effect comparable to that of high concentrations of antigens in producing late reactions. Late reactions are generally less reversible than are immediate ones and are inhibited by cromolyn sodium, corticosteroids, and corticosteroid aerosols [47, 52] but not by β-adrenergic agonists and antihistamines [53, 54].

Combined immediate and late responses: In some patients the aerosol inhalation of antigen causes immediate and late reactions. Fig. 48.1 shows an immediate and late response as well as medication that modified the response of subject AF. Late reactions are usually, but not invariably, preceded by an immediate response [47, 55]. It has been suggested that the immediate reaction is caused by pollen fragments, for example, and a late reaction caused by absorption of the pollen grains [56]. However, Mihalas and Loren [56] could not provoke symptoms or changes in pulmonary function in nine asthmatic children given antigens sublingually at 2.5 to 50 times the dose to which they were sensitive by bronchial challenge. Gwynn and colleagues [57] performed antigen inhalation challenge in asthmatic patients and found two patients with allergen-specific IgE with an early response, three with specific IgG_4 with a late response, and three with both IgE and IgG_4 antibodies with both an immediate and a late reaction. They used concentrated antigens to produce the late reactions. Lee and co-workers [58] could not reproduce these findings and suggested that IgG_4 is unlikely

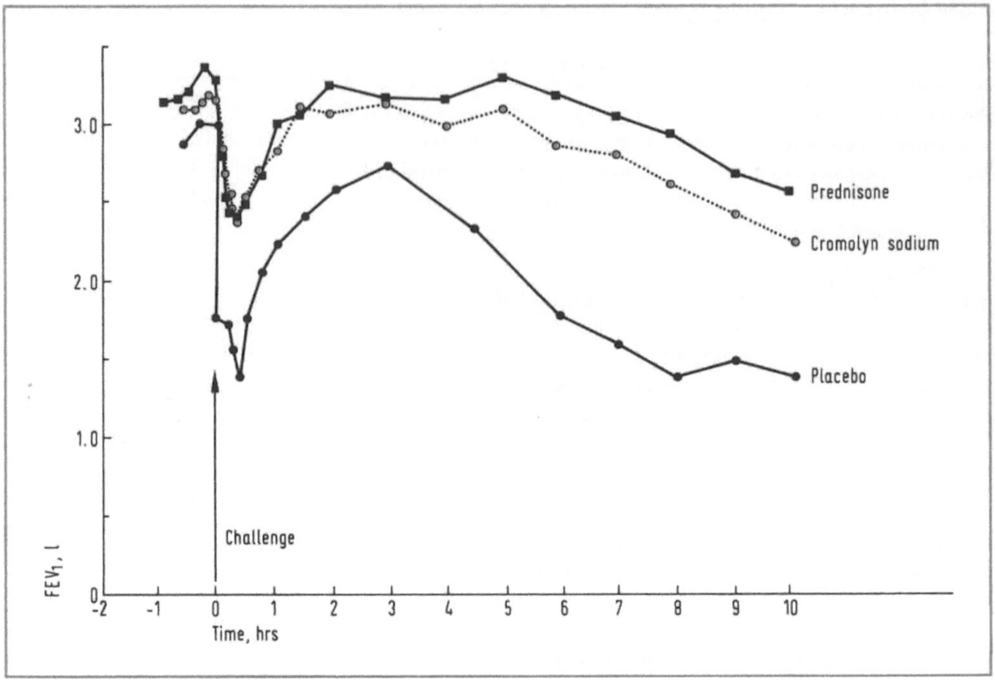

Fig. 48.1. The effect of prednisone, cromolyn sodium and placebo on an antigen inhalation challenge with ragweed in patient AF

to play an important role. I have tested a few persons who have experienced both an immediate and a late bronchial reaction to an antigen. The patients ingested increasing concentrations of the antigen but no obstruction occurred [59].

48.5 Purpose of Performing Bronchial Inhalation Challenge with Antigens

Clarification of the role of specific allergens in asthma: The indications and precautions for bronchial inhalation challenges with antigens have been outlined in Table 48.4. Advocates of bronchial inhalation challenge with allergens assume there is an advantage in testing the primary organ of involvement with allergens. With respect to asthma, this is the lung rather than the secondary organ, such as skin. There are extensive data to support the idea that bronchial inhalation challenges with antigens provide different information than a skin test or *in vitro* test does [3, 50].

Table 48.4. Indications and precautions for bronchial provocation challenge with antigens

Indications:

1. Clarification of the role of specific allergens in asthma
2. Substitution for or comparison with skin tests or *in vitro* tests
3. Clarification of mechanisms, e.g., release of mediators
4. Determination of new or provocative allergens in pulmonary disease
5. Evaluation of new treatment modalities and blocking agents
6. Establishment of the rationale for immunotherapy
7. Convince the patient of a cause-and-effect relationship

Special precautions necessary for antigen challenge:

1. No upper respiratory infection should be present
2. No ongoing asthmatic attack
3. Not if patient is unstable or reacts to a control substance
4. Not if patient lacks sufficient pulmonary reserve to tolerate the procedure

Table 48.5. Comparison between skin tests and bronchial challenge with antigens

Skin test findings	No. of patients studied	No. (%) with positive response to bronchial challenge[a]
Spector and Farr [62]		
Intradermal[b]		
Positive with 0.00001 wt/v	54	33 (61)
Positive with 0.0001 wt/v	102	36 (36)
Positive with 0.001 wt/v	131	35 (27)
Negative with 0.001 wt/v	245	9 (4)
Prick (puncture) test (1:10 or 1:20 wt/v)		
Wheal greater than 9 mm	32	16 (50)
Wheal greater than 5 mm	68	24 (35)
Wheal greater than 2 mm with erythema of 14 mm	101	25 (25)
Wheal less than or equal to 2 mm	77	2 (3)

wt/v = weight per volume
[a] With 0.001 wt/v antigen
[b] Positive response defined as wheal 6 mm in diameter larger than that produced by diluent alone

Only one study supported the conclusion that bronchial challenge offered no more than skin (or other) tests in confirming the diagnosis of allergic asthma [39]. This investigation looked at ragweed hay fever patients and asthmatic patients with comparable skin test reactivity and leukocyte histamine release. It showed no difference in the mean PD 35% (i.e., 35% fall in SGaw) antigen inhalation challenge response; i.e., antigen challenge did not differentiate the two groups, nor did skin test reactivity or *in vitro* testing [39]. The PD35 procedure itself partly explains their results, since it is a highly variable test, susceptible to suggestion and other factors [40].

Comparison of or substitute for skin tests or in vitro tests: Skin tests may not be practical if severe eczema or other skin disorders are present in an area to be tested. *In vitro* testing is a more expensive alternative to skin testing.

Bronchial challenges have been employed when there is insufficient information or discrepancies between history and skin tests or *in vitro* test results.

As stated, certain *in vitro* tests may yield negative results with the same antigen that causes a positive skin test or inhalation challenge response [60]. Also skin tests may not measure locally concentrated IgE attached to mast cells in a particular organ [61].

Although provocation tests have been touted as an absolute standard to which other tests should be compared, provocation testing also has its limitations, as will be discussed later.

Table 48.5 summarizes the relationship between skin test reactivity and bronchial inhalation challenge to these antigens [62]. In this case, two types of skin tests were used; the prick or puncture test and the intradermal skin test [62]. With the latter, if dilute antigens produced a positive reaction (defined by a wheal diameter 6 mm greater than that of the diluent control), the chance for a subsequent positive bronchial inhalation challenge was relatively great. Only 4% of the subjects tested had a positive bronchial inhalation challenge, despite a negative skin test.

This study was done with subjects who usually gave a history of perennial symptoms, so that the historic relationship to certain antigens was often unclear. If a patient has a positive skin test that accompanies a strong history of reaction to the antigen, then a bronchial inhalation challenge may not be necessary, since the history allows for a reasonable prediction of a subsequent bronchial inhalation challenge response. For example, 25 of 27 patients had a predictably positive inhalation challenge response in a previous study [50].

References

1. Spector SL, Farr RS (1976) Bronchial provocation tests. In: Weiss EB, Segal MS (eds) Bronchial Asthma: Mechanisms and Therapeutics. Little Brown, Boston, p 639
2. Spector SL (1985) Bronchial inhalation challenge procedures. In: Weiss EB, Segal MS (eds) Bronchial Asthma: Mechanisms and Therapeutics, 2nd edn. Little Brown, Boston, p 360
3. Aas K (1975) The bronchial provocation test. Thomas, Springfield
4. Boushey HA, Holtzman MJ, Sheller JR, Nadel JA (1980) Bronchial reactivity: State of the art. Am Rev Respir Dis 121:389
5. Eggleston PA (1979) A comparison of the asthmatic response to methacholine and exercise. J Allergy Clin Immunol 63:104
6. Kiviloog J (1973) Bronchial reactivity to exercise and methacholine in bronchial asthma. Scand J Respir Dis 54:347
7. Lilker ES, Jauregui R (1981) Airway response to water inhalation: A new test for "bronchial reactivity." N Engl J Med 305:702
8. Schoeffel RE, Anderson SD, Altounyan REC (1981) Bronchial hyperreactivity in response to inhalation of ultrasonically-nebulized solutions of distilled water and saline. Br Med J 283:1285
9. Spector SL, Farr RS (1975) A comparison of methacholine and histamine inhalations in asthmatics. J Allergy Clin Immunol 56:308
10. Schoeffel RE, Anderson SD, Gillam I, Lindsay DA (1980) Multiple exercise and histamine challenge in asthmatic patients. Thorax 35:164
11. Itkin IH (1967) Bronchial hypersensitivity to Mecholyl and histamine in asthmatic subjects. J Allergy 40:245
12. Holtzman MJ, Sheller JR, Dimeo M, Nadel JA, Boushey HA (1979) Effect of ganglionic blockade on bronchial reactivity in atopic subjects. Fed Proc 38:1110
13. Woenne R, Kattan M, Orange RP, Levison H (1978) Bronchial hyperreactivity to histamine and methacholine in asthmatic children after inhalation of SCH 1000 and chlorpheniramine maleate. J Allergy Clin Immunol 62:119
14. Makino S (1966) Clinical significance of bronchial sensitivity to acetylcholine and histamine in bronchial asthma. J Allergy 38:127
15. Popa V, Douglas JS, Bouhuys A (1974) Airway responses to histamine, acetylcholine and antigen in sensitized guinea pigs. J Lab Clin Med 84:226
16. Szezeklik A, Gryglewski RJ, Czerniawska-Mysik G (1975) Relationship of inhibition of prostaglandin biosynthesis by analgesics to asthma attacks in aspirin-sensitive patients. Br Med J 1:67
17. Thomson NC, Robert R, Bandouvakis J, Newball H, Hargreave F (1981) Comparison of bronchial responses to prostaglandin F_2 and methacholine. J Allergy Clin Immunol 68:392
18. Hajos MK (1962) Clinical studies on the role of serotonin in bronchial asthma. Acta Allergologica 17:358
19. Chatham M, Bleeker ER, Norman P (1982) A screening test for airways reactivity. An abbreviated methacholine inhalation challenge. Chest 82:1
20. Anderton RC, Cuff MT, Frith PA (1979) Bronchial responsiveness to inhaled histamine and exercise. J Allergy Clin Immunol 63:315
21. Mellis CM, Kattan M, Keens TG, Levison H (1978) Comparative study of histamine and exercise challenges in asthmatic children. Am Rev Respir Dis 117:911
22. Hargreave FE, Ryan G, Thomson NC, O'Byrne PM, Latimer K, Juniper EF, Dolovich J (1981) Bronchial responsiveness to histamine or methacholine in asthma: Measurement and clinical significance. J Allergy Clin Immunol 68:347
23. Kivity S, Souhrada JF (1981) A new diagnostic test to assess airway reactivity in asthmatics. Bull Eur Physiopathol Respir 17:243
24. O'Byrne P, Ryan G, Morris M, Mc Cormack D, Jones NL, Morse JLC, Hargreave FE (1982) Asthma induced by cold air and its relation to nonspecific bronchial responsiveness to methacholine. Am Rev Respir Dis 125:281
25. Benson MK (1975) Bronchial hyperreactivity. Br J Dis Chest 69:227
26. Chai H, Farr RS, Froehlich LA, Mathison DA, McLean TA, Rosenthal RR, Sheffer AC, Spector SL, Townley AG (1975) Standardization of bronchial inhalation challenge procedures. J Allergy Clin Immunol 56:323
27. Townley RG, Ryo UY, Kolotkin BM, Kang B (1975) Bronchial sensitivity to methacholine in current and former asthmatic and allergic rhinitis patients and control subjects. J Allergy Clin Immunol 56:429
28. Corrao WM, Braman SS, Irwin RS (1979) Chronic cough as the sole presenting mani-

festation of bronchial asthma. N Engl J Med 300:633
29. Curry JJ (1946) The action of histamine on the respiratory tract in normal and asthmatic subjects. J Clin Invest 25:785
30. Curry JJ (1947) Comparative action of acetyl-beta-methylcholine and histamine on the respiratory tract in normals, patients with hay fever, and subjects with bronchial asthma. J Clin Invest 26:430
31. Spector SL, Staudenmayer H, Kinsman RA, Fukuhara J, Westmoreland C (1979) Methacholine and histamine inhalation challenges in asthma: Relationship of age of onset, length of illness, and pulmonary functions. Allergy 34:167
32. Cockcroft DW, Killian DN, Mellon JJA, Hargreave FE (1977) Protective effect of drugs on histamine-induced asthma. Thorax 32:429
33. Staudenmayer H, Kinsman RA, Dirks JF, Spector SL, Wangaard C (1979) Medical outcome in asthmatic patients: Effect of airway hyperreactivity and symptom-focused anxiety. Psychosom Med 41:109–118
34. Muranaka M, Suzuki S, Miyamoto T, Takeda K, Okomura H, Makino S (1974) Bronchial reactivities to acetylcholine and IgE levels in asthmatic subjects after long-term remissions. J Allergy Clin Immunol 54:32
35. Bryant DH, Burns MW (1976) Bronchial histamine reactivity: Its relationship to the reactivity of the bronchi to allergens. Clin Allergy 6:523
36. Killian D, Cockcroft DW, Hargreave FE, Dolovich J (1976) Factors in allergen-induced asthma: Relevance of the intensity of the airways allergic reaction and non-specific bronchial reactivity. Clin Allergy 6:219
37. Nathan RA, Kinsman RA, Spector SC, Horton DJ (1979) Relationship between airways response to allergens and non-specific bronchial reactivity. J Allergy Clin Immunol 64:491
38. Townley RG, Dennis M, Itkin IH (1965) Comparative action of acetyl-beta-methylcholine, histamine, and pollen antigens in subjects with hay fever and patients with bronchial asthma. J Allergy 36:121
39. Bruce CA, Rosenthal RR, Lichtenstein LM, Norman PS (1975) Quantitative inhalation bronchial challenge in ragweed hay fever patients: A comparison with ragweed-allergic asthmatics. J Allergy Clin Immunol 56:331
40. Spector SL, Luparello TJ, Kopetzky MT, Souhrada J, Kinsman RA (1976) Response of asthmatics to methacholine and suggestion. Am Rev Respir Dis 113:43
41. Ryan G, Latimer K, Dolovich J, Hargreave FE (1987) Bronchial responsiveness to histamine: Relationship to diurnal variation of flow rates and improvement after bronchodilator. Thorax 37:423
42. Spector SL (1979) Use of provocation techniques for the evaluation of drug efficacy. J Allergy Clin Immunol 64:677
43. Cockcroft DW, Cartier A, Jones G, Tarlo SM, Dolovich J, Hargreave FE (1980) Asthma caused by occupational exposure to a furan based binder system. J Allergy Clin Immunol 66:458
44. Lam S, Wong R, Yeung M (1979) Nonspecific bronchial reactivity in occupational asthma. J Allergy Clin Immunol 63:28
45. Delehunt JC, Yerger L, Ahmed T, Abraham WM (1984) Inhibition of antigen-induced bronchoconstriction by methylprednisolone succinate. J Allergy Clin Immunol 73:479–483
46. Hargreave FE (1974) The late asthmatic responses. Can Med Assoc J 110:415
47. Pepys J, Davies RJ, Breslin ABX (1974) The effects of inhaled beclomethasone dipropionate (Becotide) and sodium cromoglycate on asthmatic reactions to provocation tests. Clin Allergy 4:12
48. Robertson D, Kerigan AT, Hargreave FE, Chalmers R, Dolovich J (1974) Late asthmatic responses induced by ragweed pollen allergen. J Allergy Clin Immunol 54:244
49. Salvaggio JE (1979) Occupational asthma: Overview and mechanisms. J Allergy Clin Immunol 64:646
50. Spector SL, Farr RS (1974) Bronchial inhalation procedures in asthmatics. Med Clin North Am 58:71
51. Bronsky EA, Ellis EF (1969) Inhalation bronchial challenge testing in asthmatic children. Pediatr Clin North Am 16:85
52. Booij-Noord H, Orie NGN, Berg WC, de Vries K (1970) Protection tests on bronchial allergen challenge with disodium cromoglycate and thiazinamium. J Allergy 46:1
53. Ruffin RE, Cockcroft DW, Hargreave FE (1978) A comparison of the protective effect of fenoterol and Sch 1000 on allergen-induced asthma. J Allergy Clin Immunol 61: 42
54. Schiller IW, Lowell FC (1947) The effect of drugs in modifying the response of asthmatic subjects to inhalation of pollen extracts determined by vital capacity measurements. Ann Allergy 5:564
55. Pepys J, Davies RJ (1977) Allergy. In: Clark TJH, Godfrey S (eds) Asthma. Saunders, Philadelphia, pp 126–161

56. Mihalas LS, Loren ML (1979) Oral challenges of inhalant antigens in asthmatics. Ann Allergy 42:145
57. Gwynn CM, Ingram J, Almousawi T, Stanworth DR (1982) Bronchial provocation tests in atopic patients with allergen-specific IgG_4 antibodies. Lancet 1:254
58. Lee TH, Durham SR, Merrett J, Merrett TG, Kay AB (1982) Allergen-specific IgG_4 in bronchial asthma. Lancet 2:1048
59. Spector SL (1984) Unpublished data
60. May CD, Williams CS (1973) Further studies concerning the fluctuating insensitivity of peripheral leukocytes to unrelated allergens and the meaning of nonspecific "desensitization". Clin Allergy 3:319
61. Huggins KG, Brostoff J (1975) Local production of specific IgE antibodies in allergic rhinitis patients with negative skin tests. Lancet 2:148
62. Spector SL, Farr RS (1979) Bronchial inhalation challenge with antigens. J Allergy Clin Immunol 64:580

49. Status Asthmaticus

R. Pariente

Status asthmaticus is a dramatic paroxysmic condition which occurs during the course of asthmatic illness. It necessitates emergency treatment of a specialized and rapidly effective nature.

Status asthmaticus (SA) is distinguished from other states of acute respiratory insufficiency by its unexpected occurrence among subjects who, until the moment of seizures, have enjoyed a normal respiratory function. Furthermore, recovery from SA results in respiratory figures reverting to previous levels. Finally, SA is resistant even to mechanical ventilation, and thus, there is a tendency to form a relatively reserved prognosis as to its presence [16].

Occurrences of such respiratory distress, markedly different from common asthmatic fits are rare in asthmatic illness. They can happen at any stage of the illness, some being inaugural, others occurring within a partially fixed obstructive syndrome [17].

It appears [1] that SA becomes more apparent after 40 years of age. Nevertheless in recent years emphasis has been placed on the possibility of such seizures occurring earlier in life.

The definition of SA is debatable. While once it meant a mortal fit, in current literature [3, 4, 8, 9] certain authors have since used the term *status asthmaticus* to cover fits which are only slightly more serious than usual, but which resist the usual therapy (corticoids + adrenaline). To give a broader definition we may say that SA is a prolonged, rebellious and threatening seizure. More recently [3, 11, 14, 15] we have, at least, been presented with a whole series of indications as to its clinical severity.

The most significant and constant of the tests available is the gas level test. In fact the study of blood gas levels in clinical tables compiled regularly show that in SA the PaO_2 level is far lower than during the course of a common asthmatic fit. Moreover, the latter registers hypercapnia with a $PaCO_2$ which surpasses 40 mm of mercury. Its corollary, then, taking into account the existence of acute hypercapnia is the habitual lowering of blood pH, which in certain cases is lower than the critical value of 7.20. The prognosis and predictive value of this acidic hypercapnia appears fundamental. The seriousness of the situation becomes major if metabolic acidity coexists. In fact, those patients suffering from overacidity show the absolute or relative ineffectiveness of catecholamines on the β-adrenergic receptors. Corticoids are effective, though, with delay from the vicious circle and uncertain prognosis [8].

The definition of SA can, then, be as follows: a sequence of events which, at a given moment brings about hypercapnia, fatigue of the respiratory muscles, lactic acidosis and then ventilatory failure.

The progressively increasing hypercapnia brings about an accumulation of H^+-ions and cardiac arrest occurs when pH values descend below 7.15. It therefore seems that, in order to speak of SA, it is essential that we retain the criterion of the hypercapnia, while remaining aware of its fallibility. The term can be criticized on two accounts:

1. Severe and inveterate asthmatics whose illness becomes a fixed and obstructive syndrome can put themselves into a state of chronic or subacute hypercapnia independently of SA.
2. A prolonged fit, already showing signs of severity, can fail to transform itself into hypercapnia at a given moment, thus leading to the wrong conclusions being drawn.

It is the rapidity with which this hypercapnia sets in that makes its value debatable. Its prognostic value, however, is altogether essential.

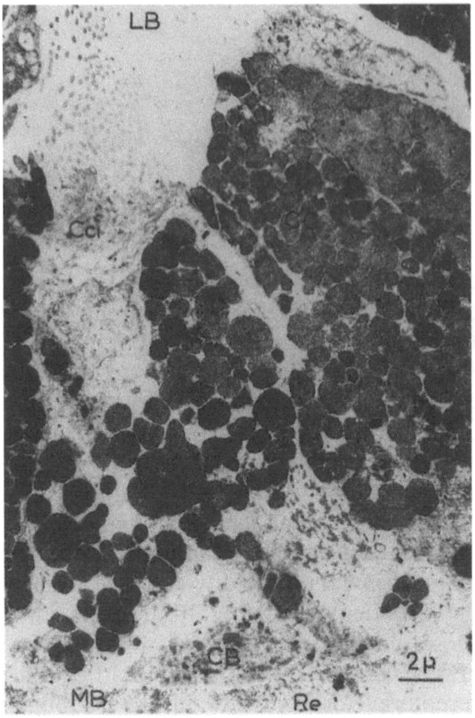

Fig. 49.1. Small bronchus showing internal diameter of 200 μ and mucous cell hyperplasia of the epithelium. LB = bronchial lumen, CC = mucous cell, Cci = ciliated cell, MB = basal membrane, CB = corpuscle body, Re = reticulin layer. (×6,500)

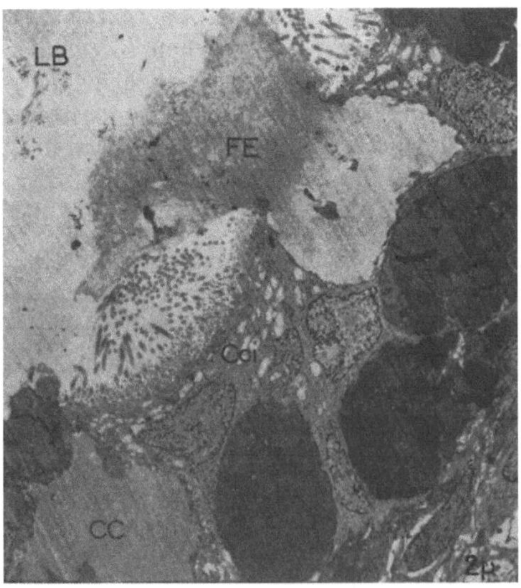

Fig. 49.2. Small bronchus showing internal diameter of 2,000 μ. LB = bronchial lumen, CCi = ciliated cell, CC = mucous cell, FE = elastic fiber. (×4,300)

One can, therefore, say that SA embraces certain clinical signs of seriousness; certain measures of resistance to habitual therapy (including corticoids) and eventually the installation of hypercapnia at a certain moment which imposes the presence or danger of potential death.

49.1 Pathology [7, 18] (Figs. 49.1–49.4)

The lesions are: 1. those of asthmatic disease (Goblet cell's hyperplasia, mucous gland's hyperplasia on submucosa, infiltration of polymorphous cells, muscle hypertrophy). 2. The main disorders are: extreme bronchoconstriction and a plug cell over the bronchial airways except in the more distal airways.

49.2 Epidemiologic Data about Status Asthmaticus

It is difficult to estimate the exact frequency with which SA occurs, but many authors have carried out retrospective research in order to know the exact mortality rate (the first was Alexander in 1963). The current figure given by the American Thoracic Society is 1 per thousand asthmatics.

The increase in the mortality rate among asthmatics during the 1960s has been attributed to:

- The increased sale of pressurized aerosols containing β_2-mimetics. It seems logical that when the patient under seizure is driven to an abuse of β_2-mimetic sprays this should be considered not a cause of grave illness but an objective indication of it [10]. The patient must be given a notion of limitation in the use of these sprays and be called upon to consult his specialist center when he is driven to an abuse of them.
- Other medicines have been put on trial as agents contributing to the occurrence of SA:
  - the abuse of several bronchodilators particularly associated with abnormally high doses of theophyllinics and β_2-mimetics;
  - the abuse of respiratory depressant sedatives;

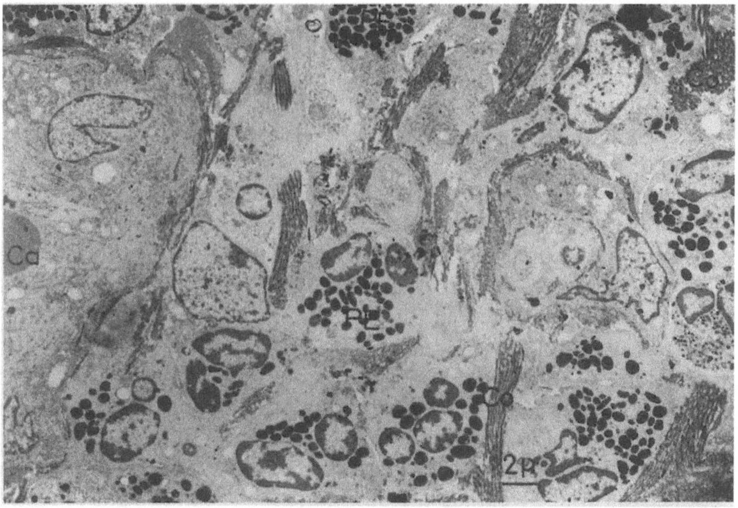

Fig. 49.3. Small bronchus showing internal diameter of 1,500 μ. Cellular infiltration of the chorion made by eosinophils. Ca = capillary, Co = collagen. (×4,300)

- corticoid treatment of long duration;
- nonsteroidal anti-inflammatory agents [5].

- A certain number of major emotional factors.
- Infection plays an extremely controversial role. It seems that bronchial and severe sinus infections contribute to asthmatic illness under certain conditions. If this infection is particularly difficult, deep-rooted or dominant then it indisputably contributes to SA.
- Personality: Certain asthmatics are predisposed towards SA though specific reasons have not been determined. In fact, the same patient may reproduce SA several times during his life, though this is a rare eventuality.

49.3 Principal Signs of Seriousness

Signs of serious illness in asthma are multiple and it is necessary to single out those found in the majority of cases [3, 4, 11]. Recent works on the subject have resulted in the proposal of a scale of seriousness with indications showing when there is a need for hospitalization under specialized care.

The symptoms currently given are as follows:

- Paleness mixed with cyanosis accompanied by severe debility.

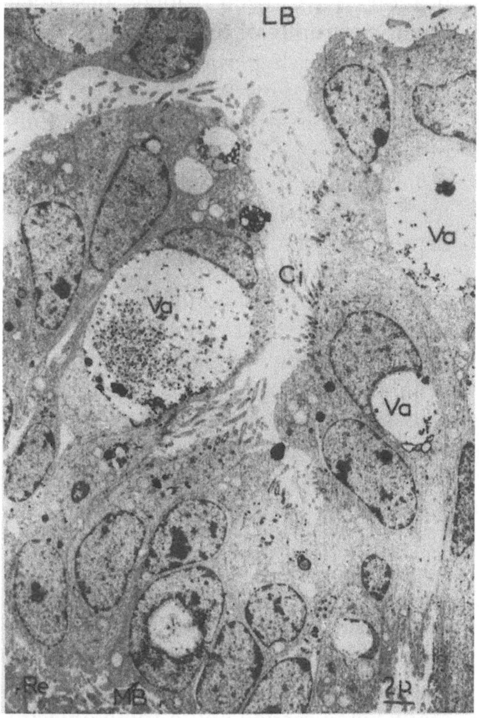

Fig. 49.4. Respiratory bronchiole. Large intracytoplasmic vacuoles (Va). LB = bronchial lumen, Re = reticulin layer, Ci = cilia, MB = basal membrane

- The *respiratory syndrome* is governed by the dyspnea, an asphyxiating polypnea. This dyspnea remains asthmatic in nature, that is to say, expiratory and as the SA becomes progressively worse, the vesicular murmur becomes fainter, like wheezing, while the dyspnea worsens [7].
- *Cyanosis.*
- Among the *cardiac signs*, emphasis must be placed on the paradoxical pulse with circulatory stoppages in the course of forced expiration (by transmural compression of the veins). This is accompanied by *tachycardia* generally in the region of 120 and sometimes higher in the more severe cases. Arterial hypotension and sweating are less important signs which develop later. Arterial pressure is, for the most part, normal. It is reduced in a certain number of more severe cases. Electrocardiographic modifications have been widely described. The hypertrophy of the right auricle and, at worst, the hypertrophy of the right ventricle are signs which can be found without necessarily implicating seriousness.
- *Neuropsychic signs:* Agitation is usual, for a while at least. This is followed by depression which, apart from anything else, is a bad prognosis. Once problems with consciousness begin, mental confusion and, at worst, coma appear. The situation is then serious and necessitates ventilatory aid.
- *Muscular syndrome:* On inspection one may notice signs of fatigue in the respiratory muscles with respiratory accessories coming into play (sign of seriousness), an alternation of abdominal respiration and upper respiration. The hollowing of the epigastrium during inspiration and especially the subjective appearance of signs of exhaustion are always a very bad prognosis. Work is currently being carried out to try to objectify the signs of muscular fatigue, with the changes of the M/L ratio of the electromyogram of the diaphragm, in particular even when the central stimuli remain high with high occlusion pressure.
- Certain studies [3, 6] have given importance to the peak flow calculated from such patients. Once this sinks to less than 120 ml/mm, the fall in peak flow should be considered a relatively reliable symptom of seriousness.
- *Hemodynamic signs:* Here pulmonary arterial hypertension is usual and, especially, considerable pulmonary vascular pressures linked with large variations of transmural pressures in the course of inspiration and expiration. These signs are given objective confirmation by angiography.
- Far more important are indications of *thoracic distension* [12]. In the course of an asthmatic seizure, radiological signs of a major distension, along with peripheral hypovascularization are considerable signs of seriousness.

In summary, symptoms of seriousness include: paradoxical pulse; the increase of dyspnea contrasting with respiratory silence; consciousness problems; and signs of respiratory fatigue. Above all, the best symptoms of confirmed SA are provided by the *blood gas level tests.* Herein we see the emergence of a vicious circle often irreversible.

49.4 The Evolution of Status Asthmaticus

Formerly SA, once defined, was almost always fatal. Since the introduction of the use of corticotherapy and artificial ventilation methods, these asphyxiating syndromes are almost always curable. They need to be tested in specialized centers. Long-term prognosis remains the real problem. If, in fact, SA can be triggered by a particular cause, then, for the most part, circumstances contributing to an attack are unknown. Reoccurrence is frequent and in the course of such a reoccurrence, prognosis is once more called into question.

Clinical forms: SA as described above can occur at any stage in the evolution of asthmatic illness and during the patient's entire lifetime. It is most frequently seen in two conditions:

1. in paroxysmic asthma, which has always been unpredictable in nature.
2. SA attacks, more often, occur in asthmatic patients aged 40 years or older who

have been asthmatic since childhood. Their obstructive syndrome is mixed and only partly reversible. Under this hypothesis, SA is generally favored by causes invoked through emotional stress and, even more so, by infections of the respiratory tracts (even the upper tract and particularly the sinuses).

This potential infection justifies the introduction of a systematic antibiotic treatment when SA enters its most acute phase.

Symptomatic forms: Attention should be given to two types of situations, occurring far more rarely and posing completely different problems.

There are patients in whom SA sets in quite brutally from one minute to the next, similar, in effect, to anaphylactic shock. These patients usually die at home or else come for consultations for repeated asthmatic fits with no free interval between the attacks. This reaction can be seen particularly in aspirin-treated asthmatics.

Other states of acute respiratory distress can be met during chronic obstructive bronchopathy following a deep rooted asthmatic illness. These patients have chronic obstructive pulmonary disease accompanied by very severe distension and have permanent dyspnea. In this case it is not rare for a state of acute respiratory distress to set in.

49.5 The Treatment of Status Asthmaticus

Treatment should always be carried out in a highly specialized department, in a thoracic department equipped with an intensive care unit [2].

The indications for assisted ventilation in such patients are rare, but when such assistance becomes necessary, it occurs at great speed.

In all patients, upon admission, it is necessary that an intravenous drip be set up in order to administer drugs and to give access to a venous path in the event of cardiorespiratory arrest.

Antibiotics should be systematically administered. Ampicillines are preferable though this is not imperative. They supply the maximum effectiveness against germs which are usually pathogenic in the lower respiratory tract; pneumococcus, Hemophilus and a certain number of negative gram and anaerobics.

Bronchodilatators: Inverse tendencies confront each other when it comes to the use of theophyllinics or of β_2-mimetics via the drip. Some authors use the association between the two therapies believing that it will eventually reach a potential result. The therapeutic plans include the following:

- *Theophyllinics administered endovenously* should be introduced via the drip and never directly intravenously. The initial dosage is 6 mg/kg in 30 min and for 24 hours about 14 mg/kg. In a continuous drip, an effective rate of theophyllinic level can be maintained.
- *β_2-mimetics* administered in the same manner in good doses (6 ampoules per 24 hours of terbutaline or an equivalent drug) have a relatively speedy effect.

These two drugs are not active on the plugs. Thus, when they are not immediately effective a certain tendency towards overdose has been noted resulting in the frequency of side effects through these means of administration. In these cases it is usual to add an anxiolytic. When confronted with severe conditions treatment with corticoids is needed.

Corticoids do not have an immediate effect, but an effect delayed by some hours. According to some authors corticoids may be given in normal doses of 600 mg of hemisuccinate of hydrocortisone per day, by venous means. For others it is preferable to give far higher doses right away after the first 24 hours, of 1,200 to 2,400 mg. There appears to be a threshold dosage which exceeds 600 mg. Their retarded effect justifies the need to be used in conjunction with bronchodilatators and not instead of them.

Injections are preferable at the beginning of the treatment; as soon as possible, administration of one corticoid through the oral channel should be employed (i.e., prednisone given as quickly as possible at 60 mg per day in the beginning, then in decreasing strength to avoid recurrence of the seizure and to diminish the frequency of post corticotherapy syndrome such as tiredness, muscular pains etc.).

In addition to this it has been proposed that in extremely severe cases adrenaline should be given by direct intravenous methods or depressive drugs for respiratory centers which allow and make assisted ventilation possible.

Medical treatment employing anxiolytics has, most frequently, led to recovery from the most severe SA. Actually, at least 90% of patients recover given such adapted medical treatment. A certain number of them, however, resist it.

Several eventualities may arise:

1. *Worsening in spite of therapy:* Clinical signs of seriousness, in particular muscle fatigue, intensify and simultaneously consciousness problems appear. The next step is assisted ventilation.
2. *The fit remains grave* in an obvious manner in which it may be necessary to use intravenous administration of basic solutions such as hypertonic bicarbonated serum or THAM. The administration of such a serum can only be carried out in a reanimation center and on a patient who is prepared to receive assisted ventilation. The doctor needs to have had a great deal of practical experience in assisted ventilation in order to administer the intravenous serum before the ventilation process even starts. If his experience is insufficient then it is better to revert to intubation before starting alcalinisation. The latter can, by depressing the respiratory system, result in a sudden worsening of the condition, urgently necessitating intubation. In most cases, however, it leads to a spectacular improvement.

There are then two possible conditions which call for assisted ventilation of a patient: worsening in spite of therapy and worsening due to the addition of bicarbonated serum.

When *assisted ventilation* is given it must be given by endotracheal intubation. The extremely dense and obstructive mucous formations which occur in conjunction with the bronchospasm, block almost completely the aerial passages. It is therefore necessary to obtain a relaxation of the spasm and a free passage for the ventilation.

In order to achieve this, ventilators are needed which are able to inject air with high pressure, in addition to medical treatment and the maintained use of bronchodilatators and corticoids. Should these be insufficient then recourse should be made to bicarbonated serum or THAM. Thanks to alcalinisation it has become absolutely exceptional to have a continued resistance to assisted ventilation, an eventuality which, should it happen, would call for a reversion to former historical techniques such as morphinisation or curarisation.

The manner of conducting this assisted ventilation, while being difficult, is at least the same as for the assisted ventilation of other respiratory failure. The relatively low V. T. with which the procedure starts must be developed to a high frequency with a high fraction of oxygen.

In the majority of cases ventilation becomes easier once the frequency can be reduced and, especially, once the tidal volume can be increased without also increasing insufflation pressure. It seems important to maintain P. I., if possible at less than 30 mmHg. In fact, it is probable that nonsusceptible stimuli brought about by high pressures of inspiration exaggerate the bronchospasm instead of helping in its reduction.

With the severing procedure, under assisted ventilation, sufferers from SA generally recover very quickly in several hours rather than days. The patient has a spontaneous respiratory frequency and a cardiac frequency which lowers as soon as wheezing and expiratory stoppage become perceptible sounds. A test of spontaneous ventilation is made by switching off the machine while leaving the tubes in place. One can ascertain whether there has been a growth in respiratory frequency and whether the capnia and shunting effect have increased. If this is not the case and if signs of seriousness have also disappeared then the need for prolonged ventilation is rare. Only patients suffering from severe and chronic bronchopathy may require prolonged assistance. In such cases the therapeutic procedure is the same as for acute obstructive bronchopathy.

Cases where free ventilation remains difficult and the hypercapnia is high for several hours or even days are exceptional. In these cases, the medical and ultimately mechanical therapy must remain unchanged for the whole duration of treatment.

49.6 Prophylactic Measures

Prophylactic measures to be taken in order to prevent the recurrence of SA are as follows: Avoid additional infections of the aerial tracts and treatment for chronic sinusitis. Research the factors which may contribute to further fits. Take the patient in charge, medically and psychologically after SA. This is absolutely essential and difficult.

Medical treatment must be maintained as long as necessary. Antibiotics should be taken for several days after the attack. Corticoids should be decreased rapidly at first and then very slowly until complete severance is achieved in the majority of cases. Bronchodilatory drugs will eventually be replaced by theophyllinics per os and spray bronchodilatators. While these sprays were shown to be less and less effective before the attack, which is also a sign of seriousness, they returned to efficacy after the attack and the patient may use them in the same manner as previously.

References

1. Arnold AG, Lane DJ, Zapata E (1983) Acute severe asthma: factors that influence hospital referral by the general practitioner and self-referral by the patient. Br J Dis Chest 1: 51–59
2. Arnold AG, Lane DJ, Zapata E (1983) Current therapeutic practice in the management of acute severe asthma. Br J Dis Chest 2: 123–135
3. Arnold AG, Lane DJ, Zapata E (1982) The speed of onset and severity of acute severe asthma. Br J Dis Chest 2:157–163
4. Benfield GF, Smith AP (1977) Predicting rapid and slow response to treatment in acute severe asthma. Br J Dis Chest 3: 249–254
5. Cohen RD, Bateman ED, Potgieter PD (1982) Near fatal bronchospasm in an asthmatic patient following ingestion of flurbiprofen. A case report. S Afr Med J 61, 21:803
6. Depeursinge C, Boutaleb AK, Willemetz JC, Depeursinge F, Dardel E, Perret C (1983) Measuring bronchial obstruction in intensive care. Schweiz Med Wochenschr 113, 33: 1128–1129
7. Derenne JP (1972) Conceptions actuelles et indications thérapeutiques de l'état de mal asthmatique. Thèse, Faculté de Médecine Paris-Sud
8. Field SB, Swartz MA, Glanz K, Francis ME (1983) Efficacy of short-term corticosteroid therapy in outpatient treatment of acute bronchial asthma. Am J Med 2:259–262
9. Luksza AR (1982) Acute severe asthma treated without steroids. Br J Dis Chest 1:15–19
10. Meurs H, Koeter GH, de Vries K, Kauffman HF (1982) The beta-adrenergic system and allergic bronchial asthma: changes in lymphocyte beta-adrenergic receptor number and adenylate cyclase activity after an allergen-induced asthmatic attack. J Allergy Clin Immunol 4:272–280
11. Rebuck AS, Braude AC, Chapman KR (1982) Evaluation of the severity of the acute asthmatic attack. Chest [Suppl 1]:289–295
12. Rushton AR (1982) The role of the chest radiograph in the management of childhood asthma. Clin Pediatr (Phila) 6:325–328
13. Tamura M, Itakura K, Sayama T, Murakami T, Suzuki Y (1983) Ventilatory response to carbon dioxide in bronchial asthma and chronic obstructive lung disease. Jpn J Med 3:190–194
14. Westerman DE, Benatar SR (1983) Ventilatory responses to carbon dioxide in asthmatics with previous carbon dioxide retention during severe asthma. S Afr Med J 63, 22: 839–842
15. Wolf B, Gaultier C, Lopez C, Boule M, Girard F (1983) Hypoxemia in attack free asthmatic children: relationship with lung volumes and lung mechanics. Bull Eur Physiopathol Respir 5:471–476
16. Zwicke DL, Donohue JF, Wagner EH (1982) Use of the emergency department observation unit in the treatment of acute asthma. Ann Emerg Med 2:77–83
17. Editorial (1982) Acute severe asthma: sacred cows under attack. Lancet 2 (8295):420–421
18. André-Bougaran J, Pariente R, Legrand M, Cayrol E, Brouet G (1972) Aspect ultrastructural de l'état de mal asthmatique. Nouv Presse Méd 1:2457–2462

I. Therapeutic Considerations

50. Physiopathological Data for the Treatment of Bronchial Asthma

R. Pauwels

The study of the pharmacological properties of antiasthmatic drugs has deeply influenced ideas concerning the pathophysiology and pathogenesis of asthma. New findings on the pathogenesis of asthma influence the hypotheses involving the mode of action of antiasthmatic drugs. A discussion on the physiopathological treatment of bronchial asthma, therefore, is based on current thinking about the pathophysiology of bronchial asthma. The main characteristic of bronchial asthma is bronchial hyperreactivity [1]. Bronchial reactivity is determined by genetic factors and by exogenous influences. Exogenous influences such as allergens, air pollutants, infection, etc. modify bronchial reactivity by causing airway inflammation. Especially illustrative is the relation between type I allergy and nonspecific bronchial hyperreactivity. The occurrence of a late phase bronchial reaction after allergen inhalation is followed by an increase in nonspecific bronchial hyperreactivity [2]. The activity of the different antiasthmatic drugs on nonspecific bronchial reactivity, airway inflammation and type I allergic reactions will therefore be discussed along with their other pharmacological effects.

50.1 Sodium Cromoglycate (SCG) [3]

DSCG is a nonbronchodilating drug that inhibits both the immediate and the late bronchoconstriction following allergen challenge. DSCG prevents the increase in nonspecific bronchial reactivity following late phase reactions. A possible clinical correlation is its effectiveness in preventing a seasonal increase in nonspecific bronchial reactivity in patients with pollen allergy. The effect of DSCG has been explained by its mast cell stabilizing effect although several data waver this hypothesis. DSCG also protects against nonspecific stimulants such as exercise, cold air, sulfur dioxide and distilled water. The involvement of mast cells in the bronchoconstriction caused by these challenges is far from being settled. Many compounds have been synthesized with equal or better mast cell stabilizing properties than DSCG, using the same pharmacological models. However, most of them have proven to be therapeutically ineffective. DSCG has, besides its mast cell stabilizing activity, other pharmacological activities which may be relevant to its therapeutic efficacy. DSCG inhibits reflex bronchoconstriction by an effect on C-fibers. It has an inhibitory effect on adenosine-induced bronchoconstriction and prevents the activation of platelets by platelet activating factor.

50.2 Ketotifen [4]

Ketotifen has no bronchodilating activity but inhibits the allergen-induced immediate and late bronchoconstriction. Ketotifen similarly reduces nonspecific bronchial reactivity following long-term treatment. Ketotifen has several pharmacological properties that may contribute to its clinical efficacy. In the human lung system ketotifen selectively inhibits the release of leukotrienes. Ketotifen has antagonistic activity against histamine, SRS and PAF. The drug has also been shown to inhibit calcium uptake in mast cells and smooth muscle. Finally, ketotifen prevented in experimental animals the development of tachyphylaxis of the β-adrenergic receptor upon chronic administration of sympathomimetic drugs. It is not clear which one of the above mentioned pharmacological properties is responsible for the clinical efficacy of the drug.

50.3 Sympathomimetic Drugs [5]

Sympathomimetic drugs have several pharmacological properties that are obviously beneficial in bronchial asthma: relaxation of bronchial smooth muscle, decrease of vascular permeability and stimulation of the mucociliary function. These properties should result in bronchodilatation and an enhanced clearance of bronchial secretions. The effects of sympathomimetic drugs on nonspecific bronchial reactivity are under investigation. Studies up to now seem to indicate no effect on this characteristic. Although sympathomimetic drugs have mast cell stabilizing properties in vitro, it has never been possible to demonstrate clearly this effect in vivo. The inhalation of sympathomimetic drugs before allergen challenge prevents the immediate bronchoconstriction but has no effect on the late reaction. This observation does not exclude an effect of sympathomimetic drugs on the late phase reaction. The lack of activity in the above mentioned challenge test could also be explained by the pharmacokinetic behavior of the drug and the absence of a sufficient amount of the drug during the critical time of the development of the late phase reaction. One can only conclude that sympathomimetic drugs given before the immediate reaction do not prevent the triggering of the late phase reaction. It is also generally said that sympathomimetic drugs have little effect on a developed late bronchoconstriction. This conclusion is based on anectodal observations rather than on a rigorous scientific protocol.

50.4 Xanthines [6]

The value of theophylline in the prophylactic treatment of bronchial asthma is well established. Theophylline is a potent bronchodilator drug with a rather narrow therapeutic margin. The possibility that theophylline may have an inhibitory activity on the allergic reaction and on the release of mediators in addition to its bronchodilating capacity has been considered by several investigators. Theophylline has been shown to inhibit the in vitro release of inflammatory mediators from rat mast cells, monkey lung fragments, human skin and lung fragments. The concentration of theophylline necessary to demonstrate an inhibitory effect on mediator release in vitro exceeds the normal therapeutic concentration by a factor of 2 to 100. Another, perhaps more relevant, in vitro finding is the observation that theophylline, at clinically relevant concentrations, exerts specific antagonism at cell surface receptor sites for adenosine and in doing so inhibits the potentiating effect of adenosine on mediator release. In vivo, in experimental animals Andersson [7] demonstrated that a low dose of aminophylline, a dose without a direct bronchodilating effect, inhibited the antigen-induced bronchoconstriction. Treatment with aminophylline for three weeks led to a decreased bronchial response to antigen in sensitized guinea pigs, even three days after treatment had ceased. The effect of theophylline on allergen-induced bronchoconstriction in man has not been extensively studied. Theophylline, at therapeutic concentrations has a slight inhibitory effect on the immediate bronchoconstriction following allergen challenge. In a recent study we demonstrated that theophylline at therapeutic concentrations clearly inhibits the late phase bronchial reaction. Enprofylline (3-propylxanthine), a new xanthine derivative with negligible ability to antagonize adenosine, has a comparable protective effect on the allergen-induced immediate and late bronchoconstriction at a five times lower plasma level. It seems, therefore, that the protective effects of xanthines on the allergen-induced bronchoconstriction are produced via mechanisms unrelated to adenosine antagonism.

50.5 Anticholinergics [8]

Anticholinergic drugs, especially when given by inhalation, have potent bronchodilating activity. They do so by a direct effect at the smooth muscle level. There is little evidence that anticholinergic drugs modify the release of inflammatory mediators but this may be due to the lack of adequate studies.

50.6 Antihistamines [9]

Antihistamines, in general, are considered to have little therapeutic benefit in bronchial asthma. Some antihistamines have bronchodilating effect when given by inhalation. Most antihistamines inhibit histamine release from sensitized human lung fragments but this in vitro observation seems to have little relevance for their in vivo effect in asthma.

50.7 Corticosteroids

Glucocorticoids have different pharmacological activities which are probably relevant to their efficacy in bronchial asthma. At low concentrations they inhibit the release of histamine from sensitized human basophils [10]. Glucocorticoids have, however, no effect on the anti-IgE-induced histamine release from purified human lung mast cells. In contrast, they clearly inhibit the release of prostaglandins from sensitized human lung fragments. Glucocorticoids also inhibit the release of prostaglandins from human neutrophils and at pharmacological doses they decrease the influx of neutrophils, mononuclear phagocytes and eosinophils into an inflammatory focus [11]. They do so by decreasing the adherence of these cells to the inflamed vessel wall and by decreasing their response to chemotactic stimuli. Glucocorticoids restore the sensitivity to β-adrenergic stimulation in cells and tissues made resistant by preincubation with a β-adrenergic stimulant. Finally, glucocorticoids produce a dose-related suppression of the spontaneous release of mucous glycoproteins from human airways [12]. The experimental pharmacological data match, to a large extent, the clinical pharmacological data. It has been known, for several years, that the previous administration of glucocorticoids inhibits the late asthmatic reaction after allergen challenge. Several investigators have recently shown that prolonged treatment with oral or inhaled glucocorticoids also has an inhibitory activity on the immediate bronchoconstriction following allergen or exercise challenge [13]. Ellul-Micallef and Fenech showed that corticosteroids, given orally, intravenously or via inhalation cause bronchodilatation in patients with chronic asthma [14]. Glucocorticoids also restore the bronchodilating activity of sympathomimetics in patients with asthma and resistance to sympathomimetic drugs [15]. Several investigators have now shown that regular treatment with oral or inhaled steroids either reduces the nonspecific bronchial reactivity or prevents the increase in nonspecific bronchial reactivity caused by prolonged allergen exposure [16]. Finally glucocorticoids produce in patients with chronic asthma a decrease in the frequency of coughing and the production of sputum [17]. Glucocorticoids therefore seem to have several interesting pharmacological effects on the airways of asthmatics. It is not possible to point out the relative importance of these pharmacological effects.

References

1. Boushey HA, Holtzman MJ, Sheller JR, Nadel JA (1980) Bronchial hyperreactivity. Am Rev Respir Dis 121:389–413
2. Cockcroft DW, Ruffin RE, Dolovich J, Hargreave FE (1977) Allergen induced increase in non allergic bronchial reactivity. Clin Allergy 7:503–513
3. Richards IM (1983) Pharmacological modulation of bronchial hyperreactivity. Eur J Respir Dis [Suppl] 129: 148–176
4. Craps LP, Ney UM (1984) Ketotifen: current views on its mechanism of action and their therapeutic implications Respiration 45: 411–421
5. Hegardt B (1981) Evaluation of the anti-allergic property of the beta-adrenoceptor agonist KWD 2131 in asthmatics. Methodological aspects and clinical trial models. Eur J Respir Dis [Suppl] 115: 1–54
6. Pauwels R, van der Straeten M (1984) The anti-allergic effect of theophylline. In: Jonkman JHG, Jenne JW, Simons FER (eds) Sustained release theophylline in the treatment of chronic reversible airways obstruction. Excerpta Medica, Amsterdam, pp 9–13
7. Andersson P, Bergstrand H (1981) Antigen-induced bronchial anaphylaxis in actively sensitized guinea pigs: effect of long-term treatment with sodium cromoglycate and aminophylline. Br J Pharmacol 74: 601–609

8. Schultze-Werninghaus G (1981) Anticholinergic versus beta-2-adrenergic therapy in allergic airways obstruction. Respiration 41:239–247
9. Eiser NM (1982) Histamine antagonists and asthma. Pharmacol Ther 17:239–250
10. Schleimer RP, MacGlashan DW, Peters SP, Naclerio R, Proud D, Adkinson NF Jr, Lichtenstein LM (1984) Inflammatory mediators and mechanisms of release from purified human basophils and mast cells. J Allergy Clin Immunol 74:473–481
11. Parillo JE, Fauci AS (1979) Mechanisms of glucocorticoid actions on immune processes. Annu Rev Pharmacol Toxicol 19:179–201
12. Marom Z, Shelhamer J, Alling D, Kaliner M (1984) The effects of glucocorticoids on mucous glycoprotein secretion from human airways in vitro. Am Rev Respir Dis 129:62–65
13. Burge PS (1982) The effects of corticosteroids on the immediate asthmatic reaction. Eur J Respir Dis [Suppl] 122:163–166
14. Ellul-Micallef R, Borthwick RC, McHardy GJR (1974) The time course of response to prednisolone in chronic bronchial asthma. Clin Sci 47:105–117
15. Ellul-Micallef R, Fenech FF (1975) Effect of intravenous prednisolone in asthmatics with diminished adrenergic responsiveness. Lancet II:1269–1270
16. Sotomayor H, Badier M, Vervloet D, Orehek J (1984) Seasonal increase of carbachol airway responsiveness in patients allergic to grass pollen. Am Rev Respir Dis 130:56–58
17. Agnew JE, Bateman JRM, Sheahan NF, Lennard-Jones AM, Pavia D, Clarke SW (1983) Effect of oral corticosteroids on mucus clearance by cough and mucociliary transport in stable asthma. Bull Eur Physiopathol Respir 19:37–41

51. Possible Therapeutic Developments

L. P. Craps

Nowadays, the proper use of bronchodilators makes the treatment of bronchial asthma safe and convenient, many patients enjoying an acceptable quality of life. However, neither the natural history, nor the prevalence, incidence, morbidity and mortality of the disease have improved [2]. This is not surprising since the pathogenesis of this disorder is poorly understood and no simple operational definition is available.

During the last twenty years, the emphasis of research and therapy has shifted from bronchospasm and its clinical triggers to inflammation and hyperresponsiveness of the bronchi, and a systematic search for nonbronchodilator, antiasthmatic drugs was initiated. The usefulness of topical corticosteroids was recognized [4]. A more specific achievement was the serendipitous discovery of disodium cromoglycate [1], whose mast cell stabilizing properties were shown afterwards [5]. Consequently, activation of mast cells within the lung was linked to allergic asthma and extensive research programs were performed, seeking orally active, selective mast cell stabilizing agents. This approach was not fruitful [15], although in many organs, including the lung, the participation of the mast cell in allergen-induced reactions is well established. Many other cells, however, like eosinophils, basophils, neutrophils, macrophages, lymphocytes and platelets, and several enzymatic systems, like the cyclooxygenase and the lipoxygenase pathways of arachidonic acid metabolism, and platelet activation, are likely to be involved in the inflammation process of asthma.

In a situation characterized by a profusion of possible mediators and mechanisms of action, aggravated by the lack of a reliable animal model of the disease, the design of nonbronchodilator, antiasthmatic compounds is a difficult task.

Ketotifen was selected due to its powerful antianaphylactic properties in several models of passive cutaneous anaphylaxis and it turned out to be prophylactic in about 70% of the patients with bronchial asthma, mainly of the extrinsic type [6, 8].

This benzocycloheptathiophene derivative (Fig. 51.1) shares, with cromoglycate, its mast cell stabilizing properties, but it has a much wider profile of pharmacological activity [7, 13], that can be summarized as follows.

Ketotifen exerts antiallergic and asthmaprophylactic effects in a large number of biological systems in vitro and in vivo:

- Prevention of lung and cutaneous anaphylaxis in the rat and guinea pig.
- Inhibition of bronchial, nasal, dermal and gastric antigen challenges in man.
- Powerful and selective histamine receptor blocking activity.
- Inhibition of mediator release from rat mast cells, human basophils, human neutrophils, and human and guinea pig lung fragments.
- Inhibition of calcium influx in the potassium-depolarized guinea pig teniae coli and through the mast cell membrane, without interaction with the binding sites for dihydropyridines nor cardiovascular effects.
- Functional antagonism of leukotriene-induced bronchospasm in the guinea pig, without a specific antagonist effect at the receptor site.
- Inhibition of platelet activating factor (PAF)-induced platelet secretion and neutrophil activation response in man.
- Prevention of PAF-induced increase in pulmonary resistance in the guinea pig.
- Suppression of PAF-induced bronchial hyperreactivity and emigration of platelets and eosinophils into lung tissue in the rabbit and guinea pig.
- Inhibition of eosinophil accumulation in the lung of the baboon after PAF exposure.

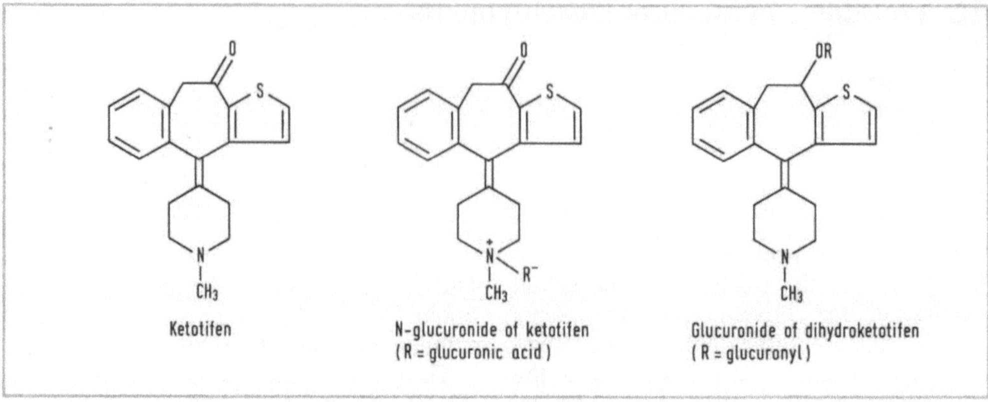

Fig. 51.1. Ketotifen and its two major metabolites in man

- Prevention and reversal of β-adrenergic tachyphylaxis in the rat.
- Accelerated restoration of responsiveness of human lymphocyte β_2-adrenoceptors after terbutaline-induced desensitization [3].

The identification of the pharmacodynamic effect(s) responsible for asthma prophylaxis allows the selection of appropriate animal models to screen further, more specific and powerful, nonbronchodilator, antiasthmatic drugs. At the present time the following assumptions can be drawn in an attempt to correlate the pharmacological properties of ketotifen and the pathogenesis of airway inflammation and increased responsiveness. Presumably, the different classes of prophylactic agents, i.e., theophylline, the corticosteroids, cromoglycate and ketotifen, possess some common properties accounting for their antiasthmatic action. Indeed, it is unlikely that pharmacological features partly shared by compounds exhibiting dissimilar clinical effects are relevant.

It has long been recognized that histamine antagonism does not confer antiasthma activity. Early controlled clinical trials with ketotifen have shown that its prophylactic effect could not be reproduced by using a specific antihistamine of equal potency [8]. The antihistaminic and antianaphylactic effects of ketotifen were also unequivocally dissociated in animal experiments [11]. The powerful H_1-receptor blocking activity of ketotifen accounts for its major side effect, sedation, and confers on this drug some additional antiallergic action, e.g., in the nasal mucous membrane and the skin. The mast cell stabilizing effect and the capacity to inhibit calcium influxes through the cell membrane are correlated, but it is very unlikely that they contribute to therapeutic efficacy, at least in asthma. By comparison with plasma levels reached during treatment, the concentrations required to inhibit mediator release from isolated cells and tissue fragments are high. In addition, a range of more or less selective mast cell stabilizing agents have proved ineffective in bronchial asthma [15].

The effects of ketotifen and other prophylactic agents in a range of test systems investigating bronchial hyperreactivity deserves closer consideration. It has been proposed recently that exacerbation of asthma symptoms and increased bronchial reactivity arise as a consequence of PAF formation within the lung [14]. Prolonged exposure to PAF induces a series of changes pertinent to asthma: sustained, nonselective bronchial hyperreactivity, emigration of platelets and eosinophils into pulmonary tissue. These effects are related to platelet activation since antiplatelet antiserum preempts PAF-mediated hyperresponsiveness. They are prevented by ketotifen (Fig. 51.2), theophylline, the corticosteroids and cromoglycate. Antihistamines, serotonin antagonists, cyclooxygenase and lipoxygenase inhibitors, leukotriene antagonists, β-adrenergic agonists, and many mast cell stabilizing agents,

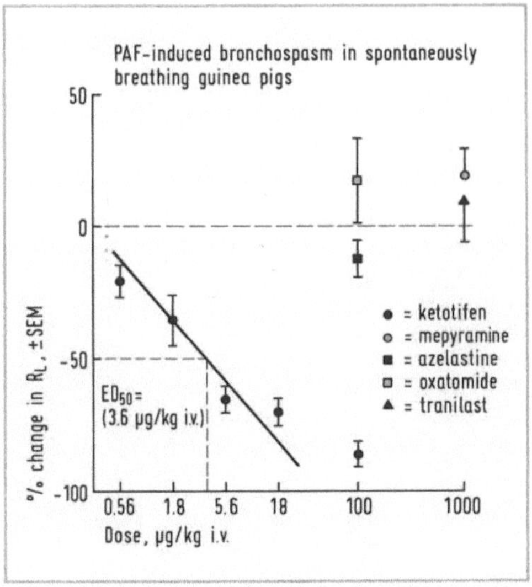

Fig. 51.2. Inhibition of PAF-induced bronchoconstriction by ketotifen (0.56–18 μg/kg i.v.), mepyramine (1,000 μg/kg i.v.), azelastine (100 μg/kg i.v.), oxatomide (100 μg/kg i.v.) and tranilast (1,000 μg/kg i.v.). The points depict the mean response (± SEM, $n \geq 5$ per dose). [From 13]

which are all nonprophylactic in clinical asthma, have no effect in this system [13].

The role of β-adrenergic tachyphylaxis both in the pathogenesis of asthma [10] and after exposure to β-adrenergic agonists [9] is not yet firmly established, the first being better documented than the second. Nevertheless, the effects of ketotifen on β-adrenoceptor expression still deserve particular attention. Ketotifen shares this property with the corticosteroids, but neither with theophylline, nor with cromoglycate, at least in the animal model. There is some recent evidence that the impaired β-adrenoceptor activity consecutive to allergen exposure may be attributed to PAF formation [12], suggesting that effects of ketotifen upon β-adrenoceptor expression are not necessarily restricted to tachyphylaxis.

In conclusion, the link between bronchial inflammation and hyperreactivity, and platelet activation provides a valuable model to screen nonbronchodilator, antiasthmatic agents. The future will show how far this new approach is successful. If its accuracy is confirmed by clinical experience, the pathogenesis of asthma would also be better understood.

References

1. Altounyan REC (1967) Inhibition of experimental asthma by a new compound, disodium cromoglycate. Acta Allergologica 22:487
2. Barbee RA, Dodge RR, Lebowitz MD, Burrows B (1985) The epidemiology of asthma. Chest 87:21S
3. Brodde OE, Brinkmann M, Schemuth R, O'Hara N, Daul A (1985) Terbutaline-induced desensitization of human lymphocyte beta-2-adrenoceptors. Accelerated restoration of beta-adrenoceptor responsiveness by prednisone and ketotifen. J Clin Invest 76: 1096
4. Brown HM, Storey G, George WH (1972) Beclomethasone dipropionate: a new steroid aerosol for the treatment of allergic asthma. Br Med J 1:585
5. Cox JSG (1971) Disodium cromoglycate: mode of action and its possible relevance to the clinical use of the drug. Br J Dis Chest 65:189
6. Craps L (1978) Expérimentation clinique d'un agent à effet antiallergique prophylactique dans l'asthme bronchique, le kétotifène. Méd Hyg 36:2561
7. Craps L (1985) Immunologic and therapeutic aspects of ketotifen. J Allergy Clin Immunol 76:389
8. Craps L, Greenwood C, Radielovic P (1978) Clinical investigation of agents with prophylactic anti-allergic effects in bronchial asthma. Clin Allergy 8:373
9. Jenne JW (1982) Whither beta-adrenergic tachyphylaxis? J Allergy Clin Immunol 70: 413
10. Koeter GH, Meurs H, Kauffman HF, de Vries K (1982) The role of the adrenergic system in allergy and bronchial hyperreactivity. Eur J Respir Dis 63 [Suppl 121]:72
11. Martin U, Baggiolini M (1981) Dissociation between the anti-anaphylactic and the antihistaminic actions of ketotifen. Arch Pharmacol 316:186
12. Mazzoni L, Morley J, Page CP, Sanjar S (1986) Prophylactic anti-asthma drugs impair the airway-hyperreactivity that follows exposure to platelet activating factor (PAF). Br J Pharmacol 86:571 P
13. Morley J, Page CP, Mazzoni L, Sanjar S (1985) Anti-allergy drugs in asthma. Triangle 24:59
14. Morley J, Page CP, Sanjar S (1984) The platelet in asthma. Lancet II:1142
15. Stokes TC, Morley J (1981) Prospects for an oral Intal. Br J Dis Chest 75:1

References

Index

agricultural asthma see under asthma
allergen avoidance 301 ff
–, drugs 303
–, food 303
–, house dust 301 f
–, inhalant allergens 302 f
–, mites 301 f
–, occupational asthma 303
allergen standardization 297 ff
–, future efforts 298
–, state of the art 297 f
allergic bronchopulmonary aspergillosis (ABPA) 58 ff
–, clinical features 59 f
–, evolution 62 f
–, incidence 58 f
–, laboratory findings 60 ff
–, –, blood eosinophilia 61
–, –, IgE 62 f
–, –, IgG 62 f
–, –, immunological tests 62
–, –, precipitins 62
–, –, pulmonary function test 62
–, –, skin test 61 f
–, –, sputum examination 60 f
–, pathophysiology 63
–, radiological features 59 f
–, treatment 63 f
–, –, antifungal therapy 64
–, –, corticosteroid therapy 64
–, –, prophylaxis 63 f
allergy, genetic factors 31 ff
–, –, atopic allergy 31
–, –, basal IgE 31 ff
–, –, HLA 31–35
–, –, HLA-associated immune hyperresponsiveness 32 f
–, –, HLA gene complex 32
–, –, specific immune response (Ir) 33 f
–, Type I 71
–, Type II 71
–, Type III 71
–, Type IV 71
alloreactive T-cell clone (ATCC) 143
alveolar macrophages (AM) 186 ff
–, bronchoalveolar lavage (BAL) 186
–, culture 186
–, immune response 189 f
–, LTB_4 191
–, membrane receptors 187 ff
–, morphology 186 f
–, putative role 192 f
–, secretion 190 f
–, –, arachidonic acid metabolites 190
–, –, enzymes 190
–, –, platelet activating factor (PAF) 190
–, –, proteins 190
–, –, reactive metabolites of oxygen 190 f
–, viability 187
arachidonic acid 212 ff
–, mediators 212 ff
–, –, hydroxyeicosatetraenoic acid (HETE) 212 ff
–, –, leukotrienes (LT) 212 ff
–, –, prostaglandins (PG) 212, 215
–, –, thromboxane A_2 (TxA_2) 212
–, metabolism 216 f
–, metabolites 213 ff
–, –, biological activity 213 ff
–, –, pro-inflammatory effects 215 f
aspergillosis see allergic bronchopulmonary aspergillosis (ABPA)
asthma
–, in adults 394 ff
–, –, natural history 394
–, –, presentation 396 f
–, –, provoking factors 394 ff
–, –, treatment 398
–, agricultural (rural) 331 ff
–, –, causes 333
–, –, –, animal allergens 333 ff
–, –, –, chemicals 338
–, –, –, food for animals 338 f
–, –, –, mites 333
–, –, –, molds 335
–, –, –, vegetal matter 336 ff
–, –, classification 331
–, –, pathophysiology 332
–, –, prevalence 331 f
–, bacterial 66 ff
–, in childhood 376 ff, 380 ff, 385 ff
–, –, clinical patterns 376 ff
–, –, diagnosis 380 ff
–, –, –, laboratory tests 382 f
–, –, –, physical examination 381
–, –, differential diagnosis 377 f
–, –, history 380 f
–, –, treatment 385 ff
–, –, –, acute exacerbations 389 f
–, –, –, drug treatment 387 ff

asthma, in childhood, treatment
–, –, –, general measures 385 ff
–, –, –, immunotherapy 390
–, –, –, inhalers 390 f
–, clinical aspects 373 ff
–, cryptogenic (intrinsic) 69
–, drug-induced 364 ff
–, –, allergic reactions 364–367
–, –, drug additives 369
–, –, eosinophilia 368
–, –, nonallergic reactions 365–368
–, exercise-induced (EIA) 77 ff, 195
–, –, arterial blood gas tension (PaO_2) 79
–, –, drugs 83
–, –, –, sodium cromoglycate 83
–, –, –, β-sympathomimetics 83
–, –, initiating stimuli 80 f
–, –, –, heat loss 80 f
–, –, –, hypertonicity 80 ff
–, –, –, water loss 80 f
–, –, lung volumes 79
–, –, pH values 79
–, –, recommendations for assessment 83 ff
–, –, refractory period 82 f
–, –, –, exercise lability index (ELI) 82
–, –, –, Jones lability index 82
–, –, role of circulating substances 81 f
–, –, –, adrenaline (AD) 81
–, –, –, cyclic adenosine monophosphate (CAMP) 81
–, –, –, histamine 81
–, –, –, neutrophil chemotactic activity (NCA) 81 f
–, –, –, noradrenaline (NAD) 81
–, –, –, sodium cromoglycate (SCG) 82
–, extrinsic 69
–, food-related 359 ff
–, –, diagnosis 361
–, –, suspicion of food intolerance 360 f
–, –, treatment 361 f
–, infectious (infective) 69
–, occupational 343 ff, 351 ff
–, –, classification 353 f
–, –, diagnosis 353 ff
–, –, low molecular weight agents 343 ff
–, –, –, anamnesis 343 ff
–, –, –, etiologic agents 343 ff
–, –, –, follow-up of affected individuals 349
–, –, –, immunological test 345 f
–, –, –, mechanism 343
–, –, –, serial functional assessments 346 f
–, –, –, skin tests 345
–, –, –, specific inhalation challenge 347 f
–, –, –, white blood cells 345
–, –, management 357
–, –, pathogenic mechanism 352 f
–, –, predisposing factors 352
–, –, prevalence 351
–, –, prevention 356 f
–, prevalence in developing countries 37 ff
–, rural (agricultural) 331 ff
–, treatment 441 ff
–, –, anticholinergics 442 f
–, –, corticosteroids 443
–, –, future aspects 445 ff
–, –, ketotifen 441, 445 ff
–, –, pathophysiological data 441 ff
–, –, sodium cromoglycate (SCG) 441
–, –, sympathomimetic drugs 442
–, –, xanthines 442
–, virus-induced 47 ff
–, –, β-adrenergic function 53
–, –, airway inflammation 48 ff
–, –, basophil mediator release 53 ff
–, –, epidemiology 47
–, –, IgE antibody production 51 f
–, –, model 55 f
atopic diseases 140 ff
–, B-lymphocytes 144 f
–, IgE production (in vitro models) 142 f
–, –, regulation by human lymphocytes 142 f
–, lymphocyte responses to allergens 141 f
–, lymphocytes 140 ff
–, –, abnormalities 140 ff
–, –, role 140 ff
–, T-cell system 140–144
autologous mixed lymphocyte reaction (AMLR) 141

bacterial agents 70 f
–, allergens 70 f
–, radioallergosorbent test 71 f
–, skin test 70 f
bacterial allergy 68, 74
bacterial antigens 73 f
–, bronchial provocation test 73
bacterial asthma see under asthma
bacterial strains 73
bacterial vaccine immunotherapy 66 ff
basophils 167 ff
–, anatomical considerations 168
–, cell-cell interactions 175 ff
–, cellular activation 168 f
–, mediators 170–173
–, –, arachidonic acid metabolites 170
–, –, histamine 170
–, –, inhibitors 174 f
–, –, leukotriene C_4 170
–, –, PAF 171
–, –, prostaglandin D_2 171
–, –, release 167 ff
–, pharmacological control mechanism 173 ff
–, physiological control mechanism 173 ff
bronchial hyperreactivity 265 ff, 276 ff
–, airway inflammation 270 f
–, autonomic nervous system 276 ff
–, –, abnormalities 276 ff
–, –, β-adrenergic hyporeactivity 276 ff
–, –, –, mechanism 278–281
–, –, –, theory 276 f

–, factors 265 ff
–, mechanism of bronchial responses 265 ff
–, –, autonomic nervous system 268 ff
–, –, mast cells 267
–, –, smooth muscles 266
bronchial hyperresponsiveness (BH) 285 ff
–, concepts 285 ff
bronchial infection 69 f
bronchial obstruction 260 ff
–, diagnostic methods 260 f
–, –, lung function tests 260 f
–, –, measuring of density dependence of airflow 261
–, –, morphology 260
–, mechanisms 224
–, site 261 ff
bronchial pathophysiology 255 ff
–, endoscopy 255 f
–, etiology 256 ff
bronchial provocation tests 421 ff
–, antigens 424–428
–, nonspecific stimuli 422 ff
–, preparatory considerations 421 f
–, responses 422 ff, 426 ff

cryptogenic (intrinsic) asthma see under asthma
cutaneous basophil hypersensitivity (CBH) 147 ff
–, basophil recruitment 148 f
–, cell-mediated immunity to allergen 148
–, chronic allergen exposure 148
–, inhalant allergens 147 f
–, mast cells 149
–, T-cells 149

disodium cromoglycate (DSCG) 195
domestic animal allergens 326 ff
–, cats 327
–, definition 326
–, diversity of allergen sources 326 f
–, dogs 327 f
–, importance 326
–, laboratory animals 328
–, multiplicity of allergen sources 326 f
–, other mammals 328
drug-induced asthma see under asthma

eosinophils 201 ff
–, eosinophil cationic protein (ECP) 206
–, eosinophil peroxidase (EPO) 206
–, leukotrienes C_4 and D_4 206
–, major basic protein (MBP) 201 ff
–, –, localization in the lung 203 f
–, –, sputum 203 f
–, role 201 ff
epidemiology 21 ff
–, analytic 21
–, criteria for diagnosis 21
–, descriptive 21
–, experimental 21
–, month of birth 24
–, morbidity rate 21
–, mortality rate 21
–, prevalence rates 21 ff
–, racial group 21
–, risk factors 24–28
–, –, air pollution 24 f
–, –, atopy 26 f
–, –, bronchial hyperreactivity 28
–, –, family history 27 f
–, –, high serum-IgE level 28
–, –, long-term exposure 25 f
–, –, meteorologic conditions 26 f
–, –, positive skin test 28
–, –, role of inhaled allergens 26 f
–, –, short-term repercussions 25
–, –, tobacco smoke 26
–, sex (male/female ratio) 23
–, social class 24
exercise-induced asthma (EIA) see under asthma
extrinsic asthma see under asthma

Fc_ε receptors see receptors
food-related asthma see under asthma

gastroesophageal reflux 89 ff
–, diagnostic methods 91
–, –, acid perfusion test 91
–, –, clinical digestive methods 91
–, –, esophageal fibroscopy 91
–, –, manometry 91
–, –, pH-metry 91
–, –, pH monitoring 91
–, –, scintiscanning 91
–, frequency 90
–, meaning in asthma 92 f
–, pathogenicity 90
–, –, abnormal production of reagins (food) 90
–, –, aspiration of gastric content 90
–, –, esophagobronchial vagal reflux 90
–, physiology 89
–, –, efficient esophageal clearing 89
–, –, glottis shutting reflex 89
–, –, lower esophageal sphincter (LES) 89
–, reflux disease (RD) 89 ff
–, –, anatomical abnormalities 89
–, –, esophageal peristalsis 89
–, –, esophagitis 90
–, –, iatrogenic factors 90
–, –, life-style 90
–, –, mechanical factors 89
–, –, pressure fall 89
–, therapeutic deductions 93 f
–, –, antireflux surgery 93
–, –, medical treatment 93
–, –, results 93 f

human major histocompatibility complex (MHC) 31 f

IgE (reagin) 100, 120, 409 ff
–, activation of inflammatory cells 110 ff
–, allergens 120 ff
–, antibodies 120
–, –, determination 410 f
–, antigens 121
–, factors affecting the production 120 f
–, immune response 121 f
–, receptors 99 ff, 107 ff
–, –, B-lymphocytes 102
–, –, basophils 100 ff
–, –, inflammatory cells 107 ff
–, –, –, IgE immune complex 111
–, –, –, presence in human diseases 111
–, –, interaction 102 ff
–, –, macrophages 102
–, –, mast cells 100 ff
–, –, T-lymphocytes 102
–, regulation of formation 120 ff
–, responders 121 f
–, serum-IgE protein 409 f
IgE-mediated mechanisms 120 ff
–, basophil blood cells 124 f
–, eosinophil cells 127
–, lymphocytes 127 f
–, mast cells 124 f
–, T suppressor cells 122 ff
IgG S-TS (short-term sensitizing IgG antibodies) 131 ff
–, Aspergillus fumigatus 133
–, budgerigar serum 133 ff
–, Dermatophagoides pteronyssinus 133
–, egg 133
–, extrinsic allergic alveolitis 135
–, grass pollen 133
–, house dust 133
–, IgE 131 ff
–, IgG blocking sensitization of human lung by IgE 136 f
–, IgG_4 137 f
–, in vitro passive sensitization of human lung 135 f
–, milk 133
–, platinum 133
–, properties 131 f
immediate-type reactions 228 ff
–, airway inflammation 228 ff
–, bronchial hyperreactivity 228 f
–, inflammation in allergic skin reactions 231 ff
–, mediator release 230 f
–, mucous hypersecretion 228
–, smooth muscle spasm 228
immune response genes (Ir genes) 121
immunology 117
–, mechanisms 117 f
infectious (infective) asthma see under asthma
inflammatory mediator release 155 ff
–, bronchial reactivity 160 f
–, mast cell 155–160
–, pharmacological control 155 ff
–, pharmacological modulation of mast cells 161 ff
–, physiological control 155 ff
–, secondary effector cells 160

late phase reactions (LPR) 237 ff
–, animal models 244 f
–, –, bronchial provocation test 245
–, –, skin tests 244
–, bronchial (LBR) 238 f, 243
–, –, bronchial hyperreactivity 242
–, –, inflammatory cells 242
–, –, trigger mechanism 242
–, clinical consequences 245
–, cutaneous (LCR) 238 f, 243
–, –, exudate from skin 239
–, –, histamine 240
–, –, IgE 239
–, –, kallikrein-kinin system 241
–, –, leukotrienes (LT) 240
–, –, mast cell mediators 239
–, –, mediators 240 ff
–, –, platelet activating factor (PAF) 241
–, –, prostaglandin D_2 240
–, –, prostaglandin E 241
–, –, prostaglandin $F_{2\alpha}$ 241
–, –, role of infiltrating cells 241 f
–, –, thromboxanes (Tx) 240 f
–, –, trigger mechanism 239
–, definitions 238 f
–, frequency 238 f
–, history 237 f
–, nasal (LNR) 238
–, –, pathogenesis 242
–, pharmacological modulation 243 f
–, –, acetylsalicylic acid 244
–, –, β-adrenergic agents 243
–, –, antihistamines 243 f
–, –, corticosteroids 243
–, –, disodium cromoglycate 243
–, –, eicosatetraynoic acid 244
–, –, indomethacin 244
–, –, ketotifen 244
–, –, onion extracts 244
–, –, thromboxane synthetase inhibitors 244
–, –, tranexamic acid 244

mast cells 167 ff
–, anatomical considerations 167
–, cell-cell interactions 175 ff
–, cellular activation 168 f
–, mediators 170–173
–, –, arachidonic acid metabolites 170
–, –, histamine 170
–, –, inhibitors 174 f
–, –, leukotriene B_4 170
–, –, leukotriene C_4 170 f
–, –, PAF 171
–, –, prostaglandin D_2 171
–, –, release 167 ff

–, pharmacological control mechanism 173 ff
–, physiological control mechanism 173 ff
mediators (release) 155 ff, 167 ff, 186 ff, 195 ff, 201 ff, 222 ff, 228 ff, 239
mite allergens 316 ff
–, biology 316 f
–, demonstration 318 f
–, ecology 316 f
–, morphology 316
–, taxonomy 316
–, treatment 318 f
mold allergens 322 ff
–, ascomycetes 322
–, atmospheric concentration 323 f
–, basidiomycetes 323
–, clinical relevance 324 f
–, deuteromycetes 323
–, fungi imperfecti 323
–, seasonal patterns 324

natural history 7 ff
–, allergy 8 ff
–, bronchial reactivity 10 f, 13
–, cure of asthma 12 f
–, genetic predisposition 14
–, immune response 11 f
–, smoking 14
neutrophils 195 ff
–, characteristics 195
–, CR 1 receptor 195
–, CR 3 receptor 195
–, IgA 195
–, IgG 195
–, leukotriene (LT) 196–199
–, –, B_4 196–199
–, –, C_4 196–199
–, neutrophil chemotactic factors (NCF or NCA) 195 f

occupational asthma see under asthma

PAF-acether (platelet activating factor) 221 ff
–, biological effects 222–225
–, detection 221
–, metabolism 222
–, source 222
–, structure 221
platelet activating factor see PAF
pollen allergens 33, 306 ff
–, atmospheric distribution 307 ff
–, chemistry 310 f
–, extraction methodology 293 f
–, –, stability 293
–, extracts 293 ff
–, mechanism 313 f
pulmonary function tests 412 ff
–, bronchodilator response 413 f, 416
–, clinical role 416 ff
–, expiratory flow rates 413
–, lung volumes 412
–, pulmonary diffusion 412 f
–, specialized sensitive tests 414 ff

Fc_ε receptors 108 ff
–, eosinophils 108 f
–, inflammatory cells 109
–, mononuclear phagocytes 108
–, platelets 109
reflux disease (RD) see gastroesophageal reflux
respiratory bacteria, antibodies 71
–, –, bacterial precipitins 72
–, –, enzyme-linked immunosorbent assay (ELISA) 72
–, –, IgE 71 f
respiratory syncytial virus (RSV) 47–52
respiratory viral infections 47 ff
respiratory viruses 47 ff
–, β-adrenergic function 53 f
–, –, experimental investigations 53
–, airway hyperreactivity 49
–, airway inflammation 48 f
–, airway obstruction 48 f
–, airway reactivity 49 ff
–, –, mechanism 49 ff
–, basophil mediator release 53 ff
–, epidemiology 47 f
–, IgE antibody production 51 f
–, upper respiratory infection (URI) 47–55
rural asthma see under asthma

short-term sensitizing IgG antibodies see IgG S-TS
sinus infection 70
skin tests 399 ff
–, factors affecting the cutaneous response 403 ff
–, interpretation 401 ff
–, methods 399 ff
–, –, diluents 400 f
–, –, intradermal reaction (IDR) 399
–, –, prick test 399 f
–, –, scratch test 400
status asthmaticus 431 ff
–, definition 431
–, epidemiology 432 f
–, evolution 434 f
–, pathology 432
–, principal signs of seriousness 433 f
–, prophylactic measures 437
–, treatment 435 ff

MIX
Papier aus verantwortungsvollen Quellen
Paper from responsible sources
FSC® C105338

If you have any concerns about our products,
you can contact us on
ProductSafety@springernature.com

In case Publisher is established outside the EU,
the EU authorized representative is:
Springer Nature Customer Service Center GmbH
Europaplatz 3, 69115 Heidelberg, Germany

Printed by Libri Plureos GmbH
in Hamburg, Germany